# ALTERNATIVE
## CURES

# ALTERNATIVE CURES

## MORE THAN 1,000
## OF THE MOST EFFECTIVE NATURAL
## HOME REMEDIES

# BILL GOTTLIEB

BALLANTINE BOOKS • NEW YORK

This book is intended as a reference volume only, not as a medical manual. The information given here is designed to help you make informed decisions about your health. It is not intended as a substitute for any treatment that may have been prescribed by your doctor. If you suspect that you have a medical problem, we urge you to seek competent medical help.

Beginning on page 704, you will find safe-use guidelines for the supplements, herbs, and essential oils recommended in this book. Please refer to the guidelines before trying any of the remedies.

Internet and street addresses given in this book were accurate at the time it went to press.

2008 Ballantine Books Mass Market Edition

Published in the United States by Ballantine Books, an imprint of The Random House Publishing Group, a division of Random House, Inc., New York.

BALLANTINE and colophon are registered trademarks of Random House, Inc.

Originally published in hardcover in the United States by Rodale in 2000.

Illustrations copyright © by Karen Kuchar are used by permission

ISBN 978-0-345-50539-2

Cover design: Gerald J. Pfeiffer
Cover photograph: Getty Images

Printed in the United States of America

www.ballantinebooks.com

OPM   19 18 17 16 15 14 13 12 11

*This book is lovingly dedicated to*

**my Dad,**
for my inheritance of responsibility, persistence, and care, without which this book couldn't have been written

**Denise,**
my dearest friend and lover, whose sweet happiness surrounded and supported me and this massive project from beginning to end

**and my Beloved Spiritual Master,**
Ruchira Avatar Adi Da Samraj, with deepest gratitude for His constant Gifts of Light, Life, and Divine True Love

# Acknowledgments

There wouldn't be an *Alternative Cures* without the gracious participation of the hundreds of alternative health practitioners who took time from their busy schedules to talk with me and tell me the secrets of their clinical successes. My conversations with them were always a pleasure. They are too numerous to name here, but to each and all, I extend my sincerest thanks and gratitude.

Heartfelt thanks to this book's stalwart editor, Jack Croft, managing editor of *Prevention* Health Books. Jack championed *Alternative Cures* from the beginning and has done everything necessary to ensure that the book's integrity and quality were never compromised. His intelligence, good judgment, professional skill, and very hard work are deeply appreciated. I extend my gratitude to a dear friend.

Gratitude to Mark Bricklin, my mentor and boss at Rodale for 12 years, who taught me how to care about the reader in every aspect of creating and writing a book, and for whom I have a unique fondness and appreciation.

To Chris Tomasino, my literary agent, for her skillful support.

To my housemates in the cooperative religious community of Adidam, Crane, Fiona, and Connie. Thank you for your kind support and practical love in maintaining a physical and emotional surround in which this book could be written.

To Michael Wood, my Annex-buddy. Thank you for your wise counsel and dear friendship.

To Kenneth Bock, M.D., and Steven Bock, M.D., for their perceptive, thorough review of the text.

To Shawn M. Talbott, Ph.D., for sharing his expertise on nutritional supplements.

To Doug and the gracious staff at Indian Springs Spa in Calistoga for keeping my "upper extremities" in shape while I transcribed hundreds of interviews and wrote dozens of chapters.

To my "computer lady," Bonnie Grasse, who rescued me when my hard drive crashed about 6 months from the finish line.

And, finally, my thanks to all the editorial staff at Rodale who worked on this project to help make it a success, including researchers Leah Flickinger, Sandi Lloyd, Kathryn Piff, Jennifer Kushnier, Nancy Zelko, Holly Swanson, Rebecca Kleinwaks, Christine Dreisbach, Debbie Pedron, Jan McLeod, Jennifer Kaas, Lois Hazel, Lucille Uhlman, Staci Sander, Mary Mesaros, Lori Davis, and Sally Reith; copy editor Jane Sherman; and cover designer Carol Angstadt, interior designer Christina Gaugler, and layout designer Jennifer Holgate.

# Contents

### Part 1
# Alternative Home Remedies

# CONTENTS

### Part 2
# Alternative Healing At-a-Glance

### Part 3
# Resources

# Introduction

# The New Direction
# of Personal Healing

While I was writing the introduction to this book, I got a phone call from my dad in Florida. He's a vigorous, optimistic, mentally sharp, can-do man in his midseventies. He still goes to work every day, managing a small start-up company. He walks the beach near his home, looking for shells to add to his extensive collection (or, better yet, to give to one of his 10 grandchildren). He loves to opine about the latest shenanigans of the politicians, the antics of his dog, and the affectionate stubbornness of his wife.

But my energetic dad also has an enigmatic health problem: Parkinson's disease, the nervous system disorder that slowly but surely robs the muscles of their power to move. The symptoms are kept pretty much under control with medications, but my dad knows the scientific facts about those drugs: They lose their effectiveness over years of use. That's why he's concerned about his health in the years to come. And that's why he called me—to ask about an *alternative cure* that he'd just heard about: a program of high-dose vitamins and minerals used by an M.D. in a nearby city to help control the symptoms of Parkinson's disease without drugs.

Well, I'll bet that this story about my dad reminds you of someone you know—your dad or mom, your son or daughter, your uncle or aunt, your friend or coworker. Someone who has turned to alternative therapies for help, even while using medications or other types of "conventional" care. There's a grassroots revolution going on in America today. It's a nationwide declaration of independence from total reliance on the treatments of conventional medicine; a millions-strong realization that those treatments are not the be-all and end-all of healing.

In short, there's a new willingness to find out about and use natural remedies—alternative home remedies, or what this book calls alternative cures—for better health. But you don't need to take my word for it. Consider these facts.

## 42 PERCENT USE ALTERNATIVES

In 1993, a study showed that 34 percent of all Americans—one in every three people—had used an alternative therapy in the preceding year (remedies like vitamins, herbs, healing foods, massage, homeopathy, relaxation techniques, and other natural treatments—exactly the kinds of remedies featured in this book).

In the same year, Americans visited primary care physicians a grand total of 388 million times—while making *425 million* visits to alternative practitioners (the kinds of practitioners interviewed for this book).

A few years later, in 1997, researchers conducted a similar study and found that 42 percent of those surveyed had used an alternative therapy during the preceding year. And my guess is that when researchers conduct the next big survey of this type a couple of years from now, they'll find that statistic has jumped another 10 percent—or even more.

Why are alternative treatments so popular? Why are millions of Americans turning to vitamins, herbs, and other natural remedies?

## PRESCRIPTION DRUGS: *One of the Top 10 Causes of Death*

Well, for the answer to that question, I had to look no further than the morning paper and this headline: *Heartburn Drug Can Harm Heart, FDA Warns.* A popular heartburn drug, used by more than 30 million people since 1993, has caused 70 deaths and 200 other incidents of heart problems, and, says the government, it should be used "only as a last resort." (*Now* you tell me!)

Of course, since millions of people have taken this drug, 70 deaths doesn't seem like such a big deal in the grand scheme of things. Unless, of course, you're one of the people who died, or one of their relatives or friends. Then a preventable, drug-related death is a very big deal. And it's even a bigger deal when you read the chapter on heartburn in this book (page 352), in which Richard Leigh, M.D., an alternative-minded doctor, says, "Taking prescription or over-the-counter antacids for months on end for heartburn is crazy." He and other practitioners recommend natural, safe remedies for this problem.

In other words, alternative-minded M.D.'s already knew that heartburn drugs are dangerous and that alternative remedies are often safer and more effective. And heartburn drugs are far from the whole story.

One study says that in a single year, *2 million hospital patients* had a serious adverse drug reaction, and about 100,000 died because of their drug treatment, making prescription drugs one of the top 10 causes of death in America! And drugs are just part of the problem. Conventional medicine also includes potentially deadly surgery and risky medical tests. Another study estimates that a total of 180,000 Americans "die every year from injuries caused by medical treatment."

This crucial point—that prescription drugs and other conventional treatments are potentially very dangerous and that alternative remedies are sometimes safer and more effective—is made again and again by the alternative-minded M.D.'s, naturopaths, herbalists, homeopaths, and other alternative practitioners quoted in the pages of *Alternative Cures*. Here's a very small sampling from the book.

From the chapter on high blood pressure (page 380):
*"Volumes of scientific research show that dietary changes can eliminate high blood pressure—or hypertension—in most patients," says Julian Whitaker, M.D. "In spite of that, the routine approach of most doctors is to immediately start a patient on drugs—and usually without any recommendation for dietary change. The dangerous side effects of high blood pressure drugs often make this approach, in my opinion, more harmful to the patient than beneficial."*

From the chapter on asthma (page 58):
*The death rate from asthma has more than doubled since 1978. After 20 years of using asthma drugs that failed to improve his condition, Richard Firshein, D.O., decided to treat his asthma himself—naturally and without excessive use of medications.*

And even where drugs are helpful, you can often boost their healing power by combining medications with alternative remedies. Here's one doctor's view, from the chapter on headaches (page 338):

> *"The treatment of chronic headache may not be successful with medications alone," says Fred D. Sheftell, M.D. "The headache sufferer needs to include a variety of other strategies, such as proper diet, nutritional supplements, stress management, and many other factors."*

It's no wonder that yet another scientific study showed that 53 percent of *physicians* interviewed used alternative therapies themselves!

## THE BODY'S NATURAL HEALING POWER

Nearly half of all Americans are choosing alternative remedies over conventional care, or combining the two, and the likely reason is that they realize that conventional treatments can be dangerous. But these folks also understand another fact about conventional treatments: They usually don't cure the problem; they only control symptoms.

More and more Americans are coming to adopt the philosophy of this book: That the body has a natural, built-in healing power. The same power that spontaneously and miraculously heals a cut can also clear up a sinus infection or relieve back pain or banish the discomforts of menopause. And one or more alternative cures can often help boost this natural healing power.

One doctor interviewed for the book, Elson Haas, M.D., put it this way: "Using a prescription drug to 'heal' is a little bit like shooting out the oil light on the dashboard when your car is low on oil. Sure, you won't know you have the problem anymore. But at a certain point, your motor is still going to burn out."

More people are also realizing that the mind and spirit—your thoughts and feelings, your desires and hopes, your sense of life's meaning and purpose—also play a major role in your physical health, and they can't be ignored.

Patricia Kaminski, a leading practitioner of flower essence therapy, which uses flower-derived tinctures to help remove blockages to a person's full expression of creativity and happiness, has this to say about the body-mind-spirit connection: "The real frontier of the new medicine will 'treat' thoughts, feelings, perceptions, and values—the soul—and by changing those realities, also improve the health of the body."

Americans are looking for practitioners like Kaminski. In one study, for example, 46 percent of those who used alternative therapies said that they did so because "the health of my body, mind, and spirit are related, and whoever cares for my health should take that into account." Dozens of the practitioners interviewed for this book do exactly that, and in the pages of *Alternative Cures*, they share the same mind-body remedies that they recommend for their patients.

## THE FEEL-BETTER MIRACLES YOU'LL FIND IN THIS BOOK

Americans want alternative remedies.

Americans want those remedies from qualified alternative practitioners.

*Alternative Cures* gives Americans what they want.

To write this book, I interviewed hundreds of America's top natural health practitioners. Alternative-minded M.D.'s, who blend the best of both conventional and alternative medicine. Naturopathic physicians, who concentrate on therapeutic foods, herbs, water therapy, and other natural means to restore health. Clinical nutritionists, who recommend the best vitamin and mineral regimens. Herbalists, who use plants to heal. Doctors of Traditional Chinese Medicine and experts in acupressure, who enhance the chi, or life-energy of the body. Psychologists, who use imagery, visualization, relaxation, and other mind-body techniques to heal. And that's only a partial listing of the types of alternative practitioners included here.

I asked them for their best home remedies for each of the 160 health conditions in this book, while always making sure that they told me when professional care is necessary and how to find the best professional care, be it alternative or conventional. In short, I've put together a compilation of remedies that you can't find anywhere else—not in any other book, not on the Internet, not in magazines. It's the best collection anywhere of cutting-edge, patient-proven alternative cures. Here's a small sample of the gems of natural healing that you'll find in the pages of this book.

The amino acids that can **banish food cravings and help you lose weight**... The super-simple postural correction that can

**clear up most cases of back pain**... A nutrient that can **stop the body-hurting side effects of the most commonly used arthritis drugs**... An herbal cocktail that can **end a case of the flu fast**... A food supplement that can prevent a hangover (just take a teaspoon before going to bed)... An aromatherapy spray that can **keep you from getting carsick**... A supplement paste that can **minimize blistering of poison ivy and poison oak,** so you hardly know you have it.

Plus: An herb that can **help stop the capillary damage of diabetes**... An acupressure "neck release" that can **help speed the healing of bursitis**... A special form of vitamin E that can **help stop the cause of heart attack if you have angina**... How to **reverse macular degeneration,** the leading cause of vision loss in America... A supplement regimen to **prevent or help reverse osteoporosis**... Why drinking lots of water may be the best remedy to **lower high blood pressure**... A simple remedy from your freezer that **short-circuits a cold sore**... The supplement for depression that a doctor says is **as powerful as antidepressant drugs**.

As you page through this book, I'm sure that you'll find plenty of ideas for improving your own health and that of your friends and family. And you'll know that you're in very good company—that of millions of Americans who, like you, have embraced alternative medicine as a true and useful option in their pursuit of better health.

*While natural remedies like nutritional supplements, herbs, and essential oils generally are safe, some can cause interactions or side effects when taken in large amounts or in certain combinations. For this reason, it's a good idea to check the safe-use guidelines beginning on page 704 before beginning treatment with these alternative therapies.*

### Part 1

# Alternative Home Remedies

# *Nutritional Supplements That Can Clear Up* Acne

Ask any number of dermatologists if poor digestion is a cause of acne, and you're likely to get the same answer from each: No.

This is precisely why dermatologists don't always cure acne, says Andrew Rubman, N.D., a naturopathic physician and founder of the Southbury Clinic for Traditional Medicine in Connecticut. "Acne has generated an entire industry of high-priced dermatologists and an incredible laundry list of very potent and expensive medications, including topical and oral antibiotics," he says.

Yes, these medications can control acne, as long as you continue to use them. But, says Dr. Rubman, many cases of acne could be cured—cleared up for good—by improving the health of the digestive tract.

The gastrointestinal (GI) tract is the body's primary organ of elimination, he explains. When your intestines are loaded with "pro-inflammatory substances"—biochemical toxins generated by the saturated fat in animal products and the hydrogenated fat in processed foods as well as by refined sugar, coffee, and alcohol—he believes that the body looks for a "second venue" to get rid of the debris. It often finds that dumping ground in the sebaceous glands, the oil-secreting glands that generate pimples when they're blocked with gunk.

When the GI tract is cooled down with anti-inflammatory fats—the fatty acids that are found in foods such as cold-water fish, nuts, and seeds—Dr. Rubman believes that it can eliminate the pro-inflammatory substances without sending them to the skin. And that can clear up adult acne.

That's why he gives all his patients with adult acne a supplement that provides a balanced combination of all the different fatty acids. What's more, he says, this supplement is especially effective in clearing up a particularly irritating form of adult

---

# GUIDE TO
# PROFESSIONAL CARE

Acne can affect self-esteem, causing problems in many areas of life, but it is not a threat to physical health, says Esta Kronberg, M.D., a dermatologist in Houston. There is, however, a very rare form of acne called acne fulminans, with fever and boils that cover the face, that is quite severe and needs immediate medical attention.

---

acne: the breakouts that happen each month right before a woman's period.

## FATTY ACIDS: *For Premenstrual Breakouts*

"Most of the adult acne patients I treat are women in their midtwenties to midthirties who have cyclical acne—who always break out 2 to 3 days before their periods," Dr. Rubman says.

He gives them a supplement called Perfect Oils, manufactured by Nutritional Therapeutics, which supplies a therapeutic balance of fatty acids from borage, fish, and flaxseed oils. Typical patients take two or three soft-gel capsules a day with food.

"I have had absolutely amazing results with this supplement," he says. "Not only does the acne go away, but as the GI tract functions better, the women's hair and nails get stronger, they have fewer problems with irregularity, they sleep better, and their libidos are stronger. They get all kinds of benefits."

## VITAMINS AND MINERALS: *An Anti-Acne Program*

Many other nutritional supplements can help heal acne and prevent outbreaks, according to Earl Mindell, Ph.D., a pharmacist and nutritionist in Beverly Hills. Here are the vitamins and minerals that he recommends.

• Beta-carotene: This form of vitamin A may help protect the skin from bacteria, which contribute to acne. Take 15 milligrams daily.

- B-complex vitamins: These are thought to help you cope with stress, which can contribute to skin problems. Take a daily high-potency B-complex supplement that supplies 100 milligrams of most of the B vitamins.
- Vitamin C: It is considered essential for the health of collagen, a component of the skin. Take 1,000 to 3,000 milligrams a day.
- Vitamin E: This nutrient can help the body assimilate vitamin A. Take 400 international units a day in a dry form, which is better absorbed, says Dr. Mindell.
- Zinc: This is believed to be one of the most important minerals for healthy skin. Take 15 milligrams daily.

## ACUPRESSURE: *Clear Up Congestion*

Traditional Chinese Medicine (TCM) sees acne as a problem with chi, the energy that keeps crucial components of the body and mind (like blood and emotions) moving freely. Acne occurs when the flow of "liver chi" is stagnant or blocked, says Jason Elias, a practitioner of Traditional Chinese Medicine in New Paltz, New York.

Four acupressure points are particularly effective for premenstrual acne, says Elias. Stimulating the points SP6 and SP9 releases congestive energy that causes menstrual problems, he says, while stimulating LV3 and LV4 helps release toxicity in the body. (For the exact locations of the points, see An Illustrated Guide to Acupressure Points on page 700.) Twice a week, sit in a chair and use your thumb to make circular movements in a clockwise direction in and around each point for about 1 minute. Press hard enough to cause slight pain, but not so much that you want to stop.

## HERBS: *A Formula to Eliminate Toxins*

Herbal remedies, both Chinese and Western, can help heal acne and prevent recurrences by cleansing the lymphatic system, Elias says. He recommends a formula that combines equal parts of the tinctures of nine herbs: red clover, burdock, yellow dock, dang gui, milk thistle, cleavers, schisandra, echinacea, and licorice.

Bring 1 quart of water to a boil and add 1 ounce of combined tinctures. Turn off the heat and steep for 30 minutes. Drink two cups a day for up to 3 months. You can refrigerate the unused portion for up to a week.

Along with lymphatic cleansers, the formula contains herbs that are thought to support the liver, nourish the blood, and fight infection—all factors that are crucial in healing acne.

**HYDROTHERAPY:** *An Herbal Steam Bath for Your Face*
A weekly steam bath for your face can open and drain the pores, helping to heal acne and prevent new outbreaks, Elias says. Adding the herb yarrow to the steaming water is very healing to the skin, he says.

Using 1 teaspoon of loose tea or a tea bag, prepare an 8-ounce cup of yarrow tea, steep for 30 minutes, and add it to a basin of steaming water. Lean over the basin for 5 to 10 minutes, holding a towel over your head as a kind of hood to keep the steam on your face. Your face should be close enough to feel the steam (about 12 inches away) but not so close that it burns.

If your acne is severe, use a steam bath two or three times a week, says Elias. If you get acne every now and then, use it once a week to help prevent outbreaks.

# *A Nutritional Plan to Kick* **Addictions**

Addictions have a root cause—a disturbance in the chemistry of the brain and body—that makes some people more likely to become dependent on alcohol, drugs, gambling, workaholism, or some other addictive substance or behavior. Some alternative practitioners believe that one thing can be dangerous to these people: It acts like a drug and triggers the addictive response that they want to suppress. That one thing is sugar.

"I believe that people with addictive personalities are sugar-sensitive," says Kathleen DesMaisons, Ph.D., president and CEO of Radiant Recovery, a treatment program for alcoholism, drug addiction, and other types of compulsive behavior, in Albuquerque, New Mexico.

# GUIDE TO
# PROFESSIONAL CARE

A person who is addicted to alcohol, drugs, gambling, or any other self-destructive behavior requires help. That help can come from a mental health professional in either an individual or group setting. It can also come from a trusted friend or advisor or a self-help group such as Alcoholics Anonymous.

Whichever route you decide to take, a good source of help is someone who has recovered from addiction, says Kathleen DesMaisons, Ph.D., president and CEO of Radiant Recovery, a treatment program for alcoholism, drug addiction, and other types of compulsive behavior, in Albuquerque, New Mexico.

"You want to work with someone who understands the issues involved and has the spiritual depth, maturity, commitment, and seriousness to guide your recovery," Dr. DesMaisons says.

Be sure to ask if the counselor or doctor that you've chosen thinks that diet plays a role in the way you feel. That way, you'll have the best of both worlds, says Dr. DesMaisons. Seeking professional help and using diet and natural remedies can support the changes you make. Do not try to heal your addiction alone.

For them, too much sugar in any form—in sweets, refined carbohydrates, or alcohol—can affect their biochemistry in two key ways.

First, it initially raises levels of serotonin, a brain chemical, or neurotransmitter, that helps control your mood and emotions, but the effect is short-lived. When this serotonin boost wears off, they feel even worse, experiencing depression and low self-esteem.

Second, it boosts levels of the "pleasure" neurotransmitters called beta-endorphins, triggering impulsive behavior and cravings for more sugar.

In other words, sugar helps to create the ideal biochemical environment for a lifetime of addiction. By changing your diet, you can begin the process of true recovery and start repairing your life.

**FOOD:** *Free Yourself From the Sugar Trap*

Dr. DesMaisons' dietary recommendations can help addictive types normalize their levels of blood sugar, serotonin, and beta-endorphins. You can implement them step by step, mastering one and then moving onto the next. And as you can see, they're very simple.

**1.** Eat breakfast every day. If you don't have food first thing in the morning your levels of blood sugar, beta-endorphins, and serotonin are disordered.

**2.** Eat lunch and dinner. "When you eat regular meals and don't snack, you teach your addictive body the new behavior of starting and stopping," says Dr. DesMaisons.

**3.** Make the change from white foods to brown. This is a major step in switching from addiction-creating sweet foods to healthy eating. Make the adjustment gradually, Dr. DesMaisons suggests. White foods include bread, cakes, cereals, and pasta made from white flour. Brown foods include the whole-grain versions of bread, cereals, pasta, flour, and so on, as well as amaranth, black beans, brown rice, lentils, soybeans, potatoes with skin, sunflower seeds, polenta, sweet potatoes, and popcorn.

**4.** Reduce or eliminate sugar. Once you've eliminated many obvious sources of sugar, it's time to eliminate hidden sources by reading food labels. Besides looking for the word *sugar*, check labels for these terms: barley malt, brown rice syrup, cane juice, fruit juice concentrate, galactose, glucose, high-fructose corn syrup, honey, lactose, corn sweetener, corn syrup, malted barley, maltodextrin, maltose, mannitol, sorbitol, xylitol, maltitol, microcrystalline cellulose, molasses, polydextrose, dextrin, dextrose, fructose, fructo-oligosaccharides, raisin juice, raisin syrup, Sucanat, and sucrose.

"Don't scare yourself about never having sugar again," Dr. DesMaisons says. "Just start with one choice at a time."

## Flower Essences to Help Reclaim Your Will

Flower essences are specially prepared tinctures that can help with your addiction by making you aware of patterns of thinking and feeling that are blocking your soul's natural expression of creativity, strength, and love, says Patricia Kaminski, co-founder and codirector of the Flower Essence Society, based in Nevada City, California. For the following remedies, take four drops four times a day for several months or until you resolve your addiction.

### BLACK-EYED SUSAN: *For Addicts in Denial*

For the addicted person who refuses to admit to a problem, this flower essence can help reveal the reality of the addiction, says Kaminski.

### RESCUE REMEDY: *Help for Detox*

Rescue Remedy (also known as Five-Flower Formula) can help a person through the difficult period of detoxifying from an alcohol or drug addiction. During the initial detoxification period, take four drops once an hour rather than four times a day to help you feel calm and stable.

### CALIFORNIA WILD ROSE: *A New Commitment to Life*

An addict is often disconnected from a commitment to life, says Kaminski—"the feeling that life is here to be lived and that he has something to say about how his life will progress." This essence helps bring a new commitment to life and new life to the will.

### NICOTIANA: *If You're Trying to Quit Smoking*

When you quit smoking, you feel tired, tense, and negative, and you have to face the emotions that you've been trying to avoid. (No wonder you reach for a cigarette!) The essence called nicotiana can help you be aware of your own life-energy and accept your feelings, says Kaminski, which helps you to avoid lighting up.

### MORNING GLORY: *For Caffeine Addiction*

This flower essence helps people overcome erratic rhythms and disturbed sleep patterns, such as staying up late at night and feeling extremely sluggish in the morning, thereby reducing the need for caffeine in the morning, says Kaminski.

# *Natural Remedies Can Reduce*
## Age Spots

They should have been called sun spots, but the name was already taken. "Age spots" had to do.

These brown spots that typically start to pepper the backs of your hands in your forties or fifties are caused by years of direct exposure to the sun's ultraviolet radiation, which damages the color-producing cells of the skin. Those cells, called melanocytes, then go into overdrive, producing too much color.

No matter what you do to lighten them, the spots will come right back if you re-expose the area to sun, says Joni Loughran, an esthetician, cosmetologist, and aromatherapist in Petaluma, California. If you're trying to fade age spots, wear a sunblock with an SPF of 15 on your hands or other exposed, spotted areas whenever you go outdoors. Then try the following alternative remedies to reduce or eliminate the spots.

---

### GUIDE TO
### PROFESSIONAL CARE

In almost all cases, age spots are a cosmetic problem, not a medical or health-threatening condition, says Esta Kronberg, M.D., a dermatologist in Houston. They can be medically removed with bleaches, liquid nitrogen, or laser surgery, if you desire.

In extremely rare cases, the area of a spot can develop a life-threatening cancer called a melanoma. If one of your age spots, or the area around a spot, has turned black and is irregular in shape (signs of melanoma), see a medical doctor immediately.

## AROMATHERAPY: *Help the Spots Fade*

The essential oils of lemon and benzoin have bleaching properties that can help age spots fade, says Barbara Close, an herbalist and aromatherapist in East Hampton, New York. Combine two to three drops of one of the oils with a vegetable carrier oil such as almond, then apply the mixture to the spot twice a day.

## LICORICE AND GLYCOLIC ACID: *A Beautiful Solution*

Although it may be hard to find, a beauty product containing glycolic acid and licorice extract can work beautifully to lighten or eliminate age spots, says Close.

Glycolic acid consists of natural sugar acids derived from citrus, papaya, or other foods. It gently exfoliates the top layer of the skin, while the licorice bleaches the spot. To apply, follow the instructions on the label.

## HONEY AND YOGURT: *A Natural Bleach*

A mixture of honey and yogurt creates a natural bleach that can help lighten age spots, says Pratima Raichur, N.D., an Ayurvedic practitioner in New York City.

To 1 teaspoon of plain yogurt, add 1 teaspoon of honey and mix thoroughly. Apply the mixture to your hands, let it dry, then wash it off after 30 minutes. Do this once a day.

## GOTU KOLA: *Encourage Cell Growth*

The herb gotu kola may help fight age spots by stimulating the growth of new, healthy cells and the production of collagen, the protein that holds skin together, says Brigitte Mars, an herbalist and nutritional consultant in Boulder, Colorado. She recommends daily use of a tincture or capsule form of the herb. Add one dropper of tincture to ¼ cup of water and take three times daily, or take one or two 60-milligram capsules a day.

# *Fast, Effective, Drug-Free Relief for*
# **Allergies**

Your immune system has decided that an everyday substance—maybe the pollen from a tree, the dander from a cat, or the dust on a bookshelf—is your enemy, an allergen. When you inhale that substance into your body, an antibody is created. This specialized protein first detects the enemy, then signals the immune system to disarm and destroy the scoundrel.

In order to neutralize the allergen, your cells must release histamine and other chemicals, causing some combination of the classic symptoms—the runny nose, the red and itchy eyes, the sneezing, the sinus headache, the scratchy throat—that you call an allergy. But if you reach for an over-the-counter antihistamine for relief, you may wind up doing more harm than good, say alternative doctors.

"Sensitivity to allergens may be concealed by taking antihistamine medications," says Jacqueline Krohn, M.D., a physician in New Mexico. This is because antihistamines treat the symptoms, not the cause. Then there are the common side effects, such as drowsiness or, with the newer "nondrowsy" products, the possibility of heart arrhythmias, Dr. Krohn says.

If you're worried that alternative home remedies won't work as well as medications, you shouldn't be. "I believe that natural remedies are strong enough that you won't have to take drugs—you'll get all the relief you need," says Mark Stengler, N.D., a naturopathic physician in San Diego.

## HYDROTHERAPY: *A Cleansing Bath for Your Immune System*

Visualize your immune system as a rain barrel, Dr. Krohn says. Many factors, such as infections, environmental toxins, and stress, can fill your barrel. When the barrel is full, one more drop—an allergen—can overflow your immune system so that

# GUIDE TO
# PROFESSIONAL CARE

The most serious aspect of an inhalant allergy is the chance that it might trigger an asthma attack, which could be fatal. If you can't get your allergies under control by yourself, seek the help of an allergist.

Some alternative practitioners believe that a traditional allergist may not be the best physician to help you control or heal inhalant allergies, says Jacqueline Krohn, M.D., a physician in New Mexico. "Traditional allergy shots and drugs provide limited control and may not give the optimal dose," she says.

Instead, she urges patients with allergies to find an allergist who provides the widest possible array of tests and treatments. She recommends that you look for an allergist whose practice includes using many of the following methods.

• Fasting and food testing to detect food allergies, since they can worsen inhalant allergies.
• Bronchial inhalation challenge testing, which detects sensitivities to chemicals and other environmental factors.
• Kinesiology testing, in which a doctor measures your muscle strength as you hold various substances. Weakness indicates that you are allergic or sensitive to the substance.
• Cytotoxic testing, a blood test to detect chemical and food allergies.
• RAST (radioallergosorbent test), a blood test to detect food, pollen, mold, dust, dust mite, and dander allergies.
• ALCAT (antigen leucocyte cellular antibody test), which measures reactions to mold, food, or chemicals.
• Patch testing to diagnose contact allergies, which are reactions to substances that touch the skin.
• EAV (electroacupuncture according to Voll) testing. Commonly used in Europe, this test uses electroacupuncture to detect a wide variety of allergies. "It is a rapid, painless, noninvasive method of screening for allergies," says Dr. Krohn.
• Serial dilution endpoint titration, which is one of the best and most accurate tests for inhalant and food allergies, says Dr. Krohn.

- Provocative neutralization therapy, a test plus therapy that "prevents, blocks, or neutralizes reactions to the problem substance," says Dr. Krohn.
- NAET (Nambudripad's allergy elimination technique), a combination of kinesiology, acupuncture, and chiropractic techniques to stop allergens from provoking symptoms.
- Enzyme potentiated desensitization, which uses enzymes and small doses of allergens to desensitize people to their allergies.
- Immunotherapy, which involves a series of injections or intake of dilute levels of an allergen to gradually desensitize you to it.

it can't deal with the invader. You experience allergic symptoms.

Some alternative practitioners believe that one of the best ways to lower the water level in your rain barrel so that your body can deal with allergens is with detoxification baths, says Dr. Krohn. She believes that the heat from the bath releases stored toxins from fat cells into the blood. They then travel to the skin and are released.

"I frequently prescribe these baths for my allergic patients," she says. "They can be very effective for decreasing and even preventing allergic symptoms, especially for people who are overloaded from chemicals." Here's how to take a detoxification bath, according to Dr. Krohn.

First, take a bath or shower to remove excess oil and dirt from your skin. Scrub with a rough washcloth or loofah, then rinse thoroughly.

Next, fill the tub with water as hot as you can tolerate without pain and deep enough to immerse your body up to your neck. (You might want to buy an overflow drain cover at a hardware store so you can fill the tub to the top.) Sit in the tub, letting the water cover your entire body, including your hands and arms (you won't submerge your head, of course). Stay in the bath for 5 minutes, then take a brief but thorough warm shower to wash the toxins off your skin so they won't be reabsorbed.

Take no more than three detoxification baths a week, gradually increasing the duration to 30 minutes. It's possible that during the bath, you'll feel slightly weak as the toxins enter your bloodstream, says Dr. Krohn. If you do, drain the water and sit in the tub until you no longer feel weak.

Don't increase the length of the baths until you can bathe comfortably without feeling weak; that is, if weakness begins after 5 minutes, take 5-minute baths. As you take detoxification baths regularly and your body purifies, you'll be able to take longer and longer ones. When you can take a bath for 30 minutes without experiencing any weakness, cut back to one a week, says Dr. Krohn. People with multiple sclerosis or severe heart disease should not use this remedy.

### NETTLE: *The Top Herbal Antihistamine*

"Seventy percent of my allergy patients who take the herb stinging nettle don't need to take any other supplement or medication for symptomatic relief," Dr. Stengler says.

To maximize the effectiveness of this herb, start taking it a couple of weeks before allergy season begins. Take two 300-milligram capsules of freeze-dried nettle three times a day.

"The freeze-dried form is more concentrated and tends to work much better," says Dr. Stengler. Taking nettle in the midst of hay fever season will still work to quiet symptoms, but it will take 3 to 4 days to kick in, he says.

### QUERCETIN: *A Nutrient Powerhouse*

"The bioflavonoid quercetin can be a potent inhibitor of histamine release," says Skye Weintraub, N.D., a naturopathic physician in Eugene, Oregon.

Taking 250 milligrams twice a day is usually sufficient to control most allergies, she says. Just don't expect to be better tomorrow. "It can take 3 to 4 weeks before quercetin becomes effective."

### BROMELAIN: *Quercetin's Best Friend*

This anti-inflammatory enzyme from pineapple helps with the absorption, and therefore the effectiveness, of quercetin, says Dr. Weintraub. Take 250 milligrams of bromelain twice a day along with quercetin.

### Hypoglycemia: The Secret Cause of Allergies?

Treating the symptoms of allergies may provide temporary relief. But Skye Weintraub, N.D., a naturopathic physician in Eugene, Oregon, believes that it may be possible to actually cure the problem by changing your diet.

"Allergens are the triggers of allergic response, but they are not the ultimate cause of the problem," she says. She believes that an unhealthy diet can leave your body so weak that it can't cope with common substances such as pollen and cat dander.

"Every time one of my patients has truly and consistently switched to a healing diet, hay fever or other respiratory allergies have either significantly diminished or vanished," Dr. Weintraub says.

She has found that many patients with allergies also have hypoglycemia, or low blood sugar. "Often, upon treating and effectively controlling the person's hypoglycemia, the original allergy also clears up," she says.

And hypoglycemia isn't hard to fix. "If all conditions were as easy to treat as hypoglycemia, the world would be an Eden of wellness," Dr. Weintraub says.

Here's how to step into your own allergy-free paradise, according to Dr. Weintraub.

First, cut out refined sugar. Eating lots of sugar, in cakes, candy, cookies, soda, and other sweet foods, floods the bloodstream with glucose, or blood sugar. The body then pumps out the hormone insulin to usher the glucose into the brain and muscles.

Refined sugar, which is a simple carbohydrate, triggers such a flood of insulin that blood sugar levels plummet 30 minutes or so after consuming the sweets. There's only one way off this roller coaster of sugary ups and downs—"all intake of refined sugar must stop," says Dr. Weintraub. That includes fruit juices and dried fruits, both of which deliver high levels of concentrated sugar.

Worried that your craving for sweets will overwhelm you? Hang in there. "Going sugar-free for 1 to 2 weeks is usually enough to knock out sugar cravings," says Dr. Weintraub.

Second, reach for complex carbohydrates. These foods, which include vegetables, whole grains, and beans, are digested slowly by the body, keeping blood sugar levels on an even keel.

"In order to avoid hypoglycemia, the majority of food in your diet should be in the form of complex carbohydrates," Dr. Weintraub says. Because fruits are too high in quickly digested sugars, she recommends eliminating all fruit at the beginning of this program. Most people can usually add some whole fruit to their diets later, she says.

Third, remember protein, which also provides a slow and steady supply of fuel. "To clear up hypoglycemia, the diet must also consist of adequate protein," says Dr. Weintraub. Aim to make protein foods like fish, lamb, turkey, chicken, brewer's yeast, tofu, nuts, and seeds about 20 to 30 percent of your diet, she advises.

Finally, eat early and often. Eating two or three big meals a day can cause the same up-and-down variations in blood sugar levels as eating refined sugars, says Dr. Weintraub. The best approach is "five or six smaller feedings, with plenty of fresh foods," she says. She recommends a small breakfast, a good midmorning snack, a light lunch, a midafternoon snack, dinner, and a small snack before bed.

## MASSAGE: *For Hands-On Relief*

A facial massage from qigong, a branch of Traditional Chinese Medicine, can help relieve the symptoms of inhalant allergies, says Glenn S. Rothfeld, M.D., regional medical director of American WholeHealth in Arlington, Massachusetts. Here's how to do it.

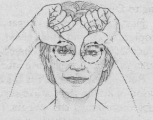

Using the pads of your thumbs, rub in small circles, starting between your eyebrows and moving down along the sides of your nose and over your cheekbones below your eyes. Next, begin between your eyebrows once again, using the flats of your thumbs to rub along your eyebrows toward your temples, then massage your temples.

"In this massage, you want to cover the temples, above the eyes, below the eyes, and alongside the nose," says Dr. Rothfeld. This helps improve circulation into the tissues and relieves the inflammation that results from allergies. Do this massage for 5 minutes two or three times a day, whenever you're suffering from allergic symptoms.

**ADRENAL GLANDULARS:** *To Strengthen Your Defense System*

The adrenal glands are known for producing adrenaline, the hormone that's pumped out when your body is under stress. But since they also produce hormones that keep your immune system revved up, weak adrenal glands can make you more vulnerable to allergies. Dr. Weintraub has noticed that when the adrenal glands are working well, the allergies get better.

One way to strengthen your adrenal glands and help prevent allergic symptoms is to take an adrenal glandular, a product made from an extract of animal adrenal glands.

"Adrenal glandulars build immunity and help defend the body against allergies," Dr. Weintraub says. She recommends taking one 180- to 200-milligram tablet two or three times a day.

**PANTOTHENIC ACID:** *Another Adrenal Aid*

Pantothenic acid, a B vitamin, also helps boost adrenal function, says Dr. Rothfeld. He recommends 200 to 500 milligrams a day.

## *Natural Treatments May Delay* Alzheimer's Disease

If you're diagnosed with Alzheimer's—the brain disease that slowly but surely devastates mental, emotional, and, finally, even physical functioning—most conventional neurologists will offer you two treatments.

One is the prescription drug donepezil (Aricept), which increases levels of acetylcholine, a brain chemical responsible for memory. The other is vitamin E, an antioxidant that slows the destruction of brain cells. Although conventional neurologists used to think that treating Alzheimer's with vitamin E was nonsense, studies have demonstrated the nutri-

# GUIDE TO
# PROFESSIONAL CARE

*Caution: You should use the alternative remedies discussed in this chapter only as part of a treatment program that is guided and monitored by a qualified medical doctor in partnership with a qualified alternative practitioner, both of whom are experienced in caring for your condition. Check with your conventional doctor before changing or stopping any conventional medical treatments or medications, and keep all of your doctors and/or alternative practitioners informed of all treatments that you are receiving.*

Dharma Singh Khalsa, M.D., president and medical director of the Alzheimer's Prevention Foundation in Tucson, suggests visiting a doctor for possible diagnosis if you notice a change in personality, recent memory loss, problems with language, or general disorientation in yourself or a loved one.

Dr. Khalsa lists the following necessary components as the foundation of any effective approach to treating Alzheimer's disease: nutritional counseling, brain-supportive nutritional and herbal supplements, physical exercise, cognitive exercise, mind-body stress-control techniques such as meditation, psychological counseling, pharmaceutical drugs, and testing for and replacement of hormones such as testosterone, growth hormone, and DHEA.

ent's effectiveness in helping to slow the progress of the disease.

Both treatments are helpful, but there's much more that you can do for Alzheimer's. Natural treatments potentially can slow the progression of the disease and perhaps even prevent its later stages, in which memory is totally eroded.

"Like the heart, the brain is an organ made of flesh and blood," says Dharma Singh Khalsa, M.D., president and medical director of the Alzheimer's Prevention Foundation in Tucson. "And just as there are many ways to slow the progression of heart disease, such as dietary changes, nutritional supplements, stress reduction, and exercise, for example, so there are many ways to slow the progression of the brain disease Alzheimer's—not just the two treatments recommended by most neurologists."

If you've been diagnosed with Alzheimer's, you need to admit that you have a serious problem and to accept the fact that you need to devote your life to caring for yourself, Dr. Khalsa says.

"You can't just take a few pills every day, whether they're prescription drugs or natural supplements, and go along with life," he says. "You must focus on the reality that your brain has a degenerative illness—possibly a progressive illness, similar to cancer—and that you must devote significant time to slowing its progress."

The remedies offered here are part of Dr. Khalsa's total program for slowing the progress of Alzheimer's. Because of the seriousness of the disease, however, you must use them only with the approval and supervision of a physician and in conjunction with the full range of medical tests and treatments needed to diagnose and treat Alzheimer's.

### HUPERZINE A: *Slow Memory Loss Without Side Effects*

Huperzine A, the active ingredient in the Chinese herb club moss, has an effect on the brain that is similar to the effect of the prescription drug donepezil, but without its expense or side effects, which can include gastrointestinal upset and liver damage, says Dr. Khalsa. "This purified ingredient of club moss blocks the breakdown of acetylcholine, the neurotransmitter important for memory," he says.

### PHOSPHATIDYLSERINE: *Boost Mental Capacity*

In his practice, Dr. Khalsa has found that the nutrient phosphatidylserine helps regenerate the outside layer of neurons, reversing the chronological age of these cells by as much as 12 years and improving the mental capacity of his Alzheimer's patients. He recommends 300 milligrams a day in three divided doses with meals.

### VITAMIN E: *Regenerate Brain Cells*

This vitamin helps shield neurons from free radicals, unstable molecules that damage cells. But, says Dr. Khalsa, it can also regenerate the areas on neurons where neurotransmitters—the chemicals that relay messages from one neuron to another—

enter. For Alzheimer's patients, he recommends 2,000 international units a day of the d-alpha tocopherol form of the nutrient, which is the most effective.

## Keep Active

Regular physical exercise can help an Alzheimer's patient form new brain cells, says Dharma Singh Khalsa, M.D., president and medical director of the Alzheimer's Prevention Foundation in Tucson. Here's how he suggests that you do it. If you have Alzheimer's and you're able to exercise on your own, you should walk every day or engage in some other exercise you enjoy. If the disease is more advanced, a caregiver should take the Alzheimer's patient for a walk, even if it's just around the patio, for example.

## COENZYME $Q_{10}$: *Protect Mental Energy*

As the disease progresses, Alzheimer's patients become less and less mentally energetic. The nutrient coenzyme $Q_{10}$ is vital for producing energy in neurons (and throughout the body), Dr. Khalsa says. It also is a "neuroprotector" that helps stop the destruction of neurons by free radicals. He recommends 200 milligrams a day.

## GINKGO: *The Underestimated Herb*

The power of this herb to protect the brain from Alzheimer's has been underestimated by conventional doctors, says Dr. Khalsa. Ginkgo maximizes the flow of blood to the brain and helps protect neurons from free radicals. He recommends 240 milligrams a day.

## DHA: *The Fat Your Brain Needs*

Docosahexaenoic acid (DHA) is a fat that is a building block of the brain and can help people with Alzheimer's retain brain function, Dr. Khalsa says. (Don't mistake this supplement for DHEA, the hormone.) He recommends taking 100 milligrams a day of DHA manufactured from microalgae.

## FISH: *Good for Neurons*

Eat plenty of cold-water fish such as tuna, trout, mackerel, and salmon, Dr. Khalsa suggests. They're rich in omega-3 fatty acids, nutrients that help protect brain cells.

# *A New Way to Beat*
# **Anemia**

If it weren't for the threat to the health of millions of American women, you might call the situation ironic. As it turns out, some alternative practitioners believe that the type of iron supplement routinely prescribed by conventional doctors for treating iron-deficiency anemia—a problem that affects one of five American women—is not the best source of iron.

"The conventional treatment is to give iron in the form of ferrous sulfate," says Jesse Lynn Hanley, M.D., a physician in Malibu, California. "This form of iron is potentially irritating to a woman's stomach, lymphatic system, and liver and is not as well-absorbed as other forms of iron."

The body needs iron to produce red blood cells. Women who don't get enough iron in their diets or who have heavy menstrual periods may have insufficient levels of either red blood cells or hemoglobin, the oxygen-carrying protein in red blood cells. Since hemoglobin is responsible for carrying oxygen, women whose levels decline feel tired and weak.

Iron-deficiency anemia also may cause dizziness, loss of appetite, diarrhea, or abdominal pain. Getting more iron is essential for relieving this condition, says Dr. Hanley.

The problem is that conventional doctors may begin and end their treatment with a recommendation for women to get more iron. This isn't enough, says Dr. Hanley. Not only are they recommending a less-than-ideal form of iron, but it's simply not enough by itself.

Why do conventional doctors routinely treat anemia with just ferrous sulfate? Because that's what is traditionally taught in medical schools, and most doctors don't question it, says Dr. Hanley. Alternative doctors, on the other hand, have asked the questions, and they have been able to come up with some better answers.

# GUIDE TO PROFESSIONAL CARE

Iron-deficiency anemia is easy to treat, but only when you know what you're dealing with. Since this condition can be debilitating, and since other, more serious problems may cause the same symptoms, you'll want to see a doctor anytime your energy levels decline and don't seem to want to come back up again for 4 to 6 weeks. Other signs of this type of anemia are a pale complexion and feeling cold much of the time.

If your menstrual flow soaks a tampon or sanitary pad every hour or your menstrual period lasts for more than 7 days, you may have what doctors call menorrhagia, an excessively heavy or long menstrual flow. You should report any heavy bleeding to your doctor.

If you're having rectal bleeding, you also need to see a doctor right away, says Jesse Lynn Hanley, M.D., a physician in Malibu, California. She recommends, however, that you see an alternative-minded doctor. This will give you the best of both worlds—authoritative advice on the best ways to correct iron deficiencies as well as advice on improving your diet and lifestyle, she says.

## IRON SUPPLEMENTS: *The Right Kind*

Unlike ferrous sulfate, forms of iron called ferrous gluconate, iron gluconate, and iron picolinate are easy for the body to digest and absorb, says Dr. Hanley. They're also less likely to irritate the stomach. Women of childbearing age, who lose blood every month through menstruation, should get 15 milligrams a day. After menopause, most women do not need supplemental iron, Dr. Hanley says. Men need 10 milligrams a day.

## IRON-RICH FOODS: *The Best Sources*

The iron found in plant foods is called non-heme iron. It's not as easily absorbed as the iron in meats, but a diet rich in plant foods is much better for you in other ways. And if you eat enough of these foods, you may get enough iron as well, says Susan Lark, M.D, a physician in Los Altos, California.

Good sources of iron include whole grains such as barley and oats; beans and peas; seeds and nuts, especially sesame seeds, sunflower seeds, pistachios, pecans, and almonds; and vegetables such as Swiss chard and kale.

## A Self-Test for Anemia

Doctors sometimes miss anemia because they confuse the symptoms with something else.

"Every symptom of anemia can be mistaken for other health conditions, including emotional problems and nervous tension," says Susan Lark, M.D., a physician in Los Altos, California. Rather than depending only on your doctor, here are two ways to see for yourself if you may have anemia.

• Press down for 2 seconds on a fingernail (unpolished) so that you're pressing against the nail bed. The area will turn white. Then stop pressing and note how long it takes for the area to turn pink again. It should happen within a second or two. The more slowly the skin turns pink, the more likely it is that you have anemia, says Jesse Lynn Hanley, M.D., a physician in Malibu, California.
• Gently pull down your lower eyelids and look at the color of the blood vessels underneath your eyes. If they're very pale, you may have anemia, says Dr. Hanley.

### VITAMIN C: *To Enhance Absorption*

Vitamin C is acidic, which helps the body absorb the non-heme iron in plant foods, says Beverly Yates, N.D., a naturopathic doctor in Seattle. She recommends squeezing the juice of half a lemon into a glass of water and drinking it before meals.

Alternatively, you can take a supplement of 1,000 to 2,000 milligrams of vitamin C with each meal, says Dr. Hanley.

### CALCIUM-RICH FOODS: *When You Limit Dairy*

Just as some foods put more iron into your body, others make it harder to get enough. Dairy foods, for example, will decrease iron absorption in women with anemia, says Dr. Lark.

To make sure that you get enough calcium when you're cutting back on dairy foods, she recommends increasing your intake of beans, peas, soybeans, sesame seeds, soup stocks made with chicken or fish bones, and leafy green vegetables.

## ALCOHOL AND SUGAR: *Cut Back to Preserve Nutrients*

Beer, wine, and other alcoholic beverages deplete the body of B-complex vitamins and some minerals, which can worsen anemia, says Dr. Lark. She recommends having no more than 4 ounces of wine, 10 ounces of beer, or 1 ounce of hard liquor once or twice a week. You'll want to reduce your sugar intake as well, since this also depletes the body of B-complex vitamins.

## CAFFEINE: *Less Means More Iron*

You'll want to go easy on coffee, black tea, soda, chocolate, and other caffeine-containing foods when you're trying to recover from anemia because caffeine inhibits iron absorption, Dr. Lark explains.

## HERBS: *Relieve Heavy Bleeding*

Blood loss through heavy menstrual bleeding is a common cause of iron-deficiency anemia, says Dr. Lark. There are a number of herbs that can help control this problem.

With anemia and heavy menstrual bleeding, be sure that your diet and supplement program—vitamins, minerals, and herbs—provides the extra nutrients that your body needs. You can take these supplements indefinitely as part of your high-nutrient diet, but never use them as an excuse to continue poor eating habits, says Dr. Lark.

Keep in mind that herbal treatments should be used by women who have a menstrual flow that's somewhat heavier than usual, says Dr. Lark. Women who have excessive blood flow need to see a doctor.

Dr. Lark recommends the following herbs in tincture form. Begin with one-quarter to one-half dropper and slowly work up to a full dropper if you need it. You may find that you feel best with slightly more or less of certain herbs, she says.

The herb goldenseal contains berberine, a compound that can help calm the muscles of the uterus. Another herb, shepherd's purse, aids in blood clotting. Taken together, these herbs may help reduce excessive bleeding, says Dr. Lark.

Yellow dock, turmeric, and milk thistle are all good choices for strengthening the liver. A healthy liver more easily breaks down estrogen, which is important for treating anemia because excess estrogen can cause heavy bleeding.

**AROMATHERAPY:** *Soothe the Symptoms*

You can use essential oils to relieve discomfort while you're trying to get your iron levels back to normal, says DeAnna Batdorff, a clinical aromatherapist and Ayurvedic practitioner in Forestville, California.

If your doctor says that you're constipated because of anemia, for example, you can use blue cypress and ginger essential oils. Once a day, put two drops of cypress oil and one drop of ginger oil on the web between your big toe and second toe, Batdorff suggests.

If your skin is cold and clammy, put one drop of rose geranium oil on your stomach once a day.

# *Learn to Release Your*
# **Anger**

They come to the workshop to pound on pillows with their fists. They twist and bite towels. They scream and yell.

Why? Because they want relief from the anger that they too often feel. They get that relief by releasing their anger, by allowing themselves to physically express it, safely and harmlessly.

Weeks later, many write or call the workshop leader, expressing delight with the results: "I don't have migraines anymore." "My back pain is gone." "I feel serene and confident most of the time instead of upset and confused."

Most conventional psychologists would say that expressing your anger in any fashion, including physically, just leads to more anger. They might add that anger is really a self-deluding mask over deeper emotions, such as sorrow and fear. In this

# GUIDE TO
# PROFESSIONAL CARE

Some psychologists may lack the training or personal experience to help you deal with anger, says John Lee, director of the Facing the Fire Institute in Asheville, North Carolina. If you're considering a therapist, ask some questions.

• What do you believe about anger?
• Have you been trained to help me deal with my anger in ways other than just talking about it?
• Have you done your own anger work?

If the therapist doesn't think that anger is a feeling in the body that needs to be released, he hasn't been trained in body-based anger-release techniques, and he hasn't done personal anger-releasing work, find another therapist, says Lee.

Most people wait too long to address their anger issues. There are some obvious signs to help you identify when you need to seek professional care, including screaming, yelling, or withdrawing from certain people on a regular basis; people going out of their way to avoid you; or the people closest to you pointing out your problem.

More subtle but equally important are the possible physical manifestations of your anger, including indigestion, insomnia, migraines, and chronic tension in your jaw.

view, the best way to deal with anger is by getting underneath it to understand your true feelings.

Well, those conventional psychologists are wrong, says John Lee, director of the Facing the Fire Institute in Asheville, North Carolina. Lee, a veteran workshop leader, has trained more than 10,000 therapists and counselors and received thousands of letters and calls from people whom he taught to use his alternative, "body-centered" psychotherapeutic techniques.

Anger is an energy that gets into your body in many different ways, says Lee. It got into your body in the past when Mom or

Dad yelled at you, for example, and you felt angry but didn't express it. It gets into your body in the present when a car cuts you off in traffic, for example, or you get four telemarketing calls during dinner.

If you don't get the anger out, it can poison your thoughts and feelings. It can even cause physical illness, from headaches to back pain to heart disease.

If you release your anger, however, you'll experience profound physical, mental, and emotional relief, Lee says. You get that relief not by yelling at or in any way hurting another person or yourself but by doing safe, energetic exercises that get anger out of your body. Here's how.

### POUNDING A PILLOW: *Let Your Anger Have It*

Find a place where you can be alone and undisturbed. Then punch a pillow or hit it repeatedly with a tennis racket while yelling and cursing and moaning and hollering. Do it for as long as you feel like doing it.

"The sounds that you let out are very important," Lee says, "because they help articulate the preverbal anger and pain that you carry from deep in your childhood."

### SCREAMING IN YOUR CAR: *Perfect for a Traffic Jam*

"Get in your car, roll up the windows, and scream as loudly as you can," says Lee. Keep screaming for as long as you have the energy for it. Lee uses this exercise himself to release the anger that he stores in his throat and gut.

"I scream until I don't feel the need pressing on me to scream anymore at that time, because that wave of anger is used up," he says.

What should you scream? "When you're screaming in a car, it's completely appropriate for you to say anything that you need to say to get your anger out." Lee says. "Use blaming, hurtful, or accusatory words, obscenities, curses—whatever."

### TWISTING A TOWEL: *Wring Out the Anger*

"Take a bath towel in both hands and twist it as tightly as you can," says Lee. "As you twist your anger into the towel, let out any sighs, moans, or grunts that come up. Or repeat 'I'm angry.'"

If you store anger in your jaw, which is a problem among 20

to 30 percent of the people in his workshops, says Lee—bite the towel as you twist and make growling sounds.

## Don't Vent Anger on Others

The remedies in this chapter are all about releasing your anger, but aiming your anger at another person is something else entirely. John Lee, director of the Facing the Fire Institute in Asheville, North Carolina, says that 10 such inappropriate expressions of anger are shaming, blaming, demeaning, name-calling and put-downs, demoralizing, criticizing, judging, preaching, teaching, and analyzing.

Such inappropriate behavior might surface when someone "pushes a button" about something that made you angry in the distant past. And, Lee says, there are actually physical signs that your anger is based on past emotional experiences: a dry mouth; a knotted stomach; shoulders thrust up to your ears; sweaty, clammy, cold hands; and a lump in your throat. If you notice one or more of those signs, do the techniques in this chapter to release your anger.

Finally, says Lee, it's crucial to understand that rage—a verbal or physical attack—is never an appropriate way to release anger. In fact, rage is not even the same as anger.

"Rage is an action and a behavior used to cover up and numb other painful emotions," Lee says. "Anger is simply a feeling in the body that needs to be expressed."

A "rageoholic" who regularly vents anger on other people should see a professional instead of using the remedies in this chapter, says Lee.

## BREAKING DISHES: *For the Auditory Person*

Some people need to hear something outside themselves to feel that their anger is being expressed. If you fit that description, Lee suggests that you go to a yard sale and spend a couple of bucks on 100 or so plates for tossing.

Put a sheet on the side of a garage or other wall to protect against ricochets, stand back far enough from the wall so that you can't possibly be hurt as the dishes shatter, and throw those plates as hard as you can, one by one, against the wall.

"While you do this," Lee says, "concentrate on your anger and on forcing it up into your arms and torso and mouth and face so that you can expel it into the world."

**AEROBIC ANGER:** *The Secrets Are Focus and Speech*

"Any form of exercise will release anger if the exercise is consciously done with that end in mind," says Lee. You could hit a racquetball as hard as you can, for example, while focusing on how angry you are and saying what you need to say. Or you could ride a stationary bicycle, pumping hard, all the while saying, "I'm angry, I'm angry."

**BREATHING:** *Make Lots of Noise*

To use breathing to release anger, breathe in slowly and deeply through your nose, filling your entire torso from the lower abdomen to the upper chest, and exhale through your mouth, sighing and groaning.

"Breathing is crucial to emotional-release work," says Lee. "By itself, breathing is often sufficient to release mild, present angers. If you're hitting every traffic light, or if the man ahead of you in the 9-item express line at the grocery has 13 items, try breathing in and out deeply a few times (you can skip the groaning and sighing in public) and see if your anger doesn't seep away."

## Three Flower Essences for Three Types of Anger

It's thought that flower essences work by increasing your self-awareness, by revealing mental and emotional patterns that you don't ordinarily notice so that you can see them, understand them, and choose to outgrow them. "I believe that flower essences have many of the attributes of good psychotherapy," says Patricia Kaminski, cofounder and codirector of the Flower Essence Society, based in Nevada City, California. For each of the following essences, take four drops four times a day for about a month.

**HOLLY:** *Break Down the Barriers*

Holly is a unifying essence that helps break down the barriers between you and another person. That allows you to stop seeing the other person as an enemy and to start seeing and even appreciating his point of view, says Kaminski. "It is quite specific for anger, hostility, envy—for all the ways in which we oppose or separate ourselves from another person," she says.

## SCARLET MONKEYFLOWER: *When You Keep Your Anger Inside*

This remedy is for sensitive and loving people who don't know how to express anger appropriately and let it build up inside until it explodes, says Kaminski. And after they do explode, they usually feel worse about themselves. They think, "I really hurt that person," or "I let the demon out."

"This type of person is typically unable to communicate his needs," says Kaminski. Scarlet monkeyflower helps you express why you're angry in an appropriate way and then simply and without hostility ask for what you need, whether it's having a teenager turn down loud music or having your spouse remember to put the cap back on the toothpaste tube.

## BLACK COHOSH: *For the Angry Person and the Target*

Kaminski recommends this remedy when two people are "locked in a pattern of victimizer and victim, with one person using anger to have power over another, to actually make the other person afraid of his anger." In this case, both the angry person and the one who is more typically passive should take the remedy.

## *Effective Supplements for Easing*
# Angina

Heart disease has you in its grip—and it's squeezing.

That's what a bout of angina feels like: A pressurelike pain in your chest, perhaps flaring to your left shoulder blade and arm, neck, jaws, or back. The pain tends to be more constant for men, while women may experience chest discomfort that comes and goes or have shortness of breath.

Angina occurs when the heart muscle temporarily doesn't get enough blood and oxygen. It's usually triggered by emotional stress, extreme temperatures, heavy meals, alcohol, cigarette smoking, or physical exertion, all of which increase the heart's demand for oxygen.

# GUIDE TO
# PROFESSIONAL CARE

*Caution: You should use the alternative remedies discussed in this chapter only as part of a treatment program that is guided and monitored by a qualified medical doctor in partnership with a qualified alternative practitioner, both of whom are experienced in caring for your condition. Check with your conventional doctor before changing or stopping any conventional medical treatments or medications, and keep all of your doctors and/or alternative practitioners informed of all treatments that you are receiving.*

Angina is a potentially life-threatening condition that always needs to be treated by a physician. At the very least, you may need to take nitroglycerin (Nitrolingual) or other prescription drugs. For an angina attack, the usual recommendation is to place one tablet of nitroglycerin under the tongue every 5 minutes until the pain is gone, taking up to a maximum of three tablets. If the pain is severe when it begins or continues after taking three tablets (or more than 15 minutes), have someone take you to the nearest hospital.

Doctors who specialize in natural medicine, however, believe that with natural remedies, it's often possible to gradually reduce your reliance on medications or, in some cases, to eliminate angina entirely. That's why they recommend seeing a nutritionally oriented doctor to treat angina.

When angina persists, many alternative doctors recommend a treatment called EDTA chelation therapy, which they say is safer, less expensive, and much more effective (because it may cure the problem) than coronary bypass surgery or other invasive cardiac procedures.

EDTA chelation therapy consists of a series of intravenous treatments with ethylenediaminetetraacetic acid, an amino acid–like molecule that binds with and removes excess metals from the arteries. This may be important, says Michael Janson, M.D., consultant physician at Path to Health in Burlington, Massachusetts, because these metals are thought to trigger the formation of free radicals, unstable oxygen molecules that play a role in coronary artery disease. Chelation treatments are

administered two or three times a week and usually last 3
hours, with most patients receiving a total of 25 to 40 treatments. Be sure that the doctor you choose has experience in
using chelation therapy.

The oxygen supply is limited, however, when the arteries leading to the heart are narrowed by buildups of plaque, the substance that signals heart disease. The result is pain—1 to 20
minutes of scary discomfort, as if a heart attack were sending
you a telegram from the future.

Angina is the edge of a cliff, and you need a guardrail. In
other words, medical treatment is a must. You will probably
need to take a prescription drug such as nitroglycerin (Nitrolingual) to keep your angina attacks under control. But alternative
doctors say that you should also use nutritional remedies that
can gradually reduce angina attacks by improving blood flow to
the heart and infusing the heart muscle with extra energy, says
Julian Whitaker, M.D., founder and director of the Whitaker
Wellness Institute in Newport Beach, California.

## COENZYME $Q_{10}$: *A Heart-Rejuvenating Supplement*

Alternative practitioners believe that the first and most important natural remedy for angina is probably coenzyme $Q_{10}$
($coQ_{10}$). It's found in every cell and is as essential as oxygen.
Without it, you'd quickly die, because it helps the body manufacture ATP, the chemical that generates most of the energy that
powers the cells of the body, including those of the heart muscle.

Stephen T. Sinatra, M.D., a cardiologist and director of the
New England Heart Center in Manchester, Connecticut, also
strongly recommends $coQ_{10}$. He cites a study in which the
supplement allowed people with angina to decrease their nitroglycerin intake. Dr. Sinatra treats people with angina with a
daily dose of 90 to 180 milligrams of $coQ_{10}$, taken with or after
meals.

"There are no significant adverse effects from $coQ_{10}$," he adds.
"It's an exciting additional strategy for patients with angina
that they should utilize indefinitely."

## CARNITINE: *Boosts the Power of CoQ₁₀*

People with angina who take carnitine (a vitamin-like amino acid) along with $coQ_{10}$ are much more likely to have reductions in angina pain and frequency of attacks than those who take $coQ_{10}$ alone, says Michael Janson, M.D., consultant physician at Path to Health in Burlington, Massachusetts.

Alternative practitioners believe that without enough $coQ_{10}$ and carnitine, the cells of the heart can't make energy from fats. Instead, they burn sugar, or glucose, for energy. This, in combination with narrowed vessels that deprive the heart of oxygen, leads to lactic acid buildup, which in turn causes the pain of angina.

So, along with $coQ_{10}$, Dr. Janson advises his angina patients to take anywhere from 500 milligrams of carnitine twice a day to 1,000 milligrams three or four times a day, depending on the severity and frequency of their angina.

## TOCOTRIENOL: *Strong Protection Against Heart Attack*

Tocotrienol is a super-powerful form of vitamin E. Study after study shows that vitamin E can help prevent or reverse heart disease, says Donald Carrow, M.D., founder and director of the Florida Institute of Health in Tampa.

Vitamin E actually refers to a variety of chemically similar nutrients, the tocopherols and the tocotrienols. Scientists used to think that the tocotrienols were the weaker of the two groups. Now they've begun to realize they're stronger.

In fact, based on his experience, Dr. Carrow believes that the tocotrienols are 30 to 60 times more powerful than tocopherol-containing vitamin E, making the nutrient one of the best ways to treat and reverse angina.

Tocotrienols, he explains, are thought to act like a blood-thinning drug. They help stop the formation of blood clots at the spot where an artery is clogged—the usual cause of heart attacks in people with angina.

Dr. Carrow advises his angina patients to take 50 milligrams of mixed tocotrienols (a product that includes forms of tocotrienol called alpha, beta, delta, and gamma) three times a day.

### Shower Away the Pain

Taking a very warm shower or bath dilates blood vessels throughout your body, including the arteries leading to the heart. This can help stop the pain of repeated episodes of minor angina, says Donald Carrow, M.D., founder and director of the Florida Institute of Health in Tampa.

"I tell all of my patients with angina to take very warm showers or baths when they're having minor attacks, and many of them get instant relief," he says.

One caution, however: Be sure that the bathroom has a good exhaust fan, and turn it on before you get in the shower or tub. Steam can reduce the amount of oxygen in a room, making angina worse.

If angina pain persists for more than 5 to 10 minutes after trying this remedy, go to the nearest hospital immediately. While this treatment may temporarily relieve angina pain, it should never take the place of prescribed medications.

## MAGNESIUM CITRATE: *Instantly Improves Blood Flow*

Magnesium citrate is an inexpensive liquid product often used as a laxative. It also works for angina because magnesium opens the arteries of the heart and strengthens the heart muscle, Dr. Carrow says. He recommends that people with angina take 1 ounce of magnesium citrate (a nonlaxative dose) once a day on an empty stomach.

People in the midst of minor angina attacks may even be able to abort the attacks by taking an extra ounce of magnesium citrate, says Dr. Carrow. Talk to your doctor before using magnesium citrate for angina, however, and never use it as a substitute for any prescribed drug treatment.

## HOMEOPATHY: *Cactus Stops Pain Fast*

This homeopathic remedy works well to stop the pain of an angina attack, says Mark Stengler, N.D., a naturopathic physician in San Diego.

But, he adds, homeopathic Cactus must be taken with—not instead of—any drug prescribed by a physician for treating angina. Take a 30C potency of the remedy, dissolving two pellets in your mouth every 5 minutes until the pain is gone.

# *Techniques to Help Control*
# **Anxiety and Panic Attacks**

Prescription benzodiazepine tranquilizers such as alprazolam (Xanax) and diazepam (Valium) aren't all bad. They can help you cope with overwhelming acute anxiety, such as may occur when there's a sudden death in the family.

When you take tranquilizers day after day to control chronic anxiety, however, as many Americans do, they can actually cause the very problem they're supposed to treat.

That's because tranquilizers are addictive, says Edward Drummond, M.D., associate medical director of the Seacoast Mental Health Center in Portsmouth, New Hampshire. Your brain and body may develop a physical dependence on tranquilizers within 4 weeks of daily use. Then, if you try to stop using the drug, the inevitable period of physical withdrawal produces—you guessed it—anxiety.

Tranquilizers have another drawback. They convince you that you need a medication to control anxiety rather than being able to tap your own inner resources to deal with the problem through alternative home remedies such as deep breathing and relaxation techniques.

"Using tranquilizers interferes with the pursuit of treatment that is truly effective," says Dr. Drummond.

Before you start using those methods, though, you should know that there's nothing abnormal about being a high-anxiety person. "High-anxiety people tend to be more intuitive, great listeners, and very sympathetic," says Reneau Z. Peurifoy, a marriage and family therapist and anxiety specialist in the Sacramento area. "They just need to learn how to manage their anxiety better."

# GUIDE TO
# PROFESSIONAL CARE

Anxiety that qualifies as an anxiety disorder requires professional care, says Edward Drummond, M.D., associate medical director of the Seacoast Mental Health Center in Portsmouth, New Hampshire. You may have an anxiety disorder if your anxiety seems out of proportion to the actual situation that triggered it or has continued for months beyond the event.

Seek a therapist who specializes in anxiety disorders, says Elke Zuercher-White, Ph.D., a psychologist at Kaiser-Permanente in the San Francisco area. And, she says, your therapist should be one who uses cognitive-behavioral treatment, which is scientifically proven to be the most helpful approach to chronic anxiety and panic attacks.

Also, if you have been taking prescription tranquilizers daily for more than 4 weeks, you need a program to help you stop taking the drugs, says Dr. Drummond, since the symptoms of sudden withdrawal can be overwhelming.

## RELAXATION: *A Response to Calm You Down*

Techniques that create the relaxation response—a calmer mind and a more relaxed body—are great for high-anxiety people, says Peurifoy. A common and effective one is the focal-point technique.

Sit quietly and comfortably in a place where you won't be disturbed and repeat a word, such as *calm* or *relax*, each time you exhale. When your mind wanders (as it inevitably will), don't worry; just bring it back to your breathing and the word. Do this technique for 10 to 20 minutes every day.

## RELAXATION: *Take Your Cue*

The only problem with relaxation response techniques is that they don't help you much when you really need them, when you're out and about and feeling anxious. That's why Peurifoy recommends cue-controlled relaxation, which is a means of practicing your relaxation technique so that you can produce the same results even when you can't do the technique. Here's how it works.

As you're practicing the focal-point technique, also perform your cue. It could be simply placing your thumb and index finger together. Then, when you experience anxiety during the day, perform the cue. Over time, you'll notice that your body and mind will start to relax on cue.

## KAVA KAVA: *Take Your Anxiety to the South Pacific*

The South Pacific herb kava kava may be as effective as a prescription tranquilizer for reducing anxiety, says Hyla Cass, M.D., assistant professor of psychiatry at the University of California, Los Angeles, School of Medicine. In fact, she says, it may actually be more effective, since low doses often enhance alertness rather than making you feel sedated the way a tranquilizer often does.

Dr. Cass recommends taking 135 to 250 milligrams of the herb in capsule or tablet form. Look for a standardized product that contains 30 percent (40 to 75 milligrams) kavalactones, the active ingredient, and take it two or three times daily as long as you find it helpful. To help you get a good night's sleep, take two doses at bedtime.

## YOGA: *A Revitalizing Visualization*

"Yoga poses provide effective relief of anxiety," says Susan Lark, M.D., a physician in Los Altos, California. They work, she says, by relaxing tense muscles and oxygenating your entire body, which quiets and calms your mood.

The following pose is known as the sponge. Do it three times a week or even daily if you notice that your anxiety symptoms respond particularly well to it.

First, says Dr. Lark, lie on your back with a rolled towel under your knees and your arms at your sides, palms up. Close your eyes and relax your whole body. Inhale slowly, breathing from your diaphragm.

As you inhale, says Dr. Lark, visualize the energy in the air around you being drawn through your entire body. Imagine that your body is porous and open like a sponge so it can draw in this energy to revitalize every cell.

Exhale slowly and deeply, allowing every ounce of tension to drain from your body. Stay in the pose as long as you're comfortable.

## Accentuate—and Affirm—the Positive

Your anxious feelings about any situation are usually based on habitual, automatic thinking patterns, says Reneau Z. Peurifoy, a marriage and family therapist and anxiety specialist in the Sacramento area. Those thoughts may sound something like "This is terrible," "I can't handle even this simple thing," or "I'm never going to get any better."

By deliberately changing these to what Peurifoy calls coping self-statements, you can deal with any situation.

The affirming statements may not immediately reduce your anxiety, but with practice, Peurifoy says, you'll create a set of positive messages to replace the old negative ones, thereby reducing chronic anxiety.

Here are some examples of coping self-statements. Memorize them and use them as needed.

• I've survived feelings like this, and worse, before.
• I don't have to do this perfectly.
• I always have options. I'm free to come and go according to my comfort.
• This will only take a short time. Soon it will be over, and I will be very pleased with myself.
• It doesn't matter what others think.

## BREATHING: *Short-Circuit Those Panic Attacks*

High-anxiety people may start worrying that they'll lose control, because they don't understand the cause of their anxiety symptoms. When those symptoms occur, these people can become so flustered, jittery, and physically upset that they precipitate a full-fledged panic attack. Soon, the mere anticipation of a panic attack can trigger one.

Many people who have panic attacks are hyperventilating—taking short, rapid breaths that produce such classic symptoms as dizziness or faintness; difficulty swallowing; shaking or muscle spasms; numbness and tingling of the mouth, hands, or feet; heart palpitations; and a feeling that they can't get enough air.

"In those situations, it is particularly helpful to do deep, diaphragmatic breathing," says Elke Zuercher-White, Ph.D., a psychologist at Kaiser-Permanente in the San Francisco area. "It is an effective technique for controlling anxiety symptoms. To overcome panic disorder, however, you must also work toward a change in your thought process so you no longer fear the symptoms of anxiety and panic attacks."

Dr. Zuercher-White recommends a very systematic method of learning this breathing, which she calls breathing retraining. Practice each of her phases for 5 minutes twice a day until you've mastered it. Then move on to the next phase.

• Phase one: Lie on your back on a bed or carpeted floor. Place one or two pillows on your stomach. Watch the tops of the pillows from the corner of your eye. As you breathe in, your diaphragm should expand, raising the pillows. When you breathe out, the pillows should move down again.
• Phase two: Lie on your back without the pillows and put one hand over your navel. Look at the ceiling or close your eyes. Take deep breaths. With your hand, feel your stomach moving up and down.
• Phase three: Repeat phase two, but keep your attention on your diaphragm and feel it move up and down. "Become one with your breathing," says Dr. Zuercher-White.
• Phase four: Sit on a sofa, leaning back so that you can watch your stomach area. Watch your diaphragm move up as you breathe in and down as you breathe out.
• Phase five: Sitting straight, repeat phase four. Be sure that your upper chest and shoulders are perfectly still; that's a sign that you're doing the exercise correctly.
• Phase six: While standing, repeat phase five.

# *Take Heart with Drug-Free*
# *Treatments for*
# **Arrhythmia**

Stress can cause your heart to skip a beat. Literally. In medical circles, it's called an arrhythmia, a big, hard-to-spell word that means an irregular heartbeat.

If you have benign arrhythmia, the kind that is not a life-threatening heart problem, your doctor may suggest a heart-calming drug such as a beta-blocker or a calcium channel blocker. While those drugs may help stop benign arrhythmia, they can also leave you impotent, constipated, and fatigued, to name just a few of the possible side effects.

"I believe the allopathic, medicine-based approach to curing benign arrhythmia is often ineffective," says Seth Baum, M.D., an integrative cardiologist and founder of the Baum Center for Integrative Heart Care in Boca Raton, Florida. There are other ways to deal with benign arrhythmia besides potentially harmful drugs, he and other alternative practitioners say.

## MAGNESIUM: *The Mineral That Relaxes Your Heart*

"One natural and important treatment for arrhythmias, whether life-threatening or benign, is the mineral magnesium," says Julian Whitaker, M.D., founder and director of the Whitaker Wellness Institute in Newport Beach, California.

Too little magnesium in the system jangles the electricity that controls muscles and nerves, possibly leading to an arrhythmia. Enough magnesium can help keep the electricity stable and your heart calm.

For benign arrhythmia, Dr. Whitaker recommends 250 milligrams of magnesium four times a day or 500 milligrams twice a day with food. Continue taking this dose for about 2 months in order to build up your reserves, he advises, then lower the dose to 500 to 800 milligrams a day. Whatever product you buy,

# GUIDE TO
# PROFESSIONAL CARE

*Caution: You should use the alternative remedies discussed in this chapter only as part of a treatment program that is guided and monitored by a qualified medical doctor in partnership with a qualified alternative practitioner, both of whom are experienced in caring for your condition. Check with your conventional doctor before changing or stopping any conventional medical treatments or medications, and keep all of your doctors and/or alternative practitioners informed of all treatments that you are receiving.*

If you have coronary artery disease (which often has no symptoms), an arrhythmia or heart palpitation can kill you. If you notice any type of arrhythmia—a skipped beat, a racing heart, a flutter in your chest—you must see a medical doctor as soon as possible, says Glenn S. Rothfeld, M.D., regional medical director of American WholeHealth in Arlington, Massachusetts.

Most arrhythmias, however, are what doctors call benign. They are about as harmless as hiccups, although more physically and emotionally disturbing.

The fact that they are harmless, though, doesn't mean that people with benign arrhythmias don't want to get rid of them. They do. Seth Baum, M.D., an integrative cardiologist and founder of the Baum Center for Integrative Heart Care in Boca Raton, Florida, treats them with natural means such as nutritional supplements instead of with drugs, which he says can have many unpleasant side effects. He advises people who experience arrhythmias to see a nutritionally oriented physician.

A useful medical test used by some alternative practitioners for those with benign arrhythmias is the Salivary Adrenal Stress Index, Dr. Rothfeld says. It helps the doctor determine whether arrhythmias are being caused by hormones generated by the adrenal glands in response to stress. If it's found that they are due to stress, they can be treated with stress-reduction techniques.

be sure the label says that it contains elemental magnesium, Dr. Whitaker advises.

You should take this supplement only if you have been diagnosed with benign arrhythmia. If you have any other heart problem or a kidney problem, check with your doctor before taking it.

## YOGA: *Strike a "Dead Pose"*

"I feel stress is a major cause of benign arrhythmia, and stress reduction is the key treatment," says Virender Sodhi, M.D. (Ayurved), N.D., an Ayurvedic and naturopathic physician and director of the American School of Ayurvedic Sciences in Bellevue, Washington.

One of the easiest ways to reduce stress is with a yoga pose called the dead pose. "In one scientific study, medical students who practiced the dead pose before and after exams did not have anxiety or heart palpitations during the exams," says Dr. Sodhi.

To perform the dead pose, lie on your back on a bed, rug, or other comfortable flat surface. Put your arms by your sides, with your palms facing up. Breathe easily and normally, and keep your attention on your breath. If your mind wanders, easily bring it back to your breath. Practice this pose for 5 minutes a day, says Dr. Sodhi, or whenever you feel assaulted by stress.

## HAWTHORN: *Look for the Right Kind*

Scientific studies show that the herb hawthorn can help control benign arrhythmia, says Dr. Baum. The studies used the flowers and leaves of the hawthorn plant rather than its berries, which have not been studied as extensively, so be sure that the herbal product you use contains the flowers and leaves.

Dr. Baum advises his patients with benign arrhythmia to take 80 to 300 milligrams of hawthorn twice a day. If you have a cardiovascular condition, however, do not take hawthorn regularly for more than a few weeks without medical supervision.

### Rubbing Out Stress

Some alternative practitioners believe that the source of most everyday or benign arrhythmias (the kinds of heart palpitations

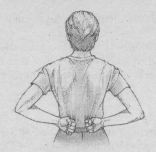

that aren't life-threatening) isn't your heart. It's your adrenal glands, says Glenn S. Rothfeld, M.D., regional medical director of American WholeHealth in Arlington, Massachusetts.

When you're feeling stressed, these glands pump out hormones that can irritate and overstimulate your heart so that it races, flutters, or skips a beat. But you can calm your adrenal glands and help prevent benign arrhythmias with qigong, a type of Chinese medicine that shows you how to send healing energy (chi) to any part of your body.

To bring chi to your adrenal glands, make fists with both hands and bend your arms behind you. Put the flat of one fist (the back of the hand) on each adrenal gland; you'll find one on each side of your back near your kidneys, just above your waist and below your ribs. Slowly and gently rub your hands up and down, feeling them warm that area of your back. Do this every day for 2 to 3 minutes, says Dr. Rothfeld.

### TAURINE: *Calm Your Nerves*

This amino acid can help stop your nerves from overstimulating your heart, which is a must in controlling benign arrhythmia, says Glenn S. Rothfeld, M.D., regional medical director of American WholeHealth in Arlington, Massachusetts. He recommends 500 to 1,000 milligrams twice a day between meals.

### KAVA KAVA OR PASSIONFLOWER: *Herbs That Calm*

Both kava kava and passionflower are thought to help calm your sympathetic nervous system, which is the part of your nervous system that initiates the "fight-or-flight" response.

For kava kava, take either a 200-milligram capsule (standardized to 30 percent kavalactones) or 40 drops of tincture three times a day, says Mark Stengler, N.D., a naturopathic physician in San Diego. For passionflower, take 250 to 500 milligrams in capsule form or 40 drops of tincture three times daily. Continue with either remedy until symptoms subside.

**COENZYME Q$_{10}$:** *For Skipped Heartbeats*

Also known as coQ$_{10}$, this compound is found in every cell of the body, where it helps manufacture energy. It may also stabilize the body's electrical system and can help prevent arrhythmias, says Stephen T. Sinatra, M.D., a cardiologist and director of the New England Heart Center in Manchester, Connecticut.

Dr. Sinatra believes that coQ$_{10}$ is particularly effective in preventing a common type of benign arrhythmia called PVCs, or premature ventricular contractions, which are usually experienced as skipped heartbeats. PVCs have many possible causes, including drinking too much coffee or alcohol and a deficiency of the mineral potassium.

A deficiency of coQ$_{10}$ is another possible cause; the supplement cures the problem in 20 to 25 percent of his patients with PVCs, says Dr. Sinatra. He recommends that people who have been diagnosed with PVCs take a daily dose of 120 to 240 milligrams of coQ$_{10}$ or use Q-Gel, a brand that he says is the best absorbed (and therefore the most effective) product on the market. Follow the label directions.

# *Beware of Treatments That Actually Accelerate* **Arthritis**

Sloths may have served as the model for one of the Seven Deadly Sins, but at least they've managed to avoid one of the most debilitating diseases—arthritis.

And James Braly, M.D., an allergy specialist in Boca Raton, Florida, thinks that he may know why. These tree-dwelling creatures sleep upside down, relieving the pressure on their bones for hours at a time, he says.

Many of the other creatures in the animal kingdom, however—including humans—almost inevitably develop some degree of this wear-and-tear disease if they live long enough.

# GUIDE TO
# PROFESSIONAL CARE

*Caution: You should use the alternative remedies discussed in this chapter only as part of a treatment program that is guided and monitored by a qualified medical doctor in partnership with a qualified alternative practitioner, both of whom are experienced in caring for your condition. Check with your conventional doctor before changing or stopping any conventional medical treatments or medications, and keep all of your doctors and/or alternative practitioners informed of all treatments that you are receiving.*

The primary symptoms of arthritis are pain, stiffness, swelling in and around the joints, and limited movement that lasts more than 2 weeks. If you have these symptoms, see a medical doctor.

There are many medical treatments that can help control arthritis pain, such as medications and surgery. But those treatments may be "ineffective and even damaging," says Gus Prosch, M.D., a physician in Birmingham, Alabama.

Dr. Prosch has treated thousands of arthritis patients with alternative therapies and says that he has an 80 percent success rate, eliminating pain and reversing the disease process.

"Conventional medical treatments address only the symptoms of the disease, not its cause," he says. Here are the steps he recommends for the professional care and relief of arthritis.

• Controlling stress through relaxation techniques and lifestyle changes
• A complete program of diet and nutritional supplements designed to alleviate arthritis pain and also reduce weight, if necessary
• Detecting and eliminating food allergies that may be causing or complicating the disease
• Testing for and treating fungal, bacterial, and viral microorganisms, such as the fungus candida, that may be causing or complicating the disease
• Removing toxic overload, including heavy metals, from the body

One of the numerous reasons is that a lifetime of moving breaks down the cartilage that forms a cushion between the ends of bones. Eventually, bone rubs on bone, resulting in pain and stiffness that can range from mild to crippling. Pain and stiffness in knees. In hips. In fingers. In shoulders. In toes. In spines. In millions and millions of Americans (about 20 million, at last count).

In fact, by the year 2020, when all the members of the Baby Boom generation will be at least 60 years old, the Centers for Disease Control and Prevention in Atlanta estimates that almost 60 million Americans will have arthritis.

More specifically, they will have osteoarthritis, the most common form of the disease (there are more than 100 different types). Rheumatoid arthritis is another very common form.

Unlike the mechanical destruction that causes osteoarthritis, the joint damage from rheumatoid arthritis occurs because of an inflammatory process that conventional medicine attributes to an autoimmune response. This means that the immune system misidentifies a part of the body as a foreign invader and attacks it. (As you'll see, some alternative healers have other opinions about the actual causes of rheumatoid arthritis.)

Rheumatoid arthritis affects about 2 million Americans, about 70 percent of whom are women. And because it's an inflammation, rheumatoid arthritis not only produces pain and stiffness but also makes joints swollen, red, and hot. Moreover, the disease doesn't limit its damage to joints. It can also harm the eyes, lungs, heart, kidneys, and other parts of the body.

There are many different medical treatments for the inflammation that osteoarthritis and rheumatoid arthritis produce, but the most common involves using nonsteroidal anti-inflammatory drugs, or NSAIDs. These include aspirin, ibuprofen, indomethacin (Indocin), naproxen (Aleve), and many others. And, while NSAIDs may reduce symptoms today, in the long run, they all make arthritis worse, says Dr. Braly.

"The single most important message that you could give to people with arthritis is that the type of drug most commonly used to treat over 20 million arthritis sufferers in the United States is actually accelerating the destruction of joint tissue," Dr. Braly says.

Fortunately, there are many alternative treatments for arthritis—some of which, say alternative healers, have the power to not only relieve arthritis symptoms but to actually reverse them.

## Help Stop the Harmful Side Effects of Painkillers

Aspirin, ibuprofen, and naproxen may offer fast relief from arthritis pain, but they also can batter the digestive tract, causing bleeding or perforation.

These nonsteroidal anti-inflammatory drugs, or NSAIDs, are the most commonly used medications for arthritis. (In addition to over-the-counter NSAIDs, prescription versions include a stronger form of naproxen as well as indomethacin, nabumetone, diclofenac, piroxicam, and oxyprozin.)

What's worse—at least for people with arthritis—is that over time, NSAIDs accelerate the destruction of joint tissue, warns James Braly, M.D., an allergy specialist in Boca Raton, Florida. In other words, they can actually aggravate the disease that they're intended to treat.

Maybe you feel that you don't have any choice but to take an NSAID because you're in too much pain without it. If so, there is a way to protect your gastrointestinal tract, Dr. Braly says. Try glutamine, an amino acid. This nutrient is a primary fuel for the lining of the small intestine, where NSAIDs do most of their damage.

If you take NSAIDs regularly, he says, you should mix 2 to 4 grams of powdered glutamine (about a rounded half-teaspoon) in 6 to 8 ounces of filtered water and take it 30 minutes before each dose of an NSAID. Take these therapeutic doses of glutamine for as long as you take NSAIDs, he advises. Glutamine is completely without toxicity in amounts up to 60 grams a day, he adds.

## GLUCOSAMINE SULFATE: *Stop the Pain of Osteoarthritis*

"Some nonsteroidal anti-inflammatory drugs, such as ibuprofen, aspirin, and indomethacin, may worsen or accelerate joint destruction by preventing new, healthy connective tissue in the joints from being formed," says Dr. Braly.

Some studies suggest, however, that glucosamine sulfate, a nutritional supplement, may build cartilage and slow the progression of the disease instead of merely masking its symptoms.

According to Walter Crinnion, N.D., a naturopathic doctor and director of Healing Naturally in Kirkland, Washington, 500 milligrams of glucosamine sulfate, taken three times a day before meals, "works great" among his patients who have osteoarthritis. But don't expect to be pain-free tomorrow; this is a slow, natural process of rebuilding a damaged body part.

Dr. Crinnion advises his patients to take 1,500 milligrams of the supplement daily for about 6 months, then lower the dosage to between 500 and 1,000 milligrams a day, according to how their bodies feel. If you don't feel relief at a maintenance dose of 500 milligrams, go back to 1,000 milligrams, he suggests.

And here's a consumer tip from Dr. Crinnion: Be sure the label says glucosamine *sulfate*. "There are other forms of glucosamine being sold, and they don't work as well," he says.

## TURMERIC: *Boost the Healing Power of Glucosamine*

In therapeutic dosages, turmeric, the yellow spice from India, works as well as NSAIDs to reduce the pain and inflammation of arthritis, says Dr. Braly. And, unlike NSAIDs, it has no side effects.

One of the anti-inflammatory substances in turmeric is curcumin, which is available in capsules. Taken together, curcumin and glucosamine sulfate reduce pain and inflammation far better than either one alone, Dr. Braly says. (And here's an extra benefit: Some studies show that curcumin may block the formation of some types of tumors.)

Follow the dosage recommendations on the label, says Dr. Braly, and take the supplement until your arthritis symptoms subside.

## GINGER: *Fresh or from a Bottle*

Ginger is another spice with scientifically proven anti-inflammatory powers, says Dr. Braly. One of its active ingredients is gingerol. People with arthritis should eat plenty of fresh ginger (raw is best); he suggests chopping it and adding as much as you're comfortable eating to salads and other foods.

Alternatively, you can take a ginger supplement. Look for a standardized ginger product and follow the dosage recommendations on the label, says Dr. Braly. Take it until your arthritis symptoms subside completely, he advises.

## MAHANARAYAN OIL: *For Immediate Pain Relief*

"I treated a woman in her eighties who had severe osteoarthritis," says Swami Sada Shiva Tirtha, director of the Ayurveda Holistic Center in Bayville, New York. "She rubbed the mahanarayan oil on her skin in the area of pain and, for the first time in 30 years, her pain went away. Of course, it came back in a few hours, but when she put the oil back on, the pain went away again."

The oil penetrates the skin and immediately softens pain-causing deposits in the bone, says Swami Tirtha. And it's completely safe, so you can use as much of it as you want for pain relief, he says. Because it's not greasy, you can rub a light coating of it into your skin as you would a massage oil.

## GUGGUL: *For Long-Term Pain Relief*

"This herb can relieve the pain of arthritis within a day or two," says Swami Tirtha. Take $\frac{1}{4}$ teaspoon of guggul tincture with $\frac{1}{2}$ teaspoon of water 30 minutes before meals three times a day, he says. You can take guggul (sometimes called guggulu) for many months, he adds. If the pain goes away, he suggests that you stop taking the herb for a month to let your body adjust. You can then take it again as a preventive or if the pain returns.

"The herb travels to the arthritic bone and removes the imbalances that are causing the stiffness, swelling, and inflammation," he says.

### Lubricate Your Joints with Dietary Oils

A deficiency of fatty acids, which are components of fat, is a major contributing factor to arthritis and arthritis pain, says Gus Prosch, M.D., a physician in Birmingham, Alabama.

There are almost as many fatty acids as there are vitamins. And, like vitamins, each one has a different role in your body. Four fatty acids—alpha-linolenic acid (LNA), eicosapentaenoic acid (EPA), docosahexaenoic acid (DHA), and gamma-linolenic acid (GLA)—help reverse some of the symptoms and complications of both osteoarthritis and rheumatoid arthritis, including inflammation, pain, a weakened immune system, and low resistance to stress of all kinds. That's why Dr. Prosch puts all of his arthritis patients on a dietary regimen (including fatty acid supplements) that guarantees that they won't have a deficiency.

"It is almost unbelievable how important these recommendations are to relieving arthritis," he says. "If patients don't follow them, they are not going to get better." Here's how to maximize your intake of anti-arthritis fatty acids.

## FISH OIL: *From the Sea or from a Bottle*

Include cold-water fish such as sardines, salmon, mackerel, halibut, herring, trout, and tuna in your diet three times a week, Dr. Prosch recommends. They are rich in EPA and DHA, which are part of a group of fatty acids commonly known as omega-3's.

If fish isn't your favorite dish, you can take fish-oil capsules. Research has shown that fish-oil supplements can sometimes reduce the pain, swelling, and stiffness of rheumatoid arthritis, says Dr. Prosch.

Take 6 grams, or six 1,000-milligram capsules, a day for 4 to 6 months, he recommends. The capsules provide 1,080 milligrams of EPA and 720 milligrams of DHA, which is the average amount needed by most patients, he says. You can take them all at once or in divided doses, according to Dr. Prosch.

As with most natural treatments for chronic disease, don't expect the pain to vanish overnight. For most people, it takes 3 to 4 months before the treatment begins to soothe aching joints. After about 5 months, Dr. Prosch recommends reducing the dosage to three capsules, or 3,000 milligrams, daily. You can take this dosage indefinitely, he says.

One slight problem with fish-oil capsules is that they can make you burp a fishy burst of air. To prevent that problem, Dr. Crinnion advises keeping the capsules in the freezer and taking them frozen.

Dr. Prosch says that if you take your full dosage at bedtime, you will not notice the fishiness during the night.

## FLAXSEED OIL: *On Your Food or in a Capsule*

Take 1 tablespoon of flaxseed oil daily, suggests Lauri Aesoph, N.D., a naturopathic doctor in Sioux Falls, South Dakota. It's a good source of LNA, another omega-3 fatty acid. Include it in your daily diet just as you would any other oil—in salad dressings, for example, or as an ingredient in recipes that don't involve heating. Store it in the refrigerator. Flaxseed oil is also available in supplement form. Follow the dosage recommendations on the label, she says.

You can take these supplements indefinitely, says Dr. Braly. They contain "essential nutrients that are profoundly deficient in the Western diet." Shoot for about 5,000 milligrams of LNA in your supplements.

## EVENING PRIMROSE: *Another Oily Option*

This supplement, made from the seeds of the evening primrose plant, is rich in GLA, the fatty acid in which people are most deficient, says Dr. Prosch. He suggests taking six capsules (containing 240 to 270 milligrams of GLA) of evening primrose oil daily.

You can cut that dose in half after 4 to 6 months, he says. He adds that there are cheaper forms of GLA on the market but cautions that they do not yield the same results as GLA from evening primrose oil.

## HYDROGENATED OILS: *A Must to Avoid*

Hydrogenated oils interfere with the metabolism of fatty acids, says Dr. Prosch. These oils are found in margarine, peanut butter, most cooking oils, and many other processed products, such as snack chips, baked goods, and salad dressings. (Natural peanut butter that is freshly ground at health food stores is okay, he says.) Avoid foods whose labels include the word *hydrogenated*, he advises.

### Acupressure for Joint-by-Joint Pain Relief

You can use some simple, press-here techniques to provide quick relief of joint pain. The remedies of Jin Shin Do Bodymind Acupressure combine traditional acupressure with breathing and visualization, says Deborah Valentine Smith, a licensed massage therapist and senior teacher of Jin Shin Do in West Stockbridge, Massachusetts.

"These powerful techniques can provide short- and long-term relief for arthritis by bringing chi, or life-energy, into the area of the joint," Smith says. "This encourages the flow of blood, which lubricates the joints, carries away toxins, and reduces pain, swelling, and inflammation." (For the exact locations of the points, see An Illustrated Guide to Acupressure Points on page 700.)

If you have trouble finding any of the points in these exercises, she says, don't worry about it. Just put your palm over the area.

Pressing the exact point has stronger effects, but the body also responds to where and how you put your attention and your breath.

Although these techniques can help relieve pain as it occurs, they are most beneficial when you add them to your daily routine, advises Smith.

## HARA BREATHING: *To Build Your Chi*

In Chinese medicine, the source of the philosophy and practice of acupressure, the hara is an area below the navel that acts as a reservoir for the body's chi.

"Arthritis is often caused by a combination of factors that includes a depletion or blockage of chi, usually caused by what we in the West call tension or stress," says Smith. "Hara breathing builds reserves of chi in your body."

First, place your hand, palm down, right below your navel. Next, inhale, expanding your belly into your hand. Imagine breathing vitality, or a life force, down into your belly with the breaths and concentrating it there as you exhale, feeling your belly flatten.

"Just doing this simple technique for a few minutes a day can build chi, making it available to circulate in your body and soothe joint pain," Smith says.

## SI3: *To Let Your Chi Flow*

In acupressure, the spine is a major crossroad for meridians, the pathways or lines along which chi circulates in the body.

"If you increase the flow of chi in the spine, you increase the flow of chi in the entire body and thus can ease the pain of arthritis all over the body," says Smith.

Roll a hand towel lengthwise into a tube (Smith says it should be long enough to extend the length of your spine). Lie on a bed with the towel underneath your back on the right side of your spine, parallel to your spine and directly under the ridge of muscle that borders it.

As you lie there, breathe deeply and press a point on the outside edge of your right hand (the side you would use to do a karate chop). The point, known as SI3, is located underneath the knuckle below the little finger; press up toward the knuckle and at a slight angle toward your fourth finger. Acupressure points are more sensitive than the areas around them, says Smith. Press until you feel distinct sensitivity.

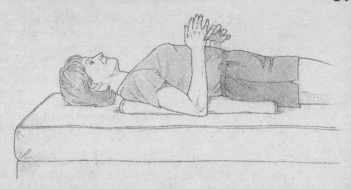

Hold the pressure for four or five breaths or as long as you'd like, says Smith. (You should only use the towel as long as you can comfortably breathe into the area.) Then move the towel to the left side of your spine and press the point on your left hand.

### KI6 AND BL62: *To Relieve Pain and Tension in the Spine or Hips*

The following simple technique circulates spinal chi and is particularly good for arthritis of the spine or hips, although it will enhance the flow of chi to the entire body. Since you determine your own comfort level, assures Smith, you can use the technique even if arthritis limits your movements.

Sit in any comfortable chair and let your head drop forward. The eventual aim is to bend from your hips until your chest meets your upper thighs and you can hold acupressure points in your ankles. Stay with what is comfortable for you, advises Smith, even if you can bend only your head at first. (If you feel dizzy at any time during this exercise, sit upright and wait for the feeling to pass.)

Breathe into the hara area just below your navel, sending the breath from there to any areas of stiffness or pain in your spine. As you exhale, gradually bend farther, extending and stretching your spine, and imagine sending the breath to your toes, says Smith. (You may also begin by resting your arms on your thighs to support your torso. Gradually, drop your arms to the sides of your thighs and then down your legs.)

When you are able to bend over far enough to reach your ankles, use the tip of one finger or your thumb to press the acupressure point (called KI6) an inch below the peak of the inside anklebone. Smith suggests that you do this on both ankles simultaneously. As you press, you will feel a tender spot at the pressure point and eventually feel warmth in your spine or toes, she adds.

Hold these points with steady pressure for four or five deep breaths or for as long as you feel comfortable, says Smith.

Next, locate the points on the outsides of your ankles (called BL62), about ½ inch below the peaks of the anklebones and right under the edges of the bones. Again, press both points at the same time and for the same length of time, says Smith.

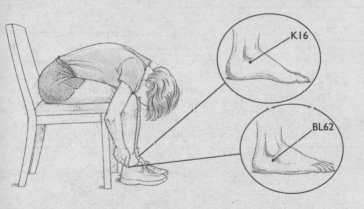

If possible, reach around the fronts or backs of both ankles with your hands and apply pressure to all four points at once, as shown above. (If you're doing this exercise with someone else, you could have your partner hold the four points while you sit in the chair and bend over, says Smith.)

## TW5: *To Soothe Pain in Your Fingers, Wrists, and Arms*

One of the best points for providing relief to this area of the body is TW5, says Smith. To locate it, use what she calls a body inch—the width of your thumb at the knuckle.

The point is on the outside of your upper arm, two body inches from the wrist crease and right in the middle of your arm, between the two bones. Hold the point for 1 to 2 minutes, or longer if it feels comfortable, says Smith.

Press hard enough to feel the pressure but not so hard that you feel tension in your hand. "People with arthritis may not be able to apply strong pressure," she says. "That's fine; they can just hold the area lightly." If you also have pain in the other arm, repeat the technique on that arm.

## Use Relaxation to Ease Stress— and Arthritis Pain

Stress—feeling tense in response to problems or difficulties— increases arthritis pain by tightening muscles, says Hope Gillerman, a certified teacher of the Alexander Technique (a type of posture and movement re-education) in New York City.

You don't have to have a massage in order to relax your muscles and break the cycle of stress and pain, however. Here's a super-simple technique to help you relax and provide some much-needed pain relief any time of the day or night, says Gillerman.

Lie on your back on an exercise mat, blanket, or rug. Bend your knees so that your feet are flat on the floor, hip-width apart and about 12 inches away from your hips. Keep your shoulders on the floor but elevate your head slightly with either a firm pillow or two or three paperback books. Rest your hands comfortably on your ribs, with your elbows out to the sides.

This posture lets your lower back drop onto the floor—and the lower back is one spot where most people hold a lot of tension. The position also helps relax the neck muscles, another tense area. As you lie on the floor, focus on your neck and lower back, thinking of them as becoming softer and softer.

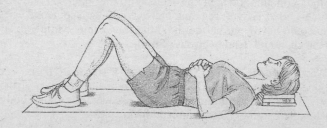

"This exercise is very good for any kind of arthritis pain, particularly for arthritis in the spine, shoulders, arms, or hands," says Gillerman. She recommends doing it for 15 minutes each morning as part of a stretching routine or at night to wind down from the day. "Don't wait for the tension to build up," she says. You can do it during the night if you wake up in pain (just get out of bed and lie on the floor) or anytime your joints are achy.

## GB41: *To Relieve Pain in Your Feet or Toes*

The GB41 point is on top of your foot between your fourth and fifth toes (your big toe is your first toe).

Starting at the web between your toes, slide your fingers between the bones (the metatarsals) toward your ankle. You'll find a notch where those bones meet; the point is in that notch and will usually be quite sensitive. Press for 1 to 2 minutes, says Smith. Again, if both feet hurt, repeat on the other foot.

## TW5 OR GB41: *To Ease Pain in Your Large Joints*

If you experience pain in your shoulders, elbows, knees, or hips, begin by holding your palm over the painful area. Then hold either of two "distal points"—TW5 or GB41—described above, says Smith. If you can hold the specific painful area and the distal point at the same time, do so. If not, you can hold one and then the other, breathing into each for four or five breaths.

If you cannot reach an area or point with your hands, you can always reach it with your breath. Imagine breathing space, ease, light, joy, warmth, or coolness into the area of discomfort, dispelling any pain or tension. As you exhale, imagine sending the breath to the relevant distal point or out your fingers or toes.

"This technique is like connecting the dots," says Smith. "By having your awareness on both the site of the pain and the point, the pain-relieving chi is moved along the meridians and through the joints."

# *Natural Inflammation Fighters for*
# **Asthma**

If you turn to conventional medicine for the answer to asthma, the "cure" may be worse than the condition, says Richard Firshein, D.O., an osteopathic physician in New York City.

"I believe that the approach of modern medicine to this disease has been woefully inadequate and misguided," Dr. Firshein says. "Asthma medications have often worsened the condition over the long term, since they treat the symptoms and not the problem, and few doctors have developed the kind of comprehensive treatment program that emphasizes healing and prevention."

Dr. Firshein's approach is a total program, and some aspects of it require medical tests and the supervision of a doctor. But many of his powerful asthma-controlling methods are alternative home remedies that almost anyone with asthma can use safely and effectively.

## MAGNESIUM: *Opens the Airways*

"If I had to recommend one nutrient for people with asthma, it would be magnesium," says Dr. Firshein. The mineral acts as a natural bronchodilator, meaning that it relaxes and opens the bronchial tract, the airway to the lungs that becomes constricted during asthma attacks. He recommends taking a daily 500-milligram supplement of either magnesium aspartate or magnesium citrate. You can take this supplement every day for 6 months, he suggests.

## FATTY ACIDS: *Reduce Lung Inflammation*

The lungs become inflamed during asthma attacks, which makes it harder to breathe. To reduce inflammation naturally, turn to the omega-3's found in fish and flaxseed oil.

# GUIDE TO
# PROFESSIONAL CARE

*Caution:* You should use the alternative remedies discussed in this chapter only as part of a treatment program that is guided and monitored by a qualified medical doctor in partnership with a qualified alternative practitioner, both of whom are experienced in caring for your condition. Check with your conventional doctor before changing or stopping any conventional medical treatments or medications, and keep all of your doctors and/or alternative practitioners informed of all treatments that you are receiving.

Asthma is a chronic and complicated condition that requires professional care from a physician who is experienced in its treatment, says Richard Firshein, D.O., an osteopathic physician in New York City. This is especially true because people with asthma need to keep track of many things simultaneously: the effects of medications, asthma triggers such as allergies, and a proper diet to ensure that they're getting all the nutrients they need.

If you experience shortness of breath, severe coughing spells, wheezing, tightness in your chest, excessive yawning, or extreme fatigue, contact your physician right away, Dr. Firshein says. If you are having an asthma attack, use your doctor-prescribed inhaler immediately, then get away from whatever triggered the attack, if possible. If you still can't breathe easily, call 911 or have someone take you to the emergency room immediately.

"Asthma involves both an acute inflammatory response and a secondary, late-phase inflammatory reaction that can occur up to 24 hours later and lasts for weeks," explains Dr. Firshein. "The late-phase response is now believed to be the cause of chronic asthma and tissue damage, and it can be halted by omega-3 fatty acids."

He recommends eating cold-water fish that are rich in omega-3 oils, such as salmon, tuna, and mackerel, three or four times a week. It's also a good idea to take six fish-oil capsules (the capsules are usually 1,000 milligrams each) a day.

If you don't eat fish, increase the dose to 12 fish-oil capsules daily. If you're a vegetarian or simply don't want to consume fish oil (many people don't like the fishy belch that sometimes occurs after swallowing the capsules), you can try flaxseed oil, which is also rich in omega-3's. Take 3 tablespoons a day. You can continue this regimen for up to a year, Dr. Firshein suggests.

There are a couple of cautions, however. About 10 percent of people with asthma (those who are sensitive to aspirin) get worse after taking fish oil. If you're aspirin-sensitive, take fish oil only with the supervision and approval of your physician. Also, if you have a high risk of stroke as well as asthma, talk to your doctor before taking fish oil, says Dr. Firshein, as fish oil may increase the risk of stroke in some people.

## ANTIOXIDANTS: *Fight Body-Damaging Free Radicals*

Your body naturally produces unstable, cell-damaging molecules called free radicals, and the level of free radicals rises when there's inflammation in the body. Since asthma is an inflammatory disease, Dr. Firshein theorizes that free radicals do much of the damage.

One way to control free radicals and limit their damage is to take supplements containing antioxidants such as beta-carotene and vitamins C and E. Dr. Firshein recommends taking daily supplements containing 400 international units of vitamin E, 3,000 milligrams of vitamin C (split into three doses), and 15 milligrams of beta-carotene. These supplements can be taken for a year, and you can talk to your doctor about reducing the doses depending on your individual progress.

## NAC: *Scoops Up Free Radicals*

The amino acid n-acetylcysteine (NAC) is a powerful scavenger of free radicals, says Dr. Firshein. "It is also a building block for glutathione, one of the most powerful free radical quenchers available to the body," he says. NAC even helps prevent mucus from accumulating in the lungs. He recommends taking 500 milligrams of NAC twice a day.

## QUERCETIN: *Help for Allergies*

Allergies often worsen asthma, says Dr. Firshein. If you have allergies, he recommends taking quercetin, a compound in the bioflavonoid family. "Quercetin has been scientifically well-documented for its anti-allergic and antihistamine properties," he says. He advises taking 100 milligrams of quercetin three times a day. He recommends that you take quercetin for up to 6 months, especially during allergy season.

## The Physician Who Healed Himself

The doctor almost died of asthma.

Richard Firshein, D.O., had just left the emergency room, where he had gone after his medicated spray failed to stop an asthma attack. The doctors had stabilized his condition and released him. He was standing on a corner outside the hospital when a bus stopped in front of him and spewed exhaust in his face. He took a breath—and stopped breathing.

Back in the emergency room, he was hooked to an IV full of steroids and other powerful drugs. His breathing was so limited that he wasn't even wheezing; there was virtually no air in his lungs.

Dr. Firshein, an osteopathic physician in New York City, survived that near-fatal asthma attack, but he almost became part of a scary statistic. The death rate from asthma has more than doubled since 1978.

After 20 years of using asthma drugs that failed to improve his condition, Dr. Firshein decided to treat his asthma himself—naturally and without excessive use of medications.

It worked. He got his asthma under control using nutritional supplements, whole foods, herbs, exercise, and breathing and mind-body techniques, as well as by avoiding allergens that could trigger attacks. Then he began to offer his alternative program (some of which is described in this chapter) to his asthma patients, a group that now numbers in the thousands.

## COLEUS: *Relaxes Bronchial Muscles*

The herb coleus has been used for centuries by practitioners of Ayurveda, the ancient system of natural healing from India, to relax the airways. Dr. Firshein recommends getting a product standardized for 18 percent forskolin, the active ingredient in coleus. Take 50 milligrams two or three times a day for up to a year, he says. Because coleus may enhance the effects of some asthma medications, you should discuss taking it with your doctor.

## LICORICE: *Similar to Steroids*

In its pure form, licorice is anti-inflammatory, providing "a cortisol-like effect," says Dr. Firshein. (Cortisol is a drug commonly used to control the inflammation of asthma.) He advises using the deglycyrrhizinated form of licorice (labeled "DGL"), which won't raise blood pressure the way some forms of licorice do. Three times a day, add 20 to 40 drops of licorice tincture to a cup of hot water and let it cool to room temperature before drinking, he advises.

## NETTLE: *Relief from Allergies*

"I use nettle for asthma patients with sinus problems or nasal allergies," says Dr. Firshein. The herb contains a form of histamine that helps control allergic reactions. He recommends taking two 400-milligram capsules three times a day.

"You have to be careful to obtain a good brand of nettle, which, hopefully, has been properly harvested in the spring," he adds. "That's when the potent constituents of the stinging leaves are present."

## BREATHING: *To Stop an Attack*

Concentrating on breathing properly can help stop an asthma attack. This works in several ways. By drawing more air into your lungs, relaxing your body, and controlling anxiety and panic, you can significantly reduce the severity of attacks. Here's what Dr. Firshein recommends.

Sit down as soon as an attack begins. Put one hand on your stomach, with the palm open and flat against your stomach. Use the thumb and forefinger of your other hand to feel for the pulse point on the opposite wrist. Let yourself relax. Next, synchronize your breathing with your heart rate. For every seven beats, breathe in. After nine beats, breathe out. Blow out through pursed lips until your air is gone. Let your body feel the rhythm of the breath and your heart. Continue to breathe this way for 10 to 15 minutes. This exercise is very calming and can help keep an attack from getting worse, Dr. Firshein says.

### The Anti-Asthma Diet

"As an asthma sufferer myself, and as a physician who treats people with asthma, I've found that certain foods can have significant benefits," says Richard Firshein, D.O., an osteopathic physician in New York City. Here are his recommendations.

• Fish, which contains oil that reduces the airway inflammation of asthma.
• Onions, ginger, and garlic, which strengthen the immune system, and cayenne, which thins mucus.
• Fruits and vegetables, which contain a hefty dose of phytochemicals. These healing components in foods help control harmful free radical molecules in the body. Try to eat at least 6 servings of each every day.
• Sea vegetables, which deliver lots of protein and minerals. They include arame, dulse, hijiki, kombu, and nori and are available at health food stores, gourmet markets, and Asian groceries.
• Whole foods, which, unlike refined and processed foods, supply the best assortment of nutrients, complex sugars, starches, and fiber, says Dr. Firshein.
• Asian green tea, which contains substances that dilate the bronchial tubes. Avoid green tea if you're sensitive to molds, however.
• Magnesium-rich foods, such as tofu, wheat germ, Swiss chard, spinach, amaranth, beets, spinach, okra, and bean sprouts. Magnesium relaxes the bronchial tubes.
• Foods high in vitamin C and beta-carotene, such as dark green, leafy vegetables; cantaloupe; and squash. These two vitamins help fight inflammation.
• Healthy condiments, such as gomasio (roasted sesame seeds and sea salt), lemon juice, fresh spices, Dijon mustard, and low-sodium, preservative-free tamari, which is similar to soy sauce. High-fat, high-salt condiments are unhealthy for people with asthma (and everybody else!).

## EXERCISE: *Keep It Short and Sweet*

People with asthma almost always benefit from regular aerobic exercise. But Dr. Firshein believes that "pulsed exercise"—brief, intense spurts—is the best approach. "I find that brief, intense cycles of exercise and relaxation are often beneficial for asthmatics, whose lung capacity may not be great and who may be afraid to exercise for extended periods of time," he says.

• First, use your peak flow meter (a device that measures breathing capacity) to check your numbers. Your doctor can help you decide what type and size is best for you and what numbers you should be looking for, Dr. Firshein says.

• Exercise for 5 minutes by walking, jogging, riding a stationary bike, jumping rope, or whatever aerobic exercise you prefer, then check your numbers again. Relax until they return to normal. This counts as one cycle.

• Then start another cycle. You can do as many cycles as you like in any exercise session, but aim for a minimum of four 5-minute cycles, says Dr. Firshein. That will give you the maximum aerobic benefit, he says.

Some people with asthma may find that they need to use an inhaler before exercise. Others may need to take intal (Cromolyn) or tilade (Nedocromil), drugs that are used to control exercise-induced asthma, says Dr. Firshein. Check with your doctor to see what's best for you, he advises.

## MEDICATIONS: *Learn to Manage Them*

Many people with asthma will eventually need to take steroids, either inhaled or taken orally, to control inflammation in the lungs. These medications are the so-called drugs of choice for treating asthma. But what a choice.

"Steroids, taken long-term, may irreversibly harm, destroy, or disrupt virtually every organ in the body," says Dr. Firshein. As part of that damage, they rob the body of a variety of nutrients.

People who follow a lifestyle approach to treating asthma may be able to stop taking steroids entirely (with their doctors' approval, of course). Before that happens, however, you need to replace the nutrients that steroids steal. "I can't emphasize enough the importance of this step," says Dr. Firshein.

• Potassium: Take three 100-milligram capsules a day (with your doctor's supervision), and eat fruits that are high in potassium, such as bananas.

• Protein: Eat more fish, milk, and soy, and consider a daily drink made with protein powder, following the directions on the label.

• Calcium and magnesium: Take 500 milligrams of calcium citrate and 500 milligrams of magnesium citrate or magnesium aspartate a day.

You should also be sure to take some of the other supplements recommended in this chapter, particularly fish or flaxseed oil, vitamins C and E, and beta-carotene.

## *Gold-Medal Cures for* Athlete's Foot

You wouldn't want to live between your toes. The space is too small. Too dark. Too damp. Too stuffy. But to the fungus that causes tinea pedis, or athlete's foot, which usually has to camp out in shower stalls, on locker room floors, and on pool decks, your toes are prime real estate. They're the perfect place to settle down, multiply—and cause the hot, red, burning, itchy, flaking, peeling skin that is this troublesome tenant's trademark.

Eviction isn't easy. The fungus can penetrate the skin, burrowing too deep for topical fungus-killing medicines to work quickly and easily, but not deep enough for prescription oral fungicides to clean house. And even after weeks or months of daily treatment, when you think the fungus is gone for good, it can suddenly reappear.

If you're prone to athlete's foot, you should never wear the same pair of shoes 2 days in a row, and you should change socks during the day if your feet sweat. Here are some alternative remedies to help you get comfortably back on your feet.

### YOGURT: *A Little Dab'll Do You*
Dabbing regular, plain yogurt on the infected areas can help reduce the symptoms of athlete's foot, says Morton Walker, D.P.M., a former podiatrist in Stamford, Connecticut. The yogurt is soothing to the skin, he says, and you can apply it as often as you need to for relief.

# GUIDE TO
# PROFESSIONAL CARE

If you've been treating athlete's foot with self-care methods for more than 6 months with no results, see a podiatrist, a dermatologist, or your family physician, who may recommend a prescription oral antifungal medication or treat you for chronic fungal infection of the toenails, which can continually reinfect the rest of your feet.

## GARLIC: *Rub Out Fungus with Oil*

Rub two to three drops of garlic oil on the affected areas of your feet, says Stephanie Tourles, a licensed esthetician, reflexologist, and herbalist in West Hyannisport, Massachusetts.

"In my experience, this treatment works extremely well to kill athlete's foot fungus," she says. "It is absorbed underneath the skin, where the fungus has penetrated."

But, she cautions, don't use the treatment if you're planning a romantic evening—unless, of course, your partner loves the smell of garlic. "The oil is absorbed into the bloodstream, so you'll have garlic odor on your breath approximately 30 minutes after you apply the oil," Tourles says.

For maximum sociability, she recommends using the oil before bedtime: Pierce two or three garlic capsules, squeeze the oil onto the fungus, rub it into the skin, put on a pair of socks (so the oil doesn't get on the sheets), and go to bed. You can use this treatment each night for 2 to 4 weeks.

## GARLIC: *The Real—and Raw—Thing*

Garlic is one of the most potent antifungal herbs, Tourles says. The raw form is most effective, she says, because none of the fungus-killing allicin (the most active ingredient in the herb) has been removed by processing.

She recommends eating four small cloves once a day and drinking lots of water (12 to 16 ounces) with the garlic to reduce stomach upset. Continue for 4 to 6 months or until you see results. Just be aware that treating yourself with garlic may upset others, since the garlic odor will permeate your entire body, warns Tourles.

If you (or your nearest and dearest) can't handle raw cloves, take the herb in capsule form, using four to eight capsules a day in three divided doses (three with breakfast, three with lunch, and two with dinner, for example). Continue for 4 to 6 months, or as long as you like, to ward off infection.

Tourles recommends the brand Kyolic, which, she says, has a standardized, reliable amount of allicin. And be sure to take the capsules with an 8-ounce glass of water to avoid intestinal upset.

## ASTRAGALUS: *The Herbal Fungus Killer*

Take astragalus, a potent antifungal herb, three times a day for maximum effectiveness, recommends Steven Subotnick, D.P.M., a podiatrist in Berkeley and San Leandro, California.

Divide the dosage recommendation on the label by three and take the herb with each meal. If the label recommends four capsules a day, for example, take two with breakfast, one with lunch, and one with dinner. Take this dose until your immune system is up to par, which should be in about 6 to 8 weeks.

### Immunity Boosters

If you have recurring athlete's foot, it may be because your immune system isn't strong enough to beat it once and for all, say podiatrists who specialize in alternative medicine.

"Chronic athlete's foot indicates that the fungus-fighting T-cells of your immune system are weak," says Dr. Subotnick. Here's how to boost your immune system's fungus-fighting power.

### Try This Natural Antifungal Treatment— It's Chemical-Free and Good for Your Skin

Over-the-counter remedies for athlete's foot may work, but they don't nourish or help heal the skin that's been traumatized by the fungal infection, says Stephanie Tourles, a licensed esthetician, reflexologist, and herbalist in West Hyannisport, Massachusetts. That's why she recommends using the following natural mixture of an herb and two essential oils. It not only kills the fungus but also soothes and heals your skin, she says.

Combine 2 teaspoons of tincture of benzoin, made from the resin of a tree grown in the tropics, with five drops of lavender essential oil and five drops of thyme essential oil.

The tincture of benzoin or benzoin resin helps heal the fungal infection, reduces redness and burning, and dries skin that's too moist, says Tourles. Lavender essential oil also helps heal skin, and thyme essential oil is a powerful antifungal.

Each evening before bedtime, massage the mixture into the area of the infection and then over your entire foot. Let your feet dry for 3 to 5 minutes before walking around or getting into bed. Since the mixture is thin and watery, says Tourles, you may want to put a blow-dryer on the low setting and dry your feet for a minute or two.

A mild case of athlete's foot should heal in 2 to 3 months, says Tourles, while a severe case may take up to 6 months.

## REFINED SUGAR: *A Must to Avoid*

Refined sugar is a toxin for the immune system, and eating too many sweets and other sugar-rich foods allows athlete's foot fungus to flourish, says Gregory W. Spencer, D.P.M., a podiatrist in Renton, Washington. Thus, if you have a case of athlete's foot that you can't kick, he recommends cutting way back on your intake of refined sugar.

## ECHINACEA: *But Not Too Much*

Echinacea is one of the best herbs for invigorating your immune system, says Dr. Subotnick. But if you take it every day, it can actually weaken immunity. Following the dosage recommendations on the label, take it for 3 weeks in a row, then take a week off.

## VITAMIN C: *For Supplemental Strength*

Vitamin C is one of the best nutrients for strengthening the immune system, says Dr. Subotnick. To defeat athlete's foot, though, you need to keep blood levels constant, which is why he recommends taking the nutrient six times a day.

Start with 250-milligram capsules for the first week (for a total of 1,500 milligrams a day), increase to 500-milligram dosages the second week (for a total of 3,000 milligrams), then to 1,000 milligrams per dose the third week (for a total of 6,000 milligrams).

If you develop diarrhea or loose bowel movements at either the 3,000- or 6,000-milligram level (a possible side effect of large doses of vitamin C), go back to the level at which you didn't have the problem.

## *A Drug-Free Approach to* **Attention Deficit Hyperactivity Disorder**

For as long as you can remember, you've been easily distracted, chronically forgetful, restless, disorganized, and impulsive. Your work and relationships have suffered. In short, you're an adult with attention deficit hyperactivity disorder, or ADHD.

Since this is a problem that out-of-control kids are famous for, you go to your doctor seeking the medication that's prescribed for millions of youngsters with ADHD. The obliging physician writes you a prescription for . . .

Cocaine.

Well, actually, it's methylphenidate (Ritalin), a drug so nearly identical to cocaine that the two are used interchangeably in medical research. And, like cocaine, the "benefits" of Ritalin are a mirage.

"Ritalin and similar stimulant-type drugs used to treat the symptoms that are called ADHD simply snuff out vitality, curiosity, imagination, and sociability—all the higher mental functions—and replace them with narrowly focused obsessive behavior," says Peter R. Breggin, M.D., director of the International Center for the Study of Psychiatry and Psychology in Bethesda, Maryland.

In other words, Ritalin helps you focus—by turning you into a robot.

There are better, natural ways for adults to deal with the symptoms of ADHD (also called ADD, for attention deficit disorder). Dr. Breggin looks for the cause of the person's distraction,

---

# GUIDE TO
# PROFESSIONAL CARE

People with symptoms of attention deficit often have an un-diagnosed underlying health problem that is the true cause, says Mary Ann Block, D.O., an osteopathic physician at the Block Center in Dallas-Fort Worth.

To uncover the problem, Dr. Block recommends that a health professional test for the following conditions that can lead to ADHD symptoms: food allergy, nutritional deficiencies, and yeast infection. Also, have your doctor check your thyroid function and take a blood test for anemia.

If you are currently taking medication for ADHD or are un-der a physician's care, consult your doctor before making any of the changes suggested in this chapter.

---

which could be anxiety, lack of confidence, a brain injury, or other factors.

And Mary Ann Block, D.O., an osteopathic physician at the Block Center in Dallas-Fort Worth, believes that diet holds the key.

## FOOD: *Eat Every 2 Hours*

Aggression. Nervousness. Agitation. Anxiety. Those typical ADHD symptoms are also symptoms of hypoglycemia, or low blood sugar, says Dr. Block.

"Blood sugar, or glucose, is the body's primary fuel, and low blood sugar is the most significant problem I find in people with the behavioral symptoms of ADHD," she says.

There is, however, an easy way to avoid low blood sugar and help clear up the symptoms of ADHD. Just follow this rule: Never let yourself get hungry.

"Always carry food with you and eat every 2 hours," says Dr. Block. By eating often during the day, you keep blood sugar on an even keel. She recommends breakfast, a midmorn-ing snack, lunch, a midafternoon snack, dinner, and a bedtime snack.

And be sure to include some protein with each meal and

snack. "Protein will break down slowly in the body and help keep blood sugar levels stable," she says. Good-for-you protein foods include chicken, turkey, fish, low-fat dairy products, beans, and nuts and seeds.

## SUGAR: *How Sweet It Isn't*

High-sugar foods such as candy, cake, pie, and soft drinks pour excess glucose into your blood, which triggers the release of insulin, a hormone that lowers glucose. Thus, eating a lot of sugar actually ends up lowering blood sugar.

If you have ADHD, you should eliminate refined carbohydrates from your diet, says Dr. Block. That means not only sugar but also white flour, which quickly turns into glucose.

## Stop Procrastinating:
## Imagine a New Internal Voice

Procrastination is a common characteristic of people with ADHD, says Thom Hartmann, a psychotherapist in Montpelier, Vermont. He says, however, that getting control of it can be as simple as changing the way you talk to yourself.

Procrastinators hear obnoxious and aggressive internal voices yelling at them in a tone that implies dire consequences if they don't do something right away. "What a great voice to ignore!" says Hartmann. Here, in his words, is a quick way to change that voice.

"Imagine something that you need to do in the near future. Next, imagine a sexy, curious, soft, nurturing voice inviting you to accomplish the task and pointing out to you all the warm, wonderful, pleasant things that will result from your action.

"If the old, obnoxious voice is still there, grab it with a loving hand and adjust its tone, pace, and volume to be sexy, curious, soft, and nurturing (or whatever adjectives work best for you). The very same words said in a different tonality will have dramatically different results."

## MULTIVITAMIN/MINERAL SUPPLEMENT:
*For Better Biochemistry*

"I have seen many of the symptoms of ADHD improve in my patients when they supplement their diets with high levels of nutrients," says Dr. Block. That's because vitamins and minerals improve the biochemistry of the body and the brain so that your nervous system (and every other system) can work as nature intended: A-OK, not ADHD.

Take a high-potency nutritional supplement only with the approval and supervision of your physician, says Dr. Block. Look for a multivitamin/mineral supplement that contains the following levels of nutrients.

- Thiamin: 25 milligrams
- Vitamin $B_6$: 100 milligrams
- Pantothenic acid : 50 milligrams
- Folic acid: 400 micrograms
- Beta-carotene: 15 milligrams
- Vitamin C: 1,000 milligrams
- Vitamin E: 400 international units
- Calcium: 500 to 1,000 milligrams
- Magnesium: 100 to 400 milligrams
- Zinc: 15 milligrams

## MAGNESIUM: *A Calming Mineral*

Extra magnesium (more than what's in most multivitamin/ mineral supplements) will help calm ADHD symptoms, says Dr. Block. In addition to a multivitamin/mineral supplement, she recommends 500 milligrams a day of magnesium.

## FATTY ACIDS: *Nutrients for the Brain*

Supplementing the diet with fatty acids has been shown to help brain cells function better. "I have seen them reduce the symptoms of ADHD," says Dr. Block. She recommends 500 milligrams a day of evening primrose oil and 3 teaspoons a day of flaxseed oil, both of which are rich in fatty acids.

## *Gentle, Nonsurgical Alternatives to Relieve* **Back Pain**

Eighty percent of Americans have back pain—usually lower-back pain—at some time in their lives. And 45 percent of those folks will have repeated "back attacks," says Jerome F. McAndrews, D.C., a chiropractor in Claremore, Oklahoma, and national spokesperson for the American Chiropractic Association.

If you're currently experiencing back pain, and you're thinking about having surgery to solve the problem, a surgeon who has performed thousands of spine surgeries says, "Think again."

"If you can recover from back pain without surgery, you're much better off," says Stephen Hochschuler, M.D., an orthopedic surgeon in Plano, Texas. Surgery, he says, can have unforeseen complications, from infections to nerve damage. Surgery can fail, leaving you with more pain than you had before. And, most important, surgery is usually not necessary.

Most people with back pain have a problem with short, tight, rigid back muscles, says Dr. Hochschuler, and it can be relieved by improved posture while sitting, standing, and working; regular aerobic exercise; stretching; and exercises to strengthen the back muscles.

Twenty percent of people with back pain have spinal injuries, usually involving the rupture of one or more disks, the gel-filled shock absorbers between the vertebrae, or bones of the spinal stack. Before opting for surgery, people with that type of injury should wait at least 3 months after being diagnosed by a doctor and use alternative remedies during that time, says Dr. Hochschuler, unless there is an emergency situation. "Many times," he says, "disks get better with the same types of nonmedical treatments that repair back muscles."

Want to start relieving your pain today with alternative home remedies? Well, sit up and notice the way you're sitting.

# GUIDE TO
# PROFESSIONAL CARE

You should see a medical doctor immediately if you have intense pain that travels down your leg or radiates from your spine, sudden weakness in your leg or foot, or loss of control of your bowels or bladder.

These symptoms are indications of a ruptured disk or other spinal problem, says Stephen Hochschuler, M.D., an orthopedic surgeon in Plano, Texas.

Once your problem has been diagnosed by a medical doctor, there are many options for nonsurgical professional care of back pain, says Dr. Hochschuler, including back specialty clinics, chiropractic, physical therapy, therapeutic massage, movement therapies such as the Alexander Technique, acupuncture (including techniques using electrical stimulation, such as electroacupuncture and Craig PENS acupuncture), gentle exercise therapies such as tai chi and qigong, and natural medical systems such as Traditional Chinese Medicine and Ayurvedic medicine.

"Shop around and make sure that whoever you see is going to treat you comprehensively, looking at your lifestyle, your posture, your habits, how fit you are, how you relax, how you handle stress, and what your diet is like," says Pamela Adams, D.C., a chiropractor and yoga instructor in Larkspur, California. "Whether you go the allopathic or the alternative route to relieve back pain, see a professional who doesn't have a narrow focus."

## Make Back Pain Take a Seat

"One of the main culprits in chronic, nontraumatic lower-back pain is sitting and leaning back," says Pamela Adams, D.C., a chiropractor and yoga instructor in Larkspur, California.

Leaning back flattens the lower, or lumbar, area of your back, depriving the lower back of its natural curve. "The weight of your body then pulls down on the lower lumbar vertebrae in the spine, stressing the ligaments and disks," says Dr. Adams. "After many years of sitting this way, you may develop lower-back pain."

Leaning back while sitting also puts your weight in the middle of your buttocks, right where your sciatic nerve passes into your legs. "If you sit this way year after year, you may pinch your sciatic nerve, and you'll start developing shooting pains down one or both legs," Dr. Adams warns.

Practicing correct posture, she says, is an effective way to prevent and relieve muscular back pain. And it's easy to do in any situation.

## SITTING: *Lift Your Breastbone*

The proper position for sitting is "just a smidgen" in front of your "sit bones," or the ischium bones of the pelvis, says Dr. Adams. Those are the big bones that you can feel pressing against the chair right where your thighs end and your buttocks begin. At least, you can feel them when you are sitting correctly. Lean slightly forward from your hips, then, keeping your pelvis in place, move your upper back slightly back. That means don't slouch forward, don't round or hunch your back and shoulders, and keep your feet flat on the floor. "You should be conscious of the curve in the small of your back," she says.

The key to this pain-relieving, pain-preventing sitting posture is to lift your breastbone as you sit, says Dr. Adams. "Pretend that a string is attached to the middle of your chest and is nudging your breastbone upward,"
she says. "You want to lengthen the space between your belly button and your breastbone. This 'corrected' sitting posture will feel awkward for a few days, however, because sitting incorrectly for so long can change the configuration and tone of your muscles," says Dr. Adams.

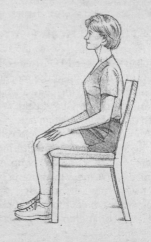

Do this breastbone-lifting exercise whenever you notice that you are leaning back or slumping over. The resulting posture not only will position your body correctly on your sit bones, says

Dr. Adams, it will also position your head correctly on top of your spine, putting your spine in a natural alignment that supports your musculature and gives the overworked muscles of your lower back some much-needed relief.

## DRIVING: *On the Road Back to Health*

"Many people who drive for a living have terrible back pain," says Dr. Adams. That's because car seats seem designed to hurt your back, she says. Your knees are higher than your hips, throwing the weight of your body onto your sciatic nerve. And you're leaning back with your head forward and your arms extended, which stresses your lower back (and your neck).

To minimize the damage, your car seat should be as flat as possible so that your knees and hips are at the same level, says Dr. Adams. "You want to drive the same way you sit."

If your car seat doesn't adjust automatically, you can build up the dip in the seat by sitting on a folded towel, a foam wedge, or a small pillow. Put a small pillow behind your lower back as well.

Next, position the seat so that you aren't reaching for the steering wheel or leaning forward to grasp it. The wheel should be close enough that your arms can hang naturally from your shoulders and your shoulders feel relaxed.

Just be sure that your breastbone is about 10 inches from the center of the steering wheel. That way, you'll lessen the possibility of injury from your seat belt or air bag if you're in an accident.

### A Physician Heals Himself—With Magnet Therapy

Julian Whitaker, M.D., *used* to have lower-back pain.

"I used to get up in the morning, let my legs flop out of bed, and then limp around for quite a while," he recalls. Now, he says that he doesn't notice any back pain. What made the difference? A corset with magnets inserted in it.

A magnetic field may help relieve pain by increasing blood flow to the injured area or by altering the transmission of pain in nerve fibers, says Dr. Whitaker, who is the founder and director of the Whitaker Wellness Institute in Newport Beach, California.

"I wear my corset under my clothes, I sleep in it—I wear it everywhere except for the shower," he says.

He recommends using magnets of 3,000 to 4,000 gauss,

although magnets with strengths as low as 500 gauss have been shown to relieve back pain. (Gauss is a measure of a magnet's strength; a refrigerator magnet is a little less than 300 gauss.)

Since magnets can cause skin irritation, it's best to give your skin a rest from them, perhaps while you sleep or when you're in the shower. If you do notice irritation, remove the magnets for a couple of hours to a day, then reapply them.

## STANDING: *Ask for a Second Opinion*

For pain-free posture when you're standing, do the breastbone-lifting exercise, says Dr. Adams, then have a friend look at you from the side. If you're standing correctly—that is, in a posture that can prevent or relieve back pain—a vertical line could pass directly through your ear, the middle of your shoulder, the middle of your hip bone, and the outside of your anklebone.

"Correcting posture induced back pain is very logical and very simple," says Dr. Adams, "but people make it so difficult. The body is a perfect mechanism. All we have to do is remove whatever imbalances are in the way of the body performing the way it is supposed to—and this easy exercise does just that."

## LIFTING: *Even If You Don't Know Squat*

You probably know how not to lift: Never bend over at the waist. And, says Dr. Hochschuler, maybe you've also learned the commonly prescribed method of correct lifting to prevent back pain: Squat with your knees apart, with the object between your knees and as close as possible to your body. Using your legs, stand up and lift, bringing the object closer to your body as you stand. Be sure to keep your back straight.

For people who can't manage a squat, however, there's another way. Put one knee on the floor, says Dr. Hochschuler. Then,

using your arms, move the object onto your opposite thigh
and, with a firm grip on the object, simply stand up.

## BODY AWARENESS: *Do a Check*

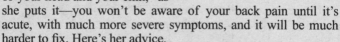

Your body is always giving
you messages, says Dr. Adams:
"This position hurts," "Get up
and stretch," "Time to quit
and rest." If you ignore the
messages—if you "go through
the day living between the top
of your head and your chin," as
she puts it—you won't be aware of your back pain until it's
acute, with much more severe symptoms, and it will be much
harder to fix. Here's her advice.

If you have a watch alarm, set it to go off every hour while
you're awake. For 15 to 30 seconds after the alarm sounds, consciously notice how your body feels. (If you're already in pain,
make this "appointment with your body" every 15 minutes.)

Are you sitting correctly? If not, lift your breastbone. Are
your shoulders up around your ears? Lower them. "Pretty soon,
checking on your body throughout the day will become automatic, and you won't need the alarm," says Dr. Adams.

## Getting Back to Sleep

Sleep time can be a chance to realign a back that's been
stressed all day, says Dr. Adams. Here are two tips to help you
do just that.

## ON YOUR BACK: *The Pain-Free Way to Snooze*

Don't sleep on your side. "Sleeping on your side puts your
head forward, hunches your shoulders, and collapses your chest
area, which means that your back can't extend and arch," says
Dr. Adams. Instead, she says, sleep on your back. "The body
opens up and you stretch, extend, and lengthen your back," she
says.

Also, sleep with a thin pillow, Dr. Adams advises, so that your head is not pushed too far forward. She recommends buying an inexpensive feather pillow (if you aren't allergic), opening one end, and removing about a third of the feathers. (Be sure to sew up the opening, and either throw the feathers away or use them to make another pillow, she suggests.)

Shape the pillow so that it fits comfortably under your neck, making it thinner under your head and thicker under your neck for support. You should also put a folded or rolled towel in the small of your back for support, says Dr. Adams. The thickness of the towel depends on your body. "It should be a little uncomfortable, but not much," she says.

If you're pregnant, however, don't sleep on your back after the first trimester. As an alternative, Dr. Adams suggests lying on your side, but not in the fetal position. Align your spine as best you can, then use a pillow that's as high as the distance between your shoulder and your neck so that it can support your head without pushing it too high or letting it sag.

## ON YOUR STOMACH: *The Perfect Pose for Sciatica Relief*

"For years, people have been told that they should never sleep on their stomachs if they have bad lower backs," says Dr. Adams. If you have sciatica, though, that could be bad advice. Sciatica is caused by overstretching ligaments and muscles in the back until they're pressing on the sciatic nerve. It's usually marked by shooting pains down one or both legs and is a condition that should be checked by a doctor.

If you sleep on your stomach when you have sciatica, Dr. Adams says, gravity can restore a natural curve to your back, relaxing those ligaments and muscles so the nerve can heal itself.

## Easy Exercises for Quick Pain Relief

These simple exercises "can be effective home remedies for a simple attack of back pain," says Stephen Hochschuler, M.D., an orthopedic surgeon in Plano, Texas. You can do these exercises as many times during the day as necessary. Here are a few guidelines.

Don't hold your breath; stretch slowly, with steady movements— don't bounce or jerk; and count the duration of each exercise as "one, Mississippi, two, Mississippi," and so on, advises Dr. Hochschuler. Finally, if doing any of these exercises causes more pain, see a physician or physical therapist.

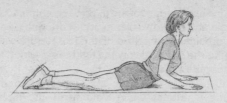

## Press Up

Lie on your stomach on a mat or carpeted floor with your elbows bent and your hands on the floor by your shoulders. Press up slightly, straightening your arms somewhat. Raise your head to look straight ahead but keep it in line with your spine. Keep your pelvis in contact with the floor and don't tighten your lower back or arch your neck. The intent is not to do a push-up with a straight back. Hold for 10 seconds, then return to the starting position. Repeat 5 to 10 times.

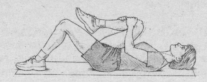

## Knee Lift

Lie on your back with both knees bent and your feet flat on the floor. With your hands on your shin, lift your right knee toward your chest, being careful not to force it any closer than is comfortable. Hold for 10 seconds, then return to the starting position. Repeat with the other leg.

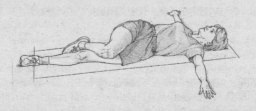

## Lumbar Rotation

Lie flat on your back with your arms extended to the sides, forming a T with your body. Raise your right leg and slowly cross it over your body, trying to touch your knee to the floor on the opposite side, but go only as far as is comfortable for you. Try to keep your shoulders flat against the floor. Hold for 10 seconds, then return to the starting position and repeat with the other leg. Do this 10 times with each leg.

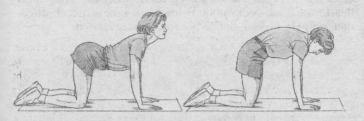

## All-Fours Arch

Start on your hands and knees on the floor. Keep your shoulders over your hands and align your hips with your knees. Arch your lower back slightly and hold for 10 seconds. Alternate between rolling upward like a cat and arching downward, but be sure that you don't arch your neck and head along with your spine. Repeat up to 20 times.

### Stretch—and Prevent Back Pain

These three simple stretching exercises (all done while sitting in a chair) can keep your spine flexible and help prevent back pain, says Michael D. Pedigo, D.C., a chiropractor in San Leandro, California, and president of the American Chiropractic Association.

"It's very important to do these exercises on an ongoing basis—even when you're pain-free—to counteract stresses and strains in the muscles of the back and prevent recurrent episodes of back pain," says Dr. Pedigo.

Do them three times a day—in the morning, at midday, and in the early evening. Don't worry if you hear some snapping and popping as your joints move through their full ranges of motion, "as long as it causes no sharp pain. If it does, stop the exercise and see a chiropractor," he says.

## ARCHING AND BENDING: *Loosening Up*

Sit in a chair in a normal, upright sitting position with your legs hip-width apart and your hands on your knees. First, slowly lower your head toward your chest as far as you can without forcing it (*a*). Then, in one smooth, continuous motion, slowly bend your neck back as far as you comfortably can (*b*). Repeat this forward-and-back motion slowly 10 times in each direction, says Dr. Pedigo, but do not force either motion.

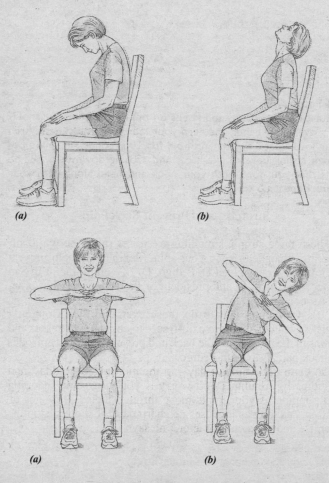

*(a)*                    *(b)*

*(a)*                    *(b)*

## SIDE-TO-SIDE: *Increasing Flexibility*

In the same sitting position, hold your hands palms down in front of you and lace your fingers together. Point your elbows to the sides, horizontal to the floor (*a*). Slowly bend to the left from the waist, tilting so that your left elbow points toward the floor and bending your spine as far as you comfortably can (*b*). Return to the upright position and repeat on your right side. Do this 10 times in each direction. "Your spine should move like a willow tree," says Dr. Pedigo.

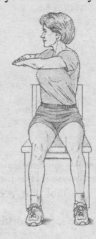

## FULL TWIST: *For Your Whole Spine*

In the same position, with your fingers laced and your elbows out, turn your head and shoulders to the right, letting your spine comfortably twist as far as it can. Repeat in the other direction. Do 10 twists on each side, says Dr. Pedigo.

## YOGA: *For Strong Back Muscles*

To prevent or relieve back pain, you need to strengthen the muscles of your back. One of the best ways is to swim regularly, Dr. Adams says, using a freestyle or crawl stroke with a regular scissors kick. But there is also a yoga pose called the half-cobra that, when done each day, is a wonderful way to strengthen your back, she says.

Lie flat on your stomach on either a carpeted floor or a mat, with your leg muscles completely relaxed and your forehead resting on the floor (*a*). Take a deep breath as you slowly push your head and torso off the floor, keeping your hips in place, then rest on your elbows (*b*), says Dr. Adams. (You probably used this position as a kid while watching television.) Keep your back relaxed and hold for about a minute. If your neck becomes sore, you can cup your chin in your hands, she says. Then breathe out; lower your arms, head, and chest back to the floor; and relax. Repeat two more times.

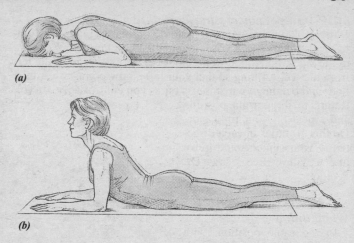

*(a)*

*(b)*

Dr. Adams suggests doing the half-cobra several times a day. The more you do it, the longer you can hold the stretch, as long as it is comfortable for you.

### Nondrug Pain Relief

Yes, you can use anti-inflammatory medications for pain relief. But if you'd rather not cope with their side effects, including digestive upset, there is a natural "medicine" that may work just as well.

### MSM: *From Nature's Pharmacy*

The nutritional supplement MSM (methylsulfonylmethane) is very effective for treating chronic back pain, says Stanley W. Jacob, M.D., professor of surgery at Oregon Health Sciences University in Portland.

"I have seen several hundred patients for back pain secondary to other problems, such as arthritis, disk degeneration, and accidents," he says. "For such pain-related conditions, MSM is usually beneficial. In fact, there may be no pharmaceutical therapy that is better."

For back pain, Dr. Jacob recommends taking up to 8 grams of MSM a day in divided doses with meals. Because the supplement may cause loose stools, start with 2 grams daily and increase by 2 grams every 7 days, if necessary, until you reach 8 grams. (Increase the dosage only if the lower dosage does not help.) This should help you avoid bowel problems, says Dr. Jacob.

Also, if you're being treated with a blood-thinning drug, take MSM only with your doctor's approval and supervision, since it may thin the blood slightly. Otherwise, says Dr. Jacob, MSM is a safe supplement with no serious side effects.

# A Fresh Approach to Banishing
# Bad Breath

Yes, brushing and flossing your teeth regularly can clean up some of the oral bacteria that commonly cause bad breath. But routine oral hygiene isn't enough to banish a malodorous mouth.

Neither are the mints and mouthwashes that line drugstore and supermarket shelves. At best, they temporarily mask the problem. What's more, the sugar in mints and the alcohol in many mouthwashes make them less than healthy options in the quest for fresh breath.

That's where natural remedies come in—and the best alternative remedy may not even be available at your drugstore (although you can find it at most health food stores). It's a tongue scraper.

## TONGUE SCRAPING: *A Grate Solution to Bacteria*

A lot of odor-producing bacteria (and maybe some smelly, decaying food particles, too) hide out in the nooks and crannies of the papillae, the microscopic, mushroom-shaped stalks that cover the surface of your tongue, says Michael Olmsted, D.D.S., a biocompatible dentist in Del Mar, California.

"Brushing won't clean those bacteria and particles from your tongue," Dr. Olmsted says. You have to scrape them off, and the best tool for the job is a tongue scraper, a U-shaped, typically

---

### GUIDE TO
### PROFESSIONAL CARE

Chronic bad breath can be caused by many different types of diseases, such as cancer, kidney failure, and diabetes. If you have a case of halitosis that doesn't quit, see a medical doctor.

Dental problems, ranging from crowns and dentures that don't fit to broken fillings, can also cause bad breath. If you do not have a serious disease and home remedies haven't eliminated your bad breath, see a dentist for professional care, says Flora Parsa Stay, D.D.S., a dentist in Oxnard, California.

---

metal device that you hold at both ends and gently drag over the length of your tongue.

"Most of the world relies on tongue scraping to keep bad breath in check and has done so for thousands of years," he says. Here's how to join the clean-tongue crowd.

Your goal is to remove the creamy-looking, white, brown, or orange layer of gunk on your tongue. To do that, says Dr. Olmsted, scrape both the top and sides of your tongue (but not the underside) from back to front. Go over the same area more than once if necessary. Start scraping as far back on the tongue as you can without gagging, since the papillae at the rear of the tongue are longest and harbor the most odor-causing bacteria and food. Scrape right after each tooth brushing.

In Ayurveda, the ancient system of natural healing from India, the tongue scraper most recommended to remove odor-causing organisms and particles is made of silver.

"The silver gives off ions that kill bacteria on the tongue," explains Edward M. Arana, D.D.S., a retired dentist in Carmel Valley, California, and past president of the American Academy of Biological Dentistry. According to Ayurveda, silver also reduces pitta, a body-heating factor that can worsen bad breath.

If silver is too rich for your taste, try copper. According to Ayurveda, a copper scraper cleans your tongue and tones up your taste buds, helping you to enjoy healthful, natural foods even more. And, says Dr. Arana, natural foods help prevent intestinal problems, which are another common cause of bad breath.

Does a tongue scraper seem like an unnecessary expense? Use a spoon instead, says Dr. Olmsted, and scrape with the edge. Just be sure that the edge isn't sharp, and don't use that spoon for any other purpose.

## HOMEOPATHY: *Fostering Freshness*

If your tongue is very heavily coated, accompany the scraping with the homeopathic remedy Mercurius vivus, says Flora Parsa Stay, D.D.S., a dentist in Oxnard, California. This remedy alleviates excess salivation, thus limiting the odor-causing coating on the tongue. Take two tablets of the 30X potency a day until symptoms improve, or for 10 days.

## CHLOROPHYLL: *A Green Alternative*

"A variety of digestive problems in the stomach and intestinal tract can cause mouth odor," Dr. Olmsted says. With many of those problems, food isn't being digested properly, and vapors from the undigested food waft into (and out of) your mouth.

Solving digestive problems can be difficult, but that doesn't mean that you have to worry about bad breath in the meantime. You can deodorize your digestive tract with chlorophyll, the same chemical that makes leaves green. When you get up in the morning, take three chlorophyll capsules or tablets on an empty stomach, says Dr. Olmsted. Then take three before or after every meal. (Regular intake of chlorophyll has the unusual but harmless side effect of giving your stools a green tint.)

## ACTIVATED CHARCOAL: *A Natural Breath Sweetener*

Another supplement that can clean out your insides and sweeten your breath is activated charcoal, says Dr. Arana. He says to take one capsule a day until the problem is solved. If you don't notice results after 10 days, seek advice from your dentist.

## DIGESTIVE ENZYMES: *Breaking Down Bad Breath*

Another possible cause of poor digestion (and bad breath) is a lack of digestive enzymes, the special chemicals that break down food in your intestines. But you can replace the missing enzymes with an enzyme supplement.

Dr. Olmsted says to look for gelatin capsules that contain the four most important digestive enzymes: protease (for protein), amylase and cellulase (for carbohydrates), and lipase (for fat).

Don't swallow the capsules, though. "Your digestion may not be strong enough to dissolve them," he says. Instead, before each meal, open a capsule, pour the contents into a 4-ounce glass of water, stir it thoroughly, and drink. Follow this regimen until your symptoms improve.

**HERBS: *Four to Freshen Breath***

Ginger, coriander, cumin, and fennel are four common herbs that can deodorize your intestinal tract, says Dr. Olmsted. For maximum effectiveness, he recommends opening one gelatin capsule of each herb, putting the contents in a tablespoon, and taking the spoonful of herbs with a little water after each meal.

# *Fast, Natural Relief from*
# Belching

Traditional doctors don't always take belching seriously, so they may advise patients simply to take antacids.

According to alternative nutritionists and physicians, however, excessive belching usually occurs when the digestive system isn't working right. If you don't have enough stomach acid and digestive enzymes, the food you eat is likely to just sit in your stomach and small intestine rather than being digested properly. When this happens, the food may produce gases that cause bloating and constant, uncomfortable belching.

How do you stop it? If you want temporary relief, you can take an over-the-counter product with the ingredient simethicone. It causes gas bubbles to come together and combine so that they're more easily expelled, says William B. Salt II, M.D., clinical associate professor of medicine at Ohio State University College of Medicine and Public Health in Columbus.

---

### GUIDE TO
### PROFESSIONAL CARE

If you have chronic belching—that is, it happens all the time, you can't control it, and you feel abdominal discomfort—you should see a gastroenterologist to rule out more serious prob-lems, such as gastroesophageal reflux disease, an ulcer, or other stomach disorders.

---

If you want to solve the problem and get permanent relief, however, alternative practitioners say that you should try herbal and dietary supplements. They may actually eliminate excess belching by helping your digestive tract do what it's designed to do.

**GINGER:** *Nearly Instant Relief*

The herb ginger stimulates digestion and is good for both relieving and preventing belching, says Mark Stengler, N.D., a naturopathic physician in San Diego.

He recommends taking one or two 550-milligram capsules of powdered ginger or 30 drops of tincture right before each meal. Or you can drink a cup of ginger tea with each meal. If you still have symptoms after a week, see a doctor, he adds.

**DIGESTIVE ENZYMES:** *A Package of Protection*

A lifetime of poor diet, such as eating too many processed foods and not enough fruits, vegetables, and whole grains, may damage the body's ability to manufacture normal levels of diges-tive enzymes. This can lead to excessive belching, says Teresa Rispoli, Ph.D., a licensed nutritionist and acupuncturist in Agoura Hills, California.

You can make up for this deficiency by taking a combination supplement that includes the full complement of digestive en-zymes. She recommends looking for a supplement that includes as many of the following enzymes as possible: protease and pancreatin for protein digestion, amylase for starches, lipase for fat, cellulase for vegetable fibers, lactase for milk sugar, and maltase and sucrase for other types of sugars.

Take the supplement before meals, following the dosage recommendations on the label. It's safe to take it indefinitely.

## CARDAMOM: *Calms the Stomach*

Cardamom may help reduce muscle spasms in the stomach, which are one cause of belching, says Dr. Rispoli. It also increases the production of digestive fluids so that food in the digestive tract is less likely to "rot" and produce gas.

You can prepare it as a tea by adding 1 teaspoon of cardamom to 8 ounces of water and boiling for 10 minutes. Drink it hot.

## HINGWASTIKA: *An Herbal Formula for Better Digestion*

In Ayurveda, the ancient system of natural healing from India, belching is a vata condition, meaning that there is an excess of air in the system. Taking the herbal formula Hingwastika can relieve excess vata, says Light Miller, an Ayurvedic practitioner in Sarasota, Florida. She recommends taking two capsules after each meal. It's safe to take this until your belching is relieved, but you should take it only with the guidance of a qualified Ayurvedic practitioner.

## TEAS: *Calming Cures*

Folk treatments for belching include clove tea and citrus peel tea, says Andrew Gaeddert, a professional member of the American Herbalists Guild and director of the Get Well Clinic in Oakland, California. To make the tea, add 1 teaspoon of cloves or finely grated citrus peel to 8 ounces of water and boil for 10 minutes. Drink the tea hot.

### Break the Belching Cycle

Maybe you don't just belch after meals. Maybe you belch all the time, throughout the day, over and over again. This condition is called aerophagia, and it probably means that you're swallowing air, says William B. Salt II, M.D., clinical associate professor of medicine at Ohio State University College of Medicine and Public Health in Columbus.

Here's what happens. When gas accumulates in your stomach, you may feel bloated, so you swallow some extra air in hopes of provoking a burp. But you probably swallow more air than you belch. This starts a cycle in which you feel bloated, swallow air to relieve yourself, belch, feel more bloated, swallow more air, and on and on. Soon, this process becomes unconscious, and you're belching all the time.

Dr. Salt believes that the best way to cure aerophagia isn't with drugs or professional treatment. It's with your mind.

"First, you must understand that constant, unconscious swallowing is the cause of your constant burping," he says. "Then, you must develop the mindfulness to observe yourself. Mindfulness is awareness of the moment and what is occurring in it. Once you understand that constant swallowing is the cause of the problem, and you observe yourself swallowing, you can usually stop it, and your belching will go away."

# Be Kind to Yourself, and You Can Stop
# **Binge-Eating Disorder**

Picture a woman alone in her kitchen, uncontrollably eating 2 pints of ice cream followed by six slices of cold pizza, a box of cookies, and a half-dozen doughnuts. Why would she do that?

Because she's been on a strict, low-fat diet, and she just can't stand the deprivation anymore?

Because she hates her "failure" to have the "perfect" body and be "perfect" in dozens of other ways, and she's unconsciously punishing herself with food?

Because she started to have a feeling that was unacceptable to her, and, without knowing why, she immediately began to eat a huge quantity of food to numb herself?

The answer, as you probably suspected, is all of the above.

"The personal issues that are expressed through binge eating— or what I call emotional eating—usually have nothing to do with food," says Geneen Roth of Santa Cruz, California, an expert on the relationship between emotions and overeating. "Food is just the substance of choice that people use at that moment to act out or repress or avoid their feelings."

# GUIDE TO
# PROFESSIONAL CARE

To break out of the diet-binge cycle, you need outside support, says Geneen Roth of Santa Cruz, California, an expert on the relationship between emotions and overeating. That support can take the form of one-on-one professional counseling; a support group that is either professionally led, led by peers, or leaderless; or even regular use of a chat group on the Internet.

If you decide on a therapist, choose one who specializes in eating disorders, says Deirdra Price, Ph.D., a psychologist in San Diego and president of Diet Free Solution. "Individual therapy needs to focus mainly on unhealthy eating behaviors and the underlying reasons that you turn to or deny yourself food," she says.

All of which means that the alternative to the self-hating, self-punishing diet-binge cycle is not another diet.

"The fourth law of the universe is that for every diet, there is an equal and opposite binge," says Roth. Besides, she adds, dieting is useless. Only 5 percent of people who lose weight on diets keep it off.

One answer to binge eating is to deal with the underlying emotional issues by learning how to be kinder to yourself. The alternative remedies in this chapter can help you to do just that.

**BINGE-FREE EATING:** *Follow These Seven Guidelines*

You can start to discover the personal feelings and beliefs about yourself that lead to binge eating if you follow some eating guidelines.

"Whatever you believe about food, you believe about yourself and your life," Roth says. She suggests the following eating guidelines as a great way to start to discover who you are, accept who you are, and begin to understand and outgrow the self-destructive patterns of binge eating.

• Eat only when you are hungry.
• Eat sitting down in a calm environment (this does not include the car).

- Eat without distractions, including radio, TV, newspapers, books, intense or anxiety-producing conversations, and music.
- Eat only what you want.
- Eat until you are satisfied.
- Eat as if you were in full view of others.
- Eat with enjoyment, pleasure, and gusto.

## MEDITATION: *Make Your Presence Known*

"All of us are walking around looking for an elusive something and missing the very thing that could fill us," says Roth. "Every day, in every moment, we spend our lives thinking about what we already did or are going to do, and we completely miss what we are doing."

This can lead to tremendous hunger, which you may try to fill by binge eating. By putting all your attention on whatever you're doing, however—by being "present"—you satisfy that hunger.

"For 5 minutes a day, bring your full attention to whatever you are doing," she says. "Walk while you walk. Talk while you talk. Eat while you eat."

Roth suggests a specific presence exercise as a daily meditation for binge eaters. Do it in the morning before you get out of bed.

Begin focusing your attention on the sensations that arise in the arch of your right foot. Then, as if you were squeezing a tube of toothpaste, move your attention up through your calf, your shin, and your knee. Proceed in the same way to your right hip, then up your right arm from your hand to your shoulder. When you get to your shoulder, move to your left shoulder, down your arm to your hand, and from your left hip to your left foot.

"During the day, each time you remember, sense your arms and legs again," says Roth. "Presence enables you to see that this body, your home, the place you've spent years trying to change, is a pretty cool place to be."

## CHOCOLATE: *Savor the Taste*

One of the best presence exercises is to carry a chocolate bar with you at all times and eat one (and only one) square of it after each meal. This will be a piece of chocolate that you're really going to taste.

When Roth asks people in her workshops to eat just one chocolate kiss, the typical reaction is "One's not going to be enough!" But, says Roth, when you eat a piece of chocolate with presence, you may be surprised at what happens. "You may find that you don't even like the taste, that it's too sweet," she says, "or that one is truly enough and that you feel satisfied."

Any number of positive things can happen when you're actually present as you're eating, when you're not thinking about something else as you eat that chocolate or not eating it as a mere prelude to the next six bars or not feeling guilty that you're eating it at all, Roth says.

You may realize that you can enjoy a small amount of typically "forbidden" food without triggering a binge. You may see that you can actually tell when you're hungry and when you're satisfied. And you may learn to trust yourself to follow the eating guidelines that will help take you beyond the self-destructive diet-binge cycle.

## Let Affirmations Guide You to Self-Acceptance

Self-hatred is one of the causes of binge eating. Someone who keeps telling herself that her body is fat, her actions despicable, and her personality flawed is likely to punish herself—with a binge.

If you can free yourself of negative thinking, however, you'll be much less likely to binge. One of the best ways to do that is with affirmations, positive phrases that you say to yourself many times a day.

"Affirmations are an effective way to counter your negative internal dialogue," says Deirdra Price, Ph.D., a psychologist in San Diego and president of Diet Free Solution. "By owning and accepting all of your characteristics, you can recognize your humanness and learn to like yourself, creating a sense of inner peace." Here are four kinds of affirmations recommended by Dr. Price.

• Self-acceptance: "I accept myself exactly how I am today. I may change my mind tomorrow, but for today, I accept myself."
• Self-acceptance for feelings: "I accept how I'm feeling right now. It may not be particularly comfortable, it may even be painful, yet I accept how I feel at this moment. I may decide to ignore my feelings tomorrow, but for today, I am accepting them."

• Self-acceptance for body image: "I accept my body the way it is today. I may decide to change my mind tomorrow and hate my body, but for today, I accept it."
• Self-acceptance for making mistakes: "I accept myself even though I made a mistake. Everyone makes mistakes from time to time. I may choose to hate myself tomorrow for many mistakes I make then, but for today, I accept that I made a mistake and I am still okay."

Memorize these self-acceptance affirmations or write them down on index cards or sticky notes and put them where you'll see them every day. Start using them as soon as you wake up.

Don't stop using them if they don't work right away. If a negative thought comes up in response to the affirmation, Dr. Price suggests that you say to yourself, "Not today. I'm not going there today."

## VISUALIZATION: *Give Back Your Unhealthy Beliefs*

The negative self-images that can cause you to binge are often the result of negative beliefs that you learned in childhood and adolescence, usually from hearing your parents or other significant people in your life criticize you, says Deirdra Price, Ph.D., a psychologist in San Diego and president of Diet Free Solution.

Common beliefs and attitudes among binge eaters include "I must be perfect or I am nothing"; "I must please everyone all the time"; "Other people's needs are more important than mine"; "I need to be thin to be happy"; "No one will want me or love me if I'm fat"; "I am a weak person"; and "I don't deserve good things."

You can free yourself from these negative beliefs, says Dr. Price, by "giving them back" to the person from whom you got them. Do this with the following three-part visualization (mental imagery) exercise.

**1.** Sit or stand in a comfortable position and imagine that you are surrounded by white light. Think about the belief that you no longer want to have. Shut your eyes and see the person who gave you the belief standing in front of you.
**2.** Cup each of your hands as if you're going to scoop water from a stream to drink. Place your cupped hands behind your

back, waist high, with the cupped part facing your back.
Scrape your hands around your body as if gathering
something off your waist.

"You are gathering the 'energy' attached to the beliefs that
are connected to you," says Dr. Price. "When you come to the
front of your body, you will have in your cupped hands the
belief, symbolically held."

**3.** With your eyes shut, see the person to whom you are
returning the belief. Say, "I give you back to you," pushing
your cupped hands out and toward the person as if you were
releasing a bird. Repeat this five or six times.

Since this visualization takes only a few seconds, you can do
it many times a day, says Dr. Price.

# *Natural Relief from Pain and Swelling of* **Bites and Stings**

You take your daily stroll around the block, and one of your
neighbors has a new (unchained! big! growling!) dog who's
decided that your middle name is Purina. You go for a dip
in the ocean while on vacation and discover that dozens of jellyfish have picked that exact spot to practice their new syn-
chronized swimming routine. You decide to clean the outside
windows on a warm spring day and literally stir up a hornet's
nest, making yourself the target of a well-executed sting
operation.

Although it's easy to joke about bites and stings, the truth
is, they're never a laughing matter. When the injury is minor,
though, alternative practitioners offer a wide variety of drug-
free home remedies for fast relief of pain and swelling.

# GUIDE TO
# PROFESSIONAL CARE

Any animal bite, even if it's superficial, should be thoroughly cleaned to prevent infection. If you're bitten by a dog or other domestic animal, especially if it was an unprovoked attack or the animal is obviously sick, and the bite breaks the skin, the animal must be checked for rabies.

If the bite is from a squirrel, raccoon, or other wild animal, assume that the animal is rabid and seek medical attention immediately. And while bites from a large animal, such as a horse or camel, may look benign, they should be examined by a physician.

You should also see a doctor if the bite causes infection; if it causes loss of function in an extremity, such as a bite over a tendon that makes it impossible for you to lift a hand or foot; if it is on your face or groin or over a joint; or if it causes a gaping wound that may require stitches. Signs of infection are fever, expanding redness, or red streaks radiating up or down from the site of the injury. These usually occur within 24 to 48 hours after the bite.

Most insect bites and stings can be treated at home, but there are certain situations that call for medical attention. If you're stung by an insect or marine animal and you start to have trouble breathing; if you develop hives that travel up your arm, leg, or whole body; or if you feel faint, vomit, or have a swollen mouth or tongue, you may be having a body-wide allergic reaction that may cause your airways to swell shut. Get to a hospital emergency room immediately.

You should also see a doctor if the injury shows signs of infection, if you develop significant swelling that home remedies don't help, or if you have repeated local allergic reactions to bug bites. If the bite or sting is from a marine animal and it punctures your skin, you run the risk of getting an infection from bacteria in the seawater or a tetanus infection, so it's a good idea to see your doctor.

## The Plant to Pick First

"My favorite herbal remedy to instantly take the pain and itchiness out of a sting or bite is plantain," says Pamela Fischer, founder and director of the Ohlone Center for Herbal Studies in Concord, California. Plantain, a very common plant, is loaded with tannins. These chemicals, she says, act as astringents, tightening skin and other tissue so that irritation and inflammation are reduced and infection is drawn out of the skin.

Plantain is a common weed that grows just about everywhere, especially where the soil is damp, heavy, and shaded. It grows 6 to 18 inches high, although it can be flat to the ground in areas that are frequently mowed or walked on. Its roundish, waxy, dull green leaves are 3 to 4 inches long with deep parallel veins that run from top to bottom. The leaf stem cups inward like a trough. From early summer through midfall, the plant sprouts green, pipe cleaner–like flower spikes.

### PLANTAIN: *Chew for Fast Relief*

If you're stung by a bee or bitten by a mosquito, and you spy some plantain nearby, Fischer says to grab some leaves and rinse them off, then put them in your mouth, chew them up, and put that wad of plantain right on the bite for instant relief. "Your bite or sting will feel much better immediately," she says. You can also rub the leaves in your hands until the juice is released, then apply them to the affected area.

### PLANTAIN: *A Poultice for Dog Bites*

First, scrub the area of the bite with soap and water to clean it as thoroughly as possible. To make the poultice, put a handful of rinsed plantain leaves in a blender, add a few drops of hot water, and blend. Put the mixture directly on the wound, says Fischer, then put gauze over the herb and a heat source (such as a hot-water bottle or heating pad) over the gauze. Apply the heat for 20 to 30 minutes. Change the poultice three or four times a day, she says.

If the bite is on a limb, she says, you can soak the bitten area in cooled plantain tea for 10 to 15 minutes three or four times a day. To make the tea, add ¼ cup of dried plantain leaves to a quart of boiled water, cover, and steep for 20 to 30 minutes.

## More Options for Fast Relief

If plantain isn't your cup of tea, here are various other ways to relieve the pain and reduce the swelling from bites and stings of all kinds.

## GOLDENSEAL: *Seal Off Infection*

Before the age of prescriptions, people often used the leaves of the herb goldenseal on a minor wound such as a cut or sting to prevent infection and hasten healing. You can do the same with goldenseal powder, says Michael Rosenbaum, M.D., an alternative physician in Corte Madera, California. Mix a small amount of water with the powder to make a paste, put the paste directly on the wound, and cover it with a bandage. Reapply the paste as necessary.

## Oil and Insects Don't Mix

Both eucalyptus and peppermint essential oils are good insect repellents, says Kal Kotecha, an aromatherapist in Waterloo, Ontario. Combine three drops of each oil with three drops of citronella essential oil, mix the oils into ½ ounce of unscented skin cream, and rub the cream on your skin before going outside.

## BENTONITE CLAY: *To Remove Toxins*

Even after a dog bite has healed, some body-hurting toxins can be left behind in your skin, says Beverly Yates, N.D., a naturopathic physician and director of the Natural Health Care Group in Seattle. To help remove them, prepare a poultice of bentonite clay (look for the words *food grade* on the label), a natural substance that helps remove impurities from the body.

To 2 tablespoons of the clay, add just enough water to make an easily moldable paste, says Dr. Yates. Cover the bite with the paste, cover the paste with gauze, and tape the gauze in place. Leave the paste on for 30 minutes. Repeat this twice a day for 4 days.

## OLIVE LEAF: *Prevents Infection*

An extract of olive leaf is thought to be an infection-preventing, natural antibiotic, Dr. Rosenbaum says. It also helps reduce inflammation, making a bite less painful. Take tablets or capsules as soon as the accident occurs and until the wound has healed, following the dosage recommendations on the label.

## HOMEOPATHY: *Crush Bee Sting Pain with Apis Mellifica*

This remedy, which is made from crushed bees, is good for a red, puffy bee sting that feels better with ice and worse with heat, says Dr. Yates. For pain and swelling, take two pellets of the 12C or 30C potency every 3 to 4 hours on the day of the sting, then repeat as needed. To take the remedy, dissolve the pellets under your tongue.

## URINE: *For Jellyfish Stings*

For a jellyfish sting, go to the bathroom—on yourself. The idea doesn't sound too appealing, right? Dr. Yates says, however, that applying your own urine to a jellyfish sting or a wound from stepping on the barbs of a sea anemone is one of the best things that you can do to stop the pain and heal quickly.

"The acidic pH of the urine immediately dissolves the barbs and venom that those animals inject into your skin, providing fast pain relief," she says. "Apply the urine in whatever way makes sense; for example, you could urinate into a glass and then sponge it on."

Dr. Yates discovered this alternative home remedy when she was living in Hawaii. "I asked the native Hawaiians what they did for marine stings, and they said this was the best remedy. I tried it, and it works great!"

# *Effective, Natural Ways to Flush Out*
# **Bladder Infections**

The standard response of a conventional doctor to a bladder infection (cystitis) is to get out a shotgun.

A "shotgun" drug, that is—a broad-spectrum antibiotic that kills off just about every type of bacteria in your body. And yes, the drug usually does clear up the infection, which is typically caused by *Escherichia coli* bacteria that have migrated up your urinary tract into the bladder. It rids you of the main symptom: burning, painful, frequent urination.

Unfortunately, the fittest *E. coli* can survive and develop into an antibiotic-resistant breed that causes recurrent bladder infections that the drug can't cure. In other words, the "solution" may bring about an even worse problem.

"Antibiotics must be given in some cases of bladder infections, particularly if there is a high fever," says Steven J. Bock, M.D., a family practitioner, acupuncturist, and codirector of the Center for Progressive Medicine in Rhinebeck, New York. He says that in many cases, however, you can successfully treat a bladder infection without antibiotics—by using a powerful array of alternative home remedies.

### CRANBERRY OR BLUEBERRY: *An Off-the-Wall Remedy*

A component of cranberry and blueberry juice stops *E. coli* bacteria from sticking to bladder walls, thus helping to heal the infection quickly, Dr. Bock says. A benefit is that the juices don't work by acidifying the urine, he says, which is good because alkaline urine (the chemical opposite of acid) is more beneficial for beating bladder infections.

He recommends drinking 24 ounces of unsweetened juice a day in three 8-ounce servings. Sugar depresses the immune system, so don't use sweetened brands.

You can also take dehydrated extracts of cranberries or blueberries in capsule or tablet form, says Dr. Bock. Follow the dosage recommendations on the label.

### WATER: *Flush Out the Bladder*

While you're drinking that cranberry or blueberry juice, you should also drink lots of water to flush out the bladder and rid it of the infection, says Dr. Bock. He recommends 64 ounces a day.

### MAGNESIUM CITRATE: *Banish the Bacteria*

This nutritional supplement creates alkaline urine, which makes it harder for *E. coli* to survive, says Dr. Bock. He recommends taking 300 to 400 milligrams a day of this supplement for as long as you have the infection.

# GUIDE TO
# PROFESSIONAL CARE

You should see a doctor immediately if you have blood in your urine, a fever that doesn't go away, or a fever and pain near one or both kidneys (a possible sign of a kidney infection). You may need treatment with antibiotics, says Steven J. Bock, M.D., a family practitioner, acupuncturist, and codirector of the Center for Progressive Medicine in Rhinebeck, New York.

Also, anyone who has recurrent bladder infections should see a doctor for a thorough checkup to detect possible structural problems—such as narrowing of the urethra, the tube that carries urine out of the bladder—that could be causing the infections.

People with recurrent bladder infections should also be tested for food allergies, which sometimes cause infections, Dr. Bock says. Postmenopausal women who have recurrent bladder infections should be evaluated for hormone imbalances, which can also cause the problem.

Dr. Bock suggests that if your doctor recommends an antibiotic for the infection, you ask to use nitrofurantoin macrocrystals (Macrodantin), a drug that is specifically intended for bladder infections, rather than a broad-spectrum antibiotic that works on your entire body. "Macrodantin is specific to the urinary tract and much less stressful on the system," he says.

## VITAMINS AND BIOFLAVONOIDS: *Strengthen the Mucosal Surfaces*

Vitamin C, vitamin A, and bioflavonoids strengthen the inner surface of the bladder, making it harder for the bacteria to stick, Dr. Bock says. To beat the infection, he recommends a daily dose of 1,000 to 4,000 milligrams of vitamin C, 300 to 600 milligrams of bioflavonoids, and 50,000 international units of vitamin A (taken under medical supervision).

Be aware, however, that although high doses of vitamin A are very effective in helping to beat bladder infections, they are also toxic over a long period of time. Take this level of vitamin A for no longer than a week, Dr. Bock says.

**ZINC:** *Power Up the Immune System*

The mineral zinc strengthens the immune system, helping it fight off the infection, says Dr. Bock. He recommends 30 milligrams a day during the infection.

**HERBS:** *A Powerful Combination*

A combination of four herbs can help beat bladder infections, Dr. Bock says. He recommends uva-ursi, which helps kill bacteria in the urine; couch grass, which cleanses and soothes the bladder; dandelion, a diuretic that increases the flow of urine to help flush out bacteria; and echinacea, which strengthens the immune system. Combine 1 ounce of a tincture of each herb in a bottle, then take ½ teaspoon of the mixture three times a day, he says.

**HOMEOPATHY:** *A Remedy for "Honeymoon Cystitis"*

If you develop honeymoon cystitis—a bladder infection that occurs after frequent intercourse—the homeopathic remedy Staphysagria can help clear it up, says Dr. Bock. Follow the dosage recommendations on the label.

### Get a New Slant On Bladder Infections

A slant board is a cushioned board positioned at an incline of 30 degrees or so, on which you lie with your feet at the top and your head at the bottom. Massaging your bladder area while in this position can help relieve a bladder infection, says Nedra Downing, D.O., an osteopathic physician who practices alternative medicine in Clarkston, Michigan.

"Just lie on a slant board and start rubbing your tummy just above the pubic bone," she says. The massage takes weight off the bladder and improves bladder circulation. It also stimulates urine flow, often allowing residual, bacteria-ridden urine to be excreted. Do the massage for 10 to 15 minutes once a day.

**PROBIOTICS:** *When You Must Take Antibiotics*

Sometimes, taking antibiotics is the only way to beat a bladder infection, says Dr. Bock. Unfortunately, these drugs also kill the "friendly" bacteria that populate your digestive tract and perform many necessary functions.

To replace the good bacteria, take a probiotic supplement while you're taking antibiotics, Dr. Bock says. It should include the bacteria *Lactobacillus acidophilus* and *Bifidobacterium bifidum*. Follow the dosage recommendations on the label.


# Reduce Pain and Speed Healing of
# **Blisters**

You hoed in the garden all afternoon. Your new shoes are too tight. You touched a hot pan.

Now you have a blister, a small area of broken cells where leaking fluid has pooled and separated the outer layer of skin from the underlying tissue. The best thing you can do is to leave it intact, because a broken blister is more likely to become infected. Just let it heal naturally. If you want to help nature take its course, though, alternative healers offer the following remedies.

## LAVENDER ESSENTIAL OIL: *Repair Skin Cells*

The essential oil of lavender is thought to regenerate skin cells, speeding healing from a blister, says Brigitte Mars, a nutritional consultant and herbalist in Boulder, Colorado.

Lavender is one of the few essential oils that you can apply directly to the skin without diluting it in a carrier oil. Just put a few drops of pure oil—not a fragrance or perfume—on the blister, then cover it with an adhesive bandage. Apply the oil two or three times a day until the blister is healed.

## HORSE CHESTNUT: *Reduce Swelling*

The herb horse chestnut can help relieve the collection of fluid in a blister, says Bradley Bongiovanni, N.D., a naturopathic physician in Cambridge, Massachusetts. Add 1 teaspoon of horse chestnut tincture to 1 cup of cool water, then soak a clean cloth in the liquid and place it over the blister for 20 minutes. Do this two or three times a day until the blister is emptied of fluid.

---

### GUIDE TO
### PROFESSIONAL CARE

The remedies in this chapter are intended for treatment of friction blisters or minor blisters from localized second-degree burns, not other types of blisters such as those from genital herpes, shingles, or contact with poison ivy or oak.

Most friction blisters or blisters from minor burns can be treated at home. If you have an open blister that is red, tender, and oozing yellow material, however, it is probably infected; see a doctor immediately.

---

## HYDROTHERAPY: *Cool It Down*

Putting a cool washcloth on the area can help relieve the pain, itching, or general discomfort of a blister, Dr. Bongiovanni says. Use this remedy as often as needed.

## DANDELION: *Fresh Stems for Faster Healing*

The "sap" of dandelion stems is loaded with vitamin A, which can speed healing of a blister, says Norma Pasekoff Weinberg, an herbal educator in Cape Cod, Massachusetts. If you have dandelions in your yard that haven't been sprayed with pesticides, pick a few, split the stems, put the white, milky juice on the blister, and cover it with a bandage. Reapply once a day until the blister heals. Some people are sensitive to the juice, however, so if you feel any itching or discomfort, wash it off immediately.

## CALENDULA: *To the Rescue*

If a blister breaks, putting the herb calendula on the area can help the skin heal more quickly, says Weinberg. You can either buy calendula oil in a health food store or get calendula tincture and combine 1 part tincture with 10 parts distilled water. Apply once or twice a day, covering the blister with a bandage until it is healed.

# A Program of Inner Cleansing Can Vanquish
## Body Odor

There's a sewage system inside your body.

It's called the intestine, of course—the interior tube where food is digested and wastes are processed.

"The only thing separating that system from the rest of your body is a membrane as thin as an eyelid," says Peter Bennett, N.D., a naturopathic and homeopathic physician in Victoria, British Columbia.

If that system is filled with toxins from a diet loaded with processed foods, from environmental chemicals, or from medications, those toxins can cross the membrane, enter the bloodstream, exit via the sweat, and create offensive body odor, he says.

Truly bad body odor—the kind that obviously offends your friends or coworkers or makes your mate ask you to see a doctor to solve the problem—is not common, he says. If you do have the problem, however, he believes that internal cleansing is the best way to correct it.

Here are suggestions from Dr. Bennett and other alternative practitioners for detoxifying your body.

### CHLOROPHYLL: *Nature's Deodorizer*

The plant chemical chlorophyll is a natural purifier, and taking it as a supplement can help detoxify and deodorize the body, Dr. Bennett says.

"Chlorophyll is absorbed from the intestinal tract into the bloodstream and has a very purifying and deodorizing effect," he says. In fact, chlorophyll is so powerful that it is typically used to reduce the odor of stool in patients who have had their colons removed and have waste routed to a bag outside the body.

---

# GUIDE TO
# PROFESSIONAL CARE

Bad body odor can be an indication of an underlying medical problem. If you've never had a problem with body odor, and you or someone close to you notices a sudden change, see a medical doctor, osteopath, or naturopathic physician for a thorough physical examination and diagnosis, says Elson Haas, M.D., director of the Preventive Medical Center of Marin in San Rafael, California.

---

"Buy a bottle and take a teaspoon two or three times a day," says Elson Haas, M.D., director of the Preventive Medical Center of Marin in San Rafael, California. Also eat more fresh, chlorophyll-rich leafy greens, such as spinach, chard, and kale.

**WATER:** *Add a Squeeze of Lemon*
Drinking lots of water every day helps the body dilute and get rid of odor-causing toxins, Dr. Bennett says. He recommends 100 ounces a day.

You may want to add a squeeze of lemon juice to each glass, says Dr. Haas. It is excellent for helping the body detoxify.

**GOLDENSEAL:** *A Killer of Bad Bacteria*
The herb goldenseal can kill toxic bacteria in the intestines and can help reduce body odor, says Dr. Bennett. Follow the dosage recommendations on the label.

**PROBIOTICS:** *More Bad News for Bad Bacteria*
Taking a probiotic, a food supplement that contains "friendly" bacteria that help maintain the health of the intestines, is a must for reducing the bad intestinal bacteria that can trigger strong body odor, says Tara Skye Goldin, N.D., a naturopathic physician in Boulder, Colorado.

Look for a product containing the bacteria *Lactobacillus acidophilus* and *Bifidobacterium bifidum* as well as FOS (fructo-oligosaccharides), which help to keep bad bacteria to a minimum. Follow the dosage recommendations on the label.

**MASSAGE:** *Try Dry Skin Brushing*

Brushing your skin with a natural-bristle dry skin brush every day stimulates the skin, improves circulation, removes old (and possibly smelly) dead skin cells, and can help the body get rid of odor-causing toxins, Dr. Bennett says.

Brush daily, using short, brisk strokes. Start with the fronts and backs of your arms, moving from the fingertips toward the armpits and always toward the heart. Then brush the fronts and backs of your legs, starting at your feet and brushing upward. Don't forget the bottoms of your feet.

Move up through the pelvic area, buttocks, abdomen, and lower back, and finish with your chest and upper back, again, always brushing toward the heart. Do your chest, abdomen, and inner thighs carefully and gently. To prevent mold, never let the brush get wet. If brushing is painful, do it lightly and persevere. The discomfort will pass, says Dr. Bennett.

## Choose a Natural Deodorant

Many commercial deodorants and antiperspirants contain aluminum or other synthetic chemicals. Alternative practitioners believe that daily exposure to those chemicals is not healthy.

"Every patient who goes through our clinic gets a thorough analysis for metals that may be damaging health, and the number one toxic metal that we find is aluminum," says Peter Bennett, N.D., a naturopathic and homeopathic physician in Victoria, British Columbia. "I don't want my patients using aluminum-containing antiperspirants."

"Aluminum and other chemicals are toxic to our own bodies and to other people," says Elson Haas, M.D., director of the Preventive Medical Center of Marin in San Rafael, California. "I encourage my patients to use natural antiperspirants and deodorants that are free of toxic chemicals." Look for chemical- and aluminum-free products in health food stores.

**FOOD:** *A Detoxification Diet*

Simplifying your diet is a must for allowing the body to cleanse itself of old, odor-producing wastes and for reducing internal toxins and poisons, says Dr. Bennett. He recommends following a 7-day purification diet that includes specific foods and avoids certain others.

Allowed foods are fruits and vegetables, olive oil or unheated flaxseed oil, herbal teas, green tea, water, lemon water, diluted fruit juices, vegetable juices, whole-grain rice and rice products (including brown, basmati, Thai, and wild rice), mung beans, bean thread noodles, and miso (a flavorful soybean paste).

Foods to avoid are meat, fish, poultry, eggs, dairy products, fats and oils (other than those listed above), chocolate, nuts, beans (other than those listed above), grains (other than those listed above), sugar, alcohol, coffee, and black tea.

# *Hydrotherapy Techniques Can Help Heal* **Boils**

Many conventional doctors will tell you that a boil is a bacterial infection of a sweat gland or hair follicle, typically on the face or in the armpit or groin, that is caused by a pore or follicle being blocked by dead skin cells and other debris. The immune system's white blood cells die in battle, creating large amounts of pus along with redness, swelling, and pain.

For a single boil, that's a likely scenario, says Peter Bennett, N.D., a naturopathic and homeopathic physician in Victoria, British Columbia. According to Dr. Bennett, however, recurrent boils are possibly caused by gastrointestinal bacteria entering the bloodstream and promoting a skin infection. They can also be caused by eating too much sugar, either refined sugar or even sugar from fruit.

Alternative medicine offers effective ways to heal small boils less than ½ inch across. You should never lance or press a boil to open it, says Dr. Bennett, as this can spread the infection and cause scarring.

## HYDROTHERAPY: *Hot Compresses to Beat Bacteria*

"Bacteria can't live where there's an adequate blood supply," Dr. Bennett says. Using hot compresses on a boil will bring blood to the area and may diminish bacteria.

# GUIDE TO
# PROFESSIONAL CARE

If you have a boil that does not improve within a few days, see a general practitioner or dermatologist for treatment, which may include antibiotics, draining, or a steroid injection. If you notice red lines radiating from the boil, if you have a fever or swelling, or if it's extremely tender or under a thick layer of skin, see a doctor right away.

For recurrent boils, you should see a naturally oriented health practitioner, who can diagnose and treat the bacterial overload in the digestive tract that is a potential cause of the problem, says Peter Bennett, N.D., a naturopathic and homeopathic physician in Victoria, British Columbia.

For an acute boil—one that pops up suddenly and is not recurrent—immerse a washcloth in hot water (as hot as you can tolerate, but not hot enough to burn), wring it out, and place it on the boil for 20 minutes twice a day.

## HYDROTHERAPY: *Hot-and-Cold Compresses to Drain Pus*

After the first day or two of treating the boil with just hot compresses, use alternating heat and cold to draw out the pus, Dr. Bennett says.

Again, soak a washcloth in hot water, wring it out, and place it on the boil for 10 minutes. Then apply another washcloth, this time soaked in ice-cold water, for 10 minutes. Repeat this cycle three times, and do the whole treatment twice a day.

## ECHINACEA AND GOLDENSEAL: *Antibacterial Herbs*

An herbal formula with echinacea and goldenseal will help kill the bacteria in the boil, Dr. Bennett says. He recommends taking 1 tablespoon of a tincture of both herbs three times a day until the boil is gone. "But beware of the taste," he cautions. "It's very bitter."

**TURMERIC:** *Cooling the Fire*

In Ayurveda, the ancient natural healing system from India, boils are seen as a "pitta" disorder—an excess of fire or heat. Turmeric is a cooling herb that can reduce the inflammation of a boil and help prevent recurrences, says Virender Sodhi, M.D. (Ayurved), N.D., an Ayurvedic and naturopathic physician and director of the American School of Ayurvedic Sciences in Bellevue, Washington.

Look for a standardized extract of turmeric and take 450 milligrams three times a day. Or use it to make a skin paste that will quickly bring a boil to a head, says Dr. Sodhi.

In a blender, combine 1 teaspoon of turmeric powder, 1 teaspoon of Epsom salts, and a baked onion with enough water to make a thick paste. Before bedtime, spread the paste on a piece of cheesecloth and put the cloth over the boil. Cover the cheesecloth with plastic wrap so the yellow coloring of the turmeric doesn't get on your bedding, then secure the poultice with a bandage. Leave the poultice on overnight; repeat for 2 nights.

# *Lifestyle Changes Can Extend Life for Women with* Breast Cancer

You've been diagnosed with breast cancer, a potentially fatal disease. That's daunting enough. But now you also have to consider all of your treatment options for removing the tumor and preventing a recurrence: mastectomy, lumpectomy, and axillary node dissection; radiation therapy, chemotherapy, and hormone therapy.

Along with these choices, however, there is one that can keep you alive longer than the average person diagnosed with breast cancer.

"A change in lifestyle is the only factor that has been scientifically proven to extend the average life span of women with breast cancer," says Charles Simone, M.D., director of the Simone Protective Cancer Center in Lawrenceville, New Jersey.

Why is lifestyle so important? "A change in lifestyle stops 'feeding' the tumor and boosts the immune system so that it can more effectively fight cancer," Dr. Simone says. The most important change, he says, is eliminating the foods that he believes contribute to 40 to 60 percent of all breast cancer.

## FOOD: *Stop Eating Red Meat and Dairy Products*

According to Dr. Simone, more than 100 scientific studies show that saturated fat—the kind in red meat and dairy products—can increase the risk of cancer.

"The saturated fat found in red meat and dairy products feeds a tumor," he believes. "If you remove that fat from the diet—and you will remove most of it by cutting out beef, pork, lamb, veal, and dairy products—you will slow the rate at which a tumor grows and perhaps even stop its growth."

All dairy products, even those such as fat-free milk, contain potential tumor-promoting growth hormones that are fed to cows to improve their milk production, believes Elizabeth Ann Lowenthal, D.O., an osteopathic physician and cancer specialist in Alabaster, Alabama. "The dairy industry uses many such hormones that promote the growth of breast cancer cells in a laboratory setting," she says.

Additionally, it is at least theoretically possible that bovine papillomavirus shed from udders of milk cows could have a tumor-promoting effect in human breast tissue. This virus is widespread in cows and is closely related to the human papillomavirus that is linked to cervical cancer in humans.

In fact, Dr. Lowenthal theorizes that the cause of the rapidly rising rate of breast cancer in Western countries may be the increasing consumption of dairy products. For this reason, she advises all of her breast cancer patients to eliminate dairy products from their diets and to take a daily 1,500-milligram calcium supplement that contains vitamin D.

## FOOD: *Don't Feed Your Tumor's Sweet Tooth*

Whether the sugar you eat is sucrose (refined white sugar) or fructose, maltose, or dextrose (natural sugars that are also used as commercial sweeteners), it all turns into blood sugar, or glucose. Some alternative practitioners believe that cancer cells rely on a metabolic process that is driven by glucose, Dr. Lowenthal says.

# GUIDE TO
# PROFESSIONAL CARE

*Caution: Cancer is a complex and life-threatening disease that requires professional medical care. Some alternative remedies may actually worsen cancer if they are not used appropriately. Therefore, use the alternative remedies discussed in this chapter only as part of a cancer treatment program that is guided and monitored by a qualified physician who is experienced in cancer care and alternative medicine. If you are being treated by a conventional doctor, check with him before changing or stopping any conventional medical treatments or medications, and keep all of your doctors and/or alternative practitioners informed of all treatments that you are receiving.*

The medical "standard of care" frequently used for Stage I or Stage II breast cancer (the two earliest stages of the disease) is lumpectomy, or surgical removal of the tumor, followed by radiation and chemotherapy, says Michael Schachter, M.D., director of the Schachter Center for Complementary Medicine in Suffern, New York.

Dr. Schachter agrees that surgery is generally a good idea for women diagnosed with Stage I or Stage II breast cancer, "but my opinion, after having treated many patients with breast cancer, is that those who use alternative therapy alone after surgery, rather than combining alternative therapies with radiation and chemotherapy, may have longer survival times."

Obviously, the choice to have conventional or alternative treatment (or both) after surgery is one that each woman with breast cancer will have to evaluate for herself.

Dr. Schachter's alternative program includes lifestyle changes; dietary recommendations that are individualized according to a person's metabolic type; oral nutritional supplements such as vitamins, minerals, enzymes, amino acids, fatty acids, herbs, and concentrated foods; a program of injections of natural anticancer substances such as high doses of vitamin C; detoxification procedures; an exercise program; stress management; body energy techniques such as acupuncture; body manipulative therapies; homeopathy; and others.

"One of the first things I ask my patients with breast cancer to do is to get off sugar," she says. You can do that by staying away from sugary desserts, not adding sugar to any food, eating a limited amount of fruit, and drinking fruit juice only once or twice a week.

## WATER: *Make Yours Distilled*

Dr. Simone urges his patients to purchase a home water distiller, which costs about $200. He contends that the distillation process removes all possible carcinogens from your drinking water—a must for anyone who has been diagnosed with cancer, he says.

## ALCOHOL: *A Must to Avoid*

Alcohol is a carcinogen. Having two or three drinks a week (a drink is one shot of distilled spirits, 4 ounces of wine, or 12 ounces of beer) increases your risk of developing breast cancer, Dr. Simone says. The same amount of alcohol can double a tumor's growth rate, he says. So, if you've been diagnosed with breast cancer, don't drink.

## TOBACCO: *Avoid Smoke—Yours and Others'*

Approximately 30 percent of all cancers are caused by inhaling tobacco smoke, which is loaded with carcinogens, Dr. Simone says. It creates free radicals, unstable molecules that can damage DNA and trigger cancer. It burns up antioxidant vitamins such as vitamin C, which are cancer protective. And it erodes your immune system, your main defense against cancer.

If you're a smoker, and you've been diagnosed with breast cancer, quit. If you smoke, your cancer is more likely to spread. Avoid secondhand smoke as well.

## EXERCISE: *Walk Four Times a Week*

Cancer thrives in an oxygen-poor environment. Mild aerobic exercise fights cancer by stimulating the immune system and oxygenating the body, Dr. Simone says.

Walking is the most inexpensive and convenient form of aerobic exercise, he says. If his breast cancer patients are over 40 or don't exercise regularly, he has them checked for cardiovascular risk factors. If their circulatory systems are normal, he has them start a walking program, gradually increasing the pace and distance until they're walking briskly for 2 miles four times a week.

## STRESS REDUCTION: *Calm Your Mind*

Mental stress (a worried, overloaded mind) weakens the immune system. Mental ease (a calm, quiet mind) strengthens it—and a stronger immune system means more resistance to cancer. Dr. Simone suggests four easy ways for his patients with breast cancer to reduce mental stress.

• Take a hot shower.
• Listen to calming music.
• Pray or meditate, repeating a single thought or process (like watching your breath) over and over.
• Be sexually intimate, either by having intercourse or just hugging and cuddling.

### Beating Cancer with Nutritional Supplements

"There are specific nutrients that have a demonstrated ability to help slow the progression of breast cancer," says Patrick Quillin, R.D., Ph.D., director of nutrition for Cancer Treatment Centers of America in Tulsa, Oklahoma. Here are his recommendations for breast cancer patients. He emphasizes that you should use these supplements only with the approval and supervision of your doctor.

### CLA: *Help for Your Immune System*

Conjugated linoleic acid, or CLA, is a component of fat that is found abundantly in animals such as "free-range" cattle, sheep, pigs, or chickens that are allowed to wander and feed freely. Scientists theorize that CLA is part of a receptor on the surface of cells that tells the immune system if the cell is a normal cell or a cancer cell. If that receptor lacks CLA and doesn't function properly, the cancer cell isn't recognized—and isn't killed.

Dr. Quillin recommends that breast cancer patients take 3,000 milligrams a day of a CLA supplement.

## Is There a Link Between Bras
## and Breast Cancer?

A study has revealed a causative factor for breast cancer that can increase your risk of getting the disease by 100 times: Wearing a bra for more than 12 hours a day.

That's the remarkable finding of Sydney Ross Singer, an applied medical anthropologist who, with his scientific assistant (his wife, Soma Grismaijer), wrote *Dressed to Kill: The Link between Breast Cancer and Bras*. Singer and Grismaijer interviewed more than 2,000 women with breast cancer and another 2,000 women without breast cancer, asking them a series of questions about their use of bras. Here's what they found.

• A woman who wears a bra 24 hours a day is 113 times more likely to get breast cancer than a woman who wears a bra less than 12 hours a day. (That statistical link is stronger than the link between cigarette smoking and lung cancer, Singer says.)
• A woman who never wears a bra is 21 times less likely to get breast cancer than a woman in the general population.

Singer hypothesizes that the straps, side panels, underwires, and other structures of the garment cut off drainage from the lymphatic system, which helps remove toxins and waste products from the cells. The longer you wear a bra, the more hours those toxins are trapped in your breasts. The end result, after many years of bra use, can be a breast tumor, Singer says.

Needless to say, the medical establishment hasn't embraced this theory. "The current medical model for the cause of breast cancer is biochemical and genetic, ignoring the simple mechanical fact of what clothing constriction can do to the body," Singer says.

There are some alternative physicians, however, who think Singer's theory might be true. "Bras and other tight clothing can impede the flow of the lymph fluid out of the breast," says Michael Schachter, M.D., director of the Schachter Center for Complementary Medicine in Suffern, New York. "Thus, wearing a bra might contribute to the development of breast cancer as a result of cutting off lymphatic drainage so that toxic chemicals are trapped in the breast. The take-home message to women from Singer's research is: Wear bras as little as possible."

Singer advises women to try his "risk-free, cost-free lifestyle experiment" for preventing the disease by either going bra-free or wearing a bra less than 12 hours a day (which definitely means not wearing it to bed).

He also says to avoid bras with underwires and other stiff, breast-shaping components, as well as push-up bras. When selecting a bra, be sure it's the right size. One tip from Singer and Grismaijer on selecting a bra that's not too tight: When you try it on, slide two fingers under the shoulder straps and the side panels. If the bra fits properly, your fingers should slide easily. The bra also should not leave marks or dents on your skin. If it does, it's too tight. "Women need to realize that wearing bras is a cultural phenomenon, not a natural one," says Singer.

## GENISTEIN: *Putting Soy's Anti-Cancer Power to Work*

Studies show that eating more soy products such as tofu (soybean curd) may lower your risk of cancer. And the most powerful anti-cancer substance in soy products may be the food chemical genistein, Dr. Quillin says.

Research shows that genistein can help kill cancer cells, stop a tumor's spread through the body, and keep a tumor from growing blood vessels.

Some doctors have told women with breast cancer not to eat more soy or take soy supplements like genistein because soy contains phytoestrogens, natural estrogens with about half the strength of the hormone manufactured by the body. But study after study shows that phytoestrogens don't increase the risk of breast cancer or accelerate the disease. In fact, genistein does just the opposite by slowing cancer growth, says Dr. Quillin. He recommends that women with breast cancer either take a genistein supplement of 6 milligrams daily or eat more soy.

## COENZYME $Q_{10}$: *To Help Stop Tumor Growth*

This supplement helps generate the cellular energy that makes your body work. When you are young and healthy, your body usually manufactures the coenzyme $Q_{10}$ ($coQ_{10}$) that it needs. But aging or illness can cause a shortage of $coQ_{10}$ that can result in a cellular environment that's favorable to tumor growth, Dr. Quillin says.

In a study of $coQ_{10}$'s cancer-fighting power, scientists gave 90 milligrams a day of the supplement to 32 high-risk patients with breast cancer. Six patients—almost 20 percent of those taking the supplement—experienced partial regressions of their tumors. When the researchers increased the dose to 390 milligrams for one of these six women, she experienced a complete remission.

"If those results were from taking a drug, there would be dancing in the streets, and the stock of the drug company would shoot up," Dr. Quillin says. "Because this was a study of a nutrient, however, there was very little attention paid to the results."

Dr. Quillin recommends that women with breast cancer take 100 milligrams of $coQ_{10}$ daily. It's safe to take this supplement for extended periods.

## *Relieve the Discomfort of*
# Breast Changes

Fibrocystic breast disease. That's how the medical establishment classifies the condition of women whose breasts are lumpy, cystic, or painful, particularly around the time of their periods.

"It's not a disease," insists Dixie Mills, M.D., breast specialist at the Women to Women health clinic in Yarmouth, Maine. "It's a normal, physiological condition that reflects the surges of the female hormones during this time of month."

In fact, says Dr. Mills, many of her patients have much less breast pain after they've been reassured that it's not a sign of disease or an omen of cancer. "Just the stress reduction from knowing her breasts are normal can eliminate a lot of a woman's physical pain," she says.

There are, however, many lifestyle factors that can aggravate benign breast changes—and a lot of alternative home remedies that can help keep the pain and lumpiness under control.

## FOOD: *Less Fat Means Less Pain*

High-fat diets raise estrogen levels in the body, and excess estrogen causes the buildup of fluid and cellular tissue in the breast that leads to lumps and pain. That's why Dr. Mills recommends eating fewer high-fat dairy products and less red meat. Besides the fat, some dairy and poultry products contain hormones that may worsen breast pain and lumps, she says.

## SOY: *To Balance Out Your Estrogen*

Soy contains natural estrogen, which balances out the excess estrogen in the body, helping to decrease breast pain and lumpiness, Dr. Mills says. "I encourage women to eat more soy—from tofu, soy milk, soy nuts, miso, tempeh, and other sources."

## FIBER: *Show Estrogen the Door*

Fiber escorts excess estrogen out of the body, says Dr. Mills, helping to decrease breast pain and lumpiness. Most vegetables and fruits are rich in fiber, as are whole grains and beans.

Dr. Mills particularly recommends high-fiber cruciferous vegetables such as cabbage, broccoli, kale, brussels sprouts, and turnips. They contain indole-3-carbinol, a chemical that helps block estrogen from binding to breast tissue.

---

### GUIDE TO PROFESSIONAL CARE

Although benign breast changes are not a risk factor for breast cancer, says Dixie Mills, M.D., breast specialist at the Women to Women health clinic in Yarmouth, Maine, you do need to rule out the possibility of cancer.

If you have breast pain each month or notice any breast lump or thickening, regardless of whether it is painful, schedule a physical exam from your doctor. If the lump is still there after your next menstrual cycle, you should be examined again.

Be sure to see a physician for yearly breast exams. Ask your doctor or nurse to teach you how to do monthly self-exams so that you can become familiar with your normal breast anatomy and are able to detect any subtle changes.

**IODINE:** *Get Relief with Ocean Plants*

Iodine blocks estrogen from sticking to its receptors in the breasts, Dr. Mills says. The best sources of iodine are sea vegetables such as kelp, wakame, and kombu. You can use kelp in granulated form as a seasoning. To use wakame or kombu, soak the seaweed until it's soft, then cut it into small pieces and add it to soups.

**CAFFEINE:** *Cut Back for a Week*

Methylxanthine, a chemical in coffee and other sources of caffeine, stretches blood vessels, irritating nerves and increasing breast tenderness, Dr. Mills says. "I recommend that women decrease their caffeine intake from sources such as coffee, tea, cola, chocolate, and over-the-counter pain relievers in the week before their periods," she says.

**VITAMIN E:** *Ex Out the Excess*

This nutrient is believed to help regulate excess estrogen, says Dr. Mills. She recommends 400 international units twice a day.

**EVENING PRIMROSE OIL:** *To Alleviate Inflammation*

Evening primrose oil, or EPA, contains a type of fatty acid that mutes inflammation and helps make breasts less painful. Dr. Mills recommends taking two 500-milligram capsules in the morning and two in the evening.

**PROGESTERONE:** *To Cut Estrogen Absorption*

The hormone progesterone may help balance the receptors in your breasts so that large quantities of estrogen can't be absorbed, says Dr. Mills. She recommends the product Pro-Gest, a cream that contains real progesterone rather than the less effective synthesized variety (such as that in products containing wild yam), which may have side effects.

Following the dosage recommendations on the label, massage the cream into your breasts, abdomen, or thighs on a daily basis. But don't expect instant results. "It takes a couple of cycles for progesterone to decrease breast lumps and pain," Dr. Mills says.

## The Most Soothing Relief: A Castor Oil Pack

A castor oil pack applied to your breasts three times during the week before your period for a month or two can decrease inflammation and eliminate breast pain, says Dixie Mills, M.D., breast specialist at the Women to Women health clinic in Yarmouth, Maine. Here are her instructions.

• Assemble all the materials you'll need: cold-pressed castor oil (castor oil that isn't cold-pressed can be used, but it contains more toxins, she says); a large, soft flannel cloth; a plastic sheet of medium thickness; a filled hot-water bottle; and a bath towel.
• Fold the cloth into two to four thicknesses so it measures about 10 inches by 14 inches after it's been folded.
• Put the plastic sheet under the cloth and pour some castor oil on the cloth; it should be wet but not dripping.
• Lie down and put the soaked cloth over your breasts.
• Place the plastic over the cloth, then put the hot-water bottle on top of the plastic.
• Fold the towel lengthwise and wrap it around the entire area. Lie on the ends to hold it all in place.
• Keep the pack in place for 1 hour. Afterward, cleanse your skin with a quart of warm water to which you've added 2 teaspoons of baking soda.

Don't wash the flannel pack. Instead, keep it in a plastic container or plastic bag to use again; refrigerate it between uses. Do the treatment three times a week for 2 to 3 months. If your breast pain is eliminated, you can begin a once-a-week maintenance program.

## MASSAGE: *A Gentle Circulation Improver*

A gentle massage can help improve circulation to the breasts and decrease pain, says Jason Elias, a practitioner of Traditional Chinese Medicine in New Paltz, New York.

"With your fingertips, make small, gentle, circular motions over the entire surface of the breasts," he says. "When you feel a cyst or a lump, massage gently around it, but never so hard that you irritate the tissue or cause any pain."

### HRT: *Talk to Your Doctor*

If you're on hormone replacement therapy (HRT), you may feel more tenderness in your breasts, says Dr. Mills. That's because hormone replacement adds estrogen and progesterone to your body. If your breasts are tender, perhaps your dosage should be adjusted, so talk to your doctor about this possibility.

# *Natural Remedies Can Shorten a Bout of* Bronchitis

You have the stuffy nose and sore throat of a cold. But the viruses that have invaded your body have decided that they'd like to travel and take in a bit more of your respiratory tract. So they journey down the road to the mucous linings of the bronchi, the tubes that shunt air from the windpipe to the lungs.

Now you have acute bronchitis—and the painful, persistent cough that goes with it.

Conventional doctors say that you have no choice but to wait out the 7 to 10 days of a typical case of acute bronchitis, perhaps taking over-the-counter medications to mute your symptoms and make you a bit more comfortable.

But Nedra Downing, D.O., an alternative doctor in Clarkston, Michigan, says that you can shorten an episode of acute bronchitis without drugs. There are home remedies that thin mucus so you can cough it up more easily and that boost the virus-fighting power of your immune system.

### NAC: *A Mucus Thinner*

The nutrient n-acetylcysteine, or NAC, can thin the mucus in your bronchi, making it watery and easy to cough up, which is the main goal in a case of acute bronchitis. Dr. Downing suggests two 600-milligram doses a day, one when you wake up and one before bed, until your symptoms subside. She suggests that you continue taking NAC for several weeks afterward to make sure all of the mucus has cleared.

## GUIDE TO
## PROFESSIONAL CARE

If your symptoms persist for more than 7 to 10 days, and you develop a fever, see a doctor immediately. You may have pneumonia.

Also, if you begin to experience shortness of breath, start coughing up larger quantities of mucus, or notice a change in the color of the mucus from clear to yellow, green, or black, see your doctor. You may have bacterial bronchitis, which requires treatment.

Finally, if you have chronic lung disease such as chronic bronchitis or emphysema or heart disease, and you develop acute bronchitis, you need to be under a doctor's supervision. The condition can be life-threatening.

## HOMEOPATHY: *Use Antiviral Engystol*

The homeopathic remedy Engystol-N, which is manufactured by BIII and available only through your health care practitioner, is a potent virus fighter.

"I recommend it to my patients for all sorts of viral problems, from colds and sore throats to viral acute bronchitis," says Dr. Downing. (Acute bronchitis is also occasionally caused by bacteria.) Follow your doctor's dosage advice, continuing until your symptoms are gone. Dr. Downing's usual recommendation is one pill dissolved under the tongue three times a day, or up to six times daily during acute episodes.

## ASTRAGALUS: *An Exceptional Expectorant*

Astragalus is what herbalists call an expectorant, which means that it helps you cough up mucus. Use six to eight drops of astragalus root tincture dissolved in water, or take one 500- to 600-milligram capsule of pure root three times a day, Dr. Downing says.

## GRAVITY: *A Slanted Approach*

Spending time on a slant board, an inclined, cushioned board that you lie on with your feet at the top and your head at the bottom, can help bronchial secretions come up. Set the board at a 30-degree angle and lie on it for 30 to 40 minutes twice a day.

"Use some astragalus, then lie on a slant board, and within 30 to 60 minutes, you should be coughing up large quantities of phlegm," Dr. Downing says. Do this for as long as your symptoms persist.

**THYME ESSENTIAL OIL:** *A Steamy Remedy*

Thyme essential oil is also helpful in bringing up bronchial mucus, Dr. Downing says. Pour water up to the fill line of the well of a vaporizer that generates hot (not cool) mist. Add a few drops of the oil and operate the vaporizer while you're in the room.

**HYDROTHERAPY:** *Speed Recovery with Mustard*

Covering your chest with a mustard plaster, made by applying mustard paste to a warm, wet towel, is another good way to thin the mucus in your bronchi, Dr. Downing says. Here are her directions.

• Mix ½ teaspoon of dried mustard powder (available at grocery stores) with 3 to 4 tablespoons of white flour.
• Add enough water to make a watery paste.
• Spread the paste on a kitchen towel (not a washcloth) and fold the towel into a rectangle about 3 by 6 inches, covering the paste. Never put the paste directly on your chest; it may burn, cautions Dr. Downing.
• Place the towel right over your breastbone (the bronchi are directly beneath that area).
• Fill a hot-water bottle with hot (but not scalding) water and put it directly over the towel.
• Leave the plaster on for at least an hour, but remove it if it becomes too hot. Repeat every 3 to 4 hours until you feel better.

**FOOD:** *Four Helpful Hints*

What you eat and drink during a case of acute bronchitis can work either for you or against you, Dr. Downing says. Here's what she recommends.

• Stay away from milk, since many people find that ingesting milk or other dairy products produces extra mucus.

If you're in that category, cut all dairy products out of your diet during a bout of acute bronchitis, she says. You can resume your normal eating habits when you're well.
• Drink plenty of water—eight 8-ounce glasses or more a day—to help thin mucus.
• Avoid refined sugar, which weakens the immune system.
• Increase your intake of spicy foods such as horseradish, garlic, onions, and hot peppers at the first sign of acute bronchitis. "These spicy foods help break up plugs of mucus in your bronchi so you can cough them out," Dr. Downing says.

# *Simple Steps to Soothe and Even Prevent*
# **Bruises**

A bruise is a sign of an injury under your skin. Broken blood vessels—from a fall, a bump, or a blow—bleed into nearby tissue, turning it that familiar shade of purple and blue (fading, of course, to brown, yellow, and green).

For everyday bruising, here's a selection of alternative home remedies to help soothe the pain and speed healing. And, if you're an easy bruiser, with a ring of purple blooming at the slightest provocation, you'll find a remedy for preventing these unsightly injuries.

### ARNICA: *Stop a Bruise before It Starts*

Arming yourself with arnica cream can save your arms—and other body parts—from painful bruising, says Pamela Fischer, founder and director of the Ohlone Center for Herbal Studies in Concord, California. "It really takes the pain away," she says. And it can also stop a bruise from forming if you use it immediately after you hurt yourself.

A few times a day, simply spread arnica cream on the area that you've injured. But don't use it if the surface of your skin is broken. "Externally, arnica is fabulous for bruising," says Fischer, "but it's poisonous internally."

## GUIDE TO
## PROFESSIONAL CARE

If a bruise appears for no apparent reason, you have one that doesn't heal, or you have blurred vision or two black eyes after being hit in the head, see a medical doctor.

You should also see a physician if you have a large bruise from a collision or injury, such as a fall, especially if the bruise is painful or limits movement in a joint; if you bruise easily and take aspirin or other over-the-counter painkillers such as ibuprofen or acetaminophen for chronic conditions such as arthritis; or if you develop a large, bruiselike clot of blood that is swollen and very painful after surgery.

### BROMELAIN: *To Minimize Bruising*

Bromelain is a protein-digesting enzyme (a natural chemical that helps break down food) found in pineapple. It may also "digest" fibrin, a substance produced after a bruise that contributes to swelling and inflammation.

"Bromelain is a very good remedy for bruising," says Holly Zapf, N.D., a naturopathic physician in Portland, Oregon. When taken with food, bromelain assists in digesting the proteins that you've eaten. When taken at other times, it actually helps digest the proteins that trigger inflammation and pain in the body, she explains.

Eating more pineapple won't work, though, because you can't get enough bromelain to do the trick. Instead, look for bromelain supplements. Take 250 to 500 milligrams in tablet or capsule form between meals until the bruising and inflammation subside.

### HYDROTHERAPY: *For Faster Relief*

All you need for fast, effective relief is a kitchen timer and two washcloths, says Beverly Yates, N.D., a naturopathic physician and director of the Natural Health Care Group in Seattle. Soak one washcloth in water that's so warm that you can barely handle it but not so hot that it burns your skin, and soak the other in very cold water. Wring out both washcloths, then put the hot one on the bruise for 3 minutes. Take it off and apply the cold washcloth for 30 seconds. Repeat this process four times, re-soaking the washcloths to keep them maximally hot and cold.

"The hot water brings blood to the area, and the cold water takes it away," explains Dr. Yates. This pumping action brings fresh nutrients to the bruise and removes waste products—the perfect combo for faster healing.

## AROMATHERAPY: *The Right Combination*

Mix three drops of peppermint essential oil and three drops of lavender essential oil with 1 ounce of sweet almond oil, says Kal Kotecha, an aromatherapist in Waterloo, Ontario. Spread the mixture on the bruise three or four times a day, covering it with gauze each time. Tape the gauze with an adhesive bandage, but not so tightly that the bruise can't "breathe." Peppermint helps reduce inflammation, and lavender helps relieve pain.

## AROMATHERAPY: *Time for a Change*

After a day or two of using the peppermint and lavender oil formula, switch to the following mixture and use it for up to 2 weeks. Combine three drops each of the essential oils of rosemary, black pepper, and juniper in 1 ounce of sweet almond oil. "These are all 'warming" oils," says Kotecha, that speed healing by increasing circulation to the bruise.

## CITRUS FRUIT: *For Those Who Bruise Easily*

If you tend to bruise easily, Dr. Yates recommends eating citrus fruits every day, especially the white part of the rinds. "They're rich in bioflavonoids, which keep platelets from clumping together and strengthen blood vessel walls, thus preventing easy bruising," she says.

# *Giving the Boot to*
# **Bunions**

When worn day after day, shoes with a narrow toe box (like most high heels, for example) can inflame the joint of the big toe, causing a red, swollen, painful knob of bone on the outer side of the foot just below the toe.

If the bone continues to thicken, which is common for someone with a bunion, it can be very pushy. It can shove your big toe to the side so that it lies like a fallen tree across your second toe. It can ruin the alignment of the bones next to your big toe so that the bottom of your foot hurts all the time. It can make your life so miserable that surgery to remove the bunion, called a bunionectomy, seems like the only way out (about 140,000 Americans choose that option each year).

Tight shoes aren't the only "risk factor" for a bunion. In fact, a genetic tendency to form a bunion, signaled by a low arch that causes the movement of the foot to be slightly off-kilter, is the hereditary fault that allows tight shoes to do their damage.

Roomier shoes and custom shoe inserts (orthotics) are the best ways to treat a bunion, but there are a number of alternative home remedies that are very effective for relieving the pain a bunion can cause.

## STRETCHING: *To Beat the Band*

Stretching your big toes is one of the best ways to reduce or eliminate bunion pain, says Stephanie Tourles, a licensed esthetician, reflexologist, and herbalist in West Hyannisport, Massachusetts.

Obviously, stretching a toe isn't the same as stretching a muscle. You need a little help—from a rubber band, says Tourles.

Sit with your legs outstretched on the floor with your heels side by side and touching. Loop a thick, fairly stiff rubber band (about 3 inches or less and ¼ inch thick, such as a heavy-duty office rubber band) around both big toes. Keeping your heels together, move the tops of your feet apart so they form a V. Hold the stretch for 5 to 10 seconds, then relax. Repeat 10 to 20 times.

If the exercise hurts, if you have arthritis, or if your bunions are very advanced, do only as many repetitions as you can. Your toes will gradually increase in strength so that you'll be able to do 10 to 20.

### ICE: *For Fast Relief*

Put some ice cubes inside a plastic sandwich bag, wrap the bag in a thin towel, and apply it to the bunion in three 10-minute cycles: 10 minutes on, 10 minutes off, and 10 minutes on. Do this two or three times a day whenever bunion pain flares up, says Gregory Spencer, D.P.M., a podiatrist in Renton, Washington. "Ice is the best and cheapest first-aid for bunion pain," he says.

### ASPIRIN: *Soak, Don't Swallow*

Crush three or four aspirin tablets into a basin of warm water and soak your feet for 10 to 15 minutes or as long as needed, suggests Dr. Spencer. This can be a very effective way to relieve the pain of an inflamed bunion. If any skin irritation results, discontinue the treatment.

### CASTOR OIL: *There's the Rub*

Castor oil can help reduce bunion inflammation, says Dr. Spencer. Rub the oil on your bunion after your foot soak, then cover the bunion with a soft bandage so the oil stays in place.

### MASSAGE: *For Long-Term Relief*

Traditional Chinese Medicine says that healing energy, or chi, runs in tracks called meridians up and down your body, from head to toe—including your big toe.

Opening or unblocking areas of stagnant chi in the meridian that runs into your big toe (the liver meridian) can help relieve bunion pain, says Dr. Spencer. The best way to unblock the flow of chi is to massage the ankle and calf, he says. Here's how to do it.

Put a few drops of massage oil on your hands and spread it

# GUIDE TO PROFESSIONAL CARE

If you have a painful big toe, see a podiatrist or orthopedic surgeon, who can tell if you have a bunion or a related problem such as arthritis, gout, or an infection.

If you have a bunion, the podiatrist will probably recommend that you wear roomier shoes and use a prescription orthotic, a custom-made shoe insert that helps prevent bunion pain and also keeps the bunion from growing larger.

Look for a podiatrist who makes his own inserts. This ensures the best care, because the orthotic is only as good as the mold that is taken of your foot, says Gregory Spencer, D.P.M., a podiatrist in Renton, Washington.

Surgery to remove the bunion should be a last resort, considered only after you've tried a prescription orthotic for at least 5 months without success, Dr. Spencer says. Therapeutic ultrasound can be very effective for relieving pain after orthotics have been used for a while, but the success rate is lower if orthotics are not used.

---

evenly on the ankle and calf of the leg with the bunion. Form a circle around your leg with both hands, with your thumbs overlapping on the inner part of your leg and your fingers on the outer part. Put one thumb on top of the other so that you can press down with both thumbs. Starting at the ankle, press with your thumbs on the inside of the ankle and leg.

Massage the area starting just above the ankle and work up the inside of the leg, probing for tender spots, which are signs of blocked chi in a meridian. If you find a tender spot, press firmly or massage the area in small circles on and around the painful area for 30 to 60 seconds, first clockwise, then counterclockwise. If going in one direction is clearly more effective for the pain, use that direction exclusively for pain relief. (Press hard enough to feel a bit of discomfort, but not so hard that the pain is unbearable.)

Next, move your hands up the leg, massaging with your overlapped thumbs as you go and concentrating on tender spots when you find them. Continue until you're just below the knee.

Repeat the massage on the other leg so your chi is balanced. Do this massage once a day until the pain is reduced or eliminated, says Dr. Spencer.

"This massage does not work on everyone, but it can banish bunion pain so that it doesn't come back for a long time—sometimes years," he says.

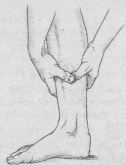

Some people may need to perform this technique on the outside and the back of the leg as well. Stretching the calf muscle is also helpful.

## *Simple Lifestyle Changes Can Banish*
# Burnout

Conventional experts tend to agree that while there are several different causes of burnout, the underlying root is psychological, not physical. Some say it's a clash between expectations and reality. The starry-eyed idealist (a nurse or social worker or teacher, for example) meets up with the harsh limitations of the job and crashes in a nosedive of frustration and disappointment.

Some say it's a problem of helplessness. You have no control over your workload or schedule. Or, no matter how much you work, your boss or the bureaucracy or some other uncontrollable factor seems to block any tangible, positive results. You start to withdraw emotionally from coworkers and clients, and you feel depressed.

But Ahnna Lake, M.D., an expert in burnout and stress-related issues who is based in Stowe and Burlington, Vermont, has an alternative view. She believes that the conventional

# GUIDE TO PROFESSIONAL CARE

If you are too tired to exercise or have persistent insomnia, you may have passed the point where you can recover from burnout just by making simple lifestyle changes.

If you experience joint or muscle pain, digestive problems, headaches, or frequent infections, you should see a physician to rule out a more serious condition. The final stage of burnout—total physical, mental, and emotional exhaustion—is very much like clinical depression and usually requires professional care, says Ahnna Lake, M.D., an expert in burnout and stress-related health issues who is based in Stowe and Burlington, Vermont.

For the most effective treatment, she recommends a physician with a mind-body orientation who understands the physical nature of burnout and can also rule out other possible medical problems.

psychological explanations of burnout don't get to the heart of the problem and often prevent people from getting the right help.

"I feel that burnout is a physical problem—a depletion syndrome," she says. "When you carry a great physical and emotional load for too long without letup, your body simply can't keep up, and it starts to show up as one or more of the symptoms of burnout."

Those symptoms include constant fatigue, irritability or depression, lack of concentration, insomnia, self-doubt, anxiety, and even becoming physically ill with stress-related problems such as frequent infections, allergies, digestive problems, or headaches.

"Overcoming burnout involves creating conditions in which the body can recuperate. Most of these are simple lifestyle changes," says Dr. Lake. As the body mends, psychological symptoms can fade completely, she adds.

Here are some of the alternative remedies that Dr. Lake and other experts suggest to repair the physical damage of burnout.

**FOOD:** *Staying Off the Blood Sugar Roller Coaster*

Diet can definitely help repair a damaged system, says Dr. Lake.

"The high-carbohydrate diet rich in pastas and breads that's commonly recommended these days doesn't work for many people who are recovering from burnout," she says. For many, a high-carbohydrate diet produces too much of a roller coaster in blood sugar levels, she adds.

Try cutting back on sugar and on starchy foods (bread, rice, and potatoes), and keep cutting back until your energy rises, advises Dr. Lake. You'll soon discover how much starch and sugar you can eat before they work against you, she says.

At the same time, emphasize the slow-burning fuel of protein and the healthy fats found in such foods as cold-water fish (salmon, mackerel, trout, and tuna), cold-pressed oils (flaxseed, olive, and safflower), and nuts and seeds. These healthy fats occur naturally in the foods we eat. Fats altered by high heat, such as in deep frying (as opposed to stir-frying), and those that are processed into solids or products with long shelf lives (hydrogenated oils) are the ones to avoid, she cautions.

Following this diet will not only help your current burnout, it will also help prevent future bouts, she says.

**REST:** *The Key to Recovery*

You need extra rest, whether in the form of more nighttime hours, a short daily nap, or simply quiet time alone, to overcome burnout naturally, says Dr. Lake. Unfortunately, she says, insomnia can be a problem with burnout. If you're experiencing difficulty sleeping, she recommends that you address this problem as well.

Since physical and emotional overload produce burnout, it's no surprise that reducing outside stressors and catching up on your rest will help your recovery. Dr. Lake suggests saying no to extra demands and avoiding situations or activities that upset or tire you.

"Learning meditation or other relaxation skills can speed the process along as well," she adds. "You will definitely feel better if you get a lot of rest."

## BREATHING: *Deep Healing*

Having anxious thoughts, such as worry about your job, about losing your job, or about not having enough money, is one of the most common causes—and symptoms—of burnout.

"One of the most effective antidotes for job-related anxiety is something that you have with you all the time—your lungs," says Barbara Bailey Reinhold, Ed.D., director of the career development office at Smith College in Northampton, Massachusetts. "You can interrupt the progression of anxious thoughts by taking deep, diaphragmatic breaths and instructing your mind to be still."

To breathe diaphragmatically, says Dr. Reinhold, inhale slowly through your nose and pull air deep into the bottoms of your lungs, feeling your belly expand. Then exhale slowly through your mouth.

She recommends deliberately inserting deep breathing into your work schedule whenever possible for about 2 minutes a session. "The calming effect is truly amazing," she says.

## EXERCISE: *An Antidote for Office Stress*

When work becomes too intense, "use some kind of physical movement or stretching to change the energy," says Dr. Reinhold. "Walking and stretching are free and easily accessible."

Keep a pair of good walking shoes at the office or in your car and take a long stroll at lunch—at least 20 minutes, says Dr. Reinhold.

## RELAXATION: *Surround Yourself with Soothing Scents*

"The right smell can instantly take you to a relaxed, restorative state of mind and body," says Ruth Luban, a counselor in Santa Monica, California.

Try testing scents to find out which is the most relaxing for you, she advises (lavender and vanilla are two common favorites). Then, she says, "put little lotions and potions" around your work area so you can smell them whenever you're feeling time-starved and deadline-driven. If a certain hand cream soothes you, keep a bottle or tube of it at work and give yourself a 1-minute hand massage with it when you're feeling stressed.

"Take the time to explore what fragrances trigger the relaxation response in you," says Luban.

**RITUAL:** *Take Time to Decompress*

It's important to separate work from the rest of our lives, says Luban. She recommends a decompression period after work, whether it's meditating, taking a hot bath, doing a jigsaw puzzle, or engaging in a hobby like woodworking.

"Whatever you do, ritualize the activity," says Luban. "Plan to do it, and do it every day at the same time, because when it becomes ritualized, you'll start to just do it naturally."


# *Quick, Natural Healing for*
# Burns


It can happen in a second, but a burn can leave a scar for a lifetime. A first-degree burn from an unexpected blast of scalding water from the shower at a motel, for example, makes skin red and painful, but the burn heals on its own in a couple of days. A second-degree burn from a careless moment at the stove, for instance, causes redness and blisters, and the pain is intense. This type is still minor, though; it heals within a couple of weeks with little or no scarring. A third-degree burn, however, such as from clothing that catches fire, destroys all layers of the skin.

A third-degree burn is a medical emergency (as are first- and second-degree burns if they cover more than 10 percent of the body). But if a first- or second-degree burn is small, and the skin isn't broken, you can safely and effectively treat it with alternative home remedies.

### ALOE: *For Minor Kitchen Burns*

"The aloe plant is by far the best remedy for minor kitchen burns," says Pamela Fischer, founder and director of the Ohlone Center for Herbal Studies in Concord, California. Keep a plant growing on your kitchen windowsill. If you burn yourself, cut off a leaf, pull off its outer skin, and put the inner part directly on the burn. Then gently pull the leaf off your skin; a

## GUIDE TO PROFESSIONAL CARE

You can use the remedies recommended here to treat first-degree burns (which look red) or mild second-degree burns (which have some minor blistering) at home.

See your doctor immediately, however, if you have a severe second-degree or a third-degree burn (the skin is usually white with red spots, wet or waxy looking, and severely blistered or charred). You should also seek medical treatment if a burn covers more than 10 percent of your body; if your face, hands, feet, or genitals are burned; if the burn causes unmanageable pain; if it becomes infected; or if you start to develop chills and a fever.

Signs of infection, which usually occur 2 to 3 days after a burn, include increased redness or pain, swelling, pus, and red streaks spreading from the burn up the extremities.

Electrical or chemical burns should always be treated by a physician because they may actually be worse than they appear.

To help speed recovery and promote wound healing, a good diet is helpful, along with supplements of vitamin E, vitamin C, zinc, and beta-carotene, says Beverly Yates, N.D., a naturopathic physician and director of the Natural Health Care Group in Seattle. These nutrients are particularly helpful in skin repair and functioning of the nervous system in the affected area, she explains. Since you may need to take doses larger than those recommended for daily use, Dr. Yates advises that you take these supplements only under a doctor's supervision.

coating of aloe "jelly" will stay behind, says Fischer. You can apply aloe as often as needed to soothe the pain.

**HOMEOPATHY:** ***For Immediate Pain Relief***

The homeopathic remedy Cantharis is best for burns, says Beverly Yates, N.D., a naturopathic physician and director of the Natural Health Care Group in Seattle.

First, she says, make sure that the burn is cleaned and dressed properly to help prevent infection. Then use the 12C potency of Cantharis, taking two pellets every 15 minutes for the first hour.

If the pain is better after this time, take the same dose every 3 to 4 hours. (Don't swallow the pellets; let them dissolve under your tongue.) If the pain isn't relieved after the first hour, however, switch to the 30C potency, taking two pellets every 15 minutes for an hour, then two pellets every 3 to 4 hours. You can take the 12C potency for up to 1 week and the 30C potency for up to 4 days, advises Dr. Yates.

## Self-Heal to the Rescue

Patricia Kaminski, cofounder and codirector of the Flower Essence Society, based in Nevada City, California, will never forget the night that Self-Heal Creme (made from the flower essence and tincture of the plant called self-heal, along with other herbal components) lived up to its name.

"There's a woodstove where I live, and one night while I was putting wood in the fire, my hand got snagged and caught—I could actually feel the flesh sizzle," Kaminski recalls. "I burned my thumb very badly. In fact, the pain was so bad that I could hardly catch my breath.

"I put cold water on it, which did nothing for the pain. I put aloe on it. Again, nothing. Then, in desperation, I opened a jar of Self-Heal Creme and stuck my whole thumb in the jar. The minute I did, the pain was completely gone, which amazed me. A couple of minutes later, I took my thumb out of the jar, and the burning sensation came right back. So I just sat around with my thumb in the jar of cream for 3 to 4 hours. I would pull it out, it would start to throb, and I would put it in again. Finally, I pulled it out and there was no pain, and I went gingerly about my activities for the rest of the evening until I went to bed.

"The next morning, I was shocked to find that the burned area never went through the various stages of a typical burn. It just went from light pink skin back to normal flesh color."

## VITAMIN E: *An Oil to Speed Healing and Avoid Scarring*

"I had a patient who always scarred when she burned herself," says Dr. Yates. "Once, she burned herself while cooking and called me 20 seconds after she did it. The first thing I told her was to take two specific homeopathics based on how she told me the burn was affecting her. Then I told her to apply vitamin E oil directly to the surface of the burn, covering the oil with gauze and taping the edges, but leaving the gauze loose enough so that air could get to the burn. Then I instructed her to change the dressing once a day until the burn healed. She healed beautifully—very quickly, and without any scarring."

Do not apply vitamin E oil to broken skin, cautions Dr. Yates, since there is a possibility of infection.

### LAVENDER ESSENTIAL OIL: *Homemade First-Aid*

"I have witnessed amazing healing of burns with the essential oil of lavender," says Colleen Dodt, an aromatherapist in Rochester Hills, Michigan.

To make the formula, combine 2 ounces of distilled water, 2 ounces of witch hazel, and 25 drops of lavender essential oil in a glass spray bottle (dark glass is best because it helps preserve the oil). Store the bottle in a cool, dry, dark place. When you need the formula, simply give the mixture a shake and spray it on. Dodt says that the spray is good not only for burns but also for stings. You can use it as often and for as long as needed, but as with vitamin E oil, do not use it on broken skin.

# *Fast Relief from the Aches and Pains of* Bursitis and Tendinitis

These two conditions are the Purple Hearts of weekend warriors.

Bursitis is inflammation of a bursa, a fluid-filled sac that provides padding between a muscle and the bony projection of a joint, such as a shoulder, hip, or knee.

Tendinitis is inflammation of a tendon, which connects muscle to bone. (Think of the Achilles tendon, which connects your calf muscle to your heel bone.)

The most common cause of both of these problems is sudden overuse: You spend Sunday painting the den, play an extra round of golf, or clean out the attic, hauling boxes all day. The next day, you wake up with a brand-new ache. Alternative prac-

# GUIDE TO
# PROFESSIONAL CARE

If you have a case of bursitis or tendinitis—perhaps from typing for hours every day or from an infection or injury—that lasts more than 4 days, you need to see a medical or osteopathic doctor, says David Edwards, M.D., a nutritionally oriented physician in Fresno, California. The doctor will find the cause and work with you to devise a long-term treatment plan.

A dietary deficiency of the mineral manganese can lead to chronic tendinitis by causing your tendons to stretch abnormally, says Dr. Edwards. He suggests that you see a doctor familiar with nutritional therapy who can test your blood for levels of the mineral. If levels are low, the doctor can prescribe a therapeutic dose of manganese to strengthen your tendons.

You should receive a high dose until your blood levels normalize, a process that may take a few weeks. At that point, you should receive a maintenance dose to prevent the problem from returning. Dr. Edwards cautions, however, that no one should take high doses of manganese except with the approval and supervision of a physician.

titioners recommend trying these gentle, natural remedies instead of reaching for over-the-counter painkillers.

## ICE: *Massage for Soothing Relief*

Ice, or specifically, ice massage, is the best treatment during the first 24 hours after the pain starts. It reduces the inflammation that is the actual source of your pain, says Rich Rieger, a licensed massage therapist in Morgantown, West Virginia.

Rieger recommends a bag of frozen peas as the best tool for the job. "The peas are like a bunch of little ice cubes inside a bag, and they can mold themselves to the exact contours of your body," he says.

Cover the bag with a thin layer of insulation such as the plastic wrap used to preserve food. The trick is to keep the bag from direct contact with your skin while keeping the actual contact cold enough to do the job. Then start your massage.

If your knee aches, gently rub the sides of the joint with the bag of peas; that's where you'll find the tendons, says Rieger. Avoid the kneecap and the back of the knee. If your elbow aches, concentrate on the back and sides of the joint and avoid the tender inside of the elbow. For your shoulder, massage all around the joint: the top, back, front, and sides.

The best technique is to rub gently and consistently just long enough for the area to become numb, approximately 5 to 10 minutes. Do the massage every other hour for the first 24 hours—except, of course, while you sleep, says Rieger. After the first 24 hours, use the ice massage three times a day.

## JIN SHIN DO: *To Alleviate—and Prevent—Problems*

Tension in the shoulders and neck is the most common cause of bursitis or tendinitis of the shoulder, arm, and wrist because those areas are some of the most tense in the body, says Deborah Valentine Smith, a licensed massage therapist and senior teacher of Jin Shin Do Bodymind Acupressure (a unique combination of acupressure, deep breathing, and visualization) in West Stockbridge, Massachusetts.

Tension in these areas, she believes, chokes off circulation to the upper limbs. With less circulation, the body can't easily repair the excessive wear and tear that come from an unusual bout of strenuous activity (which can cause an acute form of these problems) or the normal wear and tear of everyday living (which can cause the chronic form).

Smith believes that the best way to prevent or help speed the healing of bursitis or tendinitis is to regularly ease the tension in your shoulders and neck. And the best way to do that, she says, is the Jin Shin Do shoulder and neck release.

Not only will this technique help prevent or resolve bursitis in your shoulder, says Smith, it can also help prevent or heal bursitis or tendinitis in the elbow or tendinitis in the wrist, because it sends more circulation to those areas, too.

While an acupressurist would press on specific points in the neck and shoulders, you can locate "ashi" ("where it hurts") points without knowing specific acupressure points. Here's how Smith recommends doing the release.

Lie on the floor or rest your head against the back of a chair or sofa. Close your eyes and take a deep, relaxing breath. Beginning behind your ears and moving toward your spine, use

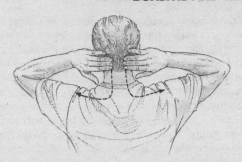

your fingertips to press into the muscles all along the base of your skull. Still breathing deeply, find the most tense or sensitive points, then press and hold those points until you feel the muscle soften or the tension ease.

Next, find the places with the most tension in the back of your neck by rubbing across the muscles, beginning under your skull and moving down to your shoulders, as shown above. When you find a tense or sensitive point, press and hold, continuing to breathe deeply, until you feel the muscle soften or the tension ease.

Cross your right arm over your chest and squeeze all the big muscles along the top of your left shoulder. Again, use all of your fingers to feel for the most tense or sensitive points; then, breathing deeply into the area, press and hold until you feel a release. Repeat on the right side.

For the next-to-last step, drop both arms to your sides, let your head rest against the chair or the floor, breathe deeply, and imagine that your skull is as heavy as a bowling ball but that it's completely cradled by the surface on which it rests. Remind your neck and shoulders that since your head is being supported for the moment, they can take a break and let go.

Finally, if you are getting up and returning to activity, imagine that your head is as light as a balloon, move your neck and shoulders around a bit, and let the balloon "lift off."

## FATTY ACIDS: THE OMEGA OF PAIN

The omega-3 fatty acids found in fish and flaxseed oil decrease inflammation, says David Edwards, M.D., a nutritionally oriented physician in Fresno, California. On the other hand, he says, the fatty acids in most polyunsaturated vegetable oils, such as corn and safflower, and in hydrogenated oils, found in margarine and many baked goods, increase inflammation. "A person who gets omega-3 fatty acids in adequate amounts will not get bursitis or tendinitis as readily," he says.

To increase your intake, eat fish twice a week, particularly salmon, herring, bluefin tuna, and mackerel, which are especially rich in omega-3's, says Dr. Edwards. You could also consider taking a supplement of flaxseed oil according to the dosage recommendations on the label, he says.

## *Enjoy More Energy When You Kick* Caffeine Dependency

Double mocha tall iced. That's the language of the Country of Caffeine.

The adult inhabitants of this country drink close to 500 million (that's right, half a billion) cups of caffeine-containing coffee every day. Younger citizens prefer their caffeine in chocolate bars and in colas served in cups the size of small buckets.

For the ailing, there is caffeine in nonprescription medications for headaches, weight loss, and menstrual cramps. For the overheated, there are almost as many varieties of iced tea— sweetened with sugar and spiked with caffeine—on supermarket shelves as there are sweat glands in the body.

Since caffeine is a central nervous system stimulant, the people in this country are electrified: always on, brains jazzy as neon, bodies humming like generators.

Unfortunately, quite a few of them also end up electrocuted.

The Country of Caffeine is America, of course. And many of its highly caffeinated citizens are nervous and irritable and can't get a good night's sleep. They have headaches, queasy stomachs, and daytime drowsiness. And they may be putting themselves at risk for osteoporosis, heart disease, and possibly even certain types of cancer. All because of caffeine.

Caffeine is a powerful drug, and it works its fatigue-banishing, brain-clearing wonders by stimulating your adrenal glands to pump out adrenaline, the hormone that launches your nervous system into action. But that hormone is pure stress—a biochemical emergency button installed by evolution for threatening situations—and the constant, unnatural overdrive can wear your body out, from your brain cells to your bones. What's worse, your body soon grows accustomed to its dose of caffeine, so you need more of the drug to produce the same energized effect.

If your body doesn't get its caffeine quota, it can go through a week or two of withdrawal symptoms, including headaches, fatigue, intense cravings for caffeine, constipation, anxiety, and a dim bulb where you used to have bright ideas.

In short, you're hooked, a condition that alternative doctors call caffeine dependency.

Now, a caffeine intake of about 250 milligrams a day (the amount in two to three cups of coffee) is probably not going to cause those kinds of problems, although some individuals are quite sensitive to caffeine and will develop caffeine-related symptoms and caffeine dependency at levels as low as 100 milligrams.

Get more than that amount, however, and your risk of developing a dependency starts to rise, says Elson Haas, M.D., director of the Preventive Medical Center of Marin in San Rafael, California.

What happens if you successfully get through the withdrawal symptoms and kick caffeine? "After 2 to 3 days, you'll feel more awake and have a more even energy level through the day than when you were using caffeine," says Dr. Haas.

So if you've had your fill of being a citizen of the Country of Caffeine—if you've decided that you want natural energy, and you don't want all the health risks from a daily fix of caffeine—here's how alternative practitioners recommend that you move to the Country of the Caffeine-Free with an absolute minimum of inconvenience.

## WITHDRAWAL: *Gradual Is Best*

If you cut back on caffeine slowly, you'll be much less likely to suffer the symptoms of withdrawal, says Dr. Haas. He recommends taking a week or two to reduce or eliminate all the sources of caffeine in your life: coffee, tea, cola, medications, and chocolate.

"If you're having 5 cups of coffee a day, for example, cut back to 4½ on the first day, to 4 on the second day, to 3½ on the third day, and so on. Or substitute tea for coffee the first week, then slowly cut back on the tea the second week."

## Kicked Coffee but Still Want a Boost?
## Try a Natural Stimulant

Alternative healers say that there are some healthy, natural stimulants that you can use instead of caffeine, both during and after the withdrawal period.

Inhaling stimulating essential oils can give you that heady feeling. Take a quick sniff of oils such as rosemary, peppermint, basil, or juniper, says Sylla Sheppard-Hanger, principal instructor at the Atlantic Institute of Aromatherapy in Tampa, Florida. "Sniffing an essential oil is the fastest route to the bloodstream and can provide an instant brain boost," she says.

Or you can try an herbal substitute. "As you move away from caffeine and caffeine-containing beverages, there are a number of substitutes that can be both stimulating and refreshing," says Elson Haas, M.D., director of the Preventive Medical Center of Marin in San Rafael, California.

He recommends drinking teas made of roasted herbal roots, such as barley, chicory, and dandelion, which are available in powders and tea bags. He also suggests grain coffees, taste-alike versions of the caffeinated variety, such as Rombouts, Postum, Pero, and Cafix.

"Herbal teas made from lemon grass, peppermint, ginger, and red clover can also be very energizing," Dr. Haas says.

## TYROSINE: *Stop Your Caffeine Cravings*

"Withdrawing from caffeine is similar to withdrawing from a central nervous system drug like amphetamine," says Michael Rosenbaum, M.D., an alternative physician in Corte Madera, California. "You're likely to feel intense craving for the stimulation of the drug during the withdrawal period."

To stop the cravings, Dr. Rosenbaum recommends taking a daily supplement of tyrosine. This amino acid can boost the level of the brain chemical dopamine, which, according to Dr. Rosenbaum, can help reduce cravings in people with all kinds of addictions during a withdrawal period.

Take the supplement on an empty stomach for maximum absorption and effectiveness, following the dosage recommendations on the label, Dr. Rosenbaum says. He recommends using tyrosine only under the supervision of a qualified alternative practitioner.

## CARDAMOM: *An Ayurvedic Antidote*

In Ayurvedic medicine, the ancient system of natural healing from India, the "antidote" to caffeine is the spice cardamom, says John Douillard, D.C., a chiropractor, expert in Ayurveda, and director of the LifeSpa in Boulder, Colorado.

To stop the craving for coffee during the withdrawal period, he recommends sucking on cardamom seeds (just as you would suck on lozenges) all day long. Cardamom is available in the spice section of most grocery stores.

"Your brain will respond to the cardamom as if you were actually drinking coffee, helping to reduce your urge to have another cup of coffee," Dr. Douillard says.

## AROMATHERAPY: *Massage Away Headaches*

A tension headache with the pain centered around the temples is the most common symptom of caffeine withdrawal. It's fine to take mild pain relievers for the first few days of withdrawal, unless they contain caffeine, says Dr. Haas. (Excedrin, Anacin, Vanquish, Empirin, and Compound are some painkillers that contain caffeine.)

But there are also alternative home remedies for handling that headache. One of the best is lavender essential oil.

"The major component of lavender is linalool, which acts as a sedative," says Sylla Sheppard-Hanger, principal instructor at the Atlantic Institute of Aromatherapy in Tampa, Florida. It helps ease mental tension and calms pain, she says.

To apply the oil, put a drop on the tip of each index finger and rub your temples with the fingertips for a minute or two.

Some people may get more headache relief from this massage by using peppermint oil, which, according to Sheppard-Hanger, relaxes the blood vessels and the muscles in the area.

Experiment with the two oils and see which one helps you most.

## ACUPRESSURE: *Use the Headache Point for Relief*

Another place to massage for headache relief is the web between your thumb and index finger.

"It's known as the headache point in acupuncture, and massaging this area provides a lot of relief from headaches," says Ben Dierauf, a licensed acupuncturist and practitioner of Traditional Chinese Medicine in San Francisco. It's also known as LI4. (For the exact location, see An Illustrated Guide to Acupressure Points on page 700.) Rub the web of each hand as hard as you can tolerate for about 30 seconds, he says.

## MASSAGE: *Relax Your Tight Scalp*

You can loosen and relax the tense neck and scalp muscles that cause headaches with two techniques recommended by Elizabeth Cornell, a licensed massage therapist and craniosacral therapist in New York City.

First, tilt your head gently toward your left shoulder and tap the muscles on the right side of your neck with the tips of your fingers for 30 to 60 seconds, Cornell says. You should tap firmly enough to soften the muscles but not hard enough to make them sore. Then tilt your head gently toward your right shoulder and repeat the procedure on the left side.

Next, grasp your hair firmly at the roots and pull gently, working from the front of your head to the back until you've covered the entire scalp, she says.

## EAR MASSAGE: *Boost Your Energy in the Morning*

Fatigue is a common symptom when you're quitting caffeine. One way to beat it is to "thoroughly rub your ears and earlobes for a couple of minutes when you wake up in the morning," says Dierauf.

Why your ears? "In Chinese medicine, the ears are considered to be mini-circuit boards that are connected to the whole body," he says. "When you massage your ears, you're pressing all these little buttons that wake up the energy, or chi, in your body and get it moving. And you need to restore the chi because it was depleted by the caffeine intake."

**HYDROTHERAPY:** *Take a Warm Bath to Stop Insomnia*

To help you beat insomnia during caffeine withdrawal, take a warm, soothing, 30-minute bath before you go to bed, says Robbie Porter, a hydrotherapist and certified massage therapist in Albany, Oregon.

# *Reducing Stress Relieves*
# **Canker Sores**

Most medical doctors and conventional dentists will tell you that no one knows the cause of canker sores. Some alternative healers, however, think that they do. It's a six-letter word with a four-letter reputation: Stress.

"The mouth is one of the first places that react to physical, mental, and emotional stress," says Michael Lipelt, N.D., D.D.S., a naturopathic physician and dentist in Sebastopol, California. "If you have a breakout in your mouth, you have extra stress in your life."

Canker sores, known to doctors as aphthous ulcers, are little white bulges that open into a stinging, red circle of pain. They take up residence for a week or so on the inside of your cheeks or lips or the loose part of your gums. (Don't confuse them with the somewhat similar-looking cold sores, which are caused by the herpesvirus and populate the outside part of your lips and the hard areas of your gums.)

Here's how to stop stress from causing canker sores—and how to soothe any sore that you may already have.

**ACTIVATED CHARCOAL:** *Stop Sores before They Start*

At the very first sign of a canker sore inside your mouth—tingling, warmth, or any other discomfort—put a tablet of activated charcoal right on the area and keep it on until the sensations go away, which should happen within about 15 to 20 minutes, says Amy Rothenberg, N.D., a naturopathic physician in Enfield,

# GUIDE TO PROFESSIONAL CARE

Canker sores are more of a nuisance than a serious medical problem. If your sores are chronic, however, meaning that you get one after another, you may want to have alternative diagnostic tests to uncover the real cause of the problem, says James Hardy, D.M.D., a holistic dentist in Winter Park, Florida.

Chemical or food sensitivity is a frequent cause of chronic canker sores, he says. There are two tests that accurately detect these sensitivities. One is an allergy test that detects the formation of an immune system component called an IgA antibody in the presence of foods and chemicals. The other is an electrodermal screening test, or EDS, which detects imbalances in acupuncture meridians and the cause of the imbalances, whether it's chemicals or foods. Dr. Hardy recommends that you see an alternative dentist, who can arrange for you to undergo one or both of these tests.

Connecticut. Don't use more than one tablet an hour. The charcoal absorbs the virus, thus stopping the eruption.

"I tell all my patients who are prone to this problem to keep tablets of activated charcoal in the house," she says. "My patients love this remedy. Literally hundreds of people have used it successfully to prevent canker sores."

There's one drawback, though: The charcoal turns the treated area black and may turn your stools slightly black as well. "There's nothing toxic or dangerous occurring," says Dr. Rothenberg. "The charcoal just dyes your stools."

## B VITAMINS: *Overcoming Deficiencies*

Deficiencies of folic acid and vitamin $B_{12}$ may cause some cases of recurrent canker sores, says Flora Parsa Stay, D.D.S., a dentist in Oxnard, California. If you have recurrent sores, she recommends taking 400 micrograms of folic acid and 200 micrograms of vitamin $B_{12}$ daily.

## ZINC: *To Speed Healing*

A canker sore is a wound, and zinc helps wounds heal faster, says Beverly Yates, N.D., a naturopathic physician and director of the Natural Health Care Group in Seattle. Zinc is particularly good for healing epithelial tissue, the type that lines your entire digestive tract, including the inside of your mouth. As soon as you notice a sore, take 30 milligrams a day, then continue with that dosage until the sore heals completely, she says.

## MYRRH: *Repairing Damaged Skin*

Myrrh is rich in tannin, a substance that dries, tones, and repairs injured skin. "I am amazed at the speed at which my patients' skin injuries recover when they use myrrh," says Dr. Yates.

Look in your health food store for an herbal tincture of myrrh. Put a whole dropper of the tincture (not just a couple of drops) on sterile cotton gauze. Four times a day, place a piece of treated gauze on the sore and leave it on for 10 to 15 minutes.

If this is more time than you're willing to spend with cotton gauze in your mouth, try this instead: Put a dropper of tincture in a 4-ounce glass of water, stir it with a spoon, swish the solution around in your mouth for a few seconds, and spit it out. Do this four times a day. "The treatment with myrrh-soaked cotton gauze is ideal, but even brief exposure to myrrh is very beneficial," says Dr. Yates.

## HERBAL WITCH HAZEL: *Common and Effective*

Myrrh isn't an easy herb to find. If you can't locate it, says Dr. Yates, use a tincture of widely available herbal witch hazel instead. (You're looking for herbal witch hazel, not the clear, alcohol-based type that you find in supermarkets. To be sure that you get the herbal product, look for the botanical name, *Hamamelis virginiana*, on the label.) Use it in the same way as you would myrrh, either on cotton gauze or in water.

## BEE PROPOLIS: *Winning the Seal of Approval*

Bee propolis helps seal in nutrients and moisture so that tissue can rebuild faster, says Dr. Yates. If you can't find pure bee propolis, look for a salve in which it's an ingredient. Other healing herbs to look for in the salve are myrrh and calendula. "All of these herbs are good for canker sores," says Dr. Yates.

## FUN: *Take It Twice a Day*

One of the best ways to protect yourself against canker sores is to reduce stress, says James Hardy, D.M.D., a holistic dentist in Winter Park, Florida. He recommends that you identify activities that you love, such as riding a bike, listening to music, making love, praying, exercising, playing with the kids, or taking a bubble bath, and be sure to do one or more of them once or twice a day, every day.

"When I see new patients with canker sores, I ask them to rate themselves 'low,' 'medium' or 'high' in stress. Then I ask them to make the same rating for fun. They often say, 'Fun?'—as if it were the first time they'd heard the word."

If their stress ratings are higher than their fun ratings, Dr. Hardy tells patients to increase the fun in their lives. "Reduce your stress by showing yourself some kindness, by doing something you love to do," he says. "This is a very important part of disease prevention, including preventing canker sores."

## IRON: *Extra Protection for Women*

Women get a lot more canker sores than men do. The reason may be fatigue (a potent form of stress) caused by a lack of iron, says Dr. Stay. If you're a woman who's prone to canker sores, she recommends a daily supplement of 18 milligrams of iron.

## LYSINE: *A Potent Stress Buster*

Fatigue and stress can also rob the body of the amino acid lysine, and low levels of lysine can trigger canker sores, says Reid Winick, D.D.S., an alternative dentist in New York City. He recommends that people who are under stress and prone to canker sores talk to their doctors about taking 1,000 milligrams of lysine a day—500 milligrams with breakfast and 500 milligrams with dinner. If you are prone to outbreaks of canker sores, take the supplement on a daily basis. If you don't, you will need to take it as soon as the problem arises to lessen the severity of the outbreak.

## R$_X$ for Canker Sores: More Fun

"I had a patient, a girl in her teens, who was very good at playing the violin," says James Hardy, D.M.D., a holistic dentist in Winter Park, Florida. "But her parents constantly pressured her to practice, and she started to develop canker sores from the stress.

When I saw her for a dental problem, I noticed the canker sores. I told her to play the violin because she loved playing, not because she was being forced into doing it, and also to add some fun activities to her life that would balance the stress and pressure of being a top-level violinist.

"I saw her a few months later, and her canker sores were completely gone. I asked her 'What did you do?' And she said, 'I took your advice, and now I do more fun things. When Mom and Dad pressure me to practice, I say, "Okay, I'll get to it. But I want to do this right now."' She increased her level of fun, decreased her level of stress, and her canker sores vanished."

## NATURAL TOOTHPASTE: *A Better Alternative*

Sodium lauryl sulfate, an ingredient in many toothpastes, is a foaming agent that has no cleansing value whatsoever, says Michael Olmsted, D.D.S., a biocompatible dentist in Del Mar, California.

It does affect your body negatively, however, by drying out the tender tissues inside your mouth and making it more likely that you'll get a canker sore. And it won't help to spend a lot of time in your drugstore or supermarket searching the shelves for a toothpaste without sodium lauryl sulfate, since nearly all commercial brands contain it, Dr. Olmsted says. His recommendation? Shop at a health food store for a brand without the additive.

# *Head Off Surgery with Natural Remedies for* Cataracts

The 7-minute surgery for cataracts is safe, painless, and effective. The clouded lens of the eye is removed, an artificial lens is inserted, and, in a few days, you can see clearly again.

There's only one problem with the operation: You probably don't need it.

"I estimate that 9 out of 10 patients in the early stages of cataracts could reverse their cataracts with natural remedies," says John D. Huff, M.D., an ophthalmologist and codirector of the Prather-Huff Wellness Center in Sugarland, Texas.

The best time to use natural remedies to stop or reverse cataracts is when they're first diagnosed, says Edward L. Paul Jr., O.D., Ph.D., an optometrist, holistic nutritionist, and director of Atlantic Eye Associates in Hampstead, North Carolina. Once cataracts are too far advanced for nutritional intervention, surgery is a must.

Even then, alternative practitioners believe that the use of nutrients has its place. "Even if the cataract is removed by surgery, the nutritional deficiencies that caused it are still present," says Marc Grossman, O.D., an optometrist, licensed acupuncturist, and codirector of the Integral Health Center in Rye and New Paltz, New York. "Unless you correct those deficiencies, I think it's just a matter of time before they'll surface in the form of a cataract in your other eye or as some other disease."

Nutritional remedies work because most cataracts are caused by oxidation. The protein in the lens of the eye is oxidized by destructive molecules called free radicals in much the same way that the transparent protein (albumin) of an egg white becomes opaque when it's fried.

But alternative practitioners say you can stop or even reverse that oxidation with the following antioxidant nutrients.

## MULTIVITAMIN/MINERAL SUPPLEMENT:
### *A Strong Foundation*

"I feel that a good, high-potency multivitamin/mineral supplement is an important foundation of any cataract treatment program," Dr. Grossman says. A high-potency supplement should supply a daily dose of at least 50 milligrams of most of the B vitamins, 15 milligrams of beta-carotene, 30 milligrams of zinc, and 200 micrograms of selenium.

## VITAMIN C: *A Must for a Healthy Lens*

"Vitamin C is the king of antioxidants and can both prevent and heal cataracts," Dr. Grossman says. He points out that the lens of the eye contains more vitamin C than any other part of the body except the adrenal glands and that vitamin C levels in the lens may be "very low and sometimes nonexistent" if a cataract is growing. He advises his cataract patients to take 1,500 milligrams of vitamin C a day.

## GUIDE TO
## PROFESSIONAL CARE

A cataract is typically diagnosed during a visit to an eye doctor for some other reason. For optimal eye care, ask your eye doctor to tell you if he finds a cataract (many doctors don't).

If a cataract is diagnosed in the early stages, you should work with an eye doctor who is willing to design a nutritional and lifestyle program that will reverse the problem, says Edward L. Paul Jr., O.D., Ph.D., an optometrist, holistic nutritionist, and director of Atlantic Eye Associates in Hampstead, North Carolina. If your eye doctor is not interested in nutritional intervention, find a doctor who is, says Dr. Paul.

## GLUTATHIONE AND NAC: *A Powerful Antioxidant and Its Helper*

"The majority of the cataracts that I see are low in the antioxidant glutathione," Dr. Grossman says. But the body needs the nutrients n-acetylcysteine (NAC) and alpha-lipoic acid (ALA) to metabolize glutathione. He recommends 50 milligrams a day of glutathione, 500 milligrams a day of NAC, and 100 milligrams a day of ALA.

## ANTIOXIDANTS: *What Eye Doctors Recommend*

Here are some other antioxidants that are necessary to stop or reverse a cataract.

• Bioflavonoids: These antioxidants help vitamin C work. Dr. Grossman recommends 500 milligrams a day.
• Beta-carotene: A low intake of this nutrient may increase the risk of developing a cataract. Dr. Paul recommends 12 milligrams daily.
• Vitamin E: Low levels can increase cataract risk. Dr. Paul advises his patients to take 400 international units a day.
• Selenium: This element gives vitamin E a jump-start, says Dr. Grossman. He recommends 200 micrograms twice a day.

• Zinc: "People with cataracts are almost always deficient in zinc, which works in the treatment of cataracts," says Dr. Grossman. He recommends 30 milligrams of zinc daily along with 2 milligrams of copper, "which may work hand in hand with zinc in cataract treatment."

## MSM: *Supplying the Sulfur Your Eyes Need*

"The nutrient sulfur is considered one of the most important elements for good vision," says Dr. Grossman. He recommends getting your sulfur from the supplement MSM (methylsulfonyl-methane) by taking ½ teaspoon of MSM powder per 100 pounds of body weight once a day.

## PAPAIN: *Stop Protein Buildup*

If you don't digest protein adequately, it can end up concentrated in the lens of the eye and possibly contribute to cataracts, says Dr. Grossman. The enzyme supplement papain (from papaya) helps digest protein. Follow the dosage recommendations on the label.

## LIFESTYLE: *These Changes Are Necessary*

A number of lifestyle changes are musts if you want a nutritional program to be effective at slowing, stopping, or reversing cataracts.

• Stop smoking. "Smoking creates more free radicals, which place a greater demand on the antioxidants and supplements to reverse the damage done to cells," says Dr. Paul.
• Wear sunglasses outdoors. "Ultraviolet radiation from the sun is a big factor in causing and worsening cataracts," says Dr. Paul.
• Eat more lightly cooked fresh vegetables. They're rich in eye-protecting antioxidants, and lightly cooking them won't deplete their nutrients. "Leafy green vegetables, like kale, spinach, parsley, and collards, and vegetables with lots of pigment, like tomatoes and carrots, are particularly good for your eyes," says Dr. Paul.
• Reduce saturated fats and fried foods. They increase the production of free radicals, "with the consequence being a greater incidence of cataracts, growing at a more rapid rate," says Dr. Paul.

• Use a relaxation technique. Whether it's deep breathing or meditation, using a relaxation technique daily is a must for healthy eyes, says Dr. Huff.

# The Natural Way to Soothe
# Chapped Lips

Rough, dry, flaking chapped lips are as natural as the weather. Why? Your lips are covered with epithelial tissue, the same sensitive mucous membrane that lines your entire digestive tract. Now, imagine for a moment what would happen if your intestines were turned inside out and exposed to hot sun, whipping wind, or blasts of cold, dry air. They might get a little chapped, yes?

When it comes to lips that are almost always chapped and dry, however, the cause may be the elements inside your body rather than those outside, says James Kennedy, D.D.S., a dentist in Littleton, Colorado.

## CALCIUM, MAGNESIUM, AND FATTY ACIDS:
### Three's Company

Calcium is the mortar that holds cells together, in your epithelial tissue and all over your body. But cells can't absorb the calcium they need without certain fatty acids, a component of a type of fat that's found in fish, flaxseed oil, and other foods that might not be regular tenants of your supermarket cart.

In fact, Dr. Kennedy believes that a deficiency of fatty acids may be the most common nutritional deficiency in America. It may also be the reason that your lips are always flaking and peeling: too little means too little calcium, which in turn means that sensitive tissues like your lips can almost literally fall apart.

To counter the problem, Dr. Kennedy recommends taking 1,000 milligrams of calcium, along with 500 milligrams of magnesium to help the body use the calcium properly, twice a day on an empty stomach.

# GUIDE TO
# PROFESSIONAL CARE

Chapped lips are rarely more than a nuisance, but there are times when you should check with your doctor to make sure that they're not something more. If you have persistent dryness, redness, or scaling, it could be a sign of precancerous activity. If your lips crack and become infected when they're chapped, the doctor may prescribe antibiotics to help them heal.

Take a tablespoon of flaxseed oil every day as well, he says. You can down the oil straight, or you can use it on salads or as a substitute for olive oil in recipes that don't involve heating. Keep it in the refrigerator.

"Calcium, magnesium, and fatty acids make an ideal remedy for chronically dry, chapped lips," says Dr. Kennedy.

## PHENOL AND CAMPHOR: *A Must to Avoid*

These two ingredients are common in lip balms. They're also common in cleaning supplies used to sterilize counters in dental offices!

"These are very strong antiseptic chemicals, and I tell people to stay away from lip balms that contain them," says James Hardy, D.M.D., a holistic dentist in Winter Park, Florida.

## COCOA BUTTER: *A Better Alternative*

Instead, Dr. Hardy recommends a lip balm containing cocoa butter, which is nontoxic and rich in the emollients and moisturizers that can protect and soothe dry, chapped lips. "Cocoa butter will help rehydrate your lips," he says.

## AROMATHERAPY: *Essential for Moist Lips*

For another all-natural, soothing lip balm, buy 2 ounces of unscented cream at any pharmacy and add healing essential oils to it, says Jade Shutes, director of the Institute of Dynamic Aromatherapy in Seattle. Use 30 drops of lavender essential oil to help reduce inflammation and redness and 16 drops of sandalwood essential oil to moisturize your lips.

## Hydrate Your Lips with Hot Water

If your lips are dry all the time, your body probably needs more water, right? But just chugging eight 8-ounce glasses of water every day won't hydrate your lips, says John Douillard, D.C., a chiropractor, expert in Ayurveda (the ancient system of natural healing from India), and director of the LifeSpa in Boulder, Colorado.

To hydrate your lips (and skin), he says, you need to sip hot water or decaffeinated tea, which gently dilates your circulatory system so that the moisture can reach the tissues. He recommends filling one or two 32-ounce insulated hot-drink containers with decaffeinated hot tea or hot water and taking one or two sips every 10 minutes or so throughout the day.

## WATER: *Stay Hydrated*

If your lips are chronically dry, drink more water, says William Payne, D.D.S., a dentist in McPherson, Kansas. The standard recommendation of 64 ounces a day may not work. Instead, try 100 ounces a day, or even more.

## MULTIVITAMIN/MINERAL SUPPLEMENT:
### *Insurance in a Pill*

Many people have diets that are so overloaded with nutrient-poor, processed foods that even though they don't have outright nutritional deficiency diseases such as scurvy or rickets, they have many minor symptoms. Like chronically chapped lips.

So, if you eat a lot of processed foods and your lips are always dry and flaky, a high-potency multivitamin/mineral supplement may correct the problem, says Dr. Payne. Take one daily until the symptoms subside.

# *Limit Side Effects of*
# **Chemotherapy and Radiation**

Nausea. Vomiting. Loss of appetite. Diarrhea. Anemia. Hair loss. Fatigue. Mouth ulcers. Yeast infections. Depression. Anxiety. Insomnia. Pain.

No, those aren't symptoms of cancer. They're some of the common side effects of two medical treatments for cancer: radiation (tumor-killing x-rays) and chemotherapy (tumor-killing medications).

"More often than not, cancer patients become very ill as a result of their treatment," says Doug Brodie, M.D., an alternative physician in Reno who has treated hundreds of cancer patients. "By using alternative remedies in addition to conventional treatment, some patients can go through radiation and chemotherapy with hardly any side effects at all."

Some alternative remedies may even improve the effectiveness of chemotherapy and radiation, says Charles Simone, M.D., director of the Simone Protective Cancer Center in Lawrenceville, New Jersey.

## MAITAKE: *Banish Nausea and Boost Energy*

This mushroom from Japan contains the food chemical beta-glucan, which can help banish nausea, sharpen appetite, and boost energy while strengthening the immune system's white blood cells that are responsible for killing cancer cells.

"An extract of beta-glucan from maitake mushrooms is one of the best home remedies to help prevent side effects from conventional cancer treatment and to beat cancer," believes Robert Rountree, M.D., cofounder of the Helios Health Center in Boulder, Colorado.

Dr. Rountree's patients take two to three droppers a day (about 30 drops) of such an extract in a product called maitake D-fraction. Other extracts of beta-glucan are available that may

## GUIDE TO
## PROFESSIONAL CARE

*Caution: Cancer is a complex and life-threatening disease that requires professional medical care. Some alternative remedies may actually worsen cancer if they are not used appropriately. Therefore, use the alternative remedies discussed in this chapter only as part of a cancer treatment program that is guided and monitored by a qualified physician who is experienced in cancer care and alternative medicine. If you are being treated by a conventional doctor, check with him before changing or stopping any conventional medical treatments or medications, and keep all of your doctors and/or alternative practitioners informed of all treatments that you are receiving.*

be derived from shiitake or reishi mushrooms as well as maitake. All three are rich in beta-glucan. Follow the dosage recommendations on the label.

### MCT AND WHEY PROTEIN: *For the Calories You Need*

Conventional cancer treatment muffles the appetite center of the brain and damages the cells of the gut. As a result, cancer patients may not feel like eating and may absorb fewer calories from the foods they do eat. That can cause severe weight loss.

To make sure his cancer patients get enough calories to maintain their weights, Dr. Rountree prescribes a highly absorbable, high-calorie oil containing a fat called medium chain triglycerides (MCT).

His favorite source of MCT is a product called Thin Oil, which comes in butter, olive oil, and garlic flavors. He advises his patients to take 1 to 3 tablespoons a day of Thin Oil, depending on their appetites, their daily calorie intakes, and their rates of weight loss. Thin Oil is available through your health care professional.

He also advocates whey protein, a product that works particularly well for people who have absorption problems. "Whey protein has lots of calories, is easily absorbed, and also boosts the immune system, helping defeat cancer," says Dr. Rountree. Follow the dosage recommendations on the label.

## GLUTAMINE: *To Protect Your Intestinal Tract*

Chemotherapy and radiation attack all of the rapidly multiplying cells in your body, not just cancer cells. To protect the cells lining your intestinal tract, Dr. Rountree recommends 5,000 to 15,000 milligrams a day of glutamine, an amino acid that fuels the intestinal cells. "Glutamine is the best remedy for shielding the intestine from the damage of chemotherapy and radiation," he says.

## The Antioxidant Debate

Cancer specialists are taught in medical school that antioxidant vitamins and minerals negate the cancer-killing power of chemotherapy and radiation, says Charles Simone, M.D., director of the Simone Protective Cancer Center in Lawrenceville, New Jersey.

Since those treatments work by generating cell-destroying free radicals, and antioxidants neutralize free radicals, it would seem logical to avoid antioxidants.

Not so, Dr. Simone says. In fact, he believes that nutritional support not only decreases the side effects of chemotherapy and radiation but also increases the "killing capacity" of the treatments.

The bottom line: According to Dr. Simone, people who take vitamin and mineral supplements along with conventional treatments recover faster from cancer and live longer than those who don't take them.

## ASTRAGALUS: *To Shield Your Immune System*

This Chinese herb strengthens the immune system, which is weakened by chemotherapy. Dr. Rountree prescribes 1,500 milligrams a day for his cancer patients.

## SIBERIAN GINSENG: *For More Energy and Stamina*

Siberian ginseng can help prevent fatigue brought on by radiation or chemotherapy, says Dr. Rountree. It also works well with astragalus to protect the immune system. He recommends 200 milligrams three to six times a day for his cancer patients.

Unfortunately, many products advertised as Siberian ginseng don't contain any of the energy-giving ingredients of the herb, so Dr. Rountree says to look for a product standardized for eleutherosides, the primary active ingredient.

## UMEBOSHI TEA: *To Prevent Nausea and Vomiting*

*Umeboshi* is a Japanese word for salt plum paste, which is one of the ingredients of this tea, along with the root of the kudzu plant and the herb ginger.

"It's the best remedy for the nausea and vomiting caused by conventional cancer treatments," Dr. Rountree says. Here's how to make it.

Buy umeboshi paste, kudzu powder (loose or in capsules), and freshly grated or powdered ginger. Put ½ teaspoon of the kudzu powder in a bowl and combine it with enough cold water to make a paste. Mash the paste, then pour 1 cup of hot water over it to dissolve it. Add ½ teaspoon of umeboshi and ½ teaspoon of ginger, pour the water into a small pot, and simmer on low heat for 30 minutes. Strain the mixture before drinking. Have it twice a day, including one cup before breakfast.

"It is very settling to the stomach of a cancer patient to have this tea first thing in the morning," says Dr. Rountree.

## GREEN TEA: *Another Nausea Stopper*

"Green tea makes people on chemotherapy feel much better and also has anti-cancer properties," says Dr. Rountree. He advises his patients to drink several cups a day or take 500 milligrams of the herb each day in capsule form. Follow the dosage recommendations on the label.

# *Internal Energy Can Beat*
# **Chronic Fatigue Syndrome**

To many conventional doctors, the initials CFS might as well stand for "certified fake sickness" instead of "chronic fatigue syndrome."

That's because many conventional doctors either don't believe that CFS exists as a disease, or they don't understand it well enough to conduct the full range of medical tests that can detect it. This is unfortunate, because CFS can plague people with daily fatigue so profound that they can't find the energy to get out of bed.

Even when people are correctly diagnosed with CFS, the medical treatments they're likely to receive won't cure it, says Jacob Teitelbaum, M.D., a physician in Annapolis, Maryland.

"Typically, a conventional doctor will tell a patient to take an antidepressant for sleep and to exercise for energy and that's it," Dr. Teitelbaum says. Not only is this treatment ineffective, he says, it can actually cause harm, since exercise may make chronic fatigue worse if the patient tries to push to exhaustion.

Dr. Teitelbaum and other alternative practitioners who have studied CFS for decades think that they know what causes the problem and the effective ways to treat it. "We suspect that the 'core defect' that underlies the disease is a defect in the energy furnaces found in each and every cell: the mitochondria," says Dr. Teitelbaum.

The mitochondria (plural for "mitochondrion") are microscopic, capsule-like structures inside the cells. They produce the energy—in the form of a chemical called adenosine triphosphate, or ATP—that powers all the functions of the body. If the mitochondria are functioning inefficiently, they may generate only one-ninth of the optimal amount of ATP, Dr. Teitelbaum says.

One secret of overcoming CFS, then, is to help the mitochon-

## GUIDE TO PROFESSIONAL CARE

You probably have chronic fatigue syndrome if you have had fatigue and at least three of the following symptoms for at least 6 months: short-term memory loss ("brain fog"), sore throats, muscle pain, joint pain, headaches, increased thirst, unrefreshing sleep, bowel dysfunction, recurrent or persistent infections, and/or tiredness after exertion that lasts for more than 24 hours. Chronic fatigue patients usually have a number of different health problems. Here are the most common.

- Disordered sleep (fibromyalgia), in which the muscles shorten and become painful
- Hormone deficiencies
- Poor immunity that leads to chronic infections, including yeast overgrowth, sinusitis, and bowel infections, among others
- Nutritional deficiencies

A holistic physician can diagnose and treat you effectively. Treatment must be tailored to your individual case, but it usually involves four steps: sleeping aids, hormone treatments, antifungal and antiparasitic medications for infections, and nutritional treatment.

dria produce more of this energy-giving substance. Here are some safe, natural, and effective ways to get your energy back again.

**MAGNESIUM AND MALIC ACID:** *Chemical Necessities*
The mitochondria in cells don't produce energy all on their own. They require the presence of many nutrients, including magnesium and a chemical called malic acid, to assist them in turning glucose (sugar) molecules into energy-giving ATP. "These nutrients can make all the difference for people with CFS," says Dr. Teitelbaum.

He recommends a magnesium/malic acid supplement called FibroCare, which includes the nutrients magnesium glycinate, vitamin B$_6$, thiamin, vitamin C, and manganese, all of which are necessary for energy production. Magnesium is particularly crucial because people with CFS are typically deficient in the mineral, Dr. Teitelbaum says.

Dr. Teitelbaum's recommended dose is six tablets of Fibro-Care a day for a total of 450 milligrams of magnesium and 1,800 milligrams of malic acid. Because of the magnesium, some people may get diarrhea at this dose, Dr. Teitelbaum cautions. If that happens, reduce the amount to one or two tablets a day. Then increase the dose by an additional tablet or two every 7 days until you're up to the full dose of six tablets. This will give your bowels time to adjust to the supplement.

After 8 months at the full dose, most people will feel better; at that point, they can cut back to two tablets a day and continue taking this dose every day, he says.

## MULTIVITAMIN/MINERAL SUPPLEMENT: *Energy Fuel*

"If I could take only the two most important nutritional supplements for CFS, they would be a magnesium and malic acid supplement and a multivitamin/mineral supplement," Dr. Teitelbaum says. Taken every day, a multivitamin/mineral supplement will provide many of the nutrients that the mitochondria need to work effectively and produce optimal amounts of energy.

Dr. Teitelbaum recommends My Favorite Multiple or My Favorite Multiple—Take One by Natrol, because he says they are the most complete. Take the supplements according to the package directions. You can take them on a long-term basis, even when you're feeling better, Dr. Teitelbaum says.

## POTASSIUM-MAGNESIUM-ASPARTATE:
### *Three-Way Protection*

The mitochondria require the nutrient aspartate in order to produce energy, says Dr. Teitelbaum. In order for it to work, however, it must be chemically combined with the minerals magnesium and potassium. In three studies, 75 to 91 percent of a total of 3,000 patients with CFS experienced some relief after taking a potassium-magnesium-aspartate supplement. You should take this supplement only under the supervision of a knowledgeable medical doctor, however.

## NADH: *The Next Step in the Energy Process*

To help your body produce and use the highest possible level of energy-giving ATP, it's helpful to take a supplement containing NADH (a form of the chemical nicotinamide adenine dinucleotide that includes hydrogen), Dr. Teitelbaum says. This compound helps the body utilize the ATP it produces, he says. In research on the supplement, 80 percent of CFS patients who took it for 2 months had a significant reduction in fatigue.

Dr. Teitelbaum recommends taking 10 milligrams a day of NADH for at least 2 months. Because NADH is destroyed by stomach acid, you must take it in a certain way. Keep the supplement by your bedside, along with a glass of water. Take it first thing in the morning, when stomach acid levels are naturally low. Then wait 30 minutes before taking other supplements or medications (except for thyroid hormones) or eating breakfast, Dr. Teitelbaum advises.

## ACETYL-CARNITINE: *Reverse the Weight Gain of CFS*

People with CFS usually have low levels of the nutrient carnitine. This deficiency contributes to the 30- to 60-pound weight gain that's often seen in the first 6 months of the disease, says Dr. Teitelbaum. Taking carnitine supplements helps the body burn fat and make energy more efficiently, which can help to stabilize or reverse this weight gain.

Dr. Teitelbaum recommends using the acetyl-carnitine form of the supplement. Take one 1,000-milligram dose twice a day for 3 months. After that, reduce the dose to 500 milligrams a day and continue taking this amount for up to 3 months or as needed.

Acetyl-carnitine is expensive, usually about $1.50 per 1,000 milligrams. To make a supply last longer, you can take a smaller amount, such as 500 milligrams daily. You will still get some benefit from taking less, and it's certainly better than not using it at all, he says.

Another option is to take the amino acid lysine in addition to the acetyl-carnitine, since the body uses lysine to produce carnitine, Dr. Teitelbaum explains. He recommends combining the two by taking 500 milligrams a day of carnitine along with 2,000 to 3,000 milligrams of lysine for 3 months, then reducing the lysine to 1,000 milligrams. Take the reduced dosage for 3 months or as needed. Lysine is particularly good for people with CFS who also have oral or genital herpes, since it may help keep the virus in check, but don't take lysine unless under the supervision of a knowledgeable medical doctor.

**COENZYME Q$_{10}$:** *For Extra Energy*
Another supplement that can help the mitochondria produce more energy is coenzyme Q$_{10}$, says Dr. Teitelbaum. He recommends 100 milligrams a day. Taking coenzyme Q$_{10}$ with a small amount of fat, such as 1 teaspoon of flaxseed oil, makes it easier to absorb, he adds.

# *Instead of Harmful Drugs, Try Supplements to Control* Chronic Pain

Alternative remedies, not prescription or over-the-counter medications, should be your first choice to control chronic pain, says James Braly, M.D., an allergy specialist in Boca Raton, Florida.

"Except in the case of extreme pain, such as the acute pain of multiple bone fractures or the chronic pain of terminal cancer, there is rarely a reason to use conventional painkilling drugs to control chronic pain to the exclusion of alternative methods," Dr. Braly states.

What's wrong with using medications to relieve chronic pain? Side effects from nonsteroidal anti-inflammatory drugs (NSAIDs) kill more than 7,000 people every year and harm thousands more, according to a national study commissioned by the American Gastroenterological Association and GD Searle and Company.

And, Dr. Braly says, there are alternative remedies that can be just as effective as prescription and over-the-counter medications in controlling chronic pain. (Check with your doctor before discontinuing any prescription medications, however.)

---

# GUIDE TO
# PROFESSIONAL CARE

There are dozens of different conditions that cause chronic pain, including arthritis, chronic headaches, back pain, fibromyalgia, and repetitive strain injury. According to James Braly, M.D., an allergy specialist in Boca Raton, Florida, you should see a doctor for any pain that doesn't respond to conventional or alternative therapies; that is associated with blood in the stool, unexplained weight loss, seizures, fever, or a stiff neck that wakes you frequently from sleep; or that changes in quality, frequency, or severity. (For more details, see the "Guide to Professional Care" in the chapter that deals with your specific problem.)

---

## 5-HTP: *Tell Your Brain to Feel Less Pain*

This natural substance (its full name is 5-hydroxytryptophan) boosts the levels of a neurotransmitter, or brain chemical, called serotonin. When you're low in serotonin, you have a lower threshold of pain. You experience pain more quickly, more severely, and for a longer period of time than people who have normal levels, says Dr. Braly.

Plus, higher levels of serotonin help you sleep more deeply. "Deep sleep is an anti-pain phenomenon," Dr. Braly says. "People who sleep poorly are more prone to chronic pain."

Doctors have used 5-HTP to end the pain of fibromyalgia, migraine headaches, and arthritis-like symptoms. "By increasing your serotonin with 5-HTP, you may be able to reduce or even eliminate chronic pain," Dr. Braly says. He recommends taking 200 milligrams or less a day. But since it is still experimental, and the long-term effects are unknown, don't take it without a doctor's guidance.

## VITAMIN B$_6$: *Another Serotonin Booster*

This vitamin is a "co-factor" for the production of serotonin, says Dr. Braly. "Scientific studies show that vitamin B$_6$ helps clear up chronic pain and chronic pain syndromes," he says. He recommends taking a high-potency B-complex supplement that

supplies a daily dose of 50 milligrams of most of the B vitamins.

## MSM: *Get the Pain-Relieving Sulfur Your Body Needs*

Do you eat lots of processed foods? Are you under constant
stress? Then you're a typical American. Those two lifestyle
factors rob your body of sulfur, a crucial anti-inflammatory,
tissue-healing, anti-pain nutrient, Dr. Braly says.

"It is my opinion that sulfur is an essential nutrient that conventional medicine has overlooked," he says. MSM (methylsulfonylmethane) helps heal connective tissue, aids in the production of
pain-relieving, detoxifying sulfur-containing amino acids, and
dramatically decreases inflammation.

Various sulfur-containing supplements can help relieve arthritis pain, "but MSM is the best sulfur donor of all supplements
and has the strongest ability to relieve pain," Dr. Braly says.
"MSM should be part of the healing therapy for anyone with
chronic pain." As a starting dose, he recommends 500 milligrams three times a day.

### For Postsurgical Pain, Try Glutamine

It's a sad scenario that's familiar to surgeons. A patient (usually
over age 60) has major surgery and heals poorly, perhaps has a
chronic infection, may have muscle wasting, and is always in pain.
The problem is called postsurgical chronic pain syndrome, and
some surgeons are preventing it with a nutrient that you can take
safely and easily on your own.

It's an amino acid called glutamine, the primary fuel for the lining
of the small intestine. Under the stress of surgery, this lining can become permeable, or leaky, triggering all kinds of problems that lead
to postsurgical chronic pain, says James Braly, M.D., an allergy specialist in Boca Raton, Florida.

"Getting supplemental glutamine in the diet protects the intestinal lining by, among other things, boosting the production of protein (which helps prevent muscle wasting), enhancing the absorption
of nutrients, increasing the amount of growth hormone (a natural
painkilling substance manufactured by the body), stimulating the
immune system, and accelerating the healing and detoxification
process," he says.

Beginning 2 weeks before surgery, patients should add a rounded teaspoon (about 4 grams) of glutamine powder to an 8-ounce glass of water and take it three to five times a day, for a daily intake of 12 to 20 grams. They should continue this dosage after surgery until any pain and inflammation are gone. Thereafter, Dr. Braly recommends a maintenance dose of 4 to 8 grams a day for those who drink alcohol, take nonsteroidal anti-inflammatory medications for any reason, exercise vigorously, are under a lot of stress, or are HIV-positive.

Glutamine has no side effects, but people who have end-stage liver failure or kidney failure should not use it, Dr. Braly says.

## BOSWELLIA: *A Powerful Anti-Inflammatory*

The herb boswellia blocks the production of inflammatory substances called leukotrienes, thus reducing inflammation and pain, says Dr. Braly. "And, unlike NSAIDs, it doesn't pose the risk of GI bleeding, ulceration, and kidney failure." He recommends taking 250 milligrams three or four times a day as long as you have pain. Look for a product that's standardized to contain 37.5 to 65 percent boswellic acids, the active ingredients in the herb.

## TURMERIC: *Mellow with Yellow*

The Indian spice turmeric, an ingredient in some kinds of mustard, is rich in a substance called curcumin, which can reduce the joint swelling, stiffness, and chronic pain of arthritis as well as or better than NSAIDs, but without the side effects, says Dr. Braly.

Curcumin relieves pain by blocking a number of inflammatory processes in the body and improving circulation to the painful area. Dr. Braly recommends taking a 200-milligram supplement two or three times a day until you are pain-free.

## BROMELAIN: *Speed Blood Flow to Injured Tissue*

Bromelain is a proteolytic enzyme, a substance that digests proteins. It also can "digest" small blood clots in the body, improving blood flow to chronically injured and painful areas, says Dr. Braly. And as a bonus, it's an anti-inflammatory.

For chronic pain, he recommends 500 milligrams a day. Look for a product with at least 1,200 mcu (milk-clotting units, a scientific measurement of bromelain's strength).

**ZINC:** *A Pain-Causing Deficiency Is Common*

Inadequate levels of zinc in the body can cause chronic pain and inflammation, a tendency toward upper respiratory infections, and delayed healing, Dr. Braly says. Such deficiencies are quite common, particularly among people over 50 (zinc levels drop as you age) and people who eat a lot of gluten cereals as found in baked goods, crackers, chips, bread, and pasta. For chronic pain, he recommends taking a daily supplement that provides 25 to 50 milligrams of zinc. Drop the daily dosage down to about 15 milligrams (which is about what is in a daily multivitamin supplement) when the pain is gone.

# Be Naturally Inhospitable to
# Cold Sores

Tiny white blisters have popped up in the corners of your mouth and around your lips. And, if you're not very careful, they'll soon pop up on the lips of your spouse, your children, and anyone else with whom you smooch or share a glass.

Unfortunately, you have oral herpes, the kissin' cousin of herpes simplex type 2, or genital herpes. And you have it for life. The herpesvirus can't be cured, and when this permanent resident isn't loitering around your mouth, it's snoozing in the nerves near your brain stem.

But it's not a sound sleeper. A lot of different factors can wake it up. Stress. Too much sunlight or heat. A weakened immune system (which is why these blisters are also called cold sores or fever blisters. They occur more easily when your immune system is distracted by fighting off a cold or fever).

Some people get cold sores every once in a while, and some get them almost nonstop. Either way, if you're prone to cold sores, you'll be glad to know that there are great natural remedies for preventing them, shortening outbreaks, and providing pain relief.

# GUIDE TO
# PROFESSIONAL CARE

In an infant or young child, a case of herpes can be dangerous because of dehydration and the spread of the infection to
the hands and eyes. If your child has oral herpes, take him to
the doctor, says Flora Parsa Stay, D.D.S., a dentist in Oxnard,
California.

In adults, conventional medicine offers no cure, but the prescription medication acyclovir (Zovirax) can help keep cold
sores under control. Those who have chronic cold sores can
take the medication daily for prevention, while those who have
occasional outbreaks can take it at the first sign of a sore to either stop or shorten the outbreak. Possible side effects of acyclovir include headache, nausea, dizziness, and itching, burning
skin.

## LYSINE: *An Effective Virus Blocker*

The herpesvirus reproduces itself by cozying up to the amino
acid arginine in the "binding site" of a cell. But if the cells'
sites are already occupied by another amino acid—lysine—the
virus has no place to call home. That's why alternative healers
suggest that you protect yourself against cold sores by increasing your intake of lysine.

If you have chronic cold sores, talk to your doctor about
preventing outbreaks with lysine, says Amy Rothenberg, N.D.,
a naturopathic physician in Enfield, Connecticut. If your outbreaks are occasional, you can most likely take lysine just
when you think you're about to have one. The usual signal is a
familiar tingling or throbbing sensation in the area.

## FOODS WITH LYSINE: *Healing Help*

During an outbreak, you may also want to eat more foods
that contain lysine, says Flora Parsa Stay, D.D.S., a dentist in
Oxnard, California. They include turkey, ricotta cheese, avocado, eggs, and chocolate.

## FOODS WITH ARGININE: *A Must to Avoid*

If you're prone to oral herpes, you should steer clear of foods that contain arginine (that advice goes double during an outbreak). Those foods include nuts (almonds, cashews, peanuts, and walnuts), seeds (sunflower and sesame), pork, milk, and cheese, says Michael Lipelt, N.D., D.D.S., a naturopathic physician and dentist in Sebastopol, California.

## YOGURT: *The Bacterial Fighter*

The acidophilus bacteria found in some brands of yogurt help counter the herpesvirus, says Michael Olmsted, D.D.S., a biocompatible dentist in Del Mar, California. He recommends 2 to 3 cups a day of acidophilus-containing yogurt, both as a preventive measure if you have chronic cold sores and to speed healing during an outbreak.

## ICE: *Freeze Out Sores*

At the first sign of a sore, cover the area where you think the outbreak is occurring with an ice cube wrapped in a napkin or washcloth. Hold it in place for as long as it's comfortable, take a break, then reapply. Keep it on your skin for a total of 15 to 30 minutes.

"Viruses don't do well in a cold environment, and the ice can stop the blisters from forming," says William Payne, D.D.S., a dentist in McPherson, Kansas.

## ASTRAGALUS: *A Virus Killer*

The herb astragalus boosts your immune system and kills viruses, which is a must in fending off cold sores, says Beverly Yates, N.D., a naturopathic physician and director of the Natural Health Care Group in Seattle. She recommends taking it in capsule or tincture form at the first sign of a sore and continuing until the outbreak is over. Follow the dosage recommendations on the label.

## CALCIUM AND MAGNESIUM: *To Prevent Problems*

These minerals help keep the body's pH alkaline, which is a necessary step in preventing cold sores, says Dr. Olmsted. He recommends taking 1,000 milligrams of calcium and 1,000 milligrams of magnesium as a daily preventive dose for those with chronic sores and the same dose during an outbreak for rapid healing.

## ZINC: *It Does Double Duty*

This nutrient builds the immune system, thus helping to resist cold sores, and also strengthens the epithelial tissue on the lips and the inside of your mouth so that sores can't get a foothold. Dr. Rothenberg recommends 15 milligrams a day as a preventive dose for those with chronic sores and the same amount during an outbreak for faster healing.

## BETA-CAROTENE: *For Fast Healing*

This vitamin strengthens the mucous membranes of the mouth and speeds the healing of a cold sore, says Dr. Rothenberg. She recommends 80 to 100 milligrams daily during an outbreak. If you have chronic cold sores, talk to your doctor about taking this amount every day as a preventive measure.

## VITAMIN E: *Building Integrity*

This nutrient also builds immunity and the integrity of the epithelium. Dr. Rothenberg recommends 400 international units a day as a preventive step for those with chronic problems and during an outbreak for speedier healing.

## VITAMIN C WITH BIOFLAVONOIDS: *For Healing and Prevention*

These nutrients also speed healing, says Dr. Stay. Look for a vitamin C product with bioflavonoids and take 2,000 milligrams daily during the entire course of the outbreak.

Dr. Rothenberg also suggests this as a maintenance dose for those with chronic cold sores.

## LEMON BALM: *Soothe the Pain*

The herb lemon balm is particularly soothing to cold sores, says Dr. Lipelt. Look for a lemon balm ointment in a health food store, he says, and use it as often as needed throughout the episode.

# *Uncommonly Strong Remedies for Common* **Colds**

You washed your hands after every handshake. When someone sneezed, you ducked. Somehow, though, you still managed to catch the common cold, and the viruses that are partying in your upper respiratory tract are making you feel uncommonly bad: feverish, headachy, tired, and coughing, with a nose so runny that Kleenex stock has gone up 20 points since you've been sick.

Conventional doctors will tell you to take cold medicine and wait it out. Alternative practitioners, however, say that a variety of nutrients, herbs, and other remedies can rev up your virus-fighting immune system, shorten your cold (to as little as 2 to 3 days), and mute the symptoms. Many of these same treatments can help prevent colds as well.

Here is a complete cold-crushing program from Kenneth A. Bock, M.D., codirector of the Rhinebeck Health Center in Rhinebeck, New York, and the Center for Progressive Medicine in Albany, New York.

"I don't put any of my patients on all of these remedies because it's too costly and there are too many pills," he says. You'll have to experiment a bit to choose the remedies that are most effective for you. If you typically get more than one cold a season, you'll have plenty of opportunities to find out what works best.

## VITAMIN C: *Maximize Immunity*

"Viral illnesses of all kinds increase your need for vitamin C," says Dr. Bock. The trick is to immediately saturate your body with vitamin C once you realize that you're getting a cold. You want to take enough of the nutrient so that you get the maximum immune activity to neutralize the infection, says Dr. Bock.

He recommends taking 6,000 to 12,000 milligrams of vitamin C a day for 1 week. Ideally, you should take some C every

# GUIDE TO
# PROFESSIONAL CARE

The vast majority of colds aren't very serious and will go away on their own. In some cases, however, what begins as a cold turns into a more serious kind of infection, such as bronchitis or sinusitis.

A cold that doesn't get better within 2 weeks and is accompanied by wheezing; pain in the ears, sinuses, or chest; or a cough that brings up greenish or bloody mucus needs to be treated by a physician, says Kenneth A. Bock, M.D., codirector of the Rhinebeck Health Center in Rhinebeck, New York, and the Center for Progressive Medicine in Albany, New York.

hour of the day to maintain saturated body levels. If that's inconvenient, take it in three equal doses, he advises.

If you develop loose bowels and gas, which are possible and harmless side effects of high doses of vitamin C, cut back on the amount by 1,000 milligrams a day until the intestinal upset goes away. Once you're feeling better, continue taking vitamin C; 3,000 milligrams a day will help keep colds from getting started, says Dr. Bock.

## VITAMIN E: *Double the Protection*

"When your immune system is fighting an infection, it generates toxic by-products that make it more difficult for you to heal quickly," says Dr. Bock. Most of those by-products come in the form of free radicals, molecules that oxidize and damage your cells.

Vitamin E works in tandem with vitamin C, helping to shield your cells from oxidative damage and allowing you to recover more quickly. Dr. Bock recommends taking 400 to 800 international units (IU) of vitamin E a day for the duration of your cold. Continue to take the same dose afterward, because vitamin E has been shown to help prevent heart disease and many other serious health problems.

### VITAMIN A: *Strengthens the Mucosa*

The respiratory tract is lined with cells that form a layer called the epithelium. This is a mucosal lining that helps trap cold viruses before they have a chance to make you sick. The surface is also lined with virus-neutralizing immune proteins.

At the first sign of a cold, take 50,000 to 100,000 IU of vitamin A a day, but take that level for only 5 days, warns Dr. Bock. The vitamin accumulates in the liver, and taking it for longer periods of time could be dangerous.

### ZINC: *Stimulate Immunity with Lozenges*

Zinc lozenges may work because many Americans are deficient in this nutrient. It's also possible that zinc directly kills the cold-causing rhinovirus. (Then again, zinc lozenges may not work at all: Some scientific studies show that they work, but some show the opposite.)

Dr. Bock recommends taking four to six zinc lozenges a day, for a total dose of no more than 120 to 140 milligrams. Again, maintain that level for no more than 5 days, since taking this much zinc for an extended period may cause an imbalance in copper levels, he explains.

### ECHINACEA: *A Time-Tested Healer*

The herb echinacea has been used for centuries to relieve colds and other upper respiratory problems. It's possible that it works by boosting the production of disease-fighting immune cells, such as phagocytes, leukocytes, and natural killer cells, explains Dr. Bock. He recommends using echinacea in capsule or tincture form.

The common advice is to take echinacea off and on—using it for a week or two, then stopping for a week or so before resuming—because of the general belief that steady use of the herb can depress immune function. Take a dose of 175 to 225 milligrams two or three times a day.

### GOLDENSEAL: *Soothes a Sore Throat*

Even though the evidence for goldenseal's effectiveness is not as strong as the evidence for echinacea, this herb does appear to strengthen the immune system. It also seems to combat localized viruses, which is why it is particularly good for a sore throat, says Dr. Bock.

You don't want to take goldenseal every day, he adds. Take 175 to 350 milligrams three or four times a day for 10 days to 2 weeks, starting at the first sign of a cold. "I recommend taking echinacea and goldenseal together for the duration of an upper respiratory illness," he says.

## Magic Mushrooms

Okay, your grandmother may say it's chicken soup. But scientists are finding that the real cold fighter may be Japanese mushrooms called maitake. These mushrooms (which some people do add to soups) contain high levels of chemicals called polysaccharides, which are believed to stimulate the immune system to unleash its arsenal of infection-fighting components, such as macrophages, natural killer cells, and T cells.

At the first sign of a cold, take 20 milligrams of a standardized liquid extract of maitake mushroom, advises Kenneth A. Bock, M.D., codirector of the Rhinebeck Health Center in Rhinebeck, New York, and the Center for Progressive Medicine in Albany, New York. Alternatively, you can take a supplement that supplies the most active ingredient in the mushrooms, beta 1,6 glucan polysaccharide, also known as maitake D-fraction.

## GARLIC: *Kills Germs Fast*

The evidence for the medical potency of garlic is irrefutable: Just eat a clove, then ask your friends if garlic is strong. That memorable smell is full of virus-killing molecules.

You can get the benefits of garlic without the strong smell by taking deodorized garlic. The odor has been removed, but not the natural medicine. Take 15 to 30 tablets or capsules providing 300 to 500 milligrams for 5 to 7 days, says Dr. Bock.

After that, you can keep taking four to six tablets or capsules a day to help keep a cold from coming back; follow the directions on the label.

## HOMEOPATHY: *Worth Trying*

"These remedies work extremely well in approximately one-third of my patients, work moderately well in another third, and have little or no effect in the final third," says Dr. Bock. But since homeopathic remedies are considered nontoxic, inexpensive, and potentially very effective, he adds, they're worth a try.

Dr. Bock recommends taking a remedy called Husteel, which contains a variety of homeopathic substances that are particularly good for colds and coughs. Follow the directions on the label and take it only for as long as you have the symptoms, he adds.

**THYMUS EXTRACT:** *Put Your Hormones to Work*

Supplements containing extracts of thymus gland are thought to stimulate the body to generate hormones that spark the formation of T cells, which are important virus killers. Take 350 milligrams of the extract according to label directions for 1 to 2 weeks, starting at the first sign of a cold, says Dr. Bock. Take this supplement only under the supervision of a knowledgeable medical doctor.

# *Natural Remedies Help Prevent Recurrence of* Colon Cancer

Alternative and conventional doctors are often like Democrats and Republicans—they can't seem to agree on anything. But whether they use chemotherapy or vitamin C, doctors who treat cancer patients seldom disagree about the best treatment for almost all of the nearly 96,000 Americans who are diagnosed each year with cancer of the colon.

Cut out the cancer.

"It is universally accepted that early surgery is the most effective treatment for most new cases of colon cancer," says Ralph Moss, Ph.D., of New York City, who is director of "The Moss Reports," a series of comprehensive guides to cancer treatment.

What should happen after the surgery is another story, however. Most conventional doctors favor some combination of radiation and chemotherapy. Alternative practitioners say, however, that to help prevent a recurrence of the disease, it is important to change the environment of the colon itself.

## YOGURT: *Regenerate Your Colon*

The colon, the large segment of the digestive tract where waste is readied for disposal, is the area of the body most exposed to cancer-causing substances, says Patrick Quillin, R.D., Ph.D., director of nutrition for Cancer Treatment Centers of America in Tulsa, Oklahoma.

"Digesting the typical American diet—low in fiber, high in fat, loaded with sugar—generates so many free radicals, a type of carcinogenic molecule, that it is as if the colon were being x-rayed twice every day," he says.

Fortunately, the colon has a natural defense against free radicals: its own "friendly" bacteria, which create a chemical environment in the colon that doesn't support tumor growth. "Establishing healthy bacteria in the colon is critical for preventing a recurrence of colon cancer," says Dr. Quillin. The best and simplest way to do that, he says, is to eat the friendly bacteria that turn milk into yogurt.

Dr. Quillin says to eat ½ cup of plain, unflavored yogurt every day. Look for a brand with "active" or "live" cultures, which means that it contains the necessary bacteria.

## COLOSTRUM: *Immune-Stimulating Mother's Milk*

Colostrum, a milk-like substance that female mammals produce soon after giving birth, is full of potent, immune-stimulating factors that jump-start a newborn's immune system. It is also thought that it can help a person with colon cancer fight off a recurrence of the disease, says Robert Rountree, M.D., cofounder of the Helios Health Center in Boulder, Colorado.

Find a concentrated, purified, nonallergenic form of bovine (cow) colostrum and follow the dosage recommendations on the label, Dr. Rountree says. It's safe to take this indefinitely.

## BROMELAIN: *An Anti-Cancer Enzyme*

Pineapples are rich in the digestive enzyme bromelain, which may help break down a tumor's protein coating, thus allowing immune cells to attack the cancer. "I believe enzyme therapy is very helpful in either preventing the recurrence of or controlling the growth of a colon tumor," says James Forsythe, M.D., medical director of the Cancer Care Center in Reno. He recommends taking bromelain supplements, following the dosage recommendations on the label. It's safe to take the supplements indefinitely.

# GUIDE TO
# PROFESSIONAL CARE

*Caution: Cancer is a complex and life-threatening disease that requires professional medical care. Some alternative remedies may actually worsen cancer if they are not used appropriately. Therefore, use the alternative remedies discussed in this chapter only as part of a cancer treatment program that is guided and monitored by a qualified physician who is experienced in cancer care and alternative medicine. If you are being treated by a conventional doctor, check with him before changing or stopping any conventional medical treatments or medications, and keep all of your doctors and/or alternative practitioners informed of all treatments that you are receiving.*

In all newly diagnosed cases of colon cancer, the tumor should be surgically removed, says Michael Schachter, M.D., director of the Schachter Center for Complementary Medicine in Suffern, New York. "If you leave the cancer there, you have a very good chance of dying from the disease," he says.

After the surgery, Dr. Schachter recommends alternative professional treatment for colon cancer, either alone or combined with conventional radiation and chemotherapy. Alternative professional treatment might consist of the following strategies.

• A diet appropriate to the person's metabolic type that emphasizes organic foods and avoids all alcohol, sugar, white flour, caffeine, and food additives
• A regimen of supplements, including vitamins, minerals, amino acids, essential fatty acids, digestive enzymes, herbs, and phytonutrients
• Concentrated supplements of therapeutic foods such as garlic, maitake mushrooms, and shark cartilage
• Special antioxidant supplements, such as coenzyme $Q_{10}$
• Intravenous treatment with vitamin C and glutathione, possibly alternated with low-dose hydrogen peroxide, a bio-oxidative treatment that stimulates the body's defenses
• A detoxification program to rebuild the gastrointestinal tract and remove cancer-causing heavy metals from the system

- Possible hormone supplements, such as DHEA and melatonin
- Depending on the individual, other alternative modalities, such as homeopathy, acupuncture, and magnetic therapy

## ANTIOXIDANTS: *The Right Combination*

Antioxidant vitamins and minerals fight the formation of cancer-causing free radicals. They help strengthen the immune system, and they can armor your body against stress, which is a must when coping with cancer. Specific antioxidants, like beta-carotene, help heal the lining of the digestive tract, where colon cancer takes root.

Dr. Forsythe recommends the following combination of supplements. It's safe to take these indefinitely.

- Selenium: 200 micrograms daily
- Zinc: 50 milligrams daily
- Vitamin E: 400 international units twice a day
- Vitamin C: 1,000 milligrams four times a day
- Beta-carotene: 30 milligrams daily

### How to Prevent Colon Cancer

Most cases of colon cancer are caused by a tumor-promoting lifestyle, says Dan Labriola, N.D., a naturopathic physician in Seattle. That makes it one of the easiest cancers to prevent. Here's how.

- Eat a high-fiber diet to hustle carcinogens through your colon before they have a chance to do any harm. Beans, whole grains, fruits, and vegetables are the best sources of fiber. How do you know if you're getting enough? "You should have at least one significant bowel movement every day," Dr. Labriola says.
- Drink plenty of water. Dehydration stalls stool in your colon, possibly exposing you to more carcinogens. You're drinking enough if you have to urinate every 2 to 3 hours, says Dr. Labriola.

• Avoid red meat, since a high intake of beef, pork, lamb, and other red meats has been linked to colon cancer. A small piece of red meat (about the size of a deck of cards) once or twice a week should be your limit, Dr. Labriola says.

• Go easy on alcohol. Studies show that the more alcohol you drink, the more likely you are to develop colon cancer. Limit yourself to a drink or two a week.

• Get enough calcium and magnesium, minerals that help protect the colon from carcinogens, Dr. Labriola says. Take a calcium-magnesium mineral supplement, following the dosage recommendations on the label, he says.

## HERBS: *These Four Fight Colon Cancer*

The following herbal supplements are thought to be most effective at combating colon cancer. Remember, though, to take them only with the approval and supervision of your doctor, says Dr. Quillin.

• Echinacea. In one European study, echinacea slowed tumor growth and increased survival time in some patients with inoperable colon cancer. Take a daily dose of 80 milligrams.

• Ginkgo. This herb may help by improving circulation to the colon, limiting one of the cellular fuels that powers the spread of a tumor, and strengthening the immune system. Dr. Quillin recommends 40 milligrams daily of a ginkgo product with 24 percent heterosides.

• Astragalus. To help prevent weight loss during chemotherapy, strengthen the immune system, and stop the spread of tumors, Dr. Quillin advises colon cancer patients to take 200 milligrams a day.

• Cat's claw. It helps friendly, anti-cancer bacteria thrive in the colon. Take 250 milligrams a day, says Dr. Quillin.

# *Hands-On Healing Can Help Shorten a Bout of*
# Conjunctivitis

Quickly—almost before you know it—one (or both) of your eyes is red, swollen, and teary; maybe it also itches and has a yellowish discharge. These symptoms mean that you have pinkeye, or conjunctivitis, an inflammation of the mucous membrane—the conjunctiva—that lines the inner eyelid and eyeball.

There are three types of conjunctivitis: viral, allergic, and bacterial. You should visit your doctor for a proper diagnosis of the type you have, because bacterial conjunctivitis needs to be treated with antibiotics. Most viral and allergic cases, however, can be treated without drugs, using alternative home remedies, says Edward L. Paul Jr., O.D., Ph.D., an optometrist, holistic nutritionist, and director of Atlantic Eye Associates in Hampstead, North Carolina.

**TRADITIONAL CHINESE MEDICINE:** *An Herbal Formula*
The Chinese herbal formula Ming Mu Di Huang Wan (Brighten the Eyes) "is a classic tonic for eye problems that involve itchy or red eyes, such as conjunctivitis," says Marc Grossman, O.D., an optometrist, licensed acupuncturist, and codirector of the Integral Health Center in Rye and New Paltz, New York. Follow the dosage recommendations on the label.

**CHAMOMILE:** *Use It As a Compress*
You can use a chamomile tea bag as a compress to reduce the inflammation of conjunctivitis, says Dr. Grossman. Put the tea bag in warm (not hot) water for 2 to 3 minutes, squeeze out the excess liquid, then place the tea bag over your inflamed eye for 2 to 3 minutes. Use this treatment three or four times a day, he says.

---

# GUIDE TO
# PROFESSIONAL CARE

Conjunctivitis is usually a viral infection that often responds to home remedies or goes away on its own, says Edward L. Paul Jr., O.D., Ph.D., an optometrist, holistic nutritionist, and director of Atlantic Eye Associates in Hampstead, North Carolina. If your red, irritated, painful eyes do not get better within a week with home remedies, if light hurts your eyes, or you notice visual changes, however, you should see your doctor.

If your eyes have a discharge of pus or mucus that is heaviest in the morning when you wake up (it may be so heavy that your eyelids are stuck together), you probably have bacterial conjunctivitis. You need to see a physician or an eye doctor immediately to get a prescription for antibiotics.

---

**REFLEXOLOGY:** *Make Conjunctivitis Toe the Line*

Pressing reflex points on your feet that send energy to your eyes is thought to help relieve conjunctivitis, says Douglas Klappich, a reflexologist and director of the Wellth Health Alternative Center in Columbus, Ohio.

Simply use your thumb to firmly press the bottom, top, and sides of the big toe, second toe, and third toe on each foot. Concentrate on the toe base, the area around the toe where it connects to the foot.

If you find a particularly sensitive spot—and it's likely that you will, since you have an eye inflammation, and these reflex points correspond to the eyes—spend 1 to 2 minutes pressing that area.

"Sometimes, you can solve the problem with just one session of reflexology," says Klappich, but he recommends repeating the sessions a couple of times each day for up to 10 days, or until the symptoms subside.

## Use Acupressure to Maximize Medication

Sometimes, when medication isn't working to clear up a case of conjunctivitis, adding acupressure will boost the power of the drug and help heal the infection, says Marc Grossman, O.D., an optometrist, acupuncturist, and codirector of the Integral Health Center in Rye and New Paltz, New York.

Here are the points to use. (For the exact locations, see An Illustrated Guide to Acupressure Points on page 700.) Do them in sequence twice a day, using the pad of your thumb to apply firm pressure to each point for 30 seconds. Don't forget to do the points on both sides of the body.

• BL1 is in the inner corner of the eye, just above the tear duct.
• GB1 is at the lateral end (closest to the ear) of each eye.
• LI4 is in the web between the thumb and index finger, at the highest point of the muscle that protrudes when the thumb and index finger are close together.
• LV2 is in the web between the first and second toes.
• ST44 is between the second and third toes about ½ inch above the point where they meet the foot.
• TB23 is in the depression at the lateral end of the eyebrow.
• BL10 is ½ inch below the base of the skull on the back of the neck, level with the space between the first and second cervical vertebrae and approximately ¾ inch from either side of the spine.

### Clearing Up Allergic Conjunctivitis

Anything that can cause an allergy can cause allergic conjunctivitis, says Dr. Paul, but natural remedies can often clear up the symptoms.

### QUERCETIN: *More Powerful Than Anti-Allergy Eyedrops*

"Quercetin, one of a class of nutrients called bioflavonoids, is more effective than anti-allergy eyedrops in stopping the symptoms of conjunctivitis," says Dr. Paul. He recommends starting with 1,000 milligrams, then increasing the dosage by

1,000 milligrams a day (to a maximum of 5,000 milligrams) until your symptoms are under control.

**HYDROTHERAPY:** *Control Itching with a Cold Compress*

A cold compress can help "short-circuit the allergic response of itching and irritation in conjunctivitis," says Daniel John Dieterichs, O.D., an optometrist in Belen, New Mexico. Here are his directions.

Fill a dish with ice cubes and water and soak a washcloth in the water. Remove it from the dish and squeeze out the excess water. Fold the washcloth and place it over both eyes, keeping it in place until it warms. Repeat the procedure until the itching subsides.

"You can control the red, sore, itchy eyes of allergy season very easily with this technique," says Dr. Dieterichs.

**VITAMIN C:** *Reduce the Inflammation*

Vitamin C helps quiet the inflammation of a case of allergic conjunctivitis, says Dr. Paul. He recommends taking 1,000 milligrams a day.

# *Drug-Free Relief from*
# Constipation

Anything from three bowel movements a day to three a week is normal. That's the word from no less an authority than the National Institutes of Health—but alternative doctors will tell you that what's generally considered normal is not necessarily *healthy*.

"A minimum of one complete, soft bowel movement a day is healthy," says Mark Stengler, N.D., a naturopathic physician in San Diego.

If you have fewer bowel movements, he says, toxins from the stool can be reabsorbed into the bloodstream, causing or complicating many different health problems.

# GUIDE TO
# PROFESSIONAL CARE

Constipation rarely requires medical care. But if you've diligently tried a high-fiber diet and other alternative remedies for 3 days or more without success, if the constipation came on suddenly, or if there's blood in your stool, you need to see a medical doctor, says William B. Salt II, M.D., clinical associate professor of medicine at Ohio State University College of Medicine and Public Health in Columbus.

Keep in mind that various over-the-counter and prescription drugs can cause constipation, Dr. Salt adds. These include non-steroidal anti-inflammatory drugs such as aspirin and ibuprofen, iron supplements, antidepressants, antihistamines, and blood pressure drugs. If you've recently begun taking medication and have developed constipation, talk to your doctor about changing your medication.

It doesn't take a doctor (conventional or alternative) to tell you that not having a daily bowel movement is just plain uncomfortable—which is why Americans spend $725 million a year seeking relief with laxatives.

Just because you can buy laxatives over the counter, however, doesn't mean that they're without risk. In fact, consistent use of a laxative weakens the muscles of the bowel so that you can actually become addicted, meaning that you'll have trouble having a bowel movement without taking one. Laxatives can also drain your body of energy-giving minerals and protein.

Most important, though, you don't need them.

"Almost everyone can clear up constipation with drug-free methods," says William B. Salt II, M.D., clinical associate professor of medicine at Ohio State University College of Medicine and Public Health in Columbus.

## FIBER: *Double Your Intake*

Most Americans get only half the daily amount of fiber that they need to prevent constipation, says Elizabeth Lipski, a certified clinical nutritionist in Kauai, Hawaii. To get what you need, she recommends a daily minimum of five servings of fruits and vegetables, three servings of whole-grain foods, and one serving of beans.

### WATER: *Stimulate the Intestines*

When you're increasing the amount of fiber in your diet, you should drink a lot of water (at least six to eight 8-ounce glasses a day). The reason fiber relieves constipation, says Dr. Stengler, is that it absorbs a lot of water, creating large, soft stools.

Hot water works better than cold because it stimulates peristalsis, the squeezing, muscular action that pushes stool through the digestive tract, says Andrew Gaeddert, a professional member of the American Herbalists Guild and director of the Get Well Clinic in Oakland, California.

### CITRUS PEEL: *Help Move Stagnant Chi*

When you drink hot water, put some citrus peel in the glass, says Gaeddert. Citrus peel stimulates chi, the life-energy of the body. Practitioners of Traditional Chinese Medicine believe that building up chi gives the body the strength to have a bowel movement.

You can also get the benefits of citrus without the peel. Lipski recommends squeezing the juice of a lemon into an 8-ounce glass of warm or hot water and drinking it first thing in the morning to help stimulate a bowel movement.

### HEALTHY OILS: *Lubricate Your Pipes*

Olive, canola, and other monounsaturated and polyunsaturated oils act as digestive lubricants and are very helpful in clearing up constipation, says Kenneth Yasny, Ph.D., a nutritionist in Beverly Hills and founder of the Colon Health Society. Put a tablespoon or two of oil on your high-fiber salad for a perfect anti-constipation meal, he says.

## When Food Isn't Enough

A high-fiber diet accompanied by plenty of water is usually enough to beat constipation. But if you can't seem to get enough fiber in your diet on a daily basis, or if your bowels still seem sluggish in spite of your efforts to eat more fiber, there are plenty of alternative remedies to help you get them moving.

Experiment with the following remedies to see which work best for you, but never use more than one at a time, Dr. Stengler cautions.

## PSYLLIUM: *Concentrated Fiber*

"Some people may need to take fiber supplements to alleviate constipation," says Teresa Rispoli, Ph.D., a licensed nutritionist and acupuncturist in Agoura Hills, California. She recommends using a supplement that contains psyllium seed, such as Metamucil or Citrucel, according to the directions on the label, and following it with a full glass of water. Psyllium supplements generally have about 5 grams of fiber per dose.

## PRUNE JUICE: *Chemical Action*

Prune juice contains compounds that appear to stimulate the intestinal action needed for bowel movements. Dr. Stengler recommends drinking two to three 8-ounce glasses of prune juice mixed half-and-half with water once a day.

Once you begin having bowel movements, cut your intake of juice in half for a day or two, then stop using it, he advises.

### Break Up the Jam with Colon Massage

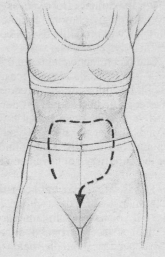

Massaging your colon, which is the final section of the digestive tract, where constipation occurs, is a "simple, completely natural, and highly effective method of helping your elimination," says Kenneth Yasny, Ph.D., a nutritionist in Beverly Hills and founder of the Colon Health Society. Here's how.

• Lie on your back with your feet flat on the floor and your knees bent.

• Beginning in the abdominal area on the right side just above your hip, use the fingertips of both hands to press as deeply as is comfortable, then move your fingertips in a circular, massaging motion.

• Continue upward to just below your ribs. Then, using the same pressing, circular motion, move across your abdomen just above your belly button. Continue to massage down to your left hip.

• Next, move to the right about 3 inches and down about 1 inch. Repeat the entire massage.

Dr. Yasny recommends doing the massage for 5 to 20 minutes a day. "You're helping to push through the fecal matter that's stuck in the colon as well as restoring circulation and muscle tone," he explains.

## CASCARA SAGRADA: *The Herb of Choice for Constipation*

A traditional remedy for constipation, cascara "is one of the few laxative herbs that improve the tone of the bowel, making it work better," says Rita Elkins, a master herbalist in Orem, Utah.

Another benefit is that it doesn't irritate the bowel like other laxative herbs, such as senna, which can cause cramping.

For maximum effectiveness, take cascara at night, after your evening meal or before bedtime. "It works while you are asleep, and you will probably have a bowel movement in the morning," Elkins says.

She recommends taking a 450-milligram capsule daily for 3 to 4 weeks, while also increasing your dietary intake of fiber. Begin by following the directions on the label. You can double the recommended dose if it doesn't seem to be working.

If a double dose doesn't work after a few days, switch brands. Either the product you're using may not be supplying enough of the active compound found in cascara sagrada bark, or the bark may not have been aged long enough to be biologically active, she says.

This is safe to take until constipation is relieved, but do not use it for more than 14 days without medical supervision. Also, do not use it if you have any inflammatory condition of the intestines, intestinal obstruction, or abdominal pain. This herb can cause laxative dependency and diarrhea.

**TRIPHALA:** *An Herb to Rejuvenate Your Digestive Tract*

Triphala is one of the best laxative herbs for long-term use, says Light Miller, an Ayurvedic practitioner in Sarasota, Florida. "It is nonaddictive, and it helps rejuvenate the digestive tract," she says. She recommends using it for 6 months, taking two 1,000-milligram tablets three times a day or six tablets at night with warm tea.

**ALOE:** *Soothing the Way*

Aloe gel lubricates the intestines, helping the bowels move more easily. It's also a natural laxative, says Dr. Miller. For someone who is very constipated, she recommends taking a tablespoon or two of the gel three times a day until the constipation is relieved. Check the label of the product you buy to be sure that it's a form intended for internal use.

**MAGNESIUM:** *You May Need Extra*

Magnesium deficiency contributes to constipation because the mineral relaxes the intestinal muscles, thus helping to keep peristalsis normal, says Lipski. She recommends taking a daily magnesium supplement of 400 to 500 milligrams to prevent constipation.

**ACETYLCHOLINE:** *Orders from the Brain*

The neurotransmitter acetylcholine affects not only the brain but also bowel function, says Dana Laake, a nutritionist in Rockville, Maryland. The nutritional precursor of acetylcholine is choline, which is found in egg yolks, legumes, meat, milk, fish, and lecithin, a food additive. Taking a 250- to 500-milligram supplement of choline citrate or bitartrate two or three times a day should relieve constipation.

## Get into Action

Putting the proper foods, herbs, and nutrients into your digestive tract is just one way to stimulate your bowels. Here are two "active" home remedies that will also help get your bowels moving.

### A REGULAR ROUTINE: *Get Your Body in the Habit*

People who are constipated need to establish a consistent time for elimination, says Gerard L. Guillory, M.D., an internist in Denver.

"Get into the habit of waking up 5 to 10 minutes earlier in the morning and spending 5 minutes on the toilet, whether or not you feel that you need to go to the bathroom," says Dr. Guillory. "A lot of people who try this technique come back to my office amazed that they're no longer constipated. They tell me, 'Hey, Doc, it sounded dumb, but I started doing it, and then I relaxed for a minute and got the urge to go. It was wonderful.'"

### EXERCISE: *Good for the Gut*

Emotional stress can worsen constipation in two ways, says Dr. Stengler. First, when you're stressed, the body steals blood from the digestive tract and sends it to the muscles. Second, stress makes the parasympathetic nervous system—the part that controls intestinal peristalsis—less effective.

Regular exercise is the best stress buster, says Dr. Stengler. He recommends getting 30 to 60 minutes of heart-pumping aerobic exercise, such as brisk walking, bicycling, jogging, jumping rope, or similar activities, three to five times a week.

# *Gentle Alternatives*
# *Soothe Painful*
# **Corns and Calluses**

Corn recipe: Take one pair of tight shoes. Wear them all day—day after day.

Too much pressure, rubbing, or pinching on the delicate skin of your feet can cause a painful corn or callus—a bump or layer of thick, hard, dead skin. Corns usually appear on the toes and calluses on the bottoms of the feet.

You'll find plenty of products on the shelf of your local drugstore that claim they soften corns and calluses. And that's just where they should stay: on the shelf. Podiatrists and other foot care professionals say that these drops are too harsh and can damage your skin.

They also say that you should never trim these hardened areas yourself with a razor or other sharp implement. That advice goes triple if you have diabetes, because poor circulation to your feet can turn a cut into a catastrophe. Ask your health care provider to trim your calluses. The American Diabetes Association recommends using a pumice stone every day to help lessen calluses. Use it on wet skin.

You should, however, switch to roomier shoes, says Gregory Spencer, D.P.M., a podiatrist in Renton, Washington. There are also many over-the-counter and prescription cushioning products for your feet that can provide plenty of comfort if you have corns or calluses.

Instead of using harsh over-the-counter products to remove corns or calluses, you can use alternative home remedies that naturally soften and regenerate the skin, helping to heal the problem and prevent its return.

## CALENDULA: *The Natural Moisturizer*

"A corn or callus is hard, dry skin, and regularly moisturizing that skin is the key to healing," says Andrea Murray, a certified reflexologist and herbalist in Portland, Maine.

A good moisturizer for softening and healing hard skin, she says, is the herb calendula. She recommends putting calendula oil or salve on the affected area twice a day and covering it with a bandage. You may need to reapply the moisturizer and bandage a third time after exercise. Keep the area continually moisturized until the corn or callus is healed. Herbal salves work best when applied after a warm foot soak.

## CASTOR OIL: *Invite It to Your Pad*

The harsh acids in medicated corn pads can irritate or even burn the skin, says Dr. Spencer. That's why he suggests that you use a nonmedicated, doughnut-shaped corn pad that surrounds and is slightly higher than the corn, protecting it from shoe pressure.

When you wear the pad (which should be every day), apply it and then coat the corn with castor oil, which is a superb moisturizer for very dry skin. (Calendula oil and vitamin E oil also

# GUIDE TO
# PROFESSIONAL CARE

If you have a chronic and painful corn or callus that has not responded to natural self-care, see a podiatrist. The doctor can custom-make an orthotic (a device that's worn in a shoe to protect your foot from pressure) or recommend custom-molded shoes. He may also trim the corn or callus, a procedure that you should never do at home.

A bunion can force the skin of your toes against the inside of your shoe, causing painful corns or calluses. One bunion treatment uses minimum-incision surgery, in which the doctor carefully inserts a tiny burr into a tiny slit in the skin. The rotating burr dissolves the bone spur, and the dissolved bone is squeezed out through the incision.

"This type of surgery is very successful for some bunions and corns and calluses caused by bunions," says Gregory Spencer, D.P.M., a podiatrist in Renton, Washington. For severe bunions, traditional bunion surgery is the better option, since minimum-incision surgery is not as corrective, he adds.

work well, Dr. Spencer says.) You may need to use a cotton swab to get the oil into the hole in the pad.

Once you've moisturized the corn, put a small piece of adhesive tape over it to keep the oil in place.

"This method moisturizes the corn all day," says Dr. Spencer. Continue wearing corn pads and using the moisturizing oil until the corn disappears.

## A Special Scrub to Smooth Calluses

Stephanie Tourles has had to deal with thick, hard calluses for most of her life. "I have extremely high-maintenance feet," says the licensed esthetician, reflexologist, and herbalist in West Hyannisport, Massachusetts.

But now she has them under control; her feet are smooth and nearly callus-free. Her secret is a special scrub that she uses to smooth and remove the calluses. Here's her five-step strategy.

**1.** Start by making her Callus Smoother Scrub. You'll need 1 tablespoon of sea salt, 1 tablespoon of calendula oil, and three drops of orange, lavender, geranium, peppermint, or spearmint essential oil.

Combine the salt, the calendula oil, and whatever essential oil you choose in a small bowl until the salt is completely covered by the oils.

Calendula oil both moisturizes the skin and helps it heal faster, says Tourles. Peppermint, spearmint, and orange oils are very stimulating. They're a great way to start the day if you use the scrub in the morning. If you're using it before bedtime, try either lavender or geranium essential oil, both of which are very relaxing.

**2.** Three times a week, fill a basin with enough warm water to cover your ankles, add 1 cup of apple-cider vinegar, and soak your feet for 10 to 15 minutes. The natural fruit acids in the vinegar will immediately soften any type of hard skin, says Tourles.

**3.** After your soak, use firm, regular pressure to massage the scrub into the calloused areas of your feet. Spend a minimum of 2 to 3 minutes on each foot, but feel free to massage your feet with the scrub for as long as you'd like.

**4.** Rinse your feet with warm water and rub them dry with a rough towel.

**5.** Massage some castor oil into each calloused area and put on a pair of socks. "Castor oil really helps to heal dry skin," says Tourles, "because it is very thick and has great staying power."

## HOMEOPATHY: *The Right Stuff*

Homeopathic remedies can sometimes help heal a corn or callus, says Steven Subotnick, D.P.M., a podiatrist in Berkeley and San Leandro, California. The trick with homeopathy is choosing the right remedy. Here are Dr. Subotnick's guidelines for treating a callus.

• If you have hard, horny calluses, painful heels, and brittle nails; if you are frequently irritable and crave pickles; and if direct sunlight makes you feel worse, try Antimonium crudum.
• If your calluses are extremely thick, your skin is dirty-looking and fissured, and you also have corns, try Graphites.

• If your calluses are hard and firm and you have cold feet, try Silicea.

• If your skin is dry, rough, and scaly; you have burning pain in the affected area; you're a typically fearful person; and your calluses feel worse when they're scratched, try Arsenicum album.

• If your calluses are very thick and they burn, try Sulphur.

• If your calluses feel worse when your feet are hanging down, try Ranunculus bulbosus.

Homeopathic remedies also may help heal soft corns, the kind that are softened by sweat and usually form between the toes, says Dr. Subotnick. Here are his recommendations.

• If your feet perspire, smell, and are raw or irritated, try the remedy Silicea.

• If they itch intensely, try Natrum muriaticum or Zinc.

• If you have athlete's foot–like cracks on your feet, but no redness or itching, and have soft corns between your toes, try Baryta carbonicum.

Take a 6C potency of the appropriate remedy, following the dosage instructions on the label. Take one homeopathic remedy at a time, and stop taking it as soon as you feel better. If your condition doesn't improve in a short time, consult a homeopathic physician.

# Stop Infection and Speed Healing of
# Cuts and Scrapes

Red alert!

The sight of blood is always alarming, particularly when it's your own. Chop your thumb along with the carrots or take a spill from your bike and scrape a knee, and the first thing you want is for the bleeding (and the pain) to stop.

If you have an inadvertent incision that needs some TLC, you can try any combination of these alternative home remedies.

## CALENDULA: *Spray-On Relief*

After washing the wound, use a nonalcoholic calendula spray, says Beverly Yates, N.D., a naturopathic physician and director of the Natural Health Care Group in Seattle. "It helps stop infection and aids in healing," she says. Apply the calendula three or four times a day, always lightly rebandaging the wound when you're finished. "You want to protect the wound but also allow as much air as possible to reach it," says Dr. Yates.

---

# GUIDE TO PROFESSIONAL CARE

If you've cut yourself, you need to see a doctor if the bleeding is severe and doesn't stop within 10 minutes or so; the cut is so deep that you can see muscle or bone; it is more than an inch long; you have multiple cuts and scrapes; or the injury is on your face or other noticeable area. If debris such as cinders or gravel is embedded in the wound, your doctor may need to numb the area and clean the wound. Also, if you haven't had a tetanus shot in the past 10 years, you may need a booster.

See a doctor as soon as possible if you develop a fever or swollen lymph nodes and there's redness, swelling, and tenderness or oozing pus at the site of the injury a day or two after you've been hurt. These are signs of infection. And, if you have mitral valve prolapse, an artificial heart valve, or a hip replacement, and you get a deep cut, you need to seek medical attention.

Cuts of all kinds usually heal more quickly if you add vitamin E, zinc, and beta-carotene to your nutritional plan, says Beverly Yates, N.D., a naturopathic physician and director of the Natural Health Care Group in Seattle. Since you may need to take larger doses of these nutrients than are usually recommended, however, do this only under the guidance of a physician, she says.

## An Herbal Cream for Your "Boo-Boo"

This homemade herbal cream is "magic" for scratches, scrapes, shallow cuts, small bites, bruises, or small first- or second-degree burns, says Pamela Fischer, founder and director of the Ohlone Center for Herbal Studies in Concord, California.

All three herbal ingredients are thought to help to soothe pain, reduce swelling, and speed healing. A cream works better than other healing mediums, says Fischer, because it lets the herbal medicine stay next to the wound.

Here are her step-by-step directions for making your own Boo-Boo Cream. Apply it three or four times a day or as needed for minor irritation and abrasions.

**1.** Combine equal parts of dried comfrey root, calendula flower, and plantain.

**2.** Grind the herbs in a clean coffee grinder. (Fischer recommends that you invest in a coffee grinder that you can dedicate to grinding herbs.)

**3.** Pour the mixture into a jar.

**4.** Add enough extra-virgin olive oil to cover the herbs, measuring the number of ounces that you use for later reference. The plant material may float to the surface, so you may have to put something on top of the herb mixture to weigh it down. Fischer suggests using a few clean stones.

**5.** Cover the jar and let the mixture sit for a week.

**6.** After a week, strain the mixture through a piece of cheesecloth or an old, clean T-shirt into another jar. There should be no plant material in the new jar.

**7.** Put a saucepan on the stove over low heat and grate beeswax into the pan until the wax is completely melted. Use ¼ to ½ ounce of wax for each ounce of olive oil that you used for the herbs.

**8.** Pour the melted wax into the jar of oil.

**9.** Pour that mixture into a small salve jar and let it "set up," or harden, for 1 hour, says Fischer. Once it's hardened, close the jar tightly. "Store the cream in your first-aid kit," she says.

## MASSAGE: *To Calm You*

A cut can shock your system, particularly if it's a little bit deep and bloody. To calm yourself (or someone else who's been cut), place the palm of one hand on your forehead and the palm of the other on the back of your head so that your palms are at the same level and facing each other. Keep your hands in place for 30 to 60 seconds while taking a few deep breaths.

"There are points on the head called emotional stress points, and this technique gently stimulates them and calms you down," says Kate Montgomery, a licensed massage therapist in San Diego. You can use this technique not just for cuts, she says, but also anytime that you've had a physical shock and need to calm yourself.

## HOMEOPATHY: *Arnica to Speed Healing*

Dissolve two pellets of the 6C potency of Arnica montana under your tongue up to four times a day for up to 4 days, says Dr. Yates. "This is the best homeopathic remedy for any kind of minor trauma to the skin, such as a cut, scrape, or bruise," says Dr. Yates. "It reduces swelling and speeds healing." She advises anyone who is physically active to carry Arnica with them at all times.

## AROMATHERAPY: *To Fight Infection*

Put three drops each of bergamot, lavender, frankincense, and lemon essential oils and one drop of myrrh essential oil in 1 ounce of a carrier oil. such as sweet almond or jojoba, says Kal Kotecha, an aromatherapist in Waterloo, Ontario. Apply the mixture to the cut or scrape.

All of the oils in this formula are thought to fight infection, says Kotecha. Lemon oil helps stop bleeding, bergamot helps relieve pain and aids the skin in regenerating, lavender also helps stop pain and speed healing, and frankincense and myrrh calm the system.

## CALENDULA: *Soften Scars with Salve*

If you're prone to the large, moundlike scars called keloids, buy some calendula salve to use on the wound. It will help to soften or possibly lessen the scar, says Dr. Yates. Apply the salve twice daily to the scar for 2 to 4 weeks after the wound has healed and a scab has formed.

# *Essential Oils Can Defeat*
# **Dandruff**

If you have dandruff, don't use dandruff shampoos. Instead, treat your scalp with the essential oils of aromatherapy.

That's the advice of Barbara Close, an herbalist and aromatherapist in East Hampton, New York. "Dandruff is not a hair problem but a skin problem," she explains. "The flaking and itchiness are the result of an overproduction of a substance called sebum from glands in the scalp, and those glands are hyperactive because the scalp is excessively dry. Most dandruff shampoos have strong medications to control the symptoms of dandruff, but they don't do anything to address the underlying disorder—the dryness and poor health of the scalp."

In fact, she points out, dandruff shampoos often contain aggressive cleansers that destroy the scalp's delicate balance of water and oil, which further irritates the glands and perpetuates the problem.

Here are the natural remedies that alternative beauty experts think are the best and most effective ways to solve the problem of dandruff.

## AROMATHERAPY: *Dandruff-Diminishing Shampoo*

Roberta Wilson, an aromatherapist based in Albuquerque, New Mexico, has created an aromatherapy formula for a shampoo that can help normalize the water- and oil-secreting glands of the scalp, thus helping to eliminate dandruff.

To 8 ounces of unscented, mild shampoo, add 10 drops of tea tree oil, 8 drops of cedarwood oil, 6 drops of pine oil, 6 drops of rosemary oil, 4 drops of clary sage oil, and 4 drops of lemon oil. "These essential oils encourage your body's systems to go into action to heal the problems that are causing the dandruff," she says.

Tea tree oil is antiseptic, helping to normalize the bacteria on

## GUIDE TO
## PROFESSIONAL CARE

There are many possible causes of dandruff, including a yeast infection of the scalp or hormone imbalances. If you have tried self-care treatments for 2 to 3 months but your dandruff persists, see a dermatologist for an accurate diagnosis and possible medical treatment with a prescription shampoo and topical steroid medications.

the scalp. Rosemary and cedarwood are thought to increase circulation to the scalp. Pine encourages elimination of toxins from the skin of the scalp. Clary sage helps regulate and balance oil production, and lemon encourages elimination of toxins and promotes internal cleansing. Use the shampoo several times a week, Wilson says.

### ROSEMARY ESSENTIAL OIL: *To Reduce Flaking*

It's believed that essential oil of rosemary can increase circulation, stimulate the scalp, and reduce flaking, according to Close. Put two to three drops of oil in a tablespoon of a rich, fatty carrier oil such as avocado oil, then massage the mixture into your scalp for 1 to 2 minutes once a day.

### EUCALYPTUS: *A Rinse to Tone the Scalp*

The leaves of the eucalyptus tree help fight infection and tone skin, and they have a long history of use by herbalists for treating dandruff, says Brigitte Mars, an herbalist and nutritional consultant in Boulder, Colorado.

To make a rinse with eucalyptus, put 4 heaping teaspoons of dried leaves in a quart of boiling water and stir. Then cover, remove from the heat, and steep for an hour. Strain the liquid into a large plastic squeeze bottle and add 1 tablespoon of apple-cider vinegar. After you've taken a shower, pour the rinse slowly over your hair. "For maximum effect, don't rinse it out—just let it dry," says Mars. Use this herbal rinse each time you shower.

## MASSAGE: *Sesame Oil for Dryness*

In Ayurveda, the ancient system of natural healing from India, dandruff is a symptom of a body-wide condition of "vata," or dryness. For that reason, Pratima Raichur, an Ayurvedic practitioner in New York City, recommends massaging the scalp twice a week with warm sesame oil, which will combat the excessive dryness.

"It is also very calming and soothing to the system, which is important, since dandruff is sometimes caused or complicated by anxiety," she says.

Massage the oil into your scalp before bed, spending about 10 minutes working it into the entire area. Then wrap your head in a hot towel and leave the towel on for 10 minutes or, for optimum moisturizing, all night. Wash it out the next day.

## SELENIUM: *Relieve Flaking and Itching*

The mineral selenium can help relieve the flaking and itching of dandruff, according to Earl Mindell, Ph.D., a nutritionist and pharmacist in Beverly Hills. Medical science doesn't know exactly why the mineral works, but Dr. Mindell says that he has seen it help people eliminate dandruff many times. He recommends taking a 200-microgram supplement daily.

## VITAMIN E: *Balance the Oils*

Dr. Raichur recommends taking a capsule of 400 international units of vitamin E a day to help balance the oils on the scalp and relieve dryness.

## ZINC: *Help Your Scalp Heal*

Dr. Raichur also recommends the trace mineral zinc, which rebuilds skin and can help your scalp heal from dandruff. She advises her clients with dandruff to take 15 to 20 milligrams daily.

# *Mood-Lifting, Drug-Free*
## *Ways to Ease*
## **Depression**

There's good news for most people with depression—the constant sad and empty feelings, the loss of pleasure in the ordinary activities of life, the disruptions of appetite and sleep. You don't need to take antidepressant drugs to start feeling better.

---

## GUIDE TO
## PROFESSIONAL CARE

There is a difference between the depressed response, which could be called a cold of the soul and can be self-treated, and clinical depression, which is like a serious, ongoing viral infection and needs professional care, says Jonathan Zuess, M.D., a psychiatrist at the Good Samaritan Regional Medical Center in Phoenix.

If your depression has lasted longer than 2 weeks and includes a mixture of symptoms such as a depressed mood most of the day, loss of interest and pleasure in life, loss of appetite, disturbed sleep, fatigue, and poor concentration, it is clinical depression, and you need to seek professional care. Thoughts of suicide at any time are another sign that you need immediate help.

Some professional care for depression consists of little more than a prescription for an antidepressant drug, Dr. Zuess says. While antidepressants can be very useful tools in some circumstances, he says, to really cure clinical depression, they should be used as part of a treatment program that emphasizes natural medicine and counseling. He recommends finding a naturally oriented medical doctor or naturopathic physician.

"If people change their lifestyles, particularly their nutritional intakes and their levels of exercise, they can often resolve depression without drugs," says Joel Robertson, Pharm.D., president of the Robertson Institute in Saginaw, Michigan.

Of course, people who are severely depressed, particularly those who are having suicidal thoughts, should see a doctor immediately and may need a period of medication to control their problem. For most people, however, alternative remedies are a good way to deal with depression, says Dr. Robertson.

### 5-HTP: *Acts like Prozac*

Are you mildly depressed? Take the supplement 5-hydroxytryptophan (5-HTP) before you try prescription antidepressants, says Othniel Seiden, M.D., a physician in Denver.

That's because this supplement is thought to work the same way as fluoxetine (Prozac) and similar antidepressant drugs such as paroxetine (Paxil) and sertraline (Zoloft): It increases levels of serotonin, a brain chemical that fights depression.

Start with 100 milligrams of 5-HTP at bedtime, says Dr. Seiden. If you don't notice any positive results after 3 days—if you're not feeling less depressed and sleeping better—increase the dosage to 200 milligrams, taking 100 milligrams when you wake up in the morning and 100 milligrams before bed.

If there is still no change in your mood after 3 days at 200 milligrams, increase the dose to 400 milligrams, divided equally between morning and night. If you still feel depressed at this point, discontinue the nutrient. It's unlikely to help you. (Although 5-HTP is very safe, Dr. Seiden says not to take dosages higher than 400 milligrams.)

It's safe to take up to 400 milligrams for several weeks after you're feeling better, then try to reduce the dosage. If your symptoms do not recur, wean yourself off completely.

### SAM-E: *An Effective Antidepressant*

The supplement S-adenosylmethionine (SAM-e) can be just as effective in treating depression as tricyclic antidepressant drugs such as imipramine (Tofranil) and amitriptyline (Elavil), says Jonathan Zuess, M.D., a psychiatrist at the Good Samaritan Regional Medical Center in Phoenix.

The supplement is synthesized from the amino acid methionine, and it is believed to improve "methylation" in the body, a process that increases the effects of neurotransmitters, including serotonin. Dr. Zuess recommends 1,600 milligrams of SAM-e a day.

### FATTY ACIDS: *Fishing for Health*

Studies show that people who eat large amounts of fish have one-tenth the rate of depression as people who don't—and the reason is probably eicosapentaenoic acid (EPA) and docosahexaenoic acid (DHA), two forms of fat (or, more technically, omega-3 fatty acids) that are present in fish, Dr. Zuess says.

Scientists don't know exactly how omega-3's protect against depression, but they do know that the fats are important to the health of neurons, or brain cells. To get sufficient omega-3's to battle depression, Dr. Zuess recommends taking approximately 10 grams a day of DHA and EPA, which usually amounts to about 30 fish-oil capsules daily. Take them in divided doses with meals. This remedy is safe for long-term use.

### ST. JOHN'S WORT: *An Uplifting Herb*

Mild and moderate depressions respond well to the herb St. John's wort, says Hyla Cass, M.D., assistant professor of psychiatry at the University of California, Los Angeles, School of Medicine.

What can you expect when you take the herb? "Within a week to 10 days, many people notice improved sleep, followed by improvements in appetite, energy levels, and physical well-being," says Dr. Cass. "By the second or third week, there may be a reduction in emotional symptoms, with less anxiety, a more positive mood, and a greater sense of peace.

"While it can work fairly quickly in some people, don't expect instant results," she says. "It can take up to 6 weeks to reach its full effect."

How much should you take? "The best dose is the lowest dose that works for you," says Dr. Cass. Start with 300 milligrams a day and increase by 300 milligrams every few days until you reach the full dose of 900 milligrams.

Take your daily dosage in three doses, one with each meal. You can continue taking St. John's wort for several months, since long-term use appears to be safe, says Dr. Cass.

St. John's wort comes in capsules, tablets, or tincture standardized to contain 0.3 percent hypericin. While there are many other compounds in the extract, this is used as a marker to ensure consistency.

## MAGNET THERAPY: *An Ancient Chinese Remedy*

Various acupuncture points are thought to help remedy depression, says Rosa Schnyer, an acupuncturist in Tucson. You can give yourself a longer treatment by taping magnets over the points and wearing them for 4 to 8 hours at a time, says Schnyer.

To help counter depression, put one magnet on the point called LI4, located on the top of the hand between the thumb and the index finger, at the highest spot on the muscle when the thumb and index finger are close together, says Schnyer.

The second point, LV3, is on the top of the foot between the first and second toes and about 2 inches from the web, toward the body. Women should use the hand point on the right side and the foot point on the left; men should use the left hand point and right foot point. (For the exact location, see An Illustrated Guide to Acupressure Points on page 700.)

"These points calm the mind and settle the spirit," says Schnyer. She says to use magnets of 400 to 800 gauss (the unit of measurement for magnets), taping them on the body with first-aid tape and leaving them on for as long as you'd like. (Refrigerator magnets aren't strong enough.)

## FLOWER ESSENCES: *Feel the Light*

Flower essences are not the same as herbal remedies, says Patricia Kaminski, cofounder and codirector of the Flower Essence Society, based in Nevada City, California. They are "soul medicine," allowing the person to become aware of and outgrow negative thoughts and feelings that can block the soul's full expression of creativity and love.

"Many of us are unable to feel light as our spiritual essence, so the soul feels dark and heavy," Kaminski says. "St. John's wort flower essence helps us to feel the light in ourselves, to feel connected to a higher source of spiritual identity." Take four drops of St. John's wort essence under your tongue four times a day. Most flower essences are used for about a month at a time, Kaminski says.

Here are some of her other recommendations for flower essences that can help relieve depression. As with St. John's wort, take four drops four times a day. You can use more than one remedy at a time.

• Scotch broom, for severe pessimism—the feeling of "What's the use?" or that the entire world is against you in some way
• Gentian, for people who experience discouragement or defeat easily, such as a student who gets a low grade and finds it hard to resume his studies
• Wild rose, to help depressed people recapture their ideals and their drive and their enthusiasm and spirit of giving

## Things to Do Today

In addition to the alternative remedies above, things that you do every day, such as how much time you spend outdoors, how much you exercise, or what music you listen to, can play a role in beating depression.

### LIGHT: *Your Day in the Sun*
Your body needs sunlight; getting too little can disturb the production of key hormones and brain chemicals, triggering depression. The solution: "Light up your life," says Dr. Zuess.
The best way is to spend 30 minutes outdoors every morning before noon, when the light is brightest. If you can't do that, at least be outside sometime during the day for a minimum of 15 minutes.

### EXERCISE: *A Universal Prescription*
The changes in brain chemistry provoked by exercise appear to parallel those of the major antidepressant drugs, says Keith W. Johnsgard, Ph.D., professor emeritus of psychology at San José State University in California.
"An hour a day of exercise 7 days a week is my universal prescription for people who are depressed," he says.
For the best antidepressant results, walk outside for an hour a day in the early morning, says Dr. Zuess.

### MUSIC: *Tune Out Unhappiness*
"Music lifts depression," says Dr. Zuess. Based on scientific research, he recommends Vienna waltzes and Mozart's piano concertos, or any gentle, melodic music with upbeat lyrics.

# *A Mineral Deficiency May Trigger Many Cases of*
# **Dermatitis**

There are many different types of dermatitis, a skin rash that can be red, itchy, swollen, oozing, crusty, scaly, or any combination of those symptoms. There is irritant contact dermatitis. Allergic contact. Photocontact. Atopic (also called eczema). Nummular. Seborrheic. Hand. Perioral.

Although a dermatologist can figure out which kind of dermatitis you have, he may not be able to do much about getting rid of it.

"Dermatologists can often accurately diagnose a dermatitis, but quite often, their therapies are terribly ineffective," says Andrew Rubman, N.D., a naturopathic physician and founder of the Southbury Clinic for Traditional Medicine in Connecticut.

Most conventional treatments fall into either of two categories. One is topical—a cream, salve, or other application that provides some degree of symptomatic relief. The other is oral—a prescription drug that suppresses bacteria or a virus that may be associated with the problem.

According to Dr. Rubman, however, most of the organisms associated with the dermatitis were living peacefully on your skin before the problem started. Somehow, the skin became less healthy, allowing the organisms to multiply and a rash to begin. The unrecognized cause of this weak skin, he says, is often a deficiency of the trace mineral selenium.

## SELENIUM: *Stop the Organism Overgrowth*

In your body, selenium hooks up with other substances to form a compound called glutathione peroxidase, which allows the immune system to "sample" the organisms that are inhabiting but not yet overgrowing the outer layer of the skin.

If the organisms are harmful in type or number, immune warriors are alerted, and they reduce or eliminate the threatening population. "Glutathione is the Rambo of the skin," says Dr. Rubman.

If you're selenium-deficient, however, the skin doesn't have that powerful advance warning system. "Without enough selenium in your diet and supplement regimen, I believe it's impossible to improve the body's resistance to many different types of dermatitis beyond a certain level," Dr. Rubman says.

To make matters worse, it's not that easy to get enough selenium from either food or supplements. Intensive farming practices have depleted the soil of the mineral, while food processing removes even more. And if you try to get your missing selenium from a supplement, you may be out of luck. Many supplements contain a form of the mineral that is poorly absorbed and therefore poorly utilized, Dr. Rubman says.

To make sure that you're getting enough selenium, he recommends an easily absorbed liquid form of the mineral, and his favored product is Aqua Sel, manufactured by T. E. Neesby. This supplement provides odorless, colorless, tasteless drops of a very bioavailable form of the mineral. Dr. Rubman recommends taking about 190 micrograms of selenium a day for the

## GUIDE TO
## PROFESSIONAL CARE

If you have any of the symptoms of dermatitis—dry, red, cracked, or thickened skin or persistent itching—for more than a few weeks, you need to see a dermatologist to determine the exact cause of the rash. Instead of dermatitis, it may be an allergy or similar sensitivity. If it is dermatitis, a dermatologist can only control the condition, not cure it.

That is why Andrew Rubman, N.D., a naturopathic physician and founder of the Southbury Clinic for Traditional Medicine in Connecticut, recommends seeing a naturally oriented health practitioner such as a naturopath, who can help you design a program that will not only relieve the symptoms of the rash but also improve your overall health and strengthen your immune system to avoid future outbreaks.

duration of the problem. If the symptoms don't improve within 6 weeks, it's time to consult a doctor.

## ANTIOXIDANTS: *Helping Injured Skin Heal*

Antioxidants can help repair damaged skin by disarming free radicals, the unstable molecules that oxidize or destroy healthy cells. Free radicals can be produced as by-products of the body's fight against the inflammation of dermatitis as well as by exposure to sunlight, smoking, eating fatty foods, and many other lifestyle factors. By muting free radicals, antioxidants not only help the dermatitis heal, they may also help prevent future flare-ups.

Here are what Dr. Rubman considers the most important antioxidants for the health of your skin. Again, if the problem doesn't clear up within 6 weeks, consult a doctor.

- Beta-carotene: 12 to 18 milligrams daily
- Vitamin C: 3,000 milligrams a day in three divided doses (at least ½ hour before or 1½ hours after meals, since stomach acid and the content of the meal can destroy C)
- Vitamin E: 600 to 800 international units daily
- Zinc: 20 milligrams a day for women; 30 milligrams a day for men (men need more because the prostate concentrates zinc in the gland and in seminal fluid)

## FATTY ACIDS: *Reduce the Inflammation*

Certain components in oils, called fatty acids, can help reduce inflammation and ease dermatitis, Dr. Rubman says. For the best combination of the full range of anti-inflammatory fatty acids, look for a supplement that contains oils from flaxseed and borage seed and omega-3, omega-6, and omega-9 oils from fish. He favors a product called Perfect Oils, manufactured by Nutritional Therapeutics. If you can't find that brand, look for a product that provides the ingredients listed above. Follow the dosage recommendations on the label.

## FOOD: *Avoid These Causes of Dermatitis*

A sensitivity to certain foods in your diet can cause dermatitis, says Bradley Bongiovanni, N.D., a naturopathic physician in Cambridge, Massachusetts. A blood test that detects food sensitivities, called an IgG (immunoglobulin G) test, is a very accurate way to discover foods that may cause an allergic reaction. You can also do a self-test by eliminating the most common dermatitis-causing culprits one by one to see if you get any relief.

The most common trigger is dairy products. To start your health experiment, cut dairy products out of your diet for 30 days. If your symptoms improve, you have very strong evidence that dairy is the cause. Then reinstate dairy in your diet for 1 week. If symptoms return, you know that these foods are responsible. If you forgo dairy products, however, it's very important to replace the calcium that you'll miss. You can do that either by taking a calcium supplement or increasing your intake of other calcium-rich foods such as nuts, seeds, and leafy green vegetables.

If eliminating dairy doesn't make a difference or doesn't completely solve the problem, use the same elimination test for the following foods, one by one: wheat, sugar, citrus fruits, corn, soy, peanut butter, chocolate, coffee, and alcohol. In this way, work through all the offenders, month by month, food by food, until you find those that are triggering the problem.

Another way to do this is to eliminate all of the potential offenders from your diet at once for 30 days, then reintroduce them one by one to find the culprit. This speeds up the detection process, but be sure to take a multivitamin supplement while you're doing the test to keep your strength (and health) up.

## Topical Relief—Naturally

Many different types of natural remedies, including essential oils, herbs, and formulations from Chinese medicine, can provide relief from the symptoms of dermatitis.

### AROMATHERAPY: *First-Rate Relief*
A combination of the anti-inflammatory essential oils German chamomile and high-Alpine lavender is considered one of the best therapies for soothing dermatitis, says Barbara Close, an aromatherapist and herbalist in East Hampton, New York.

Put three to four drops of each oil in a base of 1 ounce of borage or evening primrose oil, both of which contain nutritional factors that are thought to decrease inflammation. Apply the mixture to affected areas as needed until the irritation disappears. If the irritation worsens or does not abate after 3 days, discontinue use and see your doctor for treatment.

## To Help Control Eczema, Calm Your Emotions with Meditation

Stress can cause or contribute to flare-ups of eczema, but the ancient Indian healing system of Ayurveda offers an antidote: Sit comfortably in a quiet room where you won't be disturbed, close your eyes, and meditate for about 15 minutes.

"Meditation can help a person with eczema release the stress they've accumulated during the day," says Pratima Raichur, an Ayurvedic practitioner in New York City.

During your meditation, Dr. Raichur recommends using the mantra "Vam" (pronounce the "a" like the "e" in the word *the*).

"Let your attention go easily to the mantra," she says. "Repeat it aloud softly and at a natural pace, not too fast or too slow. As you repeat it, let your voice gradually get softer and softer, until the mantra is an unspoken thought."

If you notice that you've forgotten the mantra or been distracted in some way, gently reintroduce it into your mind. "Do not strain to focus on the sound or try to control your thought," she says. "That would create even more stress. Just maintain the attitude that whatever happens, happens. Just try to stay in the mood."

## HORSETAIL: *Relief for Eczema*

Horsetail is an ancient emollient herb that can be very helpful in soothing the discomfort of eczema, says Norma Pasekoff Weinberg, an herbal educator in Cape Cod, Massachusetts.

To make a horsetail compress, put 1 teaspoon of dried or crushed fresh horsetail stems in 1 cup of water and boil for 10 to 15 minutes. Remove from the heat and let cool until the liquid is just comfortably warm to the skin. Immerse a clean, soft, cotton kitchen towel in the boiled water, then squeeze out the excess liquid. Wrap the towel around the inflamed area and cover with another dry, heavy towel. "Keep the compress wrapped around the area for at least 10 minutes," says Weinberg.

Do this treatment at least twice a day until the symptoms disappear. After each treatment, apply a few drops of pure avocado oil. If the problem persists after a week, see your doctor.

**CHINESE HERBS:** *Reduce Redness and Swelling*
The remedy Hua Tuo is a cream containing a number of Chinese herbs that can reduce the redness and swelling of dermatitis, says David E. Molony, Ph.D., a licensed acupuncturist and director of Lehigh Valley Acupuncture Center in Catasauqua, Pennsylvania. Apply as needed until symptoms disappear.

# Breakthroughs in Treating and Preventing
# Diabetes (Type 1)

To conventional doctors, Type 1 diabetes is a classic example of an autoimmune disease. That means that the immune system mistakenly identifies part of the body as an outside invader and attacks it with substances called antibodies.

According to conventional medicine, Type 1 (insulin-dependent) diabetes occurs because the immune system attacks and kills the cells of the pancreas, the organ that produces the hormone insulin, which ushers blood sugar (glucose) out of the bloodstream and into the cells of the body. To make up for the shortfall of insulin, people with Type 1 diabetes must take insulin injections. And, since Type 1 diabetes typically begins in childhood, that means a lifetime of insulin dependency.

There are some alternative doctors, however, who believe that the cause—and treatment—of Type 1 diabetes is radically different from what conventional medicine espouses. Here are three diet-related steps that some alternative health practitioners believe can help prevent or treat this disease.

# GUIDE TO PROFESSIONAL CARE

*Caution: You should use the alternative remedies discussed in this chapter only as part of a treatment program that is guided and monitored by a qualified medical doctor in partnership with a qualified alternative practitioner, both of whom are experienced in caring for your condition. Check with your conventional doctor before changing or stopping any conventional medical treatments or medications, and keep all of your doctors and/or alternative practitioners informed of all treatments that you are receiving.*

About 5 to 10 percent of people with diabetes have Type 1. It's sometimes called juvenile diabetes because it's usually diagnosed before age 20, but it can occur at any age. Anyone who experiences frequent urination, increased appetite and thirst, fatigue, unexplained weight loss, and decreased consciousness (possibly leading to coma), should arrange for a visit to a doctor or go to the emergency room if the symptoms are severe.

## COW'S MILK: *A Must to Avoid*

"If the genes for Type 1 diabetes are in your family, meaning that any relative has had the disease, you are putting your children at risk for developing Type 1 diabetes by feeding them cow's milk instead of breast-feeding," says Jonathan Wright, M.D., a nutritionally oriented physician and director of the Tahoma Clinic in Kent, Washington.

Some international doctors and scientists in diabetes research say that cow's milk is a cause of Type 1 diabetes, Dr. Wright says. Here's why.

In a study conducted in Finland, researchers looked at blood specimens from more than 100 children with newly diagnosed Type 1 diabetes. In every child, they found "exceptionally high levels" of an antibody to a part of the protein in cow's milk. Next, the researchers discovered that the sequence of amino acids (the chemical building blocks of protein) in the cow's milk protein was exactly the same as the sequence of amino acids in the insulin-producing islet cells of the pancreas.

"In other words," says Dr. Wright, "they theorize that diabetes is not an autoimmune disease, as is commonly thought. It may be an intense allergic reaction to cow's milk, and the antibodies created during that allergic reaction also 'cross-react' with the islet cells of the pancreas, destroying them."

A group of Italian scientists who looked at the Finnish study decided to conduct additional research, investigating the correlation between their country's various levels of milk consumption and the prevalence of Type 1 diabetes. (Milk consumption is high in the north of Italy and low in the south.) They found what scientists call a direct correlation—the higher the consumption of milk, the higher the incidence of the disease.

If dairy products are the cause, cutting them out is the solution, Dr. Wright believes. "The first thing we tell the parents of a child newly diagnosed with Type 1 diabetes is 'Pour the cow's milk down the drain and throw the dairy products in the garbage,'" he says. This, he believes, stops the destruction of insulin-producing pancreatic islet cells and either helps keep children from becoming dependent on insulin injections or dramatically reduces the amount of insulin they need to take each day.

But stopping the intake of dairy foods may also prevent Type 1 diabetes, he believes. "If there is any history of Type 1 diabetes in your family, but your children have not developed the disease, my advice is to never allow them to consume any cow's milk or other dairy products," Dr. Wright says.

## GLUTEN: *A Likely Suspect*

Gluten is a protein found in wheat, rye, oats, barley, and other grains. (Buckwheat, rice, and corn are the exceptions.) Although Dr. Wright says that gluten isn't a proven cause of Type 1 diabetes, he believes it's definitely a suspect. That's because gluten can trigger another hereditary allergic condition called celiac disease, a severe intestinal illness. Certain human leukocyte antigens (HLA) that are associated with celiac disease are also associated with the development of Type 1 diabetes.

"If gluten triggers one allergic disease, it may have something to do with another, and we want to try to eliminate all the possible causes of Type 1 diabetes from the diet," Dr. Wright says.

To remove the gluten from your child's diet, you'll need to avoid all foods containing the grains mentioned above. You'll also need to steer clear of a wide variety of common gluten-containing foods and ingredients, such as distilled white vinegar, hydrolized vegetable protein, and malt extract. Fortunately, says Dr. Wright, there are many cookbooks available that will help you shop for and prepare food that's gluten-free.

## NIACINAMIDE: *To the Rescue*

Niacinamide, one of the B vitamins, is the number one nutrient for treating Type 1 diabetes, says Dr. Wright. He describes a scientific study in which experimental animals were given chemicals that kill the islet cells of the pancreas, instantly causing diabetes. When a group of the animals was given niacinamide before ingesting the chemicals, however, none of them developed diabetes; the nutrient shielded the islet cells from harm.

"If we give enough niacinamide early enough in the progress of the disease, it is possible to 'rescue' pancreatic islet cells and restore more function to the pancreas, either eliminating or decreasing the need for insulin injections," he says.

For young patients, Dr. Wright prescribes 1 gram (1,000 milligrams) of niacinamide twice a day or 0.5-gram (500 milligrams) three times a day. For adults who develop Type 1 diabetes, he prescribes 1 gram three times a day.

In the vast majority of patients, this level of niacinamide intake doesn't have side effects, Dr. Wright says. Occasionally, however, the vitamin will tax the liver slightly, causing nausea, and the dosage should be reduced. He adds that no one should take this nutrient without the approval and supervision of a doctor or other health professional experienced in the prescriptive use of supplements.

## Exercise Your Right to Less Insulin

People with Type 1 diabetes who exercise for 35 to 40 minutes 3 or 4 days a week may be able to cut their insulin needs by 20 to 25 percent, says Eric P. Durak, director of Medical Health and Fitness in Santa Barbara, California, and an expert on diabetes and exercise. Reducing insulin needs by that amount means that they may need fewer insulin shots overall, putting much less wear and tear on injection sites.

Durak suggests that for maximum enjoyment and fitness, people with Type 1 diabetes include different kinds of exercise in their sessions: a bit of aerobic exercise (such as brisk walking or jogging), a bit of strength training (working out with weights), and a bit of stretching.

# Eat Right and Exercise
## to Control
# Diabetes (Type 2)

If you're a typical American, you're also a sugarholic: One of every five calories you eat is from sugar (in the form of sucrose, fructose, and other sweeteners), for a grand total of 140 pounds of sugar a year.

For many of us, that huge quantity of sugar isn't a huge problem. When you chow down on a bowl of ice cream or chug a sugary soda, your pancreas, a digestive organ, shifts into fifth gear, secreting large amounts of the hormone insulin. The insulin quickly trucks the sugar (in the form of glucose) out of your bloodstream and into your cells for use or storage.

About 6 percent of us, however, don't have the genetic makeup to cope with a lifelong sugar overload. If you're in that group (and there's no definitive way to know who is and who isn't), eventually—usually sometime in your forties or fifties—some of the insulin receptors in your cells can go on strike and refuse to accept any more sugar deliveries, stranding excess sugar in the bloodstream. Also, the amount of insulin that your body produces is reduced. The result is Type 2 (non-insulin-dependent) diabetes, or high blood sugar.

Nearly 15 million Americans have to contend with this condition. Excess sugar in the blood damages the arteries and veins and can lead to fatal heart disease and stroke. (The death rate for middle-aged people with Type 2 diabetes is twice that of middle-aged people who do not have it.)

The glut of sugar can also cause kidney disease, eye problems, and severe nerve damage to the lower limbs and other parts of the body. (People with diabetes account for more than 50 percent of the lower limb amputations performed in the United States each year.)

If you have Type 2 diabetes, changes in the way you eat (and exercise, of course) may be your ticket back to good health, says Jonathan Wright, M.D., a nutritionally oriented physician and director of the Tahoma Clinic in Kent, Washington. Here's what he suggests.

# GUIDE TO
# PROFESSIONAL CARE

*Caution: You should use the alternative remedies discussed in this chapter only as part of a treatment program that is guided and monitored by a qualified medical doctor in partnership with a qualified alternative practitioner, both of whom are experienced in caring for your condition. Check with your conventional doctor before changing or stopping any conventional medical treatments or medications, and keep all of your doctors and/or alternative practitioners informed of all treatments that you are receiving.*

Diabetes is a serious illness that should always be monitored by a doctor. Its symptoms include increased thirst, urination, or appetite; dry mouth; vomiting; diarrhea; blurred vision; rapid or irregular heartbeat; dizziness; unintentional weight loss; and recurrent yeast or urinary tract infections. If you have any of these for longer than a week, see your physician for a diagnosis.

Once you've checked with your doctor, you may be able to control type 2 diabetes with the dietary suggestions in this chapter. A nutritionally oriented physician can also help you develop a dietary program that includes high doses of certain supplements. For example, many scientific studies have shown that the mineral chromium has the power to help normalize blood sugar levels. Most of these studies have used 200 micrograms a day of a form called chromium picolinate.

In his clinic, however, as part of an overall program, Jonathan Wright, M.D., a nutritionally oriented physician and director of the Tahoma Clinic in Kent, Washington, has found that higher doses of chromium in the form of chromium polynicotinate work much more rapidly to lessen the symptoms of Type 2 diabetes.

"By prescribing a high dosage, I've found that my patients' sugar cravings go away a lot more rapidly, so they're able to make the switch to a healthy diet much more easily and quickly," Dr. Wright says. "I've also found that their more severe symptoms disappear faster."

Dr. Wright prescribes chromium polynicotinate because it "appears to be closest to the form of chromium found in glucose tolerance factor, the body's internal regulator of blood sugar."

He also says that some preliminary research indicates that the more commonly used chromium picolinate may cause genetic damage, but that's under debate. For that reason, though, he thinks chromium polynicotinate is safer.

Dr. Wright emphasizes, however, that this level of chromium supplementation must be taken only with the approval and under the supervision of a doctor or other health care professional who is experienced in the prescriptive use of supplements.

## SUGAR AND REFINED FOODS: *Cut Back*

First, Dr. Wright believes, you should reduce sugar intake as well as minimize sugar's first cousin, the refined foods such as white bread and snack chips that contain white flour and other highly processed grains. Processed grains dump a load of glucose into the bloodstream.

### Stop the Damage with Bilberry

The smallest components of your circulatory system are the capillaries, the microscopic blood vessels that transfer nutrients and oxygen from the bloodstream into cells. In people with Type 2 diabetes, believes Jonathan Wright, M.D., a nutritionally oriented physician and director of the Tahoma Clinic in Kent, Washington, the membrane around each capillary slowly thickens.

The result can be, and frequently is, a health disaster—two to four times more heart disease and stroke than the national average for people without diabetes. Diabetic retinopathy, an eye disease that blinds up to 24,000 people with diabetes each year. Kidney disease, which causes loss of kidney function for nearly 100,000 people with diabetes yearly. And 60 percent of those with diabetes experience nervous system damage, often with numbness and pain in the feet and hands, that leads to tissue death and amputation in tens of thousands of cases.

Dr. Wright believes that one herb can help stop that capillary damage: bilberry. "Every person with Type 2 diabetes that I treat is given bilberry," he says.

In tests at his clinic, he has found that the thickened capillary membranes shrink to normal size after about 10 months of daily treatment with 80 milligrams of the herb.

"When the membrane returns to normal size, there is a much lower chance that the person with diabetes will develop heart failure, diabetic retinopathy, kidney disease, and all the other typical complications of diabetes," says Dr. Wright.

To make sure that you're getting the best-quality herb, Dr. Wright says to look for a brand with a label stating that the product is standardized to 24 percent anthocyanosides. This ensures that it contains a high concentration of the factors in bilberry, called flavonoids, that heal the capillaries.

He cautions, however, that people with Type 2 diabetes should not take bilberry on their own but should do so only with the approval and supervision of a physician or other certified health professional with experience in the therapeutic use of herbs.

## WHOLE FOODS: *Follow the Rainbow*

Add more whole foods, such as fruits, vegetables, grains, beans, nuts, and seeds, to your diet. They're rich in fiber and other nutritional factors that help stabilize blood sugar.

The simplest way to get a variety of whole foods is to try to eat every color each day, says Dr. Wright. Red tomatoes. Orange carrots. Yellow squash. Green salad. Blueberries. Brown rice. Black beans.

"If you make sure to eat a nutritional spectrum of colorful foods every day, and if you concentrate on getting those colors from whole foods, you will begin to control high blood sugar with diet," he says.

## FATTY ACIDS: *For Damage Control*

"I believe that supplements containing essential fatty acids, such as flaxseed oil, can help repair the cellular damage caused by a lifetime of consuming too much sugar," says Dr. Wright.

When shopping for a supplement, look for the words *high lignan* on the label. This indicates that the product is rich in the omega-3, omega-6, and omega-9 fatty acids, all of which are necessary for cellular healing.

Also, says Dr. Wright, if you're looking for liquid flaxseed oil instead of a capsule, look for a product that has been specially prepared using nitrogen. If that preparation method isn't used, the healthfulness of the oil is reduced during processing, he says. "A good product will tell you on the label that this was the preparation method," he says. Or look on the bottle of oil for a "use by" date. Follow the dosage recommendations on the label.

## EXERCISE: *Twice a Day, Every Day*

Studies have shown that people who exercise cut their risk of developing Type 2 diabetes by 24 percent. That's because exercise is insulin's best friend: It lends a helping hand, moving sugar out of the bloodstream and into the cells.

When muscles are fit, it takes less of the hormone to move sugar into muscle cells, says Eric P. Durak, director of Medical Health and Fitness in Santa Barbara, California, and an expert on diabetes and exercise.

If you have been diagnosed with Type 2 diabetes, you may need the insulin-regulating power of exercise, says Durak. The key to using exercise to normalize blood sugar, he believes, is to work out twice a day every day—once in the morning and once in the evening, for 15 to 20 minutes each time. If you have to eat three or more times a day to keep your blood sugar on an even keel, what makes you think that you can exercise at the often-recommended level of three times a week and still control your sugar levels? You can't, Durak says.

To create an enjoyable exercise routine that you can stay with for the rest of your life, Durak suggests that you do one type of exercise in the morning and another in the evening.

For your morning routine, he recommends doing anything that you enjoy, whether it's one of the gentler exercises like yoga or tai chi (a Chinese exercise routine of flowing movements) or a slightly more strenuous activity like working out with light weights. For your evening exercise, he suggests walking as the easiest way to get out and get going. (There's one caution, however. If you work out with weights, do it only every other day to avoid straining your muscles.)

## Restoring Energy—and Health—with Traditional Chinese Medicine

Type 2 diabetes is "an exhaustion syndrome caused by overindulging in sweet, fatty foods and wearing out the body," says Maoshing Ni, O.M.D., Ph.D., a doctor of Oriental medicine and director of the Tao of Wellness Center in Santa Monica, California.

The alternative home remedies of Traditional Chinese Medicine (TCM) are aimed at curing exhaustion by stimulating energy-restoring points on your body, eating energy-building foods, and taking energy-giving herbs.

Before using TCM remedies, however, "you should inform your allopathic physician (a doctor who uses Western or nonalternative medicine) about what you are going to be doing," says Dr. Ni. And, if you are taking insulin, "you should carefully monitor your blood sugar levels with your doctor before you adjust your medication," he says.

### Say "Ha-a-a-a-a-a"

When you're under stress, your adrenal glands pump out the hormone cortisol, which hampers insulin's ability to clear your blood of sugar. For people with diabetes, that's a lose-lose situation.

There's an easy way to counter that stress and help normalize your blood sugar, says Virender Sodhi, M.D. (Ayurved), N.D., an Ayurvedic and naturopathic physician and director of the American School of Ayurvedic Sciences in Bellevue, Washington.

"Take a deep breath through your nose, filling your lungs to capacity," Dr. Sodhi says. "Then release the air slowly with the sighing sound 'Ha-a-a-a-a-a-a.'"

This breathing technique is very helpful for ridding the body of the emotional toxins that accumulate in stressful situations, says Dr. Sodhi. "At a funeral, for example, everyone is spontaneously taking deep breaths and sighing 'Ha-a-a-a.' It's a natural way to release sorrow and other stress-caused negative emotions."

### ACUPRESSURE: *A 10-Point Plan*

In TCM, the body's energy, or chi, is said to flow throughout the body in currents called meridians. By stimulating specific spots along these currents (acupressure points) you can move the chi, sending healing energy to any part of your body.

The following points are designed to bring energy not only to your pancreas but also to all of the other parts of your body that diabetes can damage, such as your kidneys, eyes, and feet. (For the exact locations of the points, see An Illustrated Guide to Acupressure Points on page 700.)

• SP6 is four finger-widths directly above the bulge of the anklebone on the inside of your leg.
• KI3 is in a hollow area midway between the anklebone and the very back of your ankle.
• KI6 is one thumb's-width directly below the inside anklebone.
• CV4 is four finger-widths below your navel, on an imaginary vertical line running down the middle of your body and directly through your navel.
• CV12 is on the same line but above your navel, exactly between your navel and the lower edge of your sternum.
• LI11 is at the end of the skin crease on the outside of your elbow when the elbow is slightly bent.
• LU5 is on the inside of your elbow on the outer edge of the ridge of tendons that are an extension of your biceps muscle.
• LI4 is in the web between your thumb and index finger, at the highest point of the muscle that protrudes when the thumb and index finger are close together.
• LU9 is on the crease on your wrist closest to the palm, on the inside of the radial artery. (To find the artery, press on your wrist directly below the base of your thumb; you can feel your pulse in the radial artery.)
• ST44 is on the top of your foot between your second and third toes, about ½ inch above the point where the toes connect with the rest of the foot.

In each case except for the CV points, you'll press the corresponding points on both sides of your body one at a time. To activate a point, apply steady pressure for 2 minutes with your thumb or a finger. To help reverse Type 2 diabetes, press a set of three to five points each day. For example, do SP6, KI3, and KI6 on Monday, then CV4, CV12, and LI11 on Tuesday, and so on, rotating through the list.

Stop doing this routine when your blood sugar has stabilized at a normal level—a result, says Dr. Ni, that is "entirely possible" based on his experience with many patients with diabetes.

### "PUMPKIN FOOD": *Eat Some Daily*

This category includes all types of pumpkins; the entire squash family, such as winter, summer, spaghetti, and yellow squash; and cucumbers. Studies in China have shown that these foods help lower blood sugar, says Dr. Ni.

### WILD YAM: *A Herbal Helper*

People with Type 2 diabetes should use this herb daily to help maintain blood sugar within the normal range, says Dr. Ni. You can take wild yam every day for the rest of your life without harm, he says. Follow the dosage recommendations on the label. A typical dose would be equivalent to 1,500 to 3,000 milligrams a day, says Dr. Ni.

### HE SHOU WU: *Another Herbal Helper*

He shou wu, also known as fo-ti, is "very useful in lowering blood sugar and energizing the body," says Dr. Ni. He says that, like wild yam, you can take it safely every day for as long as you'd like. Follow the dosage instructions on the label.


## *Gentle, Soothing Relief from*
# Diarrhea


Believe it or not, a sudden bout of diarrhea is probably good for you.

That's because you've probably ingested something that's bad for you, such as a harmful strain of bacteria or a parasite, and your body is trying to get rid of it. For that reason, you probably shouldn't take an over-the-counter or prescription antidiarrheal drug, which will stop the cleansing process, says Mark Stengler, N.D., a naturopathic physician in San

Diego. Instead, he says, you may want to use an alternative home remedy, one that won't stop the diarrhea but will soothe your digestive tract and make the experience a little easier to bear.

## SLIPPERY ELM: *Soothing Relief*

The herb slippery elm is believed to help soothe the inflamed, irritated lining of the colon, which may help calm a case of diarrhea, says Rita Elkins, a master herbalist in Orem, Utah. You'll need fairly large quantities of the herb to do the job, but that's not a problem, because slippery elm is very safe, says Elkins.

The best way to take slippery elm for diarrhea is to open two or three 370-milligram capsules and mix the powder with water to form a gel-like paste. You'll want to take about a tablespoon of the paste, she says. You can also mix the powder with mashed banana or applesauce (both of which help calm diarrhea), says Elkins. For acute diarrhea that comes on suddenly, you'll want to triple the capsule-a-day dosage listed on the label, she adds.

## PROBIOTICS: *Balancing Intestinal Bacteria*

Your colon is filled with helpful bacteria that aid digestion. Taking a supplement of these bacteria, called a probiotic, can help normalize the colon's environment and ease diarrhea, says Elizabeth Lipski, a certified clinical nutritionist in Kauai, Hawaii.

To maximize potency and effectiveness, look for a supplement that's refrigerated in the store and that contains at least 4 billion units of the bacterium acidophilus.

Probiotics can also help prevent traveler's diarrhea. Lipski recommends taking the supplements a week before and then during your vacation abroad.

## COLOSTRUM: *Help from Mother's Milk*

Colostrum is a milk-like substance that's produced by female mammals in the first hours after giving birth. It's rich in immune-supporting factors, and some alternative practitioners believe that it can help control both acute and chronic diarrhea, says Andrew Gaeddert, a professional member of the American Herbalists Guild and director of the Get Well Clinic in Oakland, California. Look for a concentrated, purified, non-allergenic

---

# GUIDE TO
# PROFESSIONAL CARE

When diarrhea comes on suddenly, you should call your doctor if the stools are black or bloody or contain green mucus; if you have severe abdominal pain or a fever of 102°F or higher; or if you're showing signs of dehydration (such as dry skin, a dry mouth, a rapid heartbeat, confusion, weakness, thirst, or little or no urination).

You should also call your doctor if a bout of diarrhea lasts more than 3 days (sooner if your symptoms worsen). Be especially cautious with someone who is ill, children, and the elderly, who can become dehydrated from diarrhea quite quickly.

Chronic diarrhea, lasting for more than 3 months, requires professional diagnosis. It could be due to drug side effects, a food sensitivity, a parasitic or bacterial infection, inflammatory bowel disease, or even cancer.

---

form of bovine (cow) colostrum and follow the dosage directions on the label, he advises.

**HOMEOPATHY:** *To Calm the Worst Diarrhea*

For severe diarrhea, there are two homeopathic remedies that can help until you can get to a doctor, Dr. Stengler says. Try Phosphorus if you have burning, watery stools and you're very thirsty. Use Veratrum if you have violent diarrhea and your stools are very loose, with green mucus.

For either remedy, dissolve two tablets of the 6C potency under your tongue every 15 minutes until the diarrhea calms down.

**ACTIVATED CHARCOAL:** *Removes Toxins*

"Activated charcoal is an excellent remedy to help relieve diarrhea from food poisoning," says Teresa Rispoli, Ph.D., a licensed nutritionist and acupuncturist in Agoura Hills, California. It works by dragging diarrhea-causing toxins produced by bacteria out of your system. Take four to six 250-milligram capsules every 2 hours until your symptoms are relieved, she advises.

You should also take some charcoal supplements with you on your next trip outside the United States, says Dr. Rispoli, so you can use them if you develop traveler's diarrhea.

If taken regularly over a period of time, charcoal may interfere with the absorption of nutrients or increase the risk of gastrointestinal obstruction. If you take other oral medications or supplements at the same time as charcoal, the charcoal may interfere with their absorption, so take them at least 2 hours apart. At high doses, charcoal may cause stomach upset, diarrhea, constipation, or vomiting.

## Long-Term Relief

If you have chronic diarrhea—the kind that goes on for months—you need to see your doctor to find the cause. But you may also want to experiment with alternative home remedies, which can be used under a doctor's supervision, says William B. Salt II, M.D., clinical associate professor of medicine at Ohio State University College of Medicine and Public Health in Columbus.

### FIBER SUPPLEMENTS: *Adding Bulk to Loose Stools*

Taking fiber supplements with meals can be extremely helpful for chronic diarrhea, says Dr. Salt, because they help make stools firmer. Look for a product that contains psyllium seeds, without dyes or fillers. With each meal, take 2 rounded teaspoons in an 8-ounce glass of fat-free milk, water, or fruit juice, he advises.

### SIMPLE AND COMPLEX CARBOHYDRATES: *Identifying Sensitivities*

Frequently, people who have diarrhea lack the enzymes to break down disaccharides, double sugars that are simple carbohydrates, says Dana Laake, a licensed nutritionist in Rockville, Maryland.

For chronic diarrhea, she recommends a low-disaccharide diet that eliminates or limits foods with lactose (found in milk products), sucrose (table sugar found in processed foods), and maltose (found in malted milk, candies, and corn syrup). You should also avoid sugar alcohols used as artificial sweeteners, such as Sorbitol, which can contribute to gas and diarrhea, as well as starches such as corn and breads, pasta, and other flour products.

If you avoid or significantly reduce all of these for 1 to 2 weeks or more, and your diarrhea lessens or stops altogether, you've probably identified the diarrhea-causing culprit(s) in your diet, and you'll know to avoid these foods in the future, she says.

# *The Fiber Cure for* **Diverticulosis**

Surprise: Conventional and alternative practitioners are in total agreement about the most important treatment for diverticulosis, a disease of the colon, or large intestine.

Diverticulosis occurs when small areas on the colon wall pop out between the bands of muscle that encircle the organ, forming pea-size pouches called diverticula. The only solution? Increase your intake of dietary fiber.

Fiber is the indigestible material in plant foods such as grains, beans, fruits, and vegetables that helps the colon form large, soft stools. Without enough fiber to give them bulk, the stools are so small that the muscles around the colon have to squeeze extra hard to propel them from the body. This produces abnormally high levels of internal pressure that, over decades, create diverticula.

Most people with diverticulosis (approximately 50 percent of all Americans ages 60 to 80 have it) will never have symptoms. Some, however, may develop painful cramps in the lower left abdomen, along with bloating and constipation.

Adding more fiber to your diet lowers the internal pressure, reducing or eliminating symptoms. It's that simple.

# GUIDE TO
# PROFESSIONAL CARE

Anyone who has been diagnosed with diverticulosis and has recurring symptoms should be under the care of a gastroenterologist, a physician who specializes in digestive disorders, says William B. Salt II, M.D., clinical associate professor of medicine at Ohio State University College of Medicine and Public Health in Columbus.

See a doctor immediately if you develop abdominal pain, fever, and constipation (which are symptoms of infection), or if you have bright red rectal bleeding or stool that is maroon or grape-colored (a sign that a diverticulum may have broken a blood vessel in your colon). Both of these situations may require hospitalization.

In the worst-case scenario, the diverticula become infected, a condition called diverticulitis. The infection may cause a spectrum of possible symptoms, such as pain, fever, nausea, vomiting, chills, cramping, and constipation.

If these infectious attacks are frequent, or if other complications develop, such as a blocked bowel due to scarring from repeated infections, you may need surgery to remove a section of the colon.

## FIBER SUPPLEMENTS: *The Easiest Way to Get Enough*

You need 20 to 35 grams of fiber a day to help prevent problems from diverticulosis. One way to get that much fiber reliably, day after day, is with a fiber supplement, says Elizabeth Lipski, a certified clinical nutritionist in Kauai, Hawaii.

She recommends using a pure psyllium supplement, such as Konsyl, with no added sugar or flavoring. It should provide a minimum of 5 grams of fiber per teaspoon.

Since increasing your fiber intake all at once can cause gas or bloating, start with 1 teaspoon of psyllium supplement a day. Mix it with an 8-ounce glass of water, juice, or fat-free milk and take it with a meal, Lipski says.

Stay at that level for 2 days. If you don't notice any gas, increase to 2 teaspoons a day—1 teaspoon with breakfast and 1 with lunch, for example. Again, wait 2 days. If you're comfortable, increase the dose to 1 teaspoon with each meal. Always take it mixed with at least 8 ounces of liquid.

If you experience discomfort, go back to the previous level, stay there for a week, then try again. Eventually, you'll reach 3 teaspoons a day, and you should continue with that amount indefinitely, says Lipski.

One caution, however: During or right after an attack of diverticulitis, fiber can aggravate the problem. So if you've been diagnosed with diverticulitis, use fiber supplements only with the approval and supervision of your doctor.

### HIGH-FIBER FOODS: *Natural Colon Protection*

Eating at least five to nine servings of fruits and vegetables a day will provide loads of dietary fiber, with the bonus that you'll get dozens of disease-preventing phytonutrients such as vitamin C and beta-carotene, says Lipski. She also recommends adding plenty of fiber-rich whole grains and beans to your diet.

To really boost your fiber intake, read the labels on breakfast cereals and choose those that provide about 12 grams of fiber per serving. "That way, you can get about half your fiber intake for the whole day in one meal," she says.

### MSM: *Restores Elasticity to the Intestinal Wall*

While fiber is the most important healing agent for diverticulosis, it's not the only one. Diverticula are more likely to develop when the walls of the colon lose their natural elasticity, says Teresa Rispoli, Ph.D., a licensed nutritionist and acupuncturist in Agoura Hills, California.

To restore elasticity to the intestines, which will prevent new diverticula and help ensure that existing ones don't worsen, Dr. Rispoli recommends a daily dose of 1,000 milligrams of a supplement of MSM (methylsulfonylmethane). MSM has a high sulfur content, which is what helps repair and heal damaged intestinal tissue. Anyone who is prone to diverticular inflammation should stay on MSM indefinitely, she says.

She also advises taking at least 100 milligrams of vitamin C daily because it increases MSM's effectiveness.

## Put Bacteria on Your Side

When pouches in the intestine become infected, causing diverticulitis, you may need antibiotic treatment. Alternative practitioners believe that you can bolster the effectiveness of this treatment by taking a probiotic supplement of friendly colon bacteria that can help fight the infection and protect you from future episodes, says Elizabeth Lipski, a certified clinical nutritionist in Kauai, Hawaii.

She recommends using a probiotic supplement that contains at least 1 billion units of acidophilus or other beneficial bacteria, such as bifidum, bulgaricus, casei, plantarum, reuteri, salivarius, faecium, or thermophilus. The bacteria are perishable, so buy supplements that are freeze-dried and/or refrigerated at the store. You should always refrigerate them at home.

During an attack, she recommends taking two capsules three times daily. Afterward, take one capsule two or three times daily until all symptoms disappear.

### SLIPPERY ELM: *Soothing the Digestive Tract*
The herb slippery elm both strengthens and soothes the digestive system, helping to prevent diverticulosis from causing symptoms, says Andrew Gaeddert, a professional member of the American Herbalists Guild and director of the Get Well Clinic in Oakland, California. He recommends taking 3,000 milligrams of slippery elm a day, in either capsule or powder form, until symptoms subside.

# *Two Herbs Can Help Ease Nausea from* Dizziness

Sitting on the exam table in the doctor's office, you have the sensation that your body is falling, spinning, and tilting, even though you're sitting perfectly still. Your doctor has given you a diagnosis of benign positional vertigo. That's a fancy way of

## GUIDE TO PROFESSIONAL CARE

There are dozens of possible causes of dizziness, many of which are serious medical problems such as heart disease. If you feel dizzy or light-headed on a regular basis, see a doctor for a complete physical exam and diagnosis.

Specifically, you may want to see an osteopathic doctor, says Robert Dozor, M.D., president and chief executive officer of the California Institute of Integrative Medicine in Calistoga. He believes that osteopathic manipulation of the head and neck is one of the most effective treatments for chronic dizziness.

saying that your problem isn't life-threatening, but the world is spinning around you and making you feel dizzy and very nauseated.

The cause is a communication problem between the balance centers in your inner ear and your brain. The doctor writes you a prescription for a drug to stop the spinning, which also eliminates the nausea—but only by sedating you so heavily that your whole world might come to a complete halt.

"The drugs that conventional medicine uses to treat benign positional vertigo can be really disabling," says Robert Dozor, M.D., president and chief executive officer of the California Institute of Integrative Medicine in Calistoga. "Essentially, they suppress the nausea by lowering activity in the nervous system so the balance centers can't communicate with one another. But the effect is to make patients so sedated that they're not going to want to do *anything*." Alternative medicine has another answer, a way to clear up the nausea without turning off your brain.

### GINGER: *Quiet the Queasiness*

"Ginger in any form—as a capsule, as a tea, even as ginger candy, if it's actually made with the herb—can quickly calm the nausea," Dr. Dozor says. If you're taking a tablet or capsule, follow the label directions. For tea or candy, use as much ginger as you need to stop the queasiness, he says. It's safe to take this until your nausea goes away.

## GINKGO: *More Blood for Your Balance Centers*

It's thought that the herb ginkgo helps relieve dizziness by improving blood supply to the brain and to the balance centers in the inner ear, Dr. Dozor says. Look for extract standardized for 24 percent glycosides (the active ingredients), and take 40 to 80 milligrams three times a day until your nausea passes.

## ACUPRESSURE: *Thumbs Down for Nausea Relief*

An acupressure point on your wrist can help clear up nausea from vertigo, says Dr. Dozor. The point (called PE7) is on the inside of your wrist, in the center and about a finger-width below the wrist crease. (For the exact location, see An Illustrated Guide to Acupressure Points on page 700.)

"If you're suffering from vertigo, the area will feel slightly sore," says Dr. Dozor. "Put steady pressure on the point with your thumb for about 5 minutes. It's amazing how effective this is at relieving the nausea of vertigo."

### It's in Your Blood

Low blood pressure or uneven blood sugar levels are common and easily correctable—causes of dizziness, says Dr. Dozor. Here are some simple steps that will get to the root of the problem.

## LICORICE: *Keep Salt in Your Body*

One way to clear up light-headedness from low blood pressure is with the herb licorice, which helps retain sodium, Dr. Dozor says. It's available as capsules, tincture, or tea. Follow the dosage recommendations on the label.

It's safe to take this long term, but be sure that your doctor monitors your blood pressure, sodium, and potassium levels while you're taking it to ensure that your blood pressure doesn't go too high.

**FOOD:** *More Fiber, Less Sugar*

If you're feeling light-headed and dizzy a lot of the time, the problem may not be with your blood pressure but with your blood sugar, or glucose—the body's primary fuel. You may have dysglycemia, a condition in which levels of blood sugar roller-coaster up and down, taking your brain for a very unpleasant ride, says Dr. Dozor.

A simple way to stabilize blood sugar levels, he says, is to increase your intake of fiber and decrease your intake of simple carbohydrates such as white sugar and white flour.

# Natural Eyedrops Work Best for
# Dry Eyes

If you're like most Americans, when your eyes are dry, red, burning, or gritty, you reach for over-the-counter eyedrops such as Visine or Murine to make them feel better. Unfortunately, it's likely that you're making the problem worse.

"So many people use these products for dry eyes—and they shouldn't," says Daniel John Dieterichs, O.D., an optometrist in Belen, New Mexico. These products "get the red out" by constricting the blood vessels in your eyes, which doesn't do anything to effectively moisten them.

And having dry eyes is a problem that you definitely want to solve. "Dry eyes are more than a nuisance," says Edward L. Paul Jr., O.D., Ph.D., an optometrist, holistic nutritionist, and director of Atlantic Eye Associates in Hampstead, North Carolina. "Chronically dry eyes can damage the tissue of the eye, possibly even scarring the cornea and leading to irreversible loss of vision."

The first step in restoring moisture to your eyes is to use eyedrops, but they have to be the right kind of eyedrops—natural and preservative-free artificial tears.

## GUIDE TO
## PROFESSIONAL CARE

Artificial tears are the standard medical treatment for dry eyes, says Edward L. Paul Jr., O.D., Ph.D., an optometrist, holistic nutritionist, and director of Atlantic Eye Associates in Hampstead, North Carolina.

When accompanied by other symptoms, dry eyes can be a sign of infection that, untreated, can cause vision loss. See your doctor if your eyes remain pinkish red even after using artificial tears, if they hurt, if your vision changes, or if there is pus or discharge.

Dr. Paul also recommends a procedure called punctum occlusion, in which an ophthalmologist or optometrist inserts tiny plugs into the drainage ducts in the corners of the eyelids, causing tears to stay in the eye longer.

"This simple procedure is tremendously successful, dramatically improving the quality of patients' lives," he says.

### ARTIFICIAL TEARS: *Preserve Your Eyes without Preservatives*

"The first line of defense in treating dry eyes is to replace the tears that are not there with artificial tears," Dr. Paul says. Of the many dozens of different types of artificial tears available, he recommends choosing a product without preservatives, which can irritate the eyes. Of those products, he prefers either Viva-Drops or Similasan, a homeopathic product.

Viva-Drops are made of sterile vitamin A oil and other antioxidants, which may actually improve the health of the tissue of the eye so tears remain in the eye longer. The homeopathic medication in Similasan is thought to moisten the eyes and stimulate tear production.

"In my experience, these products simply work better than any of the other artificial tears available," Dr. Paul says. Use them as needed; you can't "overdose" on artificial tears, he says. If you wear contact lenses, however, be sure to remove them before using these products.

## EVENING PRIMROSE OIL: *Increase Your Production of Tears*

Nutritional support can also help relieve dry eyes. Evening primrose oil contains gamma-linolenic acid (GLA), a type of fatty acid that can increase tear production, says Dr. Paul. Take 1,500 milligrams a day. Or you can substitute the same amount of either black currant (seed) oil or borage oil, both of which are also rich in GLA.

## VITAMINS C AND B6: *Another Boost for Your Tears*

You may want to get your GLA from a product that supplies vitamins C and $B_6$, two other nutrients that can help increase tear production, says Marc Grossman, O.D., an optometrist, licensed acupuncturist, and codirector of the Integral Health Center in Rye and New Paltz, New York.

Look for a product with 1,500 milligrams of both GLA and vitamin C and 500 milligrams of vitamin $B_6$. Use as necessary, following the directions on the label.

## POTASSIUM: *Eat a Banana Every Day*

"Potassium is one of the most important minerals for relieving dry eye symptoms," says Dr. Grossman, noting that his patients with the problem are usually very low in potassium. He recommends eating a banana every day, which supplies approximately 400 milligrams of the nutrient.

### Eyes Dry After Using a Computer? Practice Blinking

To stay lubricated, the eye needs to blink about 12 times a minute, or once every 5 seconds. People who use computers, staring intently at the screen, often blink as seldom as once a minute, says Daniel John Dieterichs, O.D., an optometrist in Belen, New Mexico. Moreover, they may blink only halfway, so the lubrication that they do get is second-rate. The result is dry, red, burning eyes.

The way out of computer-caused dryness? Deliberate blinking. Practice blinking when you're at the computer, says Dr. Dieterichs. Each time, make sure that you close your eyes so that you can't see and keep them closed for just a second. If you consistently slow down your blinks, your subconscious mind will soon take over the task, and you'll be blinking the way you should.

## FOOD: *Don't Let These Hurt Your Eyes*

Eating a lot of sugar or artificial sweeteners can worsen dry eyes, says Dr. Grossman. Avoid these foods as much as possible.

You might also want to avoid dairy products, fried foods, and the hydrogenated oils in margarine and shortening. The fats in these products are thought to interfere with the metabolism of fatty acids like GLA and may be an indirect cause of dry eyes, he says.

## TRADITIONAL CHINESE MEDICINE: *An Herb for "Yin Deficiency"*

Dr. Grossman recommends a Chinese herbal formula called Lycii-Rehmannia for dry eyes. It helps treat what Traditional Chinese Medicine terms a yin-deficient syndrome, in which a part of the body is too dry or too hot. Follow the dosage recommendations on the label.

## HYDROTHERAPY: *Soak Your Eyelids*

It's very common for people with dry eyes to have blocked oil glands in their eyelids, a condition that makes tears less stable and more likely to evaporate quickly, says Dr. Dieterichs. To solve the problem, he recommends soaking and washing your eyelids twice a day. Here's how.

Each morning and evening, soak a washcloth in very warm water and place it over your lids for 3 to 4 minutes. Then, with your eyes closed, gently rub your lashes and eyelids in a left-to-right motion with the washcloth. "This technique helps a lot of people with dry eyes," Dr. Dieterichs says.

# *Natural Moisturizers Can*
# *Help Repair*
# **Dry Hair and Split Ends**

Your hair is dry—lifeless, lacking luster, and maybe brittle. Perhaps you also have the "end" result of months of dry hair—split ends. Why?

It could be genetics: You were born with curly or frizzy hair, which tends to be dry because it's overly porous. Perhaps you're using harsh shampoos that strip your sebaceous glands, the oil-generating glands in your scalp. Maybe your diet is lacking in nutritional factors that moisten hair from the roots up, or you've dried out your hair with too much sun exposure, blow-drying, or chemical treatments such as coloring and perms.

You can't do much about genetics, of course, but alternative practitioners offer many different ways to counter some of those other factors and restore luster and softness to your hair, says Mary Beth Janssen, a beauty and wellness consultant and aromatherapist in Chicago. Here are some of their suggestions.

### AVOCADO: *A Good "Food" for Dry Hair*

A conditioning hair treatment with avocado can optimize the delivery of protein to the hair shaft, thus strengthening and moisturizing dry hair, Janssen says. "A lack of protein makes hair brittle, and a lack of moisture makes it look dry," she says. Here's what she recommends.

You'll need a peeled ripe avocado, 1 teaspoon of wheat germ oil, and 1 teaspoon of jojoba oil. Combine the ingredients in a medium bowl. Then apply the mixture to your shampooed hair and scalp, massaging it into your scalp with your fingertips in small, circular motions and gently spreading the mixture from the midshaft to the ends of your hair. Finally, cover your hair with a plastic bag.

"The body heat will accentuate the conditioning," says

Janssen. Leave the mixture on for 15 to 30 minutes, then rinse thoroughly. Use this treatment once a week.

## Add Aloe to Your Shampoo

The herb aloe is incredibly healing and moisturizing and helps normalize dry hair, says Mary Beth Janssen, a beauty and wellness consultant and aromatherapist in Chicago.

She recommends adding 1 teaspoon of 99 percent pure aloe gel to your shampoo and massaging it into your scalp for 5 minutes or so when you wash your hair. Be sure to rinse thoroughly.

## AROMATHERAPY: *For More Moisture*

The essential oils of aromatherapy can help restore luster to dry hair, says Janssen. She recommends a regular scalp and hair massage with a mixture consisting of eight drops of cedarwood oil, eight drops of clary sage oil, and four drops of lavender oil in a base of 2 ounces of jojoba oil.

"Jojoba oil helps regulate oil production in the sebaceous glands," she says. The clary sage and cedarwood oils also help regulate oil production, while the lavender is thought to stimulate circulation to the scalp, improving the condition of your hair. These oils also nourish and moisturize the hair itself.

Once a week, massage the mixture into your scalp and hair, leaving it on for 35 to 40 minutes or even overnight (cover your hair with a sleeping cap to protect your pillow).

## PROTEIN: *A Post-Shampoo Treatment*

Protein treatments help fortify and strengthen the hair shaft, says Janssen. "They are particularly good for dry, fragile, or brittle hair types." She recommends using plain gelatin, combining 1 tablespoon with 1 cup of water and letting it gel slightly. "Don't let it set all the way," she cautions.

When the gelatin is partially set, add 1 teaspoon of apple-cider vinegar and two drops each of jasmine, clary sage, and rosemary essential oils, then mix well. After your shampoo, work the mixture through your hair and into your scalp and leave it on for 5 to 10 minutes. Do this treatment once a week.

**FATTY ACIDS:** *Oil Your Hair from the Inside Out*

Fatty acids found in oils such as flaxseed, evening primrose, or black currant seed oils are thought to nourish sebaceous glands, moisturizing hair from the inside out, says Earl Mindell, Ph.D., a nutritionist and pharmacist in Beverly Hills.

"A lack of essential fatty acids can contribute to dry hair," he says, so if your hair is dry, he recommends taking 1 teaspoon daily of one of the oils listed above.

# *Mouthwatering Relief for*
# **Dry Mouth**

A temporary bout of dry mouth is nothing to worry about. In fact, that's probably what's causing your problem to begin with—worry. Stress and nervousness can leave your mouth feeling like the Sahara. If that's the case, here are a couple of tips from alternative healers to help with occasional dry mouth.

**BREATHING:** *The Darth Vader Solution*

You can fix stress-caused dry mouth by breathing through your nose, says John Douillard, D.C., a chiropractor, expert in Ayurveda (the ancient system of natural healing from India), and director of the LifeSpa in Boulder, Colorado.

"Just breathe deeply in and out through your nose for about 10 minutes," he says. According to Ayurvedic principles, this method of breathing fills the lower parts of your lungs, which in turn activates the parasympathetic nervous system—the part of your nervous system that calms you down.

He also says to constrict the back of your throat a bit while you breathe so that your inhalations sound like those of the famous Darth Vader character in the *Star Wars* movies. "This tenses your lower abdominal muscles and massages the vagus nerve, which also reduces physical stress," Dr. Douillard says.

## GUIDE TO
## PROFESSIONAL CARE

Dry mouth, which is basically a lack of saliva, can be a symptom of many serious diseases, such as diabetes, leukemia, pernicious anemia, Sjögren's syndrome, Hodgkin's disease, and AIDS. It also is a common side effect of hundreds of over-the-counter and prescription drugs, says Flora Parsa Stay, D.D.S., a dentist in Oxnard, California.

Dry mouth is an oral disaster. Your tongue burns. Your breath smells. The corners of your mouth crack. Since the bacteria-produced acid that decays teeth and erodes gums isn't diluted by saliva, cavities multiply and gum disease runs rampant. And those are only some of the possible symptoms.

Obviously, a chronically dry mouth is a medical problem that needs professional attention. If you've noticed a consistent decrease in saliva for several weeks, especially after you've tried the remedies in this chapter, see a medical doctor for diagnosis and care immediately, Dr. Stay recommends.

### Relief for Chronic Dry Mouth

Many cases of chronic dry mouth are medical in origin, the result of a disease, a drug side effect, or radiation treatment for cancer. If your mouth is chronically dry, you need to seek professional care. But alternative practitioners suggest a number of ways to help prevent and relieve the symptoms of dry mouth that work as well as the moisturizers and saliva substitutes available at drugstores.

### COENZYME $Q_{10}$: *Getting You Back in Circulation*
In many people, this substance improves circulation to every area of the body, including the mouth, Dr. Stay believes. For those with chronic dry mouth, the improved circulation may help stop bad breath, cavities, and gum disease, which are three common symptoms of the problem. She recommends 60 milligrams a day if you already have these symptoms and 10 to 30 milligrams a day as a preventive dose.

## VITAMIN C: *For Tissue Repair*

All of the tissues in your mouth, including your tongue, your gums, the insides of your cheeks, and your lips, are damaged when you have chronic dry mouth. To help prevent and repair that damage, you need extra vitamin C, says Dr. Stay. She recommends a daily intake of 2,000 milligrams.

## B VITAMINS: *Beating the Bugs*

Most of the symptoms triggered by dry mouth are caused by bacteria. To battle those bugs, you need to boost the strength of your immune system, and B-complex vitamins do just that. Dr. Stay suggests talking to your doctor about taking a daily supplement with 100 milligrams of the major B-complex vitamins, such as thiamin, niacin, riboflavin, and $B_6$.

## GOLDENSEAL: *A Natural Moisturizer*

To keep your mouth moist and relieve inflamed gums, rinse before bedtime with goldenseal mouthwash, says Dr. Stay. Prepare a cup of goldenseal tea, let it cool, and stir in a teaspoon of baking soda, which also helps to reduce inflammation. Use this formulation as a mouth rinse every night, swishing it in your mouth for as long as possible before spitting it out, advises Dr. Stay.

## Homeopathy for Radiation-Caused Dry Mouth

Radiation therapy for cancer can cripple the salivary glands, causing severe dry mouth. To help relieve the problem, take a 200X potency of the homeopathic remedy called X-Ray, says Flora Parsa Stay, D.D.S., a dentist in Oxnard, California. Dissolve one tablet under your tongue every hour during the therapy, and use one tablet three times daily between treatments.

## HOMEOPATHY: *A Handy Helper*

The homeopathic remedy called Natrum muriaticum is particularly effective if you have cracks in the corners of your mouth and loss of taste, a common symptom of dry mouth, says Dr. Stay. Take a 30C potency of the remedy, dissolving one tablet under your tongue daily.

**ALOE:** *Soothes Inflamed Gums*

Aloe gel can relieve tender, burning, inflamed gum tissue, says Dr. Stay. Put some 100 percent pure aloe gel on a cotton-tipped swab and gently spread it on the inflamed areas of your gums. Don't eat or drink for at least an hour afterward. Pure aloe gel may be difficult to find. The gel from a freshly cut leaf will also work, says Dr. Stay.

**WATER:** *A Solution for Seniors*

Among those over 60, a common cause of dry mouth is simply not drinking enough water.

If you have chronic dry mouth, you need to drink at least 12 glasses of water a day (a total of 96 ounces), says Flora Parsa Stay, D.D.S., a dentist in Oxnard, California. Buy a water bottle, keep it filled, keep it with you, and sip from it throughout the day.

# *Water Is the Way to Balance*
# Dry Skin

If your skin is dry—if it feels tight, looks dull, and perhaps is flaking—you probably already know the basics of self-care. Don't wash with hot water. Don't clean with soap. Use a moisturizer a couple of times a day, and be sure to use one with no artificial fragrances, which can hurt dry, sensitive skin.

While those routines are good, however, they may not be enough. Alternative skin care practitioners have a few additional ideas for accomplishing the two tasks that are musts for normalizing dry skin: adding water and adding oil.

"Skin is dry because there is either not enough moisture or not enough oil," says Joni Loughran, an esthetician, cosmetologist, and aromatherapist in Petaluma, California.

> ## GUIDE TO
> ## PROFESSIONAL CARE
>
> If your dry skin has become widespread and uncomfortable and does not go away after 2 weeks of self-care, see a dermatologist for professional diagnosis and treatment, says Esta Kronberg, M.D., a dermatologist in Houston.

## MISTING: *Spray-On Relief*

"Misting—spraying your face with a fine mist of water—may be the single best treatment for dry skin," says Loughran.

For maximum benefit, you should always apply a moisturizer that contains humectants before misting. These ingredients attract and hold water, Loughran says, so if you mist while they're on your face, your dry skin will continue to receive moisture throughout the day. If you mist without applying the humectant moisturizer, the misting may actually start to dry your skin. Loughran suggests using natural products from the companies Penny Island, Abra, and Dr. Hauschka.

To mist, you need an 8-ounce bottle with a pump sprayer that emits a very fine spray that won't disturb makeup. Your choices of liquids and moisturizing elements to use include plain water, aloe juice, and an aromatherapy hydrosol (flower water), which is the water that's left over after a plant has been distilled to remove the essential oils.

You also can mix 10 drops of an essential oil or a blend of oils in water. If you do, though, shake the mixture vigorously before use and be careful not to spray it into your eyes, since the oils can irritate them. Some excellent oils to use for this are lavender, damask rose, chamomile, ylang-ylang, and rose geranium, says Loughran.

You should mist at least three times a day—morning, noon, and evening—but since misting is so good for dry skin, feel free to mist as often as possible, she says.

## AROMATHERAPY: *A Hydrating Facial Compress*

Daily use of a warm facial compress using aromatherapy essential oils will greatly benefit dry skin by hydrating the skin and stimulating the water and oil glands, Loughran says.

First, thoroughly rinse a clean washcloth to remove any soap or detergent residue. Next, fill a basin with warm water and add two to three drops of one of three essential oils: lavender, rose, or neroli. "These are all very gentle, harmonizing, balancing oils for the skin," says Loughran. Finally, lean over the basin, dip the cloth in the water, and hold it to your face and neck for a few moments. Do this 10 times.

## WATER: *Hydrate from the Inside Out*
Water is an internal moisturizer, helping to heal dry skin from the inside out, says Loughran. She recommends drinking a minimum of 64 ounces a day, and more if you drink coffee or alcohol, since they are diuretics that force water out of the body.

## SUPPLEMENTS: *A Program for Dry Skin*
Skin-supporting nutritional supplements can also help heal dry skin from the inside, says Earl L. Mindell, Ph.D., a pharmacist and nutritionist in Beverly Hills. Here are his recommendations.

• Black currant oil: 1,000 to 2,000 milligrams daily. This oil is a rich source of omega-6 fatty acids, which are crucial for normal skin.
• Beta-carotene: 15 milligrams a day, taking half the daily dosage with lunch and half with dinner. This nutrient is crucial for soft, smooth, disease-free skin, Dr. Mindell says.
• Zinc: 15 milligrams daily with a meal. This nutrient is important for the repair of damaged skin tissue, he says, and a deficiency can cause dry skin.
• B-complex vitamins: 100 milligrams a day after a meal. "Deficiencies of thiamin, riboflavin, pantothenic acid, or biotin can lead to dry skin problems, especially scaliness around the mouth and nose," says Dr. Mindell.
• Vitamin C: 1,000 milligrams two or three times a day. "Vitamin C helps bolster the immune system, and a stronger immune system leads to healthier skin," he says.
• Vitamin E: 400 international units once or twice a day after meals. "This nutrient helps replace cells on the skin's outer layer," he says.

## Help for Chapped Hands

Using a gentle cleansing and moisturizing routine twice a day, every day, can make chapped hands a thing of the past, says Norma Pasekoff Weinberg, an herbal educator in Cape Cod, Massachusetts.

You'll need a small cucumber, 1 tablespoon of cornmeal, ½ tablespoon of honey, some warm water, and a mild, unscented, superfatted liquid soap such as Neutrogena or Dove.

Peel the cucumber and remove the seeds, then process it in a blender or juicer for a few seconds, until smooth. In a small bowl, mix the cucumber with the honey and set aside. Put the cornmeal in a separate bowl and make a paste by slowly adding the warm water and liquid soap.

Wash your hands thoroughly with the cornmeal paste, which will cleanse gently without irritating. Rinse your hands with warm water and pat dry with a clean, soft towel.

Next, apply the cucumber mixture. Enlist someone to help you enclose your hands in plastic wrap or self-sealing plastic bags. Cover the plastic with a towel and relax for 15 to 20 minutes—the longer, the better.

Afterward, rinse your hands, blot them dry, and apply moisturizer. For extra protection, apply the moisturizer to your hands before bed and wear loose-fitting cotton gloves overnight.

## HERBS: *A Tea for Healing Parched Skin*

Herbalists call certain herbs mucilaginous, meaning that they have soothing and anti-inflammatory qualities—qualities that can help heal dry skin, says Brigitte Mars, an herbalist and nutritional consultant in Boulder, Colorado. Here's her formula for making a tea using four of the best mucilaginous herbs for dry skin: marshmallow root, fennel seed, plantain, and violet leaves.

Combine 1 part each of marshmallow root and fennel seed, then add a heaping teaspoon of the mixture to 1 quart of water and boil for 20 minutes. Add a heaping teaspoon each of dried plantain and violet leaves and simmer for 20 minutes.

Turn off the heat and let the mixture stand for 10 minutes, then strain. Drink a quart of tea daily, sipping it warm or cold throughout the day.

*Soothing the Pain of*
# Earaches

If you're reading this chapter to find out how to remedy your own earache or ear infection, you can count yourself among an unlucky few.

"While very common in children, earaches and ear infections are quite unusual in adults," says Elson Haas, M.D., director of the Preventive Medical Center of Marin in San Rafael, California.

That's because adults don't have the small eustachian tube of an infant or child, which runs horizontally from the nasal cavity to the ear and allows bacteria easy access. A fully formed tube, whose function is to equalize air pressure on both sides of the eardrum, is long and vertical, keeping bugs at bay.

While they are unlikely, however, earaches and ear infections can happen to adults, Dr. Haas says.

---

## GUIDE TO
## PROFESSIONAL CARE

In adults, some infections of the outer or middle ear should be treated by a doctor, says Elson Haas, M.D., director of the Preventive Medical Center of Marin in San Rafael, California. If your ear is extremely painful, if there's any discharge, or if you have a fever of 100°F or higher, see your doctor immediately.

Food allergies also can cause chronic earaches and ear infections, says Dr. Haas. He recommends seeing a nutritionally oriented doctor who can help you detect and eliminate the allergies.

Most earaches are the first symptom of an infection. You can get an infection of the outer ear, or ear canal. Otitis externa, commonly known as swimmer's ear, is an infection of this type. You can get an infection of the middle ear behind the eardrum, which is the type of problem that's common in children. Or you can just have a cold, allergy, or sore throat, all of which can cause ear pain. Tooth pain can also "travel" to the ear.

If the pain isn't severe, you don't have to know the exact cause of the problem, because there are plenty of alternative home remedies to soothe the ear and heal the infection that's causing your pain.

There's one caution, however: If you have ear problems and are scheduled to fly, consider taking an over-the-counter decongestant about an hour before the flight, says Janet Zand, O.M.D., a doctor of Oriental medicine and licensed acupuncturist in Austin, Texas. If your flight is longer than 3 hours, you may need to take another dose an hour before landing, depending on the strength of the decongestant. That will relieve congestion in the eustachian tube, easing ear pain during the flight and when descending.

## GARLIC: *Pierce a Capsule and Apply*

A capsule of bacteria-killing garlic oil can help get rid of an earache that's caused by an infection in the ear canal, says Linda Kingsbury, an herbalist, holistic nutritionist, and director of Earth Wisdom Holistic Services in Keene, New Hampshire.

Pierce the capsule with a pin, put a few drops of oil on a cotton ball, gently put the cotton ball in your ear, and leave it in for an hour during the day and all night. Place the cotton ball just inside your ear, being careful not to push it into your ear canal.

Taking garlic oil capsules orally will also help knock out the infection, says Kingsbury, who recommends two 500-milligram capsules a day for 7 days.

## MULLEIN: *A Good Addition to Garlic*

You may want to add some mullein flower oil to that garlic, says Dr. Haas. While the garlic oil is a natural disinfectant, the oil from mullein flower soothes the skin of the ear canal and can reduce inflammation and relieve pain.

Either add the oil to the cotton ball or put two to three drops directly in the ear every 3 to 4 hours, Dr. Haas advises.

## VITAMINS AND MINERALS: *For Healing*

The following program of supplements strengthens the immune system and can help resolve a mild ear infection, says Dr. Zand.

• Vitamin A: For best results, use the emulsified variety. Take 25,000 international units (IU) twice a day for 5 days, then 5,000 to 10,000 IU as a maintenance dose. Since the vitamin can build up in the liver and pose risks, do not take high doses without medical supervision.
• Vitamin C with bioflavonoids: Take 500 milligrams three times a day. For prevention, take the same amount once a day.
• Zinc: For both prevention and treatment of an earache, take 15 milligrams once a day at the beginning of a meal.
• Vitamin E: Take 200 to 400 IU a day for prevention.
• B-complex vitamins: For prevention, take one capsule a day of a high-potency supplement that provides at least 50 milligrams of most of the B vitamins.

## QIGONG: *Make a "V"—for Victory Over Earaches*

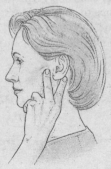

A qigong massage—a technique from Traditional Chinese Medicine—can help beat an earache, says Kingsbury. To do the massage, place your middle finger on your face in front of your ear and your index finger behind your ear near your hairline; your fingers will form a V-shape.

Starting at the base of your ear near the bottom lobe, move your fingers upward alongside the ear while pressing firmly, then release the pressure as you move them down. Do this up-and-down movement 36 times. "This massage increases circulation and improves lymph drainage," says Kingsbury. (Lymph is a fluid in your body that helps move waste material away from the cells.)

**HERBS:** *Try Echinacea and Goldenseal*

A liquid formula offering a combination of these two herbs can help clear up an ear infection, says Dr. Zand. Echinacea is thought to be an antibacterial, while goldenseal has a mild drying effect. Follow the dosage recommendations on the label.

**FOOD:** *Beware of Allergens*

Anyone who is susceptible to ear infections is probably allergic to one or more foods, says Dr. Zand. The most common food allergens are wheat, dairy products, corn, oranges, peanut butter, refined sugar, and fruit juices.

If you feel tired after eating any of these foods or notice that you feel stuffy or cough a lot or your skin itches, try removing the offenders from your diet.

**LAVENDER ESSENTIAL OIL:** *Inhale for Relief*

Essential oils can aid in healing an earache or ear infection, says Kingsbury. "One of my favorites is lavender," she says. The antiseptic properties of lavender help support the immune system and promote relaxation, two factors that are very important in healing, she says. Here's how to best reap lavender's benefits.

Fill a cereal bowl with a cup of boiling water and add three to five drops of the oil. Make a tent over your head with a towel, lean over the bowl (taking care not to burn yourself with the steam), and inhale for 5 to 10 minutes.

# *Changing Your Diet Can Reduce* Earwax Buildup

It's a lubricant. It's an antibiotic. It's a vacuum cleaner.

It's earwax, a very humble and very helpful substance produced by glands in the ear canal. This multipurpose goo lubricates the skin, helps keep bacteria and other microorganisms from taking up residence, and traps dust and dirt, moving that tiny debris away from the sensitive eardrum.

Some people, however, produce too much of this good thing—wax so plentiful that it clogs the canal, reducing hearing or causing pain, itching, or ringing in the ear. Conventional doctors don't know why certain people produce more than the average amount of wax, although genetics is one possible factor. Alternative practitioners, however, say that the foods you eat are a possible cause of earwax buildup. Here are their natural remedies to clear your ears.

## OLIVE OIL: *Loosen the Wax*

Putting a few drops of olive oil in your ear will help loosen the wax so that it can flow out naturally, says Elson Haas, M.D., director of the Preventive Medical Center of Marin in San Rafael, California. Here are his instructions.

"If you're trying to remove wax from your left ear, for example, lie on your right side and gently pull the top part of your ear up and back to straighten out the ear canal. Then, using a dropper, put three drops of olive oil in your ear, letting it ooze down the canal. Simply rest on that side for the next 10 to 15 minutes. Do this three or four times a day. The wax will gradually loosen and move out of your ear."

Although you won't actually see the earwax coming out of your ear, you'll know the oil is working because your impaired hearing and other symptoms should improve. If the earwax doesn't clear up within a few days, Dr. Haas suggests that you see your doctor.

---

## GUIDE TO
## PROFESSIONAL CARE

If nothing you do seems to reduce earwax production or effectively move it out of your ear, and if your hearing is impaired, see your doctor for an ear lavage, advises Elson Haas, M.D., director of the Preventive Medical Center of Marin in San Rafael, California. This simple procedure loosens and washes out excess wax with a stream of water.

## FLAXSEED OIL: *Reduce Inflammation*

Traditional Chinese Medicine considers excess earwax a type of inflammation, says Janet Zand, O.M.D., a doctor of Oriental medicine and licensed acupuncturist in Austin, Texas.

Since fatty acids are helpful in reducing inflammation, she recommends a supplement of flaxseed oil, which is rich in them. Take a 1,000-milligram capsule two or three times a day or have 1 tablespoon of oil with lunch and one with dinner, she suggests. (Keep the oil refrigerated because it can go rancid quickly.)

## VITAMIN C WITH BIOFLAVONOIDS: *A Natural Anti-Inflammatory*

Another way to reduce inflammation is by taking a supplement of vitamin C with bioflavonoids, Dr. Zand says. Take 500 milligrams three times a day. But don't expect less wax tomorrow. "Reducing earwax with an anti-inflammatory supplement like vitamin C takes about 6 months," she says.

## FATTY ACIDS: *Cut Back on Wax*

Eating too many "junky fats"—the saturated fats found in animal products such as meat and dairy foods and the hydrogenated fats found in packaged baked goods and many other processed foods—can create thicker, more copious earwax, Dr. Haas says.

Minimize those fats and increase your intake of the "good fats"—the omega-3 and omega-6 fatty acids that are found in fish, nuts, and seeds, says Steven Bock, M.D., a family practitioner, acupuncturist, and codirector of the Center for Progressive Medicine in Rhinebeck, New York.

## *Slow Lung Damage from*
# Emphysema and
# Chronic Bronchitis

There's no use crying over spilled milk—or smoked cigarettes. A lifetime of smoking is the main cause of emphysema and chronic bronchitis, two very similar lung diseases that doctors include under the grouping of chronic obstructive pulmonary disease, or COPD.

Both cause mild to severe shortness of breath, and both are irreversible. But it is extremely useful to slow the progress of these diseases so that you don't have to take corticosteroids, powerful drugs that ease breathing but also cause a wide range of devastating side effects, such as osteoporosis and diabetes.

Moreover, you need to decrease your risk of further lung damage from respiratory infection, because a "minor" respiratory problem can avalanche into fatal pneumonia.

Alternative home remedies can help you achieve those goals, says JoAnne Lombardi, M.D., a pulmonary specialist in Belmont, California. "You can't get back the lung function you've lost," she says. "But nutritional and other alternative remedies can be an adjunct to conventional medical care in helping to maximize lung function and prevent respiratory infections."

### PROTEIN POWDER: *It Won't Take Your Breath Away*

Many patients with COPD are malnourished, Dr. Lombardi says. "I believe it is the leading cause of declining lung function in these patients," she says.

Malnutrition, which also cripples the immune system, is a problem for those with COPD because they may find that eating is uncomfortable. It causes the stomach to press against the diaphragm, the sheet of muscle below the lungs and above the digestive organs that assists respiration. That makes shortness

# GUIDE TO
# PROFESSIONAL CARE

*Caution: You should use the alternative remedies discussed in this chapter only as part of a treatment program that is guided and monitored by a qualified medical doctor in partnership with a qualified alternative practitioner, both of whom are experienced in caring for your condition. Check with your conventional doctor before changing or stopping any conventional medical treatments or medications, and keep all of your doctors and/or alternative practitioners informed of all treatments that you are receiving.*

Emphysema and chronic bronchitis are serious conditions that require ongoing medical care, says Andrew Ries, M.D., director of pulmonary rehabilitation at the University of California, San Diego. If your symptoms seem to be worsening, or if you have congestion in your lungs, shortness or breath, or swelling in your legs, see your doctor as soon as possible.

Pulmonary rehabilitation programs at many hospitals teach patients how to maximize the effectiveness of medications, how to best use oxygen therapy, if necessary, and how to maintain a crucial program of easy aerobic and strength-training exercises.

At the same time, alternative professional treatment can help stabilize the disease, says JoAnne Lombardi, M.D., a pulmonary specialist in Belmont, California. That includes instruction in tai chi or qigong and in "mindfulness" meditation to decrease the panic of being short of breath; tests for food allergies that can complicate the disease; a comprehensive nutritional profile; and counseling on cleaning up your indoor environment to avoid additional stress on the lungs.

of breath even more severe, says Dr. Lombardi. "I believe the remedy for malnutrition has to deliver a lot of calories and protein with very little bulk," she says.

Protein drinks do exactly that, she says. Start the day with a protein powder, mixing it in a blender with fat-free milk or fruit juice, Dr. Lombardi says. Follow the dosage recommendations on the label.

## GREEN POWDER: *Maximum Nutrition, Minimum Bulk*

When you fix your protein powder drink, add a powdered, nutrition-loaded "green drink" made from barley grass, green algae, or other chlorophyll-rich plant foods. The combination will provide plenty of protein and calories as well as lots of other nutrients and enzymes, nutritional sparks that power biochemical reactions in the body.

Dr. Lombardi favors the products Green Magma and Kyogreen. Mix 1 to 3 teaspoons with the protein powder. Then, there's one more ingredient to add to that breakfast mix.

## FLAXSEED: *Decrease Inflammation*

Flaxseed is rich in omega-3 fatty acids, which may play a role in decreasing lung inflammation and easing breathing, Dr. Lombardi says. Blend up to ¼ cup of ground flaxseed with your morning drink. You can grind the seeds in a coffee grinder, she advises, and keep the leftovers from spoiling by storing them in an opaque container in the refrigerator.

## ANTIOXIDANTS: *Maximum Lung Protection*

Studies show that smokers who have higher intakes of vitamin E and other key nutrients in their diets are less prone to develop COPD. That's because these nutrients are antioxidants that block the rustlike cellular destruction of the lungs that is sparked by cigarette smoke.

Dr. Lombardi thinks that antioxidants can also help protect a patient with emphysema or chronic bronchitis from further decline in lung function. Here are her antioxidant recommendations.

- Vitamin C: 500 to 1,000 milligrams three times a day.
- Vitamin E: 400 to 800 international units (IU) daily. Look for a product with mixed tocopherols, the most effective form of the nutrient.
- Selenium: 200 micrograms daily.
- Coenzyme $Q_{10}$: 10 to 50 milligrams three times a day.

## TAURINE: *Protect Yourself from Pollutants*

This amino acid may help protect the lungs from pollutants such as ozone, Dr. Lombardi says. Follow the dosage recommendations on the label. You can take up to 1,500 milligrams a day, says Dr. Lombardi, but if you take more than 500 milligrams daily, divide the doses.

## New Help for Your Smoking-Cessation Efforts

No alternative home remedies of any kind can work for emphysema or chronic bronchitis if you don't first quit smoking, says JoAnne Lombardi, M.D., a pulmonary specialist in Belmont, California. And quitting may have just have gotten a little easier.

The nutritional supplement Sulfonil, manufactured by Thorne Research, is believed to bind with nicotine receptors in the brain to help block the craving for cigarettes, and it may do it more effectively than a nicotine patch, Dr. Lombardi says. For as long as you have cravings after you quit, whether it's 3 days or 3 months, take two capsules when you wake up, one capsule every 4 to 6 hours during the day, and two at bedtime, says Dr. Lombardi.

**MAGNESIUM:** *Strengthen Breathing Muscles*
The mineral magnesium is involved in hundreds of biochemical processes, including maintaining normal muscle contraction.

"It can strengthen the skeletal muscles involved in breathing and relax the bronchi, the tubes that lead to the lungs," Dr. Lombardi says. She recommends 300 to 500 milligrams a day in three divided doses.

**CARNITINE:** *Another Boost for Breathing*
An intake of 250 milligrams of carnitine one to three times a day can also help strengthen skeletal muscles, Dr. Lombardi says.

**CAROTENES:** *Taste a Rainbow*
Carotenes obtained from food sources may have antioxidant effects that protect against lung damage, says Dr. Lombardi. Eat highly colored foods such as red, orange, and yellow peppers; dark green, leafy vegetables; and a variety of squashes.

# *Boost Immunity to Beat*
# **Endometriosis**

Endometriosis is a ruinous disease in which cells of the uterine lining, or endometrium, grow in some other part of the pelvic area, such as the ovaries, the cervix, the bowel, or the bladder.

These runaway cells group themselves in tiny dots, layers, or cysts, and they continue to respond to hormones. They bleed during every period, inflaming, scarring, and even destroying nearby tissue. They can form a kind of glue, or adhesion, that binds organs together, creating chronic pelvic pain and severe menstrual cramps. They can also result in infertility.

Conventional doctors often dismiss the severe menstrual cramps as "normal" or prescribe powerful menstruation-stopping drugs that also shrink your breasts, lower your voice, dry your vagina, and turn your emotions into a yo-yo. Some women endure several surgeries, only to find that the pain is still there.

But Deborah Metzger, M.D., Ph.D., medical director of Helena Women's Health in San Francisco and Palo Alto, California, says that she successfully treats women with "untreatable" endometriosis by using an alternative approach.

Endometriosis, she believes, is caused by an allergy to your own hormones. Moreover, the allergy-stressed immune system often permits an internal overgrowth of the common fungus *Candida albicans*.

"With treatment for the allergy and the fungus, my patients with endometriosis become like new people," she says. "They get relief from many of their chronic symptoms, like fatigue and depression, and they have new energy and new zest for life."

Dr. Metzger says that there are many things that a woman can do on her own to strengthen her immune system, thereby reducing symptoms and speeding the healing of endometriosis.

# GUIDE TO
# PROFESSIONAL CARE

If you have any of the following symptoms, which may indicate endometriosis, you should see a medical doctor. They include painful periods with heavy, irregular flow; pain before and after your period, often accompanied by lower-back pain; pelvic pain; diarrhea; painful bowel movements during periods; painful intercourse; inability to conceive; fatigue; and low energy.

"Traditional physicians are trained to believe that only surgery or hormone therapy can treat endometriosis," says Deborah Metzger, M.D., Ph.D., medical director of Helena Women's Health in San Francisco and Palo Alto, California.

While surgery is often necessary to remove or destroy lesions, and hormone therapy helps stop the progress of the condition, Dr. Metzger suggests additional treatments to prevent the recurrence of pain and to treat associated fatigue.

Because she has found in her practice that endometriosis patients are allergic to their own hormones, Dr. Metzger treats them with a neutralization method of immunotherapy, in which drops of a specially prepared, diluted form of the hormones are taken by mouth. Also, since about half of the women with endometriosis whom she treats also have an overgrowth of the common fungus *Candida albicans*, she might prescribe the antifungal drug nystatin (Mycostatin).

Finally, Dr. Metzger has discovered that many women with chronic pelvic pain from endometriosis also have other undiagnosed conditions, such as hernias, pelvic congestion, deep nodules of endometriosis, interstitial cystitis (chronic bladder infection), and uterine retroversion (tipped uterus), which act independently to cause pain. By surgically correcting these previously undiagnosed problems, she often eliminates pain in women who have had multiple surgeries for endometriosis but still have chronic pain.

## FOOD: *Take Out the Garbage*

Dr. Metzger tells her patients that diets full of processed foods are loaded with unnatural additives and preservatives that "poison" the body and worsen the symptoms of endometriosis. "Getting away from the garbage can make a very big difference in reducing the severity of the disease," she says.

That garbage also includes "high-stress" foods, says Susan Lark, M.D., a physician in Los Altos, California. She asks her patients to minimize their intake of commercial salad dressings, ketchup, soft drinks, coffee, and alcohol, as well as red meat and dairy products.

## REFINED CARBOHYDRATES: *Save Your Energy*

Both Dr. Lark and Dr. Metzger put particular emphasis on eliminating refined carbohydrates such as sugar and white flour.

"Sugar and white flour weaken the immune system and rob the body of energy," says Dr. Metzger. She believes that by cutting those foods out of her diet, a woman with endometriosis will function much better.

## VITAMINS AND MINERALS: *To Strengthen Immunity*

"A woman with endometriosis has higher requirements for certain vitamins because she needs to repair and strengthen her immune system to help fight the disease," Dr. Metzger says.

When you take the right nutrients at the right doses, the white blood cells and other components of the immune system are revved up. She recommends taking a daily multivitamin/mineral supplement along with the following additional nutrients every day.

• Vitamin C: 1,000 to 2,000 milligrams daily in three doses
• Vitamin E: 400 to 800 international units daily
• B-complex vitamins: A supplement that supplies at least 50 milligrams a day of the major B vitamins, such as thiamin and niacin

## FATTY ACIDS: *For Pain Relief*

The omega-3 and omega-6 fatty acids, found primarily in raw nuts, seeds, oils, and fatty fish, help create hormonelike chemicals in the body called series-1 prostaglandins, which relax muscles and blood vessels, thus reducing menstrual cramps, says Dr. Metzger. They may also reduce the inflammation of endometriosis, helping to reduce pelvic pain.

Dr. Lark recommends fresh flaxseed oil as the best source of omega-3's and omega-6's; she suggests taking 3 to 4 tablespoons a day. You can add it to foods as a butter substitute, but heating it destroys the fatty acids. Another good source of both omega-3's and omega-6's is pumpkin seed oil.

It's best to use fresh oils, since the omegas have a tendency to break down after a period of time. Also, since they can be difficult to find, you may need to request a special order from your health food store. Dr. Lark says that they're also effective in capsule form, which may be more readily available.

### Defeating Candida

"The vast majority of conventional doctors do not believe in the possibility of a systemic overgrowth of the common fungus *C. albicans*, let alone know about self-care treatments for the problem," says Dr. Metzger.

She has found that half the women with endometriosis in her practice have this fungal overgrowth and that treating the fungus often helps relieve the intense fatigue that strikes most women with the disease.

Thus, in addition to avoiding refined carbohydrates and sugars, which feed the fungus, here are some home remedies that can help clear up the infection.

**GRAPE SEED EXTRACT:** *Fight the Fungus*
This is a very potent antifungal that can help kill candida, says Dr. Metzger. Because it's so potent, she cautions women not to use more than is recommended on the label. Continue treatment with capsules for 3 to 6 months, she advises.

**GARLIC:** *A Candida Killer*
Taking capsules of garlic, which is also antifungal, is very effective at killing candida, Dr. Metzger says. Take 500 milligrams three or four times a day for 4 to 6 weeks.

**PROBIOTICS:** *Normalize Your Intestinal Flora*
A probiotic supplement containing the "friendly" intestinal bacteria *Lactobacillus acidophilus* and *Bifidobacterium bifidum*

can help limit the growth of candida, says Dr. Metzger. The supplement that you'll probably find in the store is called *L. acidophilus*, with *B. bifidum* also listed on the label.

Look for a refrigerated supplement containing both bacteria and follow the dosage recommendations on the label.

# *High-Energy Secrets to Wipe Out* Fatigue

Even though fatigue is the number one complaint that general practitioners hear from their patients, it can't be solved by conventional medicine alone, says Erika Schwartz, M.D., an internist in West Chester County, New York.

Fatigue isn't a disease, she explains. It doesn't show up on diagnostic tests. No drug can cure it. There isn't an operation that will cut it out of the body. Some conventional doctors, who are trained to detect illnesses with tests and solve them with drugs or surgery, may dismiss fatigue as incurable.

"Some doctors simply tell their patients that fatigue is as natural a consequence of growing older as gray hair and wrinkles," Dr. Schwartz says. "They say to people, 'You simply have to learn to live with it.' That is sheer and utter nonsense."

Instead, says Dr. Schwartz, lack of energy is a symptom of a fatigue-causing lifestyle, particularly a nutrition style that loads (and overloads) the engines of our bodies with low-quality fuel.

"We are underfed and underfueled and unable to step up to all the tasks and opportunities at hand," says Pamela Smith, R.D., a nutritionist in Orlando, Florida. "We push our bodies through the day without the right food as though we were cars that could run without gasoline."

But, says Smith, it's easy to banish fatigue and restore energy, because high-level energy is your natural state. "Energy is scripted into every cell of your body," she says. "The question is: Are you allowing that energy to flow forth so that it literally moves fatigue out of the way?"

## GUIDE TO
## PROFESSIONAL CARE

In today's busy, high-stress world, fatigue is almost a way of life for many people. It usually doesn't mean that there's a physical problem to worry about, says Erika Schwartz, M.D., a physician in West Chester County, New York.

There are many conditions, however, including mononucleosis, low thyroid function, and hepatitis, to name just a few, that can cause very serious fatigue. So if you're eating well, getting enough rest, and taking supplements, and your stress levels are low but you're still dragging for a month or more, you should make an appointment to see your doctor for a thorough checkup, Dr. Schwartz says.

---

If you want to answer that question with a hearty "Yes," try these energy-releasing remedies.

### CARNITINE: *A True Rejuvenator*

"I call carnitine the capsule of youth," says Dr. Schwartz. This amino acid transports nutritional fuel into the mitochondria, the energy factories in every cell. It also removes waste from the mitochondria so the operation of the factories isn't slowed by toxins.

Without carnitine, the body can't produce energy, and the typical American diet doesn't supply enough, says Dr. Schwartz.

"I have seen the positive effects of carnitine supplementation in hundreds of my patients, who looked and felt reinvigorated within days," she says.

Dr. Schwartz recommends starting with 500 milligrams of carnitine in tablet form twice a day, at breakfast and at lunch. As with all supplements, she advises taking it with an 8-ounce glass of water for digestive comfort.

Dr. Schwartz advises her patients to take carnitine indefinitely, recommending a minimum of 1,000 milligrams a day for people over 40. The older you are, the more you need it, she adds.

## COENZYME Q$_{10}$: *The Perfect Complement to Carnitine*

While carnitine carries fuel into the mitochondria, coenzyme Q$_{10}$ (coQ$_{10}$) helps the mitochondria use the fuel to make energy. Scientists have focused primarily on coQ$_{10}$'s ability to revive the cells of the heart. Studies have shown that it may help reverse life-threatening congestive heart failure by restoring the energy of the muscle cells.

It appears, however, that coQ$_{10}$ energizes all the cells in the body, not just those of the heart. "Without sufficient coenzyme Q$_{10}$, you will not be able to produce enough energy to maintain optimal health," Dr. Schwartz says.

To get a truly therapeutic dose from your diet, you would have to eat huge amounts of food—more than 6 pounds of beef, 14 pounds of peanuts, and 6 pounds of sardines daily—so Dr. Schwartz recommends a supplement as the best way to get enough. She suggests taking 30 milligrams twice a day, at breakfast and lunch. You can take this supplement indefinitely, she says.

### The Fire Down Below

In Ayurveda, the ancient system of natural healing from India, fatigue is a sign of "low digestive fire." This is a signal that the stomach and the rest of the digestive tract don't have the energy to metabolize and absorb food, says DeAnna Batdorff, a clinical aromatherapist and Ayurvedic practitioner in Forestville, California.

"When people build their digestive fires, they're going to get a much better result in terms of curing fatigue than if they just try to improve their energy with nutritional means," she says.

The best way to heighten digestive fire is with a breathing technique called the breath of fire. It involves taking 20 to 30 deep, slow breaths, with all of your attention focused on your stomach. But the breath of fire isn't like typical deep breathing, in which you let your abdomen soften and expand as you inhale, says Batdorff.

When you do the breath of fire, pull your stomach in as you inhale deeply and slowly, then push it out as you exhale slowly. Double-check your shoulders during the exercise to be sure that they're relaxed and your spine is erect.

Do this exercise once or twice every day, says Batdorff. It builds fire by promoting movement in the circulatory system. You will feel heat rise in your face if you've done the exercise properly, says Batdorff. "Then the exercise is complete," she adds.

## MAGNESIUM: *Relief for Tired Bodies*

Many people with everyday fatigue would benefit from taking magnesium, a mineral that's crucial for energy production. If you have a lot to do but can't seem to rouse your body to action, try taking 400 milligrams of magnesium at lunch along with carnitine and $coQ_{10}$, says Dr. Schwartz.

## GLUTAMATE: *Beat Brain Fatigue*

If you have mental fatigue that makes it hard for you to concentrate or think clearly, you may want to start taking a glutamate supplement.

"Glutamate is an amino acid that helps stabilize blood sugar levels," says Dr. Schwartz. "This prevents the sharp dips in blood sugar that can contribute to brain fatigue." She recommends taking 800 milligrams of glutamate with breakfast and 400 milligrams with lunch.

## OMEGA-3 FATTY ACIDS: *Energize Your Mood*

Fatigue and depression often go hand in hand. To help a blue mood, Dr. Schwartz suggests taking 1,000 milligrams of omega-3 fatty acids, which are essential for normal brain function. Take the supplement every day at breakfast, she advises.

### Foods That Fight Fatigue

"When it comes to having all the energy that you want and need, eating the right foods at the right times is as basic as getting enough sleep," says Smith. But, she says, don't worry about what you shouldn't eat. Instead, focus on foods and drinks that power you with high-octane energy fuel.

## WATER: *Avoid the Main Factor for Fatigue*

Dehydration—not drinking enough water every day—is one of the main reasons that people are fatigued, says Smith. "If you do nothing else in your quest for energy but begin to drink water each day, and drink a lot of it," she says, "you will experience a phenomenal boost in your energy."

Why water? It transports energy-giving nutrients, provides a cellular environment where they can work, helps oxygenate the blood, and maintains proper muscle tone. She recommends drinking between 64 and 80 ounces a day.

## FOOD: *Eat Often for Energy*

Eating small amounts of food throughout the day helps keep blood sugar levels—and energy levels—from plummeting, says Smith. Those mini-meals should supply carbohydrates and protein for maximum energy, since the glucose from the carbohydrates and the amino acids from the protein individually will fuel you for only a few hours, she says. Plus, choose low-fat foods, since high fat translates into low energy. Here's what a day of mini-meals might include.

• For breakfast, oats cooked in fat-free milk or juice, sweetened with apple juice or white grape juice, flavored with pumpkin pie spice and vanilla, and topped with fresh or dried fruit.
• At midmorning, a piece of fresh fruit or 1 to 2 ounces of low-fat cheese.
• For lunch, a turkey sandwich on whole-grain bread with Dijon mustard, a large green salad with chickpeas and feta cheese, or a piece of chicken with broccoli and a sweet potato. ("Always look for that balance of carbohydrates and protein, allowing carbohydrates to be burned for energy and utilizing the protein for building functions," says Smith.) For dessert, fresh mango and strawberries.
• In midafternoon, a snack of baked tortilla chips with bean dip and salsa.
• For dinner, fish or chicken, brown rice or a grain, a green salad, vegetables, and fruit-sweetened yogurt for dessert.
• In the evening, a snack of whole-grain cereal with fat-free milk or soy milk.

## Fill Your Life with Energy

Which would you prefer, sunshine streaming in the window or a windowless wall? Soothing music or a refrigerator's whine? Delicious scents or the chemical smell of a copy machine? In each case, the pleasing choice is obvious. And when you choose a pleasurable, low-stress environment, you're also choosing energy.

"You may be astounded by the enormously energizing effect of modifying your environment," says Smith.

## WARM COLORS: *Energizing the Brain*

Surrounding yourself with warm colors will send impulses to your brain that can boost your energy, says Smith. If it's your workspace that you want to energize, start by cleaning up the clutter—the paperwork and newspapers—on your desk. You'll eliminate cool whites, blues, and blacks that can cause energy to dip.

Then add yellow, orange, or red, Smith advises. (The electromagnetic waves of yellow are the most energizing, followed by those of orange, then red.) Any warm color will do the trick: a plant with yellow flowers, a poster with sunny colors, a warm painting, or Mexican pottery, for example. One caution for extroverts: An excess of fiery colors can overstimulate and distract you. Choose calming blue or green.

## NATURAL SCENTS: *Stimulate Alertness*

"Pleasant scents stimulate a nerve in the body that triggers wakefulness," says Smith. You don't need fancy potpourris or an aromatherapy dispenser, though. Just keep a basket of oranges or lemons on your desk and slice one when you're feeling fatigued. (You'll also benefit from the color of the fruits.) Or keep a mint plant nearby and break off a leaf to breathe in its aroma, she suggests.

## SOUNDS: *An Earful of Energy*

"Noise is an invisible fatigue factor in today's world," says Smith. She suggests using foam earplugs if you can't eliminate energy-sapping sounds in your environment. You could also buy a "white noise" machine that generates the sounds of waves, wind, or waterfalls.

Wearing headphones and listening to energizing music of your choice is another good option. "The best brain response will come from listening to music with gentle rhythms, such as that of the piano or flute, and without lyrics or loud drums," she says.

## Eliminate Fatigue Factors

If you're feeling lifeless, you need to look at your whole life. Getting too little sleep and not enough exercise commonly causes fatigue, says Smith. But there are easy ways to remedy the situation.

### SLEEP: *Refresh Yourself*

"Restful sleep can become part of your energized lifestyle prescription," says Smith. To improve your sleep, here's what she advises.

• Try to go to bed and get up at the same time every day, since the body craves regularity.
• Don't have coffee after lunch since caffeine can sabotage sleep.
• Avoid high-fat food in the evening because fat can make it harder to get to sleep or stay asleep.
• Sleep in a cool, dark, quiet room; it's the best environment for serious snoozing.
• Sleep on your side; you'll breathe easier and reduce snoring, which can make for a restless night.

### EXERCISE: *10 Minutes Equals 2 Hours of Energy*

A brisk, 10-minute walk can energize you for 2 hours, says Smith. She recommends taking three brief walks a day to keep your energy levels constant.

"You can walk almost anytime, anywhere," she says. If you prefer a longer exercise session, add some stretching and weight lifting to your program to keep your muscles loose and toned, which is a must for maximum energy.

If you're extremely fatigued, however, you may want to start with more restful types of exercise, such as yoga or the gentle Chinese exercises of tai chi, says DeAnna Batdorff, a clinical aromatherapist and Ayurvedic practitioner in Forestville, California.

"If your body is already depleted, aerobic exercise can leave you more tired than when you started," she says. "But if you start with an exercise routine using yoga or tai chi, you'll gradually build your energy over a month or so, and then you can add aerobic exercise to your routine."

# *Alternative Ways to Shrink or Even Eliminate* **Fibroids**

Fibroids are noncancerous masses that grow from the wall of the uterus; they can be as small as the dot of an *i* or bigger than a grapefruit. You can have one fibroid or dozens.

Uterine fibroids can be symptomless, but they can also cause problems such as heavy menstrual bleeding, bleeding between periods, constant pain or pressure in the abdomen or pelvis (or both), frequent urination (as a fibroid presses on the bladder), pain during intercourse, and lower-back pain.

And they're very common—25 to 50 percent of all women eventually develop them.

Should those women have hysterectomies (surgery to remove the uterus, or womb)? Certainly not right away, says Jason Elias, a practitioner of Traditional Chinese Medicine in New Paltz, New York.

"Unless a woman is bleeding so profusely that her health or life is threatened, I believe she should ask her surgeon to wait for 3 months, and during that time she should use natural means to attempt to reduce or eliminate her fibroids," he says.

Elias has seen dozens of cases in which fibroids have stopped growing, shrunk, or disappeared when a woman used alternative remedies. Here are some self-treatments that he suggests.

### ACUPRESSURE: *10 Minutes of Hands-On Healing*

In Traditional Chinese Medicine (TCM), chi is the life-force or energy that flows in currents, or meridians, throughout the body. The "liver chi" is understood to be both the organ itself and the energy system that controls the movement of the blood.

And, according to TCM, it is primarily "stagnant" liver chi that creates any kind of tumor or mass, including fibroids, Elias says. Stimulating the following acupressure points can help un-

# GUIDE TO PROFESSIONAL CARE

You should have a gynecologist check for uterine fibroids if you experience abnormal menstrual bleeding, a lump in your lower abdomen, difficulty with urination, or chronic pressure or pain in your lower abdomen or pelvis.

If the doctor diagnoses fibroids, however, don't quickly agree to a recommendation for a hysterectomy, an operation that removes the uterus, advises Herbert Goldfarb, M.D., director of the Montclair Reproductive Center in New Jersey and Minimally Invasive Gynecology in New York City.

"When gynecologists go from diagnosis of fibroids to a hysterectomy without any other consideration, they do their patients a disservice," Dr. Goldfarb says.

Instead, he says, women who are diagnosed with fibroids should receive a full range of additional diagnostic testing, including a hysteroscopy, in which the doctor inserts a fiber-optic scope into the uterus to accurately determine the location and size of fibroids. Dr. Goldfarb also recommends a transvaginal ultrasound, which detects the presence of fibroids.

Once the extent of the problem is accurately determined, your gynecologist can work with you to decide on the right treatment, which, again, is not necessarily a hysterectomy. Available treatments include not taking any immediate measures but conducting regular exams to monitor the growth of the fibroids; synthetic hormones; a myomectomy, in which the tumors are removed but the uterus is preserved; and myolysis, in which the fibroids are destroyed with a laser or special electrical needle.

block stagnant liver chi and shrink fibroids, Elias says. For the precise locations of the points, see page 700.

• LV3 is on the upper part of the foot between the big toe and the second toe, in the depression between the bones.
• LV14 is in the space between the ribs, two ribs from and directly below the nipple.

• CV4 is in the exact middle of the body, halfway between the pubic bone and the navel.
• SP6 is approximately three thumb-widths above the inside anklebone in a depression just to the side of the shinbone.
• SP10 is on the inside of the knee, 2½ inches above the kneecap in the fleshy part of the bulge.

To work the points, sit in a chair and move from point to point, making circular movements with your thumb in a clock-wise direction in and around the point for about 1 minute. Use pressure that's slightly painful but not so much so that you want to stop.

Work each point twice a day for at least 3 months. If your doctor confirms that your fibroids have shrunk or disappeared, continue stimulating the points to keep the fibroids from coming back.

## FOOD: *Avoid Eating Estrogen*

The hormone estrogen "feeds" fibroids, says Elias, which is why they often vanish with menopause, when estrogen levels decrease. But you also feed yourself estrogen in foods such as red meat, poultry, dairy products, and eggs, which contain the synthetic estrogen routinely fed to animals that are grown for market.

"I believe high-estrogen foods should be avoided for the 3-month healing period and, ideally, thereafter," Elias says. One way to achieve this is to seek out organic, hormone-free dairy, eggs, meat, and poultry.

Elias also asks his fibroid patients to avoid refined sugar, white flour, alcohol, caffeine, and cigarettes, all of which stress the body and interfere with healing because they overwork the liver and lead to stagnation and fibroid growth.

## FOOD: *Have Lots of Fiber and Soy*

Fiber helps the liver process and excrete excess estrogen, so Elias recommends emphasizing high-fiber foods such as whole grains, beans, vegetables, and fruit. Also, concentrate on soybean products like soy milk, tofu, soy sauce, and miso (a flavorful soy paste). Soy is rich in natural estrogens called phytoestrogens, compounds that are 100 times weaker than synthetic estrogens, so they don't harm your body. But they do bind to estrogen receptor sites, preventing harmful synthetic estrogens from damaging your system, says Elias.

## MAGNESIUM: *Nourishment for the Muscle*

A deficiency of the mineral magnesium is common among Americans, and it often creates stagnation in muscle tissue, such as the walls of the uterus, Elias says. Adequate amounts of the mineral relax muscle tissue, allowing a fresh flow of blood into the area. He recommends taking 1,000 to 1,500 milligrams of supplemental magnesium a day.

## $B_6$ AND EVENING PRIMROSE OIL: *To Process Estrogen*

Elias suggests that women with fibroids take 100 milligrams a day of vitamin $B_6$ and 1,000 milligrams a day of evening primrose oil, which supplies the essential fatty acid gamma-linolenic acid (GLA). Both of these supplements help the body process estrogen, he says.

## MULTIVITAMIN/MINERAL SUPPLEMENT: *To Boost Healing*

Elias also recommends a high-potency multivitamin/mineral supplement to be sure that you're getting all the nutrients your body needs to heal. Follow the dosage recommendations on the label.

## PROGESTERONE: *To the Rescue*

Progesterone cream contains natural progesterone, and supplying the body with more progesterone so that estrogen is not dominant can help heal fibroids, Elias says. Look for a cream that specifically lists progesterone, not wild yams, as an ingredient.

"I have been recommending this to my patients for 10 years, and it is quite safe," he says. Use the cream twice a day for about 15 days a month, from ovulation to the onset of menstruation. In the morning and again in the evening, rub ½ teaspoon of the cream into areas of soft skin, such as the insides of your thighs or your lower abdomen. Continue this process for at least 3 months. If your doctor confirms that your fibroids have shrunk or disappeared by that time, keep using the cream as a preventive measure.

# *Conquer the Pain and Fatigue of* **Fibromyalgia**

Want to develop fibromyalgia syndrome in the next day or two? It's not that hard to do.

Just go to the local sleep lab, have yourself hooked up to an electroencephalograph (a machine that detects and displays brain waves), and, right before bedtime, ask the technician to wake you up every time you start producing delta waves, the brain waves of deep sleep.

"Within 1 to 2 days, you'll develop classic fibromyalgia pain," says Jacob Teitelbaum, M.D., a physician in Annapolis, Maryland.

Yes, the 3 to 6 million Americans who have the symptoms of fibromyalgia—the shifting pattern of constantly achy and tender muscles all over the body; the near-constant fatigue; the barrage of other problems that include frequent infections and bowel disorders—are suffering from a sleep disorder, alternative healers say.

Here's what typically happens: You feel exhausted all day, but when it's time for bed, your mind is racing. You eventually fall asleep, but you wake up repeatedly, sometimes as often as 3 to 15 times a night. Finally, at about 4:00 or 5:00 A.M., you wake up again—and stay awake until the alarm sounds. Then the dismal cycle of dragging days starts all over again.

Dr. Teitelbaum believes that this lack of deep sleep, caused by a malfunctioning hypothalamus, the master endocrine gland in the brain, can affect almost every part of the body. It shortens muscles, leaving them chronically tense and tender. It plays havoc with your hormones, your immune system, your brain neurotransmitters, and your digestion, triggering one or more of dozens of possible symptoms. It triples your body's levels of substance P, the chemical responsible for sensitivity to pain, so your muscles hurt—a lot. Also, since the body repairs itself dur-

# GUIDE TO
# PROFESSIONAL CARE

"Your doctor is likely to be unfamiliar with the research on effective treatment of fibromyalgia," says Jacob Teitelbaum, M.D., a physician in Annapolis, Maryland. But there *is* effective treatment. "I have treated hundreds of patients with fibromyalgia—some of whom have been to 10, 20, or even 30 doctors—and more than 85 percent are improved or cured. That is, their symptoms are no longer a problem," Dr. Teitelbaum says. Improvement usually occurs in about 3 months on his program, he says.

Dr. Teitelbaum treats the problem as a malfunction of the hypothalamus, the master endocrine gland in the brain. His treatment protocol can include some or all of the following, depending on symptoms and the results of laboratory tests.

- Hormone medications or supplements for possible deficiencies of thyroid, adrenal, and ovarian or testicular hormones
- Various drugs and herbs for sleep disorders
- Medications for low blood pressure due to a malfunction of the hypothalamus
- Antiparasitic and antifungal drugs for these types of infections
- A multivitamin supplement, magnesium glycinate, malic acid, vitamin $B_{12}$, iron, and other supplements for nutritional deficiencies

You or your doctor can find out more about the details of Dr. Teitelbaum's treatment protocol at www.endfatigue.com on the Web.

ing deep sleep, none of those problems ever gets a chance to heal.

The disease can start in many different ways, says Dr. Teitelbaum. Stopping it baffles conventional physicians, some of whom fail to even recognize that fibromyalgia exists. But Dr.

Teitelbaum has had remarkable success reducing and usually even eliminating the pain and fatigue of fibromyalgia with a combination of natural remedies and medicines.

He suggests that each of these remedies be used for 6 months. If you are sleeping through the night and feeling better at that point, he says to gradually decrease their use over a 9- to 12-month period.

### VALERIAN AND LEMON BALM: *For Deep Sleep*

At night, the herb valerian, taken in conjunction with lemon balm, can help increase the amount and depth of deep sleep, says Dr. Teitelbaum. He recommends taking the product Valerian Rest with Lemon Balm by To Your Health, containing 160 to 480 milligrams of valerian and 80 to 240 milligrams of lemon balm, before bedtime.

During the day, the valerian alone can have a calming effect. He recommends 100 milligrams three times a day for anxiety.

### KAVA KAVA : *A Reasonable Alternative*

This herb relaxes muscles, calms the mind, and deepens sleep, says Dr. Teitelbaum. He recommends taking 200 to 750 milligrams before bedtime. Look for a product standardized for at least 30 percent kavalactones, the herb's active ingredients.

Very rarely, kava causes photosensitivity. If you take it and develop a rash, Dr. Teitelbaum says to reduce your dose by 50 percent and take the herb with a high-potency B-complex vitamin containing 50 milligrams of most of the B's. This often eliminates the rash.

### MELATONIN: *Reset Your Body Clock*

Your pineal gland, a hormone-secreting gland in your brain that produces melatonin, controls your body's internal clock, or its awareness of day and night. In fibromyalgia, that clock is out of whack, says Dr. Teitelbaum. "The body doesn't know whether it's day or night—it's very confused." Taking the hormone melatonin can help reset your internal clock, so when it's time to sleep, you fall asleep.

He recommends that people with fibromyalgia take 200 to 300 micrograms before bedtime. "In most people, this dosage is every bit as effective for improving sleep as a higher amount," he says. Do not take this supplement unless under the supervision of a knowledgeable medical doctor.

## MAGNESIUM: *To Relax Muscles*

"Magnesium is involved in many different reactions in the body and is especially important for muscles to relax," Dr. Teitelbaum says. "If your intake of magnesium is low, your muscles may stay in spasm, and your fibromyalgia will not resolve."

Since much of the magnesium in food is removed by processing, the average American gets far less than the 400 milligrams that the government's official standards say your body needs. "Almost everyone is deficient in magnesium," Dr. Teitelbaum says.

He says that the form of supplemental magnesium you use to correct that deficiency is critical. There are many types of magnesium, and not all of them are well-absorbed by the body. He recommends the product FibroCare Tablets, by To Your Health, which supplies magnesium glycinate combined with malic acid, making the magnesium maximally absorbable. Follow the dosage recommendations on the label and continue to take the supplement as a preventive measure even after your fibromyalgia improves.

There's one caution, however. Supplemental magnesium can cause diarrhea. If that occurs, cut back on your intake by 75 to 100 milligrams a day until the diarrhea goes away.

## MASSAGE: *Rub Out Pain*

One of the best (and easiest) types of massage for soothing tight, aching, tender muscles is deep friction massage, says Ralph R. Stephens, a licensed massage therapist and instructor of sports massage and neuromuscular therapy at Ralph Stephens Seminars in Cedar Rapids, Iowa. Here's how to do it.

Put the middle, index, and ring fingers of one hand on an area of muscle tension or tenderness and apply enough pressure so that your fingertips won't slide over your skin or clothing. Make 5 to 10 circular motions, rubbing just hard enough to elicit mild discomfort but not hard enough to cause pain.

"The massage movement shifts the skin over the deeper muscle layers, rolling the muscle fibers across each other, improving circulation, and relaxing the nervous system," says

Stephens. Once you've massaged one spot, move over by a hand-width or so and repeat.

"You can massage your legs, arms, chest, and the back of your neck quite easily with this technique," Stephens says. Massage an area, let it rest for a few minutes, then massage it a second time. This can be done daily, and you should experience some immediate relief. If massage causes pain in an area, you are pressing too hard, working it too long, or both. Allow the area a few days of rest and then massage it again with less intensity.

## VISUALIZATION: *Watch Your Muscles Relax*

Through visualization, you can tap the power of your mind to help relax the tight, tender muscles of fibromyalgia, says Simone Ravicz, Ph.D., a clinical psychologist in Pacific Palisades, California, who has fibromyalgia.

First, sit comfortably in a chair. Let your attention go to a spot where your muscles hurt. Next, says Dr. Ravicz, visualize the muscles in that area as tied in a knot. Then, in your mind's eye, see them slowly loosening, becoming completely untied, and finally lengthening and stretching.

As you're visualizing, take slow, deep breaths and let your entire body relax. Do this visualization exercise once a day for 5 to 10 minutes to reduce pain and help prevent daily flare-ups.

## MULTIVITAMIN/MINERAL SUPPLEMENT: *To Your Health*

Fibromyalgia can cause multiple nutritional deficiencies because of digestive problems, says Dr. Teitelbaum. He recommends that everyone with this condition take a high-potency multivitamin/mineral supplement.

He recommends My Favorite Multiple or My Favorite Multiple—Take One by Natrol, which he believes are the most complete supplements on the market. Follow the dosage recommendations on the label, and take the supplement on a long-term basis as a preventive even after your fibromyalgia improves.

# *Better Digestion Is the Key to Stopping* **Flatulence**

Antibiotics come with numerous side effects, but here's one that you may not have heard about. They can give you gas, not only when you're taking them but also afterward—and maybe for the rest of your life.

Flatulence is a natural part of digestion, caused by gas-producing bacteria in the intestinal tract. But people who have taken antibiotics may have to deal with it more often because antibiotics do more than kill bacteria that cause infections. They also kill bacteria throughout the body, including the billions of helpful bacteria that normally live in the large intestine, says Pamela Sky Jeanne, N.D., a naturopathic doctor in Gresham, Oregon.

When these bacteria are destroyed, unfriendly bacteria (and other organisms, such as yeast) take their place and begin generating toxins that can lead to gas, bloating, and diarrhea. This condition is called dysbiosis—too many bad bacteria, too few good.

Restoring the body's natural bacterial balance is an essential first step for controlling flatulence. In addition, there are things you can do to help your entire digestive system work more efficiently, which will go a long way toward reducing the discomfort (and embarrassment) of flatulence.

## PROBIOTICS: *Restoring the Good Bacteria*
Since antibiotics invariably disrupt the intestine's normal bacterial balance, or what doctors call the intestinal flora, alternative practitioners believe that you can restore the balance by taking a probiotic—a supplement that contains helpful bacteria. Look for a supplement that contains 2 to 3 billion units of acidophilus, bifidum, or other organisms, says Dr. Jeanne.

Just be sure to buy supplements that are refrigerated in the

# GUIDE TO
# PROFESSIONAL CARE

Some flatulence is normal, but when it happens all the time, it may be a symptom of digestive problems that won't go away without professional treatment, says Pamela Sky Jeanne, N.D., a naturopathic doctor in Gresham, Oregon.

If you experience symptoms such as involuntary weight loss, loss of appetite, vomiting, a change in bowel habits, or rectal bleeding, you should see a physician. If you are experiencing those symptoms, you may want ask your doctor if you should consider having a comprehensive digestive stool analysis. This test can detect gas-causing problems such as dysbiosis (an imbalance of bad and good bacteria), candida (yeast) infections, and more. You may also want to see a naturopathic or alternative-minded medical doctor in order to have a test for food sensitivities, Dr. Jeanne says.

store. That way, you'll know that the organisms are alive and active, she advises. You need to take probiotics during antibiotic therapy and for a minimum of 2 weeks after finishing the antibiotic dose. Follow the dosage recommendations on the label.

"Probiotics work," adds Elizabeth Lipski, a certified clinical nutritionist in Kauai, Hawaii. "They really keep the bad bacteria under control."

## DIGESTIVE ENZYMES: *After Each Meal*

The body produces lots of digestive enzymes, chemicals that help break down food so that it can be absorbed through the wall of the intestine. Some people don't produce enough of these enzymes, however. This is especially common once you pass your 50th birthday, since levels of digestive enzymes tend to decline with age.

"A digestive enzyme supplement will help your body digest food more quickly and easily," says Lipski. She recommends taking a digestive enzyme after each meal, following the directions on the label. Many people find that they get the best results when they combine digestive enzymes with probiotic supplements, she adds.

## FOOD: *Round Up the Gashouse Gang*

Some people are sensitive to the proteins and sugars in certain foods, which results in poor digestion and gas, Lipski says. Food sensitivities can be tricky to identify because it's hard to know what's causing the problem.

She recommends experimenting with different foods by eliminating them from your diet, one by one, for 10 days. If your gas is reduced, you'll know you've found the culprit. Here are some of the worst offenders.

• Dairy foods, because many people lack an enzyme called lactase that the body needs to digest the sugar (lactose) in milk and other dairy foods.
• Fruit juices, which contain a sugar called fructose that causes gas in many people. Even people who aren't sensitive to fructose may have gas when they drink more than three glasses of juice a day, Lipski says.
• Artificial sweeteners such as xylitol and sorbitol, which are found in many candies and baked goods and can make people gassy.
• Wheat, because many people are sensitive to its protein, gluten.
• Beans, cabbage, brussels sprouts, cauliflower, and cucumber, which all contain a potential gas-producing carbohydrate called raffinose. In the long run, however, these otherwise healthful foods can actually reduce gas because the body's bacteria will undergo alterations in order to deal with the raffinose, Lipski says.

## GINGER: *A Digestive Boost*

Ginger is an excellent herb for preventing or clearing up flatulence, says Mark Stengler, N.D., a naturopathic physician in San Diego. It works by stimulating digestion and relaxing the muscles of the digestive tract so food spends less time in the intestines.

Take two capsules, or 250 milligrams, with each meal, he says. Look for a product that has been standardized for 1 percent gingerols, one of the active ingredients.

## Do You *Really* Have a Problem?

Many people who think they're passing too much gas are actually releasing normal amounts, says William B. Salt II, M.D., clinical associate professor of medicine at Ohio State University College of Medicine and Public Health in Columbus. "Normal is anywhere from 6 to 21 times a day," he says.

The easiest way to find out if your gas expulsions are in the normal range is to keep a small notebook with you and actually tally gas-passing episodes. "Many of my patients who do this find that they aren't having abnormal numbers of passages," Dr. Salt says. "More often than not, they don't have a problem; they just thought that they did."

### CHLOROPHYLL: *Deodorize Your Insides*

A chlorophyll supplement can reduce gas and odor by detoxifying partially digested food in the digestive tract, says Lipski. Chlorophyll is entirely safe, and you can take it whenever you're feeling uncomfortable, following the directions on the label.

### FENNEL SEEDS: *A Digestive Aid*

"Chewing on fennel seeds after a meal is an excellent way to relieve flatulence," says Dr. Jeanne. The oils in the herb aid the digestive process, she explains, so you may want to nibble some seeds after every meal. Chew 5 to 10 seeds well, then swallow them to get the full effect, she advises.

### ACTIVATED CHARCOAL: *For Reliable Short-Term Relief*

You're about to be in a social situation where gas is a no-no, but you're in the middle of a gas attack! What do you do? Try a supplement of activated charcoal, says Andrew Gaeddert, a professional member of the American Herbalists Guild and director of the Get Well Clinic in Oakland, California.

Charcoal works by binding with toxins and other substances in the digestive tract and ushering them out of the body—quietly. The supplement should relieve gas in about 30 minutes.

Gaeddert recommends taking one to two 200- to 500-milligram tablets before occasional social situations, but never for more than 2 weeks at a time.

# *Natural Remedies to Power Away* **Flu**

Peter Holyk, M.D., says he's never had a bout of flu that lasted overnight. Think about it: never having to suffer from one of those awful 24-hour (or longer) bugs that make you feel achy, feverish, and totally fatigued. It doesn't seem possible.

"With alternative home remedies, I believe that you can knock out the flu in less than 24 hours," says Dr. Holyk, director of the Contemporary Health Clinic in Sebastian, Florida. The reason you can beat the flu with natural medicine is that these remedies help boost the power of your immune system, allowing it to quickly and easily beat the infection that's beating on you.

Of course, many doctors suggest that you should still get a yearly flu shot if you're age 65 or over, or if you have diabetes or heart, lung, or kidney disease (or you live with anyone who fits these criteria, since you don't want to infect them). Flu is much more dangerous for people with underlying illnesses, so you don't want to take chances.

If you already have the flu, however, here are a few ways to get rid of it fast.

### DR. HOLYK'S ANTI-FLU COCKTAIL: *Power in a Glass*
There are many different herbs and foods that can help beat the flu, and you can blend quite a few of them in one flu-chasing cocktail, which Dr. Holyk recommends drinking twice a day when you have the flu. Here's what it includes.

• One or two cloves of garlic. Garlic is a potent antiviral food, sparking natural killer cells and other immune factors into action. Chop the cloves of garlic as fine as possible before putting them in the blender, which helps to release the active ingredients.

> # GUIDE TO
> # PROFESSIONAL CARE
>
> Flu usually goes away without complications, but sometimes the infection moves into the lungs, causing viral or bacterial pneumonia. That's why it's important to stop flu as quickly as you can, says Peter Holyk, M.D., director of the Contemporary Health Clinic in Sebastian, Florida.
>
> If your symptoms last more than 5 days or if your flu is accompanied by an extremely high fever (104°F or higher), chest pain, blood in your nasal mucus, or phlegm that is brown, green, or bloody, go to a doctor right away. Dr. Holyk doesn't recommend trying to suppress a fever of 99° or 100°F, however, as a low-grade fever causes your immune system to increase its activity and helps it fight the flu more effectively.
>
> There's not a lot that conventional doctors can do to stop flu, but alternative physicians have a number of very effective techniques. "If flu is severe, I will use viral neutralization, injecting a person with a series of very dilute doses of the flu vaccine," says John M. Sullivan, M.D., a physician in Mechanicsburg, Pennsylvania. "People can typically return to work in 24 hours with this treatment."
>
> Intravenous doses of vitamin C and virus-killing hydrogen peroxide can also short-circuit the flu, says Guillermo Asis, M.D., director of Path to Health in Burlington, Massachusetts.

• Three droppers of echinacea tincture. This classic herbal remedy for upper respiratory infections increases the production of white blood cells, lymphocytes, and macrophages, which are immune system factors that fight the flu virus.
• Three droppers of goldenseal tincture. It helps reduce the irritation and inflammation in the lining of your respiratory tract, soothing a cough or sore throat.
• Three droppers of cat's claw tincture. Used for centuries by people in the Andes, this herb is well-known among alternative practitioners as a powerful immune booster.
• A pinch of cayenne pepper. It helps thin mucus and improves circulation.

• The juice of ½ lemon. Lemon juice helps clean the liver so that it can more effectively process all the toxins generated by the body as it fights the flu.
• Six to 8 ounces of organic tomato or vegetable juice. This is the base of the drink.

Once you have everything ready, put the ingredients in a blender along with a couple of ice cubes to make the drink more palatable. After blending, sip it slowly for a few minutes. Drink the mixture twice a day for the duration of the flu, which, thanks to the cocktail, should be mercifully short, says Dr. Holyk.

## WATER: *You'll Need a Lot*

Fighting the flu puts your metabolism into overdrive. Your body throws off water in huge amounts, says Dr. Holyk. You have to replace that water because your body needs it to expel toxins produced by your immune system as it's destroying the virus.

To make sure that you're getting enough water, Rashid Ali Buttar, D.O., an osteopathic physician who practices emergency and preventive medicine in Charlotte, North Carolina, recommends drinking enough water (in ounces) to equal two-thirds of your body weight daily. The minimum for maintenance is about one-half your weight. If you weigh 150 pounds, for example, you'll want to drink at least 100 ounces of water a day if you're sick and 75 ounces for maintenance.

## HYDROTHERAPY: *Good for Circulation*

You don't have to take water internally to get the benefits. Applying water to the outside of your body, a technique called hydrotherapy, can improve circulation, relieve congestion, and increase the number of flu-fighting white blood cells, says Mark Stengler, N.D., a naturopathic physician in San Diego. Here's how to do it.

• Take a comfortably hot bath or shower for 5 minutes.
• Get out and dry yourself quickly.
• Place a towel in cold water, wring it out, and wrap it around your body from your armpits to your groin. Leave it in place for 20 minutes, or until it's warmed. In the meantime, cover yourself with a wool blanket to avoid getting chilled.

Doing hydrotherapy once or twice a day can help relieve many of the worst flu symptoms and make you feel a lot better, Dr. Stengler says.

**FOOD:** *Wait for Dairy until You're Better*

Dairy foods increase mucus production, which makes the nasal congestion caused by flu even worse, Dr. Stengler says. Also, since many people are sensitive to dairy products, your body may be wasting immune cells on the food instead of fighting the virus, he explains. So avoid dairy products until you kick the flu.

**GINGER:** *Good for What Ails You*

Ginger tea fights flu on a number of fronts, says Dr. Stengler. It helps relieve nasal congestion. It can improve blood flow through the muscles and the rest of the body, helping to eliminate chills and muscle aches and allowing immune cells to circulate more effectively. It even helps reduce the pain of sore throat.

Have a cup every 2 to 3 hours until your flu is better, says Dr. Stengler. "Make enough for the day and warm it up before you drink it," he adds.

You can buy ginger tea bags in health food stores, or you can make tea from scratch by boiling a 5-inch piece of fresh ginger in 2 cups of water for 5 to 10 minutes.

**ASTRAGALUS:** *Multiplies T Cells*

This potent, immune-stimulating herb from the pharmacy of practitioners of Traditional Chinese Medicine helps defeat the flu by triggering the production of virus-fighting T cells, says Nedra Downing, D.O., an osteopathic physician who practices alternative medicine in Clarkston, Michigan. She recommends taking three drops of astragalus tincture in water three times a day for 10 days.

## Why You Should Favor a Fever

Conventional medicine often views a fever as an enemy to be vanquished—quickly—with drug intervention. Alternative healers take a decidedly different view.

"We don't view most fevers as a problem," says Mark Stengler, N.D., a naturopathic physician in San Diego. "A fever is stimulating your immune system to defeat the virus. If you eliminate the fever, you can prolong the flu."

Even though fever is good, however, you don't want to get too hot, Dr. Stengler adds. If your temperature is higher than 104°F, you should see a doctor.

A quick way to reduce fever is to drink a cup of yarrow tea every few hours. "Your fever should be reduced after you've had two or three cups," says Dr. Stengler.

Both feverfew and elderberry have long been used to help calm fevers, says Rashid Ali Buttar, D.O., an osteopathic physician who practices emergency and preventive medicine in Charlotte, North Carolina. He recommends taking 250 milligrams of feverfew two or three times a day in pill or capsule form. If you choose elderberry, drink some tea every few hours.

## VITAMIN C: *Keeps Your Body Strong*

When you have the flu, your virus-fighting white blood cells need vitamin C to be most effective, Dr. Downing says. The vitamin also shores up your adrenal glands, which help your body resist the stress of the infection. She recommends 3,000 milligrams of vitamin C a day in three divided doses. It's best to use the buffered form, which is easier on the stomach, she says. You can take this for several months during flu season.

## IP-6: *A Virus Killer*

The supplement IP-6, short for inositol hexaphosphate, is thought to stimulate the natural killer cells of the immune system, which are true to their name, says Dr. Downing: They kill flu viruses. Take two capsules twice a day as long as you're sick, she advises.

## THYMUS EXTRACT: *More Help for T Cells*

Supplements of thymus gland extract are thought to help the body generate hormones that spark the formation of T cells, which work as important virus killers. Take 350 milligrams of the extract according to label directions for 1 to 2 weeks, starting at the first sign of the flu, says Kenneth A. Bock, M.D., codirector of the Rhinebeck Health Center in Rhinebeck, New York, and the Center for Progressive Medicine in Albany, New York. Do not take this supplement unless under the supervision of a knowledgeable medical doctor.

**STEAM:** *Force Out the Virus*

Coughing is essential when you have the flu. Otherwise, virus-laden mucus that isn't expelled may harden and travel to the lungs, possibly leading to pneumonia, says Guillermo Asis, M.D., director of Path to Health in Burlington, Massachusetts. Using a steamer or humidifier to keep mucus moist and moving out of your body will help prevent this, he explains.

It's best to keep a steamer or humidifier running in your bedroom until the flu is gone. Add six to eight drops of thyme, eucalyptus, or rose geranium essential oil to the water to help moisten mucous membranes, Dr. Downing says.

# *Identifying and Relieving* Food Allergies

Most conventional allergists will tell you that food allergies are relatively uncommon, occurring in less than 1 percent of the population and mainly in children.

Further, they feel that most people with food allergies are allergic to one food, or maybe two or three at the most. The allergic symptoms—mostly skin, respiratory, and digestive problems—are obvious, they say, and often start within an hour or two of eating the offending food. The immune system reacts to the food allergen in the same way it might react to other allergens such as pollen or mold: It immediately produces an antibody that causes a release of histamine, one of the many chemicals that trigger classic allergy symptoms.

There's one problem with this description, says James Braly, M.D., an allergy specialist in Boca Raton, Florida. It's just flat out wrong.

"I believe that the thinking of the majority of allergists is some 20 to 30 years out of date when it comes to food allergy," Dr. Braly says. "Mountains of scientific research show that these widely held views about allergy are distorted."

Yes, some people do have the classic type of food allergy described above, but Dr. Braly believes that's only one type of food allergy, accounting for only about 5 to 10 percent of all cases. Here's what you need to know about the other 90 to 95 percent.

Food allergies aren't rare, and they don't occur mainly in children. In fact, the majority of Americans—adults as well as children—are allergic to certain foods, Dr. Braly says. No one knows why so many people are allergic, but Dr. Braly theorizes that the major causes are excess stress, inadequate rest, a toxic environment, and an unnatural diet.

In addition, food allergies don't affect just the skin or the respiratory or digestive system. They can affect any system, tissue, or organ in the body, says Dr. Braly, and often, they do.

Many health problems are either caused or complicated by food allergies, says Jacqueline Krohn, M.D., a physician in New Mexico. These include anemia, high blood pressure, fatigue, eczema, asthma, migraines, ear infections, sinusitis, hearing loss, thyroid disease, hay fever, fibrocystic breast disease, kidney disease, diabetes, arthritis, gallbladder disease, irritable bowel syndrome, and heartburn as well as many others, she says.

Moreover, allergic reactions to foods don't always occur immediately. Your symptoms may show up anywhere from 2 hours to 3 days after eating the food, so you may never suspect that the cause of your discomfort has anything to do with food. And you may be allergic to many foods, not just 1 or 2, Dr. Braly says (3 to 10 is not uncommon, and sometimes it may be as many as 20).

The immune system reacts to food allergens (usually, undigested proteins that pass into the bloodstream through a gut wall that's been made permeable, or "leaky," by many lifestyle and biochemical factors) by producing many different types of antibodies that attach to the allergens. These food-antibody complexes trigger an array of inflammatory reactions that create various symptoms and diseases, Dr. Braly says.

There's one more thing you need to know: "Food allergies can be minimized, corrected, or eliminated," he says.

# GUIDE TO PROFESSIONAL CARE

You should seek immediate medical attention if serious symptoms of allergy develop after eating. These include severe hives, itching, swelling, light-headedness, wheezing, shortness of breath, and difficulty swallowing.

You should also see your doctor if you have any chronic illness or unexplained symptom; if you are from a family of allergy sufferers (there is a strong genetic influence in allergies); if you have a family member who has gluten sensitivity or celiac disease; or if you have Type 1 (insulin-dependent) diabetes, autoimmune thyroid disease, or osteoporosis that is not responding to conventional therapy.

If you can't figure out which foods are causing your symptoms, or if you're not even sure that foods are responsible, see an alternative-minded allergist who understands the true nature of food allergies, says James Braly, M.D., an allergy specialist in Boca Raton, Florida. Since food allergies can be so complicated, most people find that they need professional care, he explains.

Your doctor may order a highly accurate blood test that can test delayed reactions to more than 100 foods. After the test, your doctor may conduct an elimination-and-challenge test that involves removing foods from the diet, then reintroducing them one at a time. Once the tests are complete, you and your doctor can create a dietary plan to avoid the foods that trigger your allergic reactions.

## Discovering the Cause

Finding out which foods or food proteins you're allergic to can be complicated. Many people need the help of physicians to identify their food allergies and then avoid the foods that are making them sick. But here are some steps that you can try on your own to start identifying the source—or sources—of your problems.

## FOOD DIARY: *Your Personal Guide*

You need to know which types of foods you're eating all the time, that is, every day or almost every day. One (or more) of these is most likely to be your allergic food.

"When you continually bombard the body with the same foods containing the same nutrients, especially in the context of a leaky gut, it eventually cries 'uncle,'" Dr. Braly says.

Mark Stengler, N.D., a naturopathic physician in San Diego, recommends keeping a food diary. Write down everything you eat (including the ingredients in processed foods) for a week.

If you find that you're eating any food or ingredient three, four, or more times a week, eliminate it from your diet for 10 days and see whether you feel better. Then eat it again and see whether you feel worse. If not eating the food improves your symptoms, and eating it worsens them, it's very likely that you're allergic to that food, says Dr. Stengler.

## ELIMINATION DIET: *Round Up the Usual Suspects*

Most people with food allergies react to one of a small number of commonly eaten foods. The usual suspects include dairy foods, eggs, grains (especially wheat, rye, barley, oats, and corn), soybeans in any form (from tofu to soy milk), citrus fruits, and peanuts.

Thus, another strategy is to eliminate all of these foods from your diet for 10 days, then reintroduce them one by one to see if anything happens, says Dr. Stengler. Reintroduce only one food every 4 days, since it takes that long for your body to clear itself of a food allergen.

### Combating Allergies with Vitamin C

Vitamin C is good for everyone, but people with food allergies may need extra amounts. That's because this essential nutrient helps stop allergic reactions to foods, says Jacqueline Krohn, M.D., a physician in New Mexico.

It relieves symptoms and prevents inflammation. It helps in the manufacture of adrenal hormones, which are needed to combat the body-wide stress of allergic reactions. And it helps rejuvenate an immune system worn out by responding to allergens.

"Allergic people should take vitamin C daily," says Dr. Krohn. The idea is to take as much as your body can handle. That level differs from person to person, so keep taking more until you experience diarrhea, then reduce the amount slightly until the side effect disappears.

Start with 1,000 milligrams a day, taken with a meal. Increase the amount by 1,000 milligrams daily, dividing the total dosage evenly throughout the day, Dr. Krohn advises. When you develop diarrhea, reduce the amount by 1,000 milligrams. This will be your proper level, she says.

Use ascorbic acid or any of the ascorbate forms, but check the label to be sure that they're hypoallergenic. Do not use timed-release or chewable vitamins, Dr. Krohn says. You may not have enough stomach acid to digest the timed-release form, and chewables often contain allergenic substances. If you experience mild bladder irritation or burning in the stomach, switch to a different form of ascorbate.

## Living Allergy-Free

Once you've identified the food (or foods) that is causing your allergy, you obviously need to avoid it. In addition, there are a number of simple changes that will make your body less sensitive.

### ROTATION DIET: *Helps Prevent Allergies*

People who eat the same foods all the time are more likely to develop food allergies than those who eat a wide variety of foods. Dr. Braly recommends following a rotation diet, which means eating the same food no more than once every 4 days.

This can help prevent food sensitivities from getting started, he explains. And you'll certainly want to avoid eating processed foods, simply because they're loaded with common allergens and chemical additives. "Most people who are allergic to foods are sensitive to chemicals as well," he adds.

### FRESH AND ORGANIC FOODS: *Easier on the Body*

People with food allergies should emphasize lots of fresh, organically grown vegetables, noncitrus fruits, nondairy sources of lean animal protein, and oily fish. These are among the "safest" foods because they are the ones our primitive ancestors ate. They're the foods that our bodies have adapted to, Dr. Braly says.

## MSM: *Relief with Sulfur*

The nutritional supplement MSM (methylsulfonylmethane), a form of sulfur, doesn't cure food allergies. It may relieve the symptoms, however, perhaps by preventing or decreasing inflammatory reactions in the body, says Stanley W. Jacob, M.D., professor of surgery at Oregon Health Sciences University in Portland.

If you take the supplement regularly, says Dr. Jacob, you may be able to eat a food that would otherwise cause you problems. He recommends taking MSM powder twice a day, following the label instructions.

## BETAINE HYDROCHLORIDE: *Help Prevent Allergens from Forming*

"When your digestive tract doesn't break down food properly, the body can't recognize it as food and may treat the food particles as invaders, or allergens, rather than as nutrition," says Dr. Krohn.

Do you feel as though food just sits in your stomach after you eat? If so, you may have this problem, which could be caused by a lack of hydrochloric acid in the stomach, she says.

While it's best to have low stomach acid diagnosed by a doctor, Dr. Krohn says that you can test your digestion by squeezing half a lemon into a cup of warm water and drinking it with meals. If that improves your digestion, it's a sign that you have an acid deficiency. Stop drinking the lemon juice and take a supplement of betaine hydrochloride before eating. Start with a dose of 300 milligrams and see if it helps. If necessary, you can increase the dose by 50 milligrams. If your symptoms persist, see a medical doctor.

If you feel a mild, harmless burning in your stomach after taking the supplement, you may not need the extra acid, says Dr. Krohn. Drinking 12 to 16 ounces of water will quickly stop the burning.

## DIGESTIVE ENZYMES: *Help for the Pancreas*

A deficiency of stomach acid isn't the only reason that foods can turn into allergens. You may also have a deficiency of the food-digesting enzymes produced by the pancreas, says Dr. Krohn. You can replace these enzymes with supplements. She recommends choosing one that contains amylase, cellulase, protease, papain, or bromelain. Take the supplement with meals, following the directions on the label, she advises.

## MULTIVITAMIN/MINERAL SUPPLEMENT:
### *All-Around Protection*
Nearly everyone should take multivitamin/mineral supplements because there's so much overprocessed, nutrient-stripped food in our diets.

"Those with food allergies may need extensive supplementation," says Dr. Krohn, because the allergic process interferes with digestion and may cause nutritional shortages. She recommends looking for a supplement that is free of common allergy-causing ingredients such as milk, corn, wheat, eggs, soy, sugar, and yeast.

# *A Fresh Approach to*
# Foot Odor

You could call it Limburger Feet Disease. Bacteria that are similar to the type that ripens limburger into one of the smelliest of cheeses is also responsible for the smelliest of feet, says Gregory Spencer, D.P.M., a podiatrist in Renton, Washington. The bacteria feast on the fat molecules in sweat, and the odor is produced by, well, for the sake of politeness, let's just say by bacterial postmeal by-products.

Obviously, one of the best ways to get rid of the smell is to get rid of the bacteria. And, says Dr. Spencer, alternative home remedies provide easy, effective ways to do just that.

## VINEGAR AND GRAPEFRUIT SEED EXTRACT:
### *Soak Away Problems*
"My patients with smelly feet have had very good results with vinegar soaks," says Dr. Spencer.

Put ¼ to 1 cup of vinegar in a basin of warm water and add a few drops of liquid grapefruit seed extract, which is a strong

# GUIDE TO
# PROFESSIONAL CARE

If you've tried various home remedies for foot odor and your feet still smell, see a podiatrist, who may recommend other ways to relieve the problem, such as a special zinc-containing bath to shrink the size of the sweat glands in your feet, says Morton Walker, D.P.M., a former podiatrist in Stamford, Connecticut. The podiatrist may refer you to a medical doctor for a physical examination to rule out any serious health problems that may be causing the odor, such as anemia. You should also see a podiatrist if the skin on your feet is very dry and cracked.

You also may want to consider seeing a naturopathic physician to undergo a detoxification program, which will help rid your body of toxic substances that can contribute to foot odor, says Steven Subotnick, D.P.M., a podiatrist in Berkeley and San Leandro, California.

antibacterial. Soak your feet for 15 to 20 minutes a day. Don't use this soak if you have areas of broken skin on your feet, however.

You'll probably have to soak your feet daily for 1 to 2 weeks, until the bacteria are dead. You'll know they're dead when your feet stop smelling.

## THYME ESSENTIAL OIL: *An Oily Option for Soaking*

"I always recommend that clients with foot odor soak their feet daily, adding a few drops (no more than three) of thyme essential oil, which helps reduce unpleasant smells, to the water," says Andrea Murray, a certified reflexologist and herbalist in Portland, Maine. After the soak, don't forget to dry your feet thoroughly, and don't use this remedy if you have open sores.

## FOOD: *Stop Feeding Bacteria*

The smell-producing bacteria on your feet love to feast on the animal fat in beef, pork, lamb, and other types of red meat, says Steven Subotnick, D.P.M., N.D., a podiatrist and naturopathic doctor in Berkeley and San Leandro, California.

His recommendation for anyone with smelly feet is to switch to a vegetarian diet. "I see the best results in eliminating foot odor in people who begin to follow this dietary regimen," Dr. Subotnick says. You should check with a doctor before changing your diet, however, as some people may develop anemia if such diets are not properly supplemented and supervised.

## NATURAL ANTIPERSPIRANT: *Not Just for Underarms Anymore*

Look for a natural antiperspirant containing sage or coriander, two odor-stopping herbs, and apply it to the soles of your feet once or twice a day, says Stephanie Tourles, a licensed esthetician, reflexologist, and herbalist in West Hyannisport, Massachusetts.

"Most commercial antiperspirants completely block the moisture flow from the skin, which is not healthy," she says. Baking soda is another ingredient in natural antiperspirants that can help prevent odor, she says.

## HOMEOPATHY: *Choosing the Right Cure*

Homeopathic remedies can also help cure smelly feet, says Dr. Subotnick. He recommends Silicea if your feet are icy cold, sweaty, smelly, and yellow, and Graphites if your feet smell with or without sweating. Use Rumex if the sweat is very sour-smelling, and try Staphysagria for cold feet that smell like rotten eggs. Consider Pulsatilla if your feet are warm and have an offensive odor and if you tend to get sick after putting your feet in cold water.

For each of the above remedies, take a 6C potency as directed on the label. Stop taking it as soon as the foot odor is gone.

### Spray the Odor Away

A spritz of witch hazel mixed with peppermint and geranium essential oils can help relieve smelly feet, says Stephanie Tourles, a licensed esthetician, reflexologist, and herbalist in West Hyannisport, Massachusetts.

Witch hazel is an astringent, so it helps dry out skin that's too moist, a common problem in people with foot odor. Both peppermint and geranium essential oils are antibacterials that help kill odor-causing germs, says Tourles. Here's how to make and use the spray.

Combine 1 cup of commercial witch hazel, 20 drops of peppermint essential oil, and 40 drops of geranium essential oil. Put the mixture in a spray bottle and shake well before using. Spray your feet right before you put on your socks and shoes in the morning and let your feet dry completely before donning your footwear. Spray again when you get home from work and once more before you go to bed.

You can use this spray even if your feet aren't smelly. "I love to use this in the summertime when my feet get overheated, because it dries and cools them," says Tourles.

# Bone Up to Speed Healing of
# **Fractures**

Simple. Open. Hairline. Stress.

Those are all names for different types of fractures, the medical term for broken bones. Fortunately, Mother Nature (usually with a little help from a cast to immobilize the break) heals a simple fracture in 2 to 3 months.

A hot, itchy, confining cast may have you thinking about ways to speed up that process—ways to help the body build new bone faster. Well, most conventional doctors won't have many (or any) ideas to help you do that. Alternative practitioners, however, offer several home remedies that you can bone up with.

## PROBIOTICS: *Boost Your Vitamin K*

*Lactobacillus acidophilus* and *Bifidobacterium bifidum* are two kinds of intestinal bacteria that are thought to help manufacture vitamin K. This nutrient in turn helps your body synthesize osteocalcin, a protein that aids in building bone.

You can find supplements containing these bacteria in most health food stores, says Thomas O'Bryan, D.C., a chiropractor, nutritionist, and director of the Omnis Chiropractic Group in Glenview, Illinois. Look for a brand that must be refrigerated;

---

# GUIDE TO
# PROFESSIONAL CARE

If you've broken a bone, you must see a doctor to have the fracture set and a cast applied. If the limb looks deformed, if you have pain and numbness immediately surrounding the injured area, or if you can't put any weight on the limb, it's probably fractured. And the best doctor to see is a specialist in orthopedic medicine, says Thomas O'Bryan, D.C., a chiropractor, nutritionist, and director of Omnis Chiropractic Group in Glenview, Illinois.

Once the fracture is set, though, you may want to see a nutritionally oriented health practitioner who can advise you on the best foods and nutritional supplements to repair and build bone.

"Allopathic doctors aren't likely to give you advice about how to promote faster, better healing of bone tissue with food, but a nutritionally oriented practitioner will," Dr. O'Bryan says.

---

it's probably of higher quality. Follow the dosage recommendations on the label; the usual dose is 1 teaspoon of powder.

## VITAMIN D: *For Calcium Absorption*

For the first 4 weeks after your injury, take a daily supplement of 400 international units of vitamin D, a nutrient that helps the body absorb calcium, says Dr. O'Bryan.

"I also recommend that my patients get out in the direct sun for 15 to 30 minutes a day. This allows your body to make its own vitamin D," says Dr. O'Bryan. "Glass blocks ultraviolet rays, so sitting near a sunny window won't work." Be sure to use sunscreen with an SPF of at least 15, and avoid the peak sun hours of 10:00 A.M. to 4:00 P.M. when possible.

## MULTIMINERAL SUPPLEMENT: *Building Blocks for Strong Bones*

You know that calcium is crucial for healthy bones, but you may not know that the kind of calcium you take can make a big difference. And there are other key minerals that your body

needs to build strong bones, says Dr. O'Bryan. Look for a supplement that contains the following minerals.

• Calcium: When a highway is built, cement is poured on
cross-linked cables. When new bone is built, bone is "poured"
on a supporting understructure. Microcrystalline
hydroxyapatite is the best form of calcium for providing that
understructure, Dr. O'Bryan believes. He recommends 1,000
milligrams a day.
• Silicon: "This trace mineral hasn't gotten the positive press
it deserves," says Dr. O'Bryan. He cites a scientific study in
which laboratory animals with fractures were given silicon;
their breaks healed completely in 17 days. A group of animals
that did not get the mineral showed little or no healing after 17
days. Dr. O'Bryan recommends 1 milligram a day.
• Magnesium, boron, and manganese: Dr. O'Bryan suggests
250 to 500 milligrams of magnesium (which works with
calcium to help build bone), 2 milligrams of boron, and 10
milligrams of manganese.

## "Bicycle" in a Pool for Faster Recovery

Bones grow when they're stressed by activity. The bones in the
left arm of a left-handed major league pitcher are thicker than the
bones in his right arm, for example. So, if you want to heal a broken leg, broken hip, or hip replacement faster, you need to get back
on your feet as soon as possible after the cast is off.

You can do that by going for a daily 5- to 10-minute "bicycle ride"
in the deep end of a swimming pool, says Thomas O'Bryan, D.C., a
chiropractor, nutritionist, and director of Omnis Chiropractic Group
in Glenview, Illinois. Wearing a life jacket for buoyancy, move your
legs in the water as if you were riding a bicycle. The non-weight-bear-
ing movement will begin to demand stronger bone formation even
before you can comfortably put weight on the injured leg.

As you heal, move to the shallow end of the pool and put a bit
of pressure on your leg. The water will support most of your
weight, Dr. O'Bryan explains, but just that small amount of pressure will shorten the time that you spend on crutches. As your leg
starts to feel stronger, walk in even more shallow water, which will
put a little more pressure on the limb.

"You need to urge your doctor to let you do this exercise as soon as possible after your cast is off," says Dr. O'Bryan, "because the sooner you begin doing the exercise, the sooner your leg will heal completely."

## HORSETAIL: *Sip for Silicon*

If you can't find a mineral supplement with silicon, Dr. O'Bryan says to drink two to three cups a day of tea made with the herb horsetail, which is rich in the mineral. To make the tea, use 2 teaspoons of dried herb per cup of boiling water. Pour the desired amount of water over the measured amount of herb in a saucepan, boil for 5 minutes, then remove from the heat and steep for an additional 10 to 15 minutes, says Dr. O'Bryan. Be sure to use dried herb, not powdered extract.

## FOOD: *Turn Over a New Leaf*

Dark green, leafy vegetables such as collard greens, turnip greens, mustard greens, broccoli, and parsley deliver calcium and magnesium. Try to eat at least one serving of these vegetables a day, Dr. O'Bryan says.

## COFFEE: *Cut Back*

Coffee blocks your body's absorption of calcium, so try to avoid drinking it while you're healing, Dr. O'Bryan says.

## SODA: *Can It*

Did you notice the ingredient "phosphoric acid" on the label of the soda you're drinking? It sucks calcium out of your bones like a leech.

"Drinking soda every day will inhibit the formation of new bone," Dr. O'Bryan says. His advice: Drink milk, sparkling water, or fruit juice instead. In addition, research shows that when soft drinks displace milk and fruit juices in the diet, you get fewer of the nutrients found in milk and juice, such as calcium, phosphorus, and vitamin C.

## *Aloe Can Aid in Healing*
# Frostbite

Keep water in the freezer long enough, and you get an ice cube. Keep your body in the freezing cold long enough, and you get frostbite. In both cases, the mechanism is exactly the same: Fluid freezes.

Obviously, frostbite is a medical emergency. The symptoms— skin that stings and burns, then becomes numb and waxy white—call for an immediate trip to an emergency room. This is the first degree of frostbite. Following this first stage, the skin develops blisters, then turns red with blisters, and finally, becomes purple with deeper blisters.

The *common* medical treatment for frostbite includes rapid rewarming and painkillers such as ibuprofen, which is also anti-inflammatory. But this may not be the most *complete* treatment for healing and preventing permanent tissue damage, says J. P. Heggers, Ph.D., professor of surgery (plastic) and of microbiology and immunology at the University of Texas Medical Branch in Galveston.

Anyone who works or plays in the cold—that is, anyone at risk for frostbite—should know that another way to treat frostbitten tissue is to add to the standard medical approach a very generous helping of an alternative home remedy, aloe.

### ALOE: *Prevent Permanent Damage*

After you've been treated by your doctor for frostbite, spread aloe gel on the frostbitten area four times a day to speed healing and prevent permanent damage.

"Aloe does help take care of frostbite," says Pierre Brunschwig, M.D., a holistic physician in Boulder, Colorado. "You can use the gel directly from a cut leaf of the plant or buy 100 percent pure aloe gel. Simply apply it liberally to the involved

## GUIDE TO
## PROFESSIONAL CARE

Frostbite usually occurs after exposure to temperatures of −4° to −10°F for more than 6 hours. High winds can reduce higher temperatures to dangerously low levels, however, and getting wet or touching metal objects can accelerate the frostbite process.

When skin freezes, it's actually the fluid in the cells that freezes, forming small ice crystals that destroy the cells. The blood clots, cutting off circulation, the skin becomes waxy and white, and you lose all feeling in the affected area. The fingers, toes, earlobes, chin, and tip of the nose are most vulnerable. If the damage is extensive, the skin and even deeper tissue can die, sometimes necessitating amputation of the affected parts.

Anyone who develops frostbite symptoms should seek medical attention immediately. There are four degrees of frostbite. After the waxy-white stage, the skin develops clear blisters, then turns red with blisters, and finally, becomes purple with deeper blisters. But don't wait for these changes. Even less severe frostbite can lead to discolored skin, burning pain, numbness, and joint problems. Severe cases may require hospitalization.

area four times a day until the area is healed. The aloe will stop the pain, stimulate healing, and prevent infection."

Why does aloe work so well? The answer comes from Dr. Heggers.

In 1983, he was working at the burn center in the hospital at the University of Chicago School of Medicine in that windy (and chilly!) city. One day during the winter, bus service was canceled because the wind chill was −80°F, and 30 people who hadn't heard the news ended up with frostbite while waiting for the bus. They also ended up in the burn center for treatment.

Dr. Heggers and his colleagues knew that frostbite blisters contain the chemical thromboxane, the same tissue-damaging substance found in burn blisters. They also knew that a cream made from the aloe plant could inhibit thromboxane formation, speeding the healing of burns, so they decided to use aloe cream on the frostbite patients, applying it four or five times a day. The results were remarkable. "All of the patients healed without major tissue loss in the affected areas," says Dr. Heggers.

In a study conducted a few years later, Dr. Heggers and his colleagues at the burn center at the Detroit Receiving Hospital looked closely at the hospital's records of 154 patients with frostbite: 56 had been treated by the burn team with aloe and ibuprofen, and 96 had been treated by other doctors with other methods. Among the patients who received aloe and ibuprofen, there was 80 percent healing of frostbitten tissue, compared to 33 percent in those who received other treatments. And while only 7 percent of the aloe group had permanent tissue loss, 33 percent of the other group lost tissue.

Dr. Heggers emphasizes that while all cases of frostbite must be treated by a doctor, patients should feel free to add aloe to the treatment regimen with their doctors' okay. And he offers this final caution: "When you're putting it on, be sure that you don't rub the skin too hard and cause loss of tissue. Put it on very gently."

## Protect Your Feet with Cayenne Pepper

Before you head out into the bitter cold, be sure that you have cayenne pepper in your shoes.

"In third-world countries, this is a much-used folk remedy for stopping frostbite," says Pamela Fischer, founder and director of the Ohlone Center for Herbal Studies in Concord, California. Cayenne pepper and other hot chile peppers work externally by improving circulation to the areas that they touche. But don't sprinkle pepper in your socks, she says. The best way to apply it is to combine a little Chinese hot oil (which contains chile extracts) with an equal amount of olive oil, then rub the mixture into your feet before you go out in the cold. Don't apply the mixture to broken skin, however.

Taking cayenne internally will also help keep circulation moving in your extremities, says Fischer. She recommends filling empty size 00 gelatin capsules with about 1/4 teaspoon of powdered cayenne per capsule. Take one capsule once a day.

This preventive remedy is not a substitute for cold-weather common sense, however, cautions J. P. Heggers, Ph.D., professor of surgery (plastic) and of microbiology and immunology at the University of Texas Medical Branch in Galveston. Dress warmly, being extra sure to protect your head, ears, face, hands, and feet. If you get wet, get out of your wet clothing *immediately*. And stay indoors when it's bitterly windy and cold, he says.

## *No More Surgery for* Gallstones

If you care about natural health, the statistics are, well, galling.

Every year, 1 million Americans are diagnosed with gallstones, joining 20 million others who already have the problem. About 500,000 people a year have gallbladder surgery, in which the organ is removed. This is the most effective "solution" offered by conventional medicine.

According to alternative physicians, however, most of those surgeries—possibly up to 85 percent—are unnecessary. People could achieve the same results (eliminating pain and the risk of damage to the gallbladder, liver, and pancreas) with alternative remedies, says Mark Stengler, N.D., a naturopathic physician in San Diego.

"About 15 percent of those who are diagnosed with gallstones need surgery because their stones are large and dangerous," Dr. Stengler says. "But the other 85 percent—those who have small to medium gallstones—can prevent gallstone attacks or complications with dietary changes, herbs, and nutritional supplements."

To understand how alternative home remedies work, you need to know a little about the gallbladder. This small, pear-shaped organ stores bile, a liquid produced by the liver for digesting fats. When bile becomes too concentrated while sitting

# GUIDE TO
# PROFESSIONAL CARE

Many times, gallstones are silent—that is, you have them, but they're not causing symptoms and they aren't a problem. Gallstone attacks are another story. If you experience steady, severe pain in your upper abdomen—especially on your right side under your ribs—that increases rapidly and lasts from 30 minutes to several hours, you need to see a doctor immediately. (Some people who have gallstone attacks have pain between the shoulder blades or under the right shoulder, and there may be nausea or vomiting.)

Gallstones that are big enough to cause symptoms may be dangerous if not treated by a doctor. You'll probably be given an ultrasound test to diagnose the stones, and you may need surgery to remove your gallbladder.

If you've already been diagnosed with gallbladder disease, see a doctor immediately if you have sweating, chills, a low-grade fever, nausea and vomiting, clay-colored stools, or jaundice (yellowing of the skin or the whites of the eyes). These are signs that a gallbladder duct is blocked, and that's an emergency.

in the gallbladder, hard, crystal-like stones can form. (Eighty percent of gallstones are made of cholesterol; the other 20 percent are made of calcium salts and the pigment bilirubin.) People who are overweight are much more likely to form gallstones than those who are lean. In fact, for every pound of fat in your body, you produce 10 milligrams of cholesterol.

The stones can be as small as a grain of sand or as large as a golf ball, and there can be one stone or thousands. The stones may irritate and inflame the gallbladder ducts (the tubes that connect the gallbladder and the small intestine), causing the intense pain of a gallstone attack.

"Alternative remedies can't dissolve gallstones, but they can keep stones from becoming larger and also keep the gallbladder ducts from becoming inflamed," Dr. Stengler says. "With alternative remedies, you're very likely not to have any symptoms or need surgery."

## LOW-FAT DIET: *Cutting Off the Bile Pipeline*

The saturated fat in dairy foods, meats, vegetable shortening, coconut oil, palm oil, and hydrogenated oils makes bile more concentrated, says Elizabeth Lipski, a certified clinical nutritionist in Kauai, Hawaii.

People who reduce the amount of fat and sugar in their diets while at the same time increasing fiber intake may be able to stop gallstone attacks because the bile will be less concentrated, making stones less likely to form.

## FATTY ACIDS: *Keep Stones Small*

While cutting down on fat is a must for people with gallstones, increasing your intake of omega-3 fatty acids—the kind of fats found abundantly in fish, flaxseed oil, and olive oil—is recommended.

High-quality oils help improve the solubility of bile, stopping the growth of stones, says Lipski. She recommends taking 1 to 2 tablespoons a day of flaxseed, olive, canola, safflower, soy, sunflower seed, or walnut oil.

## HIGH-FIBER FOODS: *Protection against Excess Cholesterol*

Since most gallstones are made of cholesterol, getting more dietary fiber is essential. This indigestible portion of vegetables, fruits, grains, beans, nuts, and seeds helps remove excess cholesterol from the body, says Dr. Stengler.

He recommends eating five servings of fruits and vegetables every day as well as plenty of whole-grain foods, such as high-fiber breakfast cereal, and beans.

### The Gallbladder Flush

People with small gallstones may be able to get them out with a gallbladder flush, says Teresa Rispoli, Ph.D., a licensed nutritionist and acupuncturist in Agoura Hills, California. Here's how to do it.

• About an hour before bedtime, blend ¼ cup of olive oil and ¼ cup of freshly squeezed lemon juice and drink the mixture. Then take cascara sagrada, an herbal laxative, according to the label directions.
• Lie on your right side for 30 minutes, then go to bed.

• In the morning, check to see if your stools contain tiny green stones (you may see dozens). If you find some, you'll know the flush was effective.
• Repeat the flush for 2 or 3 more days.

To be safe, you should do gallbladder flushes only with the approval and supervision of a health care practitioner, Dr. Rispoli says.

## WATER: *Make an Effort to Drink More*
Bile tends to become concentrated when people are somewhat dehydrated, says Lipski. To prevent this, she recommends drinking a lot of water. A useful guide is to drink ½ ounce of water for each pound you weigh. If you weigh 150 pounds, for example, you should drink 75 ounces of water.

## SUGAR: *Less Is Best*
Eating too much sugar can inflame the gallbladder ducts, says Dr. Stengler. He recommends avoiding table sugar as well as sugary foods such as cookies, cake, and candy.

## MILK THISTLE: *Stimulation for the Liver*
Milk thistle is believed to stimulate the liver and also may help reduce cholesterol levels in the bile, Dr. Stengler says. He recommends taking 600 milligrams of milk thistle extract daily, standardized to 70 to 80 percent silymarin, the active ingredient in the herb.

# *Shorten Outbreaks of*
# Genital Herpes

Janet Zand, O.M.D., a licensed acupuncturist and doctor of Oriental medicine, prefers to use natural means—healthy food, nutritional supplements, herbs, homeopathic remedies, and acupressure—to solve health problems.

# GUIDE TO PROFESSIONAL CARE

**Caution:** *You should use the alternative remedies discussed in this chapter only as part of a treatment program that is guided and monitored by a qualified medical doctor in partnership with a qualified alternative practitioner, both of whom are experienced in caring for your condition. Check with your conventional doctor before changing or stopping any conventional medical treatments or medications, and keep all of your doctors and/or alternative practitioners informed of all treatments that you are receiving.*

If you suspect that you're having an outbreak of genital herpes, with small, irritating, fluid-filled blisters and red, burning, itchy sores on your genitals, buttocks, or thighs, see a medical, osteopathic, or naturopathic doctor immediately for an accurate diagnosis and treatment.

If you have frequent outbreaks, you may want to see a natural medicine practitioner for a drug-free, immunity-strengthening program to control them.

A herpes infection in a pregnant woman can threaten the unborn baby and must be treated by an obstetrician or gynecologist.

She's willing to make an exception, however, in the case of genital herpes, a sexually transmitted virus that can erupt repeatedly in 7- to 10-day outbreaks of itchy, burning blisters and sores in the genital area.

If you want to short-circuit an outbreak, Dr. Zand, of Austin, Texas, recommends that you see a medical doctor and take the antiviral drug acyclovir (Zovirax). "Acyclovir is generally considered a safe and well-tolerated conventional medical treatment for genital herpes, particularly to help stop a first outbreak that just keeps going and going," she says.

Like any drug, though, it has possible side effects, including headaches and nausea. Also, if you take it day after day, you may build up a tolerance to it. If you'd like to try natural remedies to help control genital herpes, alternative practitioners believe that the following regimens can help shorten an outbreak and decrease its severity.

## LYSINE: *It Works If You Use It Right*

Natural healers commonly recommend the amino acid lysine as a daily nutritional supplement to help keep herpes under control.

Although this supplement has the unique ability to fight off the virus, you can also develop a tolerance to it if you take it every day, warns Dr. Zand. "It's better to use lysine when you feel an outbreak coming on and for a few weeks after an outbreak," she says.

She recommends taking a 500-milligram capsule four times a day during the first 72 hours of an outbreak. For the next 4 days, take 500 milligrams three times a day, then 500 milligrams daily for 2 weeks. Finally, take 500 milligrams three times a week for 2 weeks.

## FOOD: *Avoid Those with Arginine*

Lysine has an evil twin named arginine, which encourages the herpesvirus. Just before or during an outbreak, avoid all foods rich in arginine, says Dr. Zand, which include whole-wheat products, brown rice, oatmeal, chocolate, carob, corn, dairy products, raisins, nuts, and seeds.

## OLIVE LEAF: *Gets Rid Of the Lesions*

A supplement of olive leaf extract is thought to be extremely effective in ending a bout of herpes, and it can help prevent new outbreaks if taken daily, says James Privitera, M.D., an allergy and nutrition specialist in Covina, California. "The extract gets rid of the lesions and helps prevent them from coming back," he says.

Look for a product with 20 percent oleuropein, the immunity-strengthening ingredient in the extract. During an outbreak, take five 500-milligram tablets a day for 3 weeks. After that, follow the dosage recommendations on the label for daily use.

## VITAMINS AND MINERALS: *For Quick Healing*

"A herpes outbreak is a sign that your body is under stress, and whenever you're under stress, you need more nutrients," Dr. Zand says. The following program may help reduce the stress, she says, thus shortening the herpes attack and reducing its severity.

- Vitamin A: 25,000 international units (IU) twice a day for 3 days, then 20,000 IU a day for 4 days
- B-complex vitamins: 50 milligrams twice a day for a month
- Vitamin C: 500 to 1,000 milligrams three times daily for 3 days, then 500 to 1,000 milligrams twice daily for 4 days, then 500 milligrams once or twice a day for a week
- Vitamin E: 400 IU twice a day for the duration of the outbreak, then one 400 IU supplement daily for 1 to 2 weeks after the initial outbreak
- Zinc: 10 milligrams twice a day for a week
- Calcium/magnesium: A supplement with 500 milligrams of calcium and 250 milligrams of magnesium twice a day for 1 month
- Selenium: 200 micrograms daily for 2 weeks

## WATER: *Double Your Intake*

Drinking a lot of water at the first sign of an outbreak helps flush toxins out of your body that are weakening your immune system and allowing the virus to reactivate, says Amy Rothenberg, N.D., a naturopathic physician in Enfield, Connecticut. Double the amount of water you typically drink, or drink a daily minimum of 64 ounces. "I've seen this stop outbreaks in my patients many times," she says.

## GOLDENSEAL: *A Symptom-Soothing Topical Herb*

Powdered goldenseal can help dry up herpes lesions, thus decreasing the burning and itching, Dr. Zand says. "Goldenseal powder works very well to lessen the discomfort of an acute attack." To use the powder, add enough water to make a paste, then apply it liberally to the lesions three or four times a day for 3 days.

## MSM: *A Super Supplement*

A supplement used to ease joint pain can also provide relief from a herpes outbreak. Dr. Zand recommends taking a 500-milligram capsule of MSM (methylsulfonylmethane) three times a day until discomfort lessens.

## Preventing Outbreaks

The following remedies can strengthen your immune system and help to prevent future outbreaks.

**REISHI MUSHROOMS:** *Naturally Antiviral*
Taking a daily supplement made from reishi mushrooms is an excellent preventive to stop outbreaks, Dr. Zand says. "It is thought to have natural antiviral properties that lessen both the severity and frequency of outbreaks." She suggests taking a 350- to 500-milligram capsule once or twice a day, or follow the dosage recommendations on the label.

**MULTIVITAMIN SUPPLEMENT:** *Added Protection*
Taking an easily digested multivitamin supplement daily will provide extra nutrients to help lessen the chance of new outbreaks.

**PROBIOTICS:** *Keep "Damp Heat" under Control*
In Traditional Chinese Medicine, a probiotic supplement containing the healthy bowel bacteria *Lactobacillus acidophilus* or *Bifidobacterium bifidum* decreases "damp heat" in the bowel so that it can't travel to the genitals and cause herpes, Dr. Zand says. "I've seen again and again in my patients with herpes that those who take a probiotic supplement of 500 milligrams twice a day are less prone to outbreaks."

**SIBERIAN GINSENG:** *One Week a Month*
Siberian ginseng is an "adaptogenic" herb that strengthens the immune system, says Dr. Zand. Use it in liquid or capsule form for 1 week each month, following the dosage recommendations on the label.

# *Reduce Your Reliance on Medication for*
# **Glaucoma**

The inside of the eye has its own plumbing. A thin, watery fluid called aqueous humor is constantly pumped in and drained out. But if the drain is clogged, fluid builds up, pressing on and destroying all or part of the optic nerve and damaging peripheral vision.

That "plumbing problem" is called glaucoma.

For people with the most common form of glaucoma, there is usually no pain or other symptoms of any kind. By the time they actually experience vision loss and are diagnosed with the disease, irreversible damage has been done. Medical treatment is a must so that continued pressure (what eye doctors call intraocular hypertension) doesn't cause even greater loss of peripheral vision. The treatment consists of eyedrops, and if they don't work, surgery is performed.

There are also alternative remedies that will help control and lower the pressure in the most common form of glaucoma—remedies that can help you reduce your reliance on medication.

**ALPHA-LIPOIC ACID:** *To Lower the Pressure*

This antioxidant can help lower the pressure and improve the visual field, says Marc Grossman, O.D., an optometrist, licensed acupuncturist, and codirector of the Integral Health Center in Rye and New Paltz, New York. He recommends 150 milligrams a day.

For the best combination of alpha-lipoic acid and other nutrients for glaucoma, Dr. Grossman favors a product that also contains 500 milligrams of magnesium and 1,500 milligrams of vitamin C.

**FATTY ACIDS:** *To Unclog the Drainage System*

One reason that the eye's drainage system, or trabecular meshwork, becomes clogged may be that it's inflamed, like an

# GUIDE TO
# PROFESSIONAL CARE

*Caution: You should use the alternative remedies discussed in this chapter only as part of a treatment program that is guided and monitored by a qualified medical doctor in partnership with a qualified alternative practitioner, both of whom are experienced in caring for your condition. Check with your conventional doctor before changing or stopping any conventional medical treatments or medications, and keep all of your doctors and/or alternative practitioners informed of all treatments that you are receiving.*

Ten percent of people with glaucoma have closed-angle glaucoma, in which drainage from the eye is blocked suddenly and completely, triggering symptoms such as blurry vision, severe pain in or behind the eyes, and nausea. This is a medical emergency and requires immediate care.

The other 90 percent have open-angle glaucoma, in which the drain slowly becomes clogged. This type has no symptoms and is typically diagnosed after vision loss occurs. Once diagnosed, you must be under the care of an eye doctor, and medication or surgery may be necessary.

Other health professionals may complement your treatment with alternative modalities, however, says Marc Grossman, O.D., an optometrist, licensed acupuncturist, and codirector of the Integral Health Center in Rye and New Paltz, New York. You might consider the following strategies.

• Detecting and eliminating any food allergies may help reduce pressure in the eye. See an allergist who treats for this type of allergen.
• An acupuncturist may be able to help reduce the pressure.
• Manipulation of the head and neck area, called craniosacral therapy, can often help glaucoma. See an osteopath, chiropractor, or other health professional who is trained in the technique.

arthritic joint. Fatty acids, such as the omega-3's in fish oil, can decrease inflammation, opening the clog and helping to control the pressure.

Dr. Grossman recommends 1,000 to 1,500 milligrams a day of fish oil, a rich source of fatty acids. Or, if fish oil doesn't agree with you (some people have fishy burps after taking the supplement), use 1,000 milligrams a day of flaxseed oil or black currant (seed) oil.

## VITAMIN B$_{12}$: *An Eyesight Saver*

This nutrient can help improve eyesight or prevent it from worsening in glaucoma patients, says Dr. Grossman. He recommends a sublingual (under-the-tongue) spray form. Follow the dosage recommendations on the label.

## VITAMIN C: *Reduce Pressure Three Ways*

"In parts of Europe and Asia, vitamin C is considered routine treatment for glaucoma," says Dr. Grossman. It is thought to help the aqueous humor flow out of the eye, decrease excess fluid production throughout the body, and increase "blood osmolarity," which allows blood to flow out of the eye. He recommends 1,500 milligrams a day.

## COENZYME Q$_{10}$ AND VITAMIN E: *A Therapeutic Combination*

Combining vitamin E and coenzyme Q$_{10}$ can help lower pressure in glaucoma patients, says Dr. Grossman. He recommends 400 international units of vitamin E and 30 milligrams of coenzyme Q$_{10}$ daily.

## MAGNESIUM: *Relax Smooth Muscles*

The so-called smooth muscles inside the eye regulate the outflow of the aqueous humor, Dr. Grossman says. The mineral magnesium helps relax those muscles, allowing more fluid out of the eye. He recommends 500 milligrams a day.

### Meditation Is a Must for Glaucoma

Stress is an important contributing factor to glaucoma that is usually overlooked by conventional physicians, says John D. Huff,

M.D., an ophthalmologist and codirector of the Prather-Huff Wellness Center in Sugarland, Texas.

And, Dr. Huff says, meditation is an excellent way of reducing pressure in the eye for those who are prone to it when they're under stress. "The person can often stop using glaucoma medications, with a doctor's approval," he says. Here are his instructions for a simple technique called breath-focused meditation.

Sit comfortably in a chair and close your eyes. Focus your attention on your abdominal muscles and let them relax. Let your breaths be full and deep.

Next, focus your attention on the movement of air in and out of your nostrils—just notice the flow in, then notice the flow out. If thoughts distract you, move your attention gently back to your breathing.

Do this for 5 to 20 minutes twice a day, in the morning after you shower and prepare yourself for the day, but before breakfast, then again in the evening before dinner.

## MELATONIN: *Sleep Better and Get Better*

The hormone melatonin is thought to reduce the rate of aqueous humor production during sleep and may also help glaucoma patients (who often sleep poorly) sleep better, says Dr. Grossman. He recommends 1 milligram of melatonin 30 minutes before bedtime.

## TRADITIONAL CHINESE MEDICINE: *Herbs to Cleanse the Liver*

In Traditional Chinese Medicine, a person with glaucoma is said to have a problem with "liver yang rising," says Dr. Grossman. That means that the energy in the liver meridian, a pathway of subtle energy in the body, is stagnant or deficient, stressing the eyes and contributing to glaucoma.

To move or increase that energy, you need to remove strain from the liver with cleansing herbs. "I'm very big on using liver herbs along with nutrition for this disease," he says.

The Chinese herbal formula for this problem is Hsiao Yao Wan (Relaxed Wanderer Pills). After consulting an herbalist, take the formula daily, following the dosage recommendations on the label.

He also recommends a formula with several herbs. Combine

1 ounce each of tinctures of bilberry, coleus, dandelion, eyebright, ginkgo, and milk thistle in a large bottle. Take 1 teaspoon twice a day for 3 to 6 months.

## Natural Remedies Have Clout with
# Gout

Imagine that some of the liquid in your body suddenly turned into glass—and the glass shattered.

That's similar to what happens when you have a gout attack. Some of your body's uric acid, a normal by-product of protein metabolism, changes from a liquid into tiny crystals. Those crystals, sharp spikes and all, can settle in your joints. (The joint of the big toe is their favorite.) The resulting pain, redness, heat, and swelling can be so intense that you can't even walk.

---

### GUIDE TO
### PROFESSIONAL CARE

Since gout is not a life-threatening condition, Gus Prosch, M.D., a physician in Birmingham, Alabama, recommends trying natural remedies for 4 to 5 days, especially if you have been diagnosed in the past. If you've never been diagnosed with gout but suspect that you're having an attack, see a medical doctor, who will administer a blood test for a high level of uric acid, which is a sure sign of gout.

If your gout attack is intensely painful, colchicine, a powerful (and very toxic) drug, can stop the pain in 10 minutes by dissolving uric acid crystals, says Jay M. Holder, M.D., D.C., Ph.D., a chiropractor and addiction specialist in Miami and Miami Beach. It can be given only by a medical doctor, usually through injection. Your doctor will probably also prescribe an 800-milligram prescription dose of ibuprofen for pain.

More than 2 million Americans, most of them men over 30, have gout, which is a form of arthritis. Scientists don't know why some people develop abnormally high levels of uric acid, which is what triggers the change from liquid to crystal form. Genetics is a possible cause, and diet and overweight are risk factors. Taking thiazide diuretics for high blood pressure has also been linked to the disease.

Whatever the cause, once you've had one attack (which can last for days if it's not treated), you're more likely to have another—and another. Plus, uncontrolled buildup of uric acid crystals over many years can destroy a joint and lead to the formation of stones in the kidneys and gallbladder.

"If you've had your first attack of gout, you want to prevent ever having another," says Jay M. Holder, M.D., D.C., Ph.D., a chiropractor and addiction specialist in Miami and Miami Beach. There are plenty of alternative home remedies to do just that.

### WATER: *Wash Away Uric Acid*
After you've had your first gout attack—in other words, after you know that you have high levels of uric acid in your system— you should drink "tremendous amounts of water on a daily basis to flush the uric acid crystals out of your system and dilute the concentration of uric acid," says Dr. Holder. By "tremendous amounts," he means about 1 gallon (128 ounces) of water a day.

"Water is one of the most important remedies for gout," Dr. Holder says. "If you don't drink large amounts of water, no other single natural remedy will work as well."

One year after your first gout attack, you can cut back on the amount of water, but continue drinking 2 to 3 quarts a day.

Also, Dr. Holder says to drink distilled water or water filtered by a reverse osmosis process, both of which are pure. Reverse osmosis filtration systems, which are installed under your kitchen sink, are available for between $300 and $500. Other types of water, including spring water, he says, may actually contribute to circulatory disease by depositing minerals in the blood vessels, thus leading to hardening of the arteries.

### CHERRIES: *To Prevent—Or Even Abort—a Gout Attack*
For those with gout, life is just a bowl of cherries. Really.

Substances in cherries, called anthocyanocides, are very effective at lowering uric acid levels, says Walter Crinnion, N.D., a naturopathic doctor and director of Healing Naturally in Kirkland, Washington.

How many cherries should you eat? According to traditional healing lore and very preliminary research, eating anywhere from ½ cup to 1 pound (about 70) of cherries a day may help people with gout, says Laurie Aesoph, N.D., a naturopathic doctor in Sioux Falls, South Dakota.

Eating a pound of cherries a day can help prevent a gout attack or abort an attack in progress, Dr. Holder says. But rather than eating all those cherries, he suggests that you pit them and blend them with distilled water to make juice. Avoid store-bought cherry juice, since pasteurization removes anthocyanin. "We use this remedy in our clinic, and it works," he says.

Wild or black cherries work best to combat gout, says Gus Prosch, M.D., a physician in Birmingham, Alabama. Because they're so hard to find, he recommends that you take wild or black cherry extract in either liquid or pill form, according to the dosage recommendations on the label.

"Old country doctors would tell patients to eat black cherries to stop having gout attacks, and the remedy usually worked," he says.

### Auricular Therapy: Instant Natural Pain Relief for a Gout Attack

Lend an ear if you want fast relief from gout.

"I don't know of any noninvasive remedy that works as quickly or as well for the pain of gout as ear acupuncture, or auricular therapy," says Jay M. Holder, M.D., D.C., Ph.D., a chiropractor and addiction specialist in Miami and Miami Beach.

In Chinese medicine, a healthy person's life-energy, or chi, flows along subtle lines called meridians. But when chi isn't flowing smoothly, such as when someone is in pain or has other disease symptoms, there are points along the meridians that can be stimulated to balance the flow and eliminate the symptoms.

Those points are usually stimulated by using needles (acupuncture) or finger pressure (acupressure) throughout the body. But in auricular therapy, you stimulate cranial nerve points on your ear with an electronic stimulator, a handheld wand that's used to detect points in your ear where chi is blocked; it costs between $150 and $300. (See Products on page 729 for more information.)

Because they do not locate and treat the blocked chi, acupuncture and acupressure are ineffective compared with electronic, or microcurrent, stimulation of cranial nerve points, says Dr. Holder.

To use an electronic stimulator, run the wand over the cranial nerve points shown below. When it buzzes, use the wand to press the point with slight pressure for 30 seconds, or until you feel relief. Continue searching for other blocked cranial points until you have tested all of them.

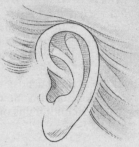

One caution: This technique is so effective that you may be tempted not to bother with trying to prevent gout attacks. That would be a big mistake, says Dr. Holder, because the disease would still progress, slowly but surely destroying your joints. If you have a gout attack, use this technique. But, he says, use alternative home remedies as well, along with a corrective diet to prevent future attacks.

## HIGH-PURINE FOODS: *A Must to Avoid*

One way to control uric acid levels is to avoid eating too many foods rich in purine, a protein-related substance that the body turns into uric acid.

"If you avoid high-purine foods, gout attacks won't be as common," says Dr. Aesoph, "and when they occur, they won't be as severe."

The foods highest in purine include organ meats such as liver, kidney, and sweetbreads; fish such as sardines, mackerel, and anchovies; vegetables such as asparagus and mushrooms; and beans of any kind.

## ALCOHOL: *Pull the Trigger*

Alcohol of all types, including beer, wine, and liquor, triggers the body to produce uric acid. To control gout, you must avoid alcohol, says Dr. Holder. The type of alcohol you drink makes no difference, he says, since they all contain ethyl alcohol, which is the culprit behind uric acid buildup.

### APPLE-CIDER VINEGAR: *A Tablespoon of Relief*

Taking a tablespoon of apple-cider vinegar each morning is very effective in helping to prevent gout attacks, says Dr. Holder. For severe cases—frequent and very painful attacks—a tablespoon morning and evening may be necessary.

### VITAMIN B$_6$ AND MAGNESIUM:
*For Better-Hydrated Tissues*

Vitamin B$_6$ helps distribute water in the body to keep all of its tissues maximally hydrated, which helps prevent uric acid from turning into crystals. Magnesium aids in the absorption of vitamin B$_6$.

Dr. Holder recommends 50 milligrams of B$_6$ once a day as a preventive dose or three times a day as a therapeutic measure, along with 400 milligrams of magnesium.

# *Moving Beyond the Pain of* **Grief**

The death of a loved one may be the most profound emotional experience that we will ever have to endure. Unfortunately, there's no quick "cure" for such grief. There are alternative approaches that can help ease your pain in a time of sorrow, however.

One key is to allow yourself to fully feel all of the painful emotions that you experience after a loss. If you don't, those emotions are stored in the body as tension and can cause physical or emotional disease, says Arthur Samuels, M.D., medical director of the Stress Treatment Center of New Orleans.

**BREATHING:** *Feel, Release, Love*

Meditating on saying goodbye can help you fully experience and relieve the pain of grief, Dr. Samuels says. Here's how to do it.

Identify where in your body you feel emotional pain, anger, sorrow, or fear. Common places are the heart, stomach, or throat, but it can be anywhere, or you may sense it in your whole body. Then imagine seeing, hearing, and touching this place. For example, you might "see" a sad expression on that part of you.

Allow yourself to breathe as if you are inhaling and exhaling from your heart. You might see yourself as a 5-year-old child looking very sad. Imagine opening the space around your heart and breathing in the painful emotion. Accept it uncritically. As you breathe out, send compassionate love to the part of you that is suffering. For the time being, let other thoughts pass and focus entirely on breathing in the painful emotion and transforming it into loving feelings.

After you have done this for a while, start to say goodbye to the person you've lost. Say goodbye in great detail and bid farewell to everything that you remember about them. Let yourself cry with each goodbye. You may want to have someone hold you as you go through this step.

If and when you start to feel more comfortable, begin to think of the essence of what you miss about your loved one. Perhaps it was the person's laughter or their affection for you. Open up to your tears and breathe in that essence. Feel it becoming part of you, a gift from your loved one, an attribute that you can now express in your life.

"Don't worry if in the first few days or weeks after your loss you don't feel any pain. You just feel numb," Dr. Samuels says. "At some point, the reality of your loss will set in, and you will be more able to do this exercise. If you do this every day, each time you miss your loved one, you'll find it a very effective experience for resolving grief."

## Flower Essences Heal the Soul Naturally

Flower essences, which are specially formulated preparations of specific flowers, can help heal emotional and mental problems by removing blockages to the full expression of the soul's

> # GUIDE TO
> # PROFESSIONAL CARE
>
> Local churches, hospitals, and social agencies as well as Hospice and other national organizations often offer support groups. You can locate them by contacting Hospice or the pastoral care office of a hospital in your area.
>
> "Individual professional counseling is often helpful to survivors as they deal with the more prominent grief responses, such as extreme sadness, guilt, anger, and fear," says Carol Staudacher, a grief consultant in Santa Cruz, California. People who are experiencing prolonged or disabling grief should consult a medical or mental health professional, she advises.

innate strength and resilience, says Patricia Kaminski, cofounder and codirector of the Flower Essence Society, based in Nevada City, California. They are particularly effective in times of grief, she says. Take four drops four times a day for several months.

**BLEEDING HEART:** *For the Loss of a Loved One*
The flower essence known as bleeding heart is a remedy for someone who has lost a loved one, even a pet, says Kaminski. The remedy helps mend the heart, she says, allowing you to deeply experience grief and feel closure about the loss.

**BORAGE:** *For the Courage to Continue*
If you feel heavy-hearted, with a weight on your soul that stops you from re-engaging the world, borage is the right remedy, says Kaminski. "It is a very uplifting remedy that allows the soul to find a buoyancy, a full-heartedness to carry on," she says.

**LOVE-LIES-BLEEDING:** *For Self-Pity*
If you feel that God and people have forsaken you, and you cannot understand why you need to suffer so profoundly, the essence called love-lies-bleeding is the right remedy, says Kaminski. "It helps the soul move with and accept loss."

### YERBA SANTA: *For Longstanding, Unreleased Grief*

Unreleased grief is stored in deeper layers of the body-soul structure, says Kaminski, particularly the lungs, where it causes health problems such as asthma, frequent colds, and concavity of the chest. For this profound type of grief, she recommends the flower essence yerba santa.

## Aromatherapy, for a Breath of Life

Try experimenting with the oils listed below to see "which one affects your heart when you smell it—which one makes you feel that you'll be able to overcome your sorrow and pain," says DeAnna Batdorff, a clinical aromatherapist and Ayurvedic practitioner in Forestville, California. To use the oil you select, put three drops in a teaspoon of a carrier oil such as almond or olive oil. Bottle an ounce of the mixture and inhale from the bottle or rub the formula on your ears whenever you like.

### ROSE GERANIUM: *A Balm for the Heart*

This essential oil helps soothe grief by relaxing and opening the heart chakra, the subtle circle of energy around your heart and chest, Batdorff says.

### BASIL: *For Improving Concentration*

Essential oil of basil is a mental stimulant, says Batdorff. It may be particularly good if you are having a hard time concentrating, which is a common problem in times of grief.

### CEDARWOOD: *If You're Feeling Tense*

This essential oil is extremely grounding and softening, says Batdorff, and can help if you're feeling tense and anxious.

# *Restore Your Soul by Banishing Unhealthy* **Guilt**

Guilt can be healthy when it serves as a natural internal feedback system that tells you when you're psychologically or spiritually offtrack. But there's also an unhealthy type of guilt that prevents you from taking the healing action you need.

"Unhealthy guilt is one of the biggest blocks to healing," says Joan Borysenko, Ph.D., a psychologist and president of Mind/Body Health Sciences in Boulder, Colorado. "It's a constant and uncomfortable sense of having done something wrong, of being deficient. It doesn't really matter what you do or don't do. *Nothing* you do is ever quite right. You never feel that you are truly a good person."

Alternative healing offers many simple ways to overcome this type of guilt. Perhaps one of the best is flower essence therapy, which uses specially prepared tinctures from various flowers to help you release or outgrow feelings and thoughts that block your strength and creativity.

Flower essences may be part of a holistic healing plan for mild guilt, but you should seek professional help if you're constantly plagued by severe guilt. "Guilt is one of the most powerful blocks to physical, emotional, and mental healing," says Patricia Kaminski, cofounder and codirector of the Flower Essence Society, based in Nevada City, California. "Flower essences can help remove that block."

For each of the following remedies, take four drops four times a day for about a month.

**PINE:** *To Forgive Yourself*

"This is the most important remedy for guilt," Kaminski says. "It's for people who, no matter how much they can forgive others, can never forgive themselves. It allows warmth toward yourself and acceptance for all life." Pine may also work for people who always feel sinful based on their religious upbringing, she says.

## MULLEIN: *For a Stronger Conscience*

Mullein as a flower essence is for people who know that they are doing something wrong (such as having an affair) but need to bring guilt to bear on their conscience and take steps to resolve the issue, says Kaminski. "This remedy helps the person come to an inner place of clarity about moral decisions," she says.

## CRAB APPLE: *For Those Who Feel Impure*

This essence is for those whose guilt is in their bodies, who feel that they have a physical stain or are impure. "The person who can benefit from this remedy very often has unusual gynecological or sexual symptoms," Kaminski says. (Another remedy for women who feel guilty about their sexuality is Easter lily.)

## PINK YARROW: *For Unproductive Guilt*

This remedy is for people who feel a level of guilt that is totally out of proportion to anything they did, such as an employee who feels guilty when the boss is angry at a coworker or a child who feels guilty because of a divorce. Such guilt is completely unproductive, Kaminski says.

### Ayurvedic Remedies for Guilt

Ayurveda, the ancient natural healing system from India, says that health is a balance of three essential elements: vata (air), pitta (fire), and kapha (water).

"Guilt is a vata imbalance," says DeAnna Batdorff, a clinical aromatherpist and Ayurvedic practitioner in Forestville, California. "The individual has too much vata, or air, in their system and needs grounding."

This vata imbalance can cause lower-back pain, dry skin, brittle nails, and kidney problems, she says. The following remedies are intended to decrease vata, helping rid you of guilt as well as preventing the physical problems that it can cause.

# GUIDE TO PROFESSIONAL CARE

If you begin to experience an overwhelming sense of anxiety related to guilt, you may need help from a mental health professional, says Joan Borysenko, Ph.D., president of Mind/Body Health Sciences in Boulder, Colorado.

"You may be tapping into traumatic experiences in your childhood that you cannot process by yourself," she says. To find the best therapist, get recommendations from friends who have seen therapists, then interview the one that you choose to see if he is someone that you feel you can work with.

## ENERGY HEALING: *Put Your Hand on Your Throat*

Guilt is usually caused by a feeling that others' needs are more important than your own. The result is that you often can't express what you need to say or do. Such guilt usually wells up in your throat, Batdorff says.

"In fact, your energy feels like it's stuck in your throat," she says. "Verbalization is down. You feel very vulnerable."

To counter this physical pattern of guilt, Batdorff suggests that whenever you feel uncomfortable about saying something because of guilt, you first put one hand, palm down, on the lowest part of your throat, at your collarbone. Announce that you have something to say, then say it.

"This simple physical gesture protects you and nourishes you and lets you know that it's okay to say or do what you need to," Batdorff says.

## VETIVER ESSENTIAL OIL: *Ground Yourself*

The essential oil vetiver is thought to stabilize the body, says Batdorff. This grounding can help eliminate guilt.

"Using this essential oil will help you feel 'in your body' rather than having your attention on everyone else because you're worried about how you're affecting them or what they're thinking about you," Batdorff says. "It builds self-awareness. It also nourishes the kidneys."

To use it, put one drop over each kidney (directly above

your waist and about 3 inches from each side of your spine)
twice a day. You can also inhale the oil whenever you're feeling guilty.

## PETITGRAIN ESSENTIAL OIL: *For Guilty Secrets*

Sometimes, people feel guilty because of something they've
done. They know that they have to talk about it to restore peace
to the relationship, but they just can't get the words out. If
you're in that situation, petitgrain essential oil can help, Batdorff says. Put two or three drops in a bath, take a few minutes
to think about the problem, and then have a chat with the person
you feel you've wronged.

## FOOD: *Don't Put More Air in Your Body*

To decrease guilt, you need to avoid vata foods, says Batdorff. They include carbonated beverages, citrus fruits, vinegar,
and pickled or fermented foods.

# *The Real Causes of, and Cures for,* **Gum Disease**

If your gums are red and puffy and bleed when you brush or
floss, you have the early stage of gum disease, called gingivitis.
It's caused by the buildup of plaque, the gum-destroying, tooth-
loosening gunk that coats your teeth faster than you can say
"periodontist."

Brushing and flossing may be helpful in removing plaque,
but there are other steps recommended by alternative practitioners that can prevent or reverse gum disease. Moreover, what
you may not hear from a conventional dentist is that even if you
faithfully brush and floss, you can still end up with gingivitis.
We'll explain how—and what to do about it—later, but first,
here are some tips to keep your gums healthy.

## SALT: *Concentrating On the Real Solution*

Even brushing and flossing can't erase all the nasty bacteria living on your gums. To do that, you have to kill those germs. One way to do it is with salt, which dehydrates the creepy critters.

Here's a salty recipe for gum health from David Kennedy, D.D.S., a dentist in San Diego.

Pour ½ pound of baking soda and ½ pound of salt into a clean, empty gallon jug. Add enough warm water to fill the jug, shake thoroughly, and set aside. A thin layer of salt and soda that has not dissolved should form on the bottom of the jug.

You should now have a concentrated salt solution, with each molecule of water bordered by a molecule of salt. If you don't see an undissolved layer, add more salt and baking soda until you do. Just before you use the rinse, add a teaspoon or two of hydrogen peroxide 3 percent solution to help kill bacteria and sterilize the gums.

Fill an oral irrigator, such as a WaterPik, with the solution.

## GUIDE TO PROFESSIONAL CARE

If you have gingivitis, you must see a dentist. Left untreated, gingivitis can become periodontitis, a condition in which receding gums and bone loss eventually start to tumble the teeth out of your mouth.

But gingivitis is also a sign that you have an underlying health problem, says Michael Lipelt, N.D., D.D.S., a naturopathic physician and dentist in Sebastopol, California. If you have gingivitis, your gums are telling you that there is an imbalance in your system from a high-fat, nutrition-poor diet; too much stress; indoor pollutants; or any number of other possible causes.

To bring balance back to your body, Dr. Lipelt recommends seeing a naturopathic physician who has been trained in whole-body healing. He recommends choosing a doctor who is a graduate of either Bastyr University or the National College of Naturopathic Medicine, both of which have rigorous 4-year training programs.

Point the tip of the irrigator at each tooth and circle it, then poke the tip gently under the gum. Don't swallow the solution while you're irrigating.

Add 1 cup of water to the jug after each use. You should have enough solution for 10 irrigations, then you'll need to start a new batch.

"When my patients floss, brush, and use this bug-killing solution once a day, they remove many of the bacteria that cause gum disease from their mouths," says Dr. Kennedy. "Over 50 percent of all Americans have gingivitis. If they followed this procedure, they would take one step toward slowing the progress of the disease."

## HERBS AND ESSENTIAL OILS: *A Healing Combo*

To help reduce inflammation and swelling of gum tissue, use a combination of herbal tinctures and essential oils, says Gary Verigin, D.D.S., a dentist in Escalon, California. Mix 2½ ounces each of echinacea, thyme, and cinnamon bark tinctures with four to six drops each of eucalyptus oil, lavender oil, peppermint oil, and vegetable glycerin.

Dip a perio-aid—a wooden toothpick with a plastic handle—into the solution and gently clean the crevice that surrounds each tooth by inserting the toothpick parallel to the tooth, as if you were cleaning your cuticles. Gently work below the gum line on each tooth, being careful not to tear the gum tissue. Do this every evening before going to bed, recommends Dr. Verigin. This type of cleaning is not painful, but the first few cleanings may be uncomfortable if your gums are inflamed, he says.

If you don't have the time, energy, or inclination to make this herbal mixture, consider buying Tooth and Gum Tonic, manufactured by the Dental Herb Company. This product, available through dentists, contains all of the above ingredients and was highly recommended by Dr. Verigin, Reid Winick, D.D.S., an alternative dentist in New York City, and James Medlock, D.D.S., a mercury-free dentist in West Palm Beach, Florida.

You can use Tooth and Gum Tonic with a perio-aid as described above, says Dr. Verigin.

Alternatively, says Dr. Medlock, you can use it as a mouth rinse, in an irrigator, or for brushing (just pour a little of the solution in the palm of your hand and dip your toothbrush in it).

## MAGNETIZED ORAL IRRIGATOR: *Take Charge of Plaque*

Regular oral irrigators clean deep inside the "pockets" of diseased gums where bacteria live. But an irrigator with a magnet in the handle does more than merely clean, says Dr. Winick. It polarizes the water so that the teeth have a positive charge and the bacteria a negative charge. One study found that patients who used a magnetized irrigator had 64 percent less calculus, the hardened layer of plaque that forms on teeth, than those who used a typical irrigator.

You can find irrigators with magnetic handles at some health food stores and through mail-order suppliers.

### Getting to the Root of Gum Disease

What if you faithfully brush and floss, but your gums are still inflamed—red, puffy, and prone to bleeding? Well, the problem may not be in your mouth. It may be in your stomach (and the rest of your digestive tract).

That's the opinion of Michael Lipelt, N.D., D.D.S., a naturopathic physician and dentist in Sebastopol, California. "Even when people do a great job with their home care, if their diets are bad—high in fat and sugar, low in fiber, and emphasizing processed rather than whole foods—they will create digestive disharmony, which will negatively affect the condition of their mouths," he says.

Lots of other alternative healers agree with him. Here are their suggestions for healing your gums by changing your diet.

## FOOD: *Turning Down the Heat*

In Traditional Chinese Medicine, poor digestion is said to turn the stomach into a kind of steamy cauldron, creating toxic gases that drift upward in the body and damage the tissues of the gums. To "cool" your stomach, Dr. Lipelt suggests eating more salads and fruits, especially seasonal produce, and fewer fatty, sugary, and spicy foods. The best cooling foods, he says, are melons, cucumber, watercress, and tofu.

## MISO SOUP: *Really Cool Cuisine*

It's a lot easier than making French onion. Boil 1 cup of water and let it cool until you can comfortably put your finger in it. Then pour the water into a soup bowl and stir in a tablespoon of miso, a soybean paste that's a staple of Asian cuisine. You can find it in most health food stores and many supermarkets. "This soup is very cooling to the stomach," says Dr. Lipelt.

## PROTEIN: *Observe the Limit*

Too much protein in your diet changes your saliva so that it's more hospitable to gum-destroying bacteria, says Dr. Verigin. He recommends limiting your protein intake to no more than 75 grams a day. (That doesn't mean that you have to be a vegetarian—just a little more cautious. A 3-ounce hamburger patty, for example, provides about 20 grams of protein.)

## CAFFEINE, SUGAR, AND ALCOHOL: *Easy Does It*

These foods beat up your immune system, making it easier for the gum-destroying bacteria to do their dirty work, says Dr. Winick. Your best bet, he says, is to eliminate them entirely.

## VITAMIN C: *For Healthy Gums*

Poor digestion can stop nutrients from being absorbed—the same nutrients that you need to keep your gums healthy. One of them is vitamin C, which helps the body create collagen, the cellular foundation of gum tissue.

To protect your gums, take 1,000 milligrams of vitamin C a day, says Dr. Verigin—but not all at once. Instead, take 500 milligrams twice a day, in the morning and evening.

## COENZYME Q$_{10}$: *Boosting Circulation*

This substance helps reverse gum disease by increasing circulation and bringing a better supply of oxygen to the gums, says Dr. Verigin. He recommends 100 milligrams a day.

Be sure to get oil-based soft-gels, which are better absorbed, says Dr. Winick.

## PYCNOGENOL: *Pining for Relief*

This antioxidant, derived from pine bark, increases circulation to the gums by dilating the blood vessels. It also has an anti-inflammatory effect, says Dr. Winick. He recommends taking 1 milligram per pound of body weight three times a day. Someone who weighs 150 pounds, for example, would take 150 milligrams three times a day.

**GLUCOSAMINE SULFATE:** *Undoing the Damage*

This substance, which can help regenerate the cartilage in arthritic joints, also can help rebuild disease-damaged gums, believes Dr. Verigin. Take a 300-milligram capsule three times daily, he says.

**ALOE:** *Rinse Away Inflammation*

If your best efforts don't stop the bleeding and inflammation, soothe your gums with pure aloe gel, says Flora Parsa Stay, D.D.S., a dentist in Oxnard, California. At the store, check the label to be sure you're getting the form that can be used internally. Then, three or four times a day, mix 1 tablespoon of the gel with ½ cup of warm water, rinse your mouth for 30 seconds, and spit it out, she says.

# *Herbal and Nutritional Remedies to Stop* **Hair Loss**

When it comes to male pattern baldness, New York City–based consumer advocate Spencer David Kobren has seen a lot of false promises.

"Almost every remedy in the hair-loss 'industry' that has not been FDA-approved is a rip-off, and there are very few places to turn for accurate, unbiased information," says Kobren.

What's more, he says, some dermatologists have a blasé attitude about hair loss and often won't work with a patient to create a program to reverse the problem.

But Kobren—who has male pattern baldness and once spent years trying to fix the problem—says that there is a scientifically proven medical solution that can actually reverse the problem in 66 percent of men who use it: the drug finasteride (Propecia), which is also used for prostate problems.

Also, he says, there are alternative remedies, such as herbs and nutritional supplements, that work very much like Propecia and can make a real difference for men who are losing their hair.

As for hair loss in women, which is a much more complex problem that often requires professional diagnosis and treatment, many experts in alternative beauty care believe that you can help the problem with natural remedies.

First, here are Kobren's self-care recommendations for men, based on his review of scientific research and clinical findings and reviewed and endorsed by doctors.

### SAW PALMETTO: *A Natural Treatment*

Medical science understands that the cause of male pattern baldness is a hormone called dihydrotestosterone (DHT), a by-product of testosterone that shrinks and eventually kills hair follicles. The less DHT that reaches the follicles, the more hair

---

# GUIDE TO
# PROFESSIONAL CARE

Hair loss in men is rarely health threatening, unless it's sudden and occurs in patches over the head (a disease of the hair follicles called alopecia areata).

Usually, men's hair loss is genetic male pattern baldness. If you have this problem, you also have many medical options, from medications such as finasteride (Propecia) to hair transplants. If you decide to seek professional medical treatment for male pattern baldness, find a dermatologist who is willing to work with you to explore your options and help you solve the problem, rather than one who uses one treatment for all hair-loss patients, says Spencer David Kobren, a New York City–based consumer advocate for people with hair loss.

Hair loss in women is often difficult to diagnose and can be caused by many factors, including alopecia areata, hormone imbalances, menopause, dietary protein and amino acid deficiency, intestinal parasites, damage from hair treatments, and stress.

"A woman with hair loss should discuss the proper treatment with a naturally oriented medical doctor or naturopathic physician. He can help you get to the bottom of what's causing the loss of hair and then prescribe the appropriate action," says Elson Haas, M.D., director of the Preventive Medical Center of Marin in San Rafael, California.

you'll have. Finasteride works by inhibiting the production of the enzyme 5-alpha-reductase, which converts testosterone to DHT.

The herb saw palmetto does almost the same thing; it stops DHT from binding to receptor sites at the hair follicles. In short, says Kobren, it may help stop and even reverse baldness.

Based on studies of the herb, Kobren advises men with hair loss to take a 160-milligram dose of saw palmetto every morning and another every evening. Look for a product that is "concentrated and purified" and has 85 to 95 percent fatty acids and sterols, which ensure its potency.

### NETTLE AND PYGEUM: *Two More Helpful Herbs*

The herb pygeum also blocks 5-alpha-reductase, and nettle is known to enhance the effects of pygeum. Use 50 to 100 milligrams of nettle and 60 to 500 milligrams of pygeum, standardized for 13 percent beta sterols, every day, says Kobren.

### ZINC: *For Follicle Protection*

Zinc cuts the activity of 5-alpha-reductase and helps stop DHT from getting to the hair follicles. "This mineral helps prevent and treat male pattern baldness," says Kobren. To stop hair loss, he advises men to take 60 milligrams a day for 6 months.

### FATTY ACIDS: *For Better Texture and Density*

"Fatty acids found in flaxseed oil, sunflower oil, black currant oil, evening primrose oil, and soy oil are effective against the processes that contribute to male pattern baldness," Kobren says. He advises men to take 1 teaspoon a day of any one of those oils.

He also recommends taking a 500-milligram capsule of black currant oil twice a day since it's particularly rich in gamma-linolenic acid (GLA), which is a must for healthy hair. "If you take black currant oil, you will probably notice an improvement in the texture, density, and quality of your hair in 6 to 8 weeks," he says.

### GREEN TEA: *Inhibits the Hair-Killing Enzyme*

Like some of the hair-helping herbs, green tea inhibits the production of 5-alpha-reductase, the enzyme that allows DHT to shrink and kill your hair follicles. Drink one to three cups every day, says Kobren.

## Combating Hair Loss in Women

In Ayurveda, the ancient healing system from India, hair loss is seen as a symptom of a whole-body imbalance caused by factors such as too much stress, poor nutrition, or unhealthful habits such as smoking or excessive drinking, says Pratima Raichur, an Ayurvedic practitioner and esthetician in New York City.

Dr. Raichur suggests that a woman with hair loss relax more often, by meditating regularly, for instance, or by receiving a relaxing treatment such as a foot massage.

"Reducing stress is the most important factor in combating hair loss," she says. The following Ayurvedic remedies may also help stop or reverse the condition.

### GOTU KOLA: *To Calm the Nervous System*

The herb gotu kola is calming and can help slow or stop stress-related hair loss, says Dr. Raichur. Follow the dosage recommendations on the label.

### FENUGREEK: *To Encourage New Growth*

A paste made with ½ teaspoon of fenugreek powder and ¾ cup of unsweetened coconut milk can energize the scalp and encourage hair growth, Dr. Raichur says. Apply the paste briskly to your scalp, she says, cover your scalp with a plastic cap for 30 minutes, then wash with a gentle shampoo. "Do this treatment twice a week for about 2 months," she says. You can find fenugreek powder in the spice section of supermarkets.

### MASSAGE: *Soothe Your Scalp with Sesame Oil*

Stress collects in the head as heat, or what Ayurveda calls pitta, says Melanie Sachs, cofounder of Diamond Way Ayurveda in San Luis Obispo, California. "When the head is hot, the hair roots become unstable, and hair loss can result," she says.

To cool the head, Sachs recommends a scalp massage with sesame oil, which penetrates the skin to lubricate not only the scalp but also the entire body. "It's just like growing grass," she says. "If you keep the head and body moist, I believe the hair will grow." The massage also releases tension and increases circulation in the scalp, which is helpful for new growth.

With 2 to 4 teaspoons of oil, use four fingertips of each hand to start massaging at the occiput, the bony ridge at the back of the head above the neck. Massage forward in firm circles and zigzags. Massage your entire scalp, and be gentle rather than vigorous if your scalp is tight.

"Urge the scalp to move over the skull," Sachs says. The more you work the scalp, the more it will loosen. You can do the massage for as long and as often as you like.

### Aromatherapy: It Worked for Her

Melanie von Zabuesnig is no stranger to hair loss. At the age of 7, the Murrieta, California, aromatherapist was diagnosed with alopecia areata, a disease of the hair follicles that causes clumps of hair to fall out. By the time she was 32, the disease had advanced to alopecia universalis, or total loss of hair, including body hair.

Von Zabuesnig discovered that many essential oils encouraged hair growth by regulating the amount of oil on the scalp, cleansing the scalp thoroughly, improving circulation to the scalp, and nourishing the roots of the hair. She eventually created her own hair-restoration formula, massaging it into her scalp each night and washing it out in the morning with a natural shampoo.

Within 3 months, she says that her entire scalp was covered with soft, new hair that soon thickened and darkened to the point that she no longer needed a wig. Here is her original recipe.

Using a wooden or plastic (not aluminum) utensil, mix the following essential oils in a glass bowl: 1 tablespoon of jojoba oil, three drops of rosemary oil, three drops of lavender oil, one drop of lemon balm (melissa) oil, and one drop of Atlas cedarwood oil.

Massage the mixture into your scalp with your fingertips. Leave it on for 30 minutes or overnight, then shampoo as usual, adding one drop of rosemary oil to each shampoo application. As a final rinse, add one drop of lavender oil and one drop of rosemary oil to a quart of cool water and pour it over your head.

# *A Simple Natural Medicine*
## *Can Prevent*
# **Hangover**

It's unlikely that you'll find an over-the-counter medicine on the shelves of your drugstore that can reliably prevent the headache, nausea, dry mouth, red eyes, and dizziness that are the mixed drink of misery called a hangover.

While drinking to excess is never a good idea, there is an alternative remedy that can help prevent a hangover from occasional overindulgence. It's a remedy that has "worked time and time again, for almost everyone I know who has tried it," says Walter Crinnion, N.D., a naturopathic doctor and director of Healing Naturally in Kirkland, Washington.

## BIFIDUS: *A Teaspoon Before Bedtime Heads Off Hangovers*

"I come from an Irish Catholic family, and enthusiastic drinking is sometimes part of our get-togethers," says Dr. Crinnion. "At the end of the evening, I get out a bunch of glasses, put a teaspoonful of bifidus powder in each one, fill them with water, stir until the bifidus is dissolved, and then hand them out to everybody as their 'nightcap.'

"They wake up the next morning feeling great; no one ever has a hangover. Bifidus is an exceptional remedy. To my knowledge, it has never failed to prevent a hangover in anyone I know who's used it."

Bifidus (also known as bifidum) is one of the helpful bacteria that inhabit the large intestine, keeping nasty bacteria at bay, manufacturing B vitamins, and helping the bowels stay regular. But, says Dr. Crinnion, it has another very handy property: It detoxifies acetaldehyde, a digestive by-product of alcohol that is theorized to cause most of the symptoms of a hangover. "The level of acetaldehyde is dramatically lowered when a person takes bifidus after drinking," he says.

He recommends the product Bifido Factor from Natren. Mix 1 teaspoon in 8 ounces of water and drink before bedtime.

## B VITAMINS: *Clear the Liver of Toxins*

Thiamin and vitamin $B_6$ help clear the liver of acetaldehyde, reducing the symptoms of a hangover, says Dr. Crinnion. Take one high-potency B-vitamin supplement, such as a B-50, before you start drinking, he advises.

## MILK THISTLE: *Help Your Liver Cope*

The herb milk thistle is believed to protect liver cells from alcohol by preventing toxins from entering the cells and helping to remove those that are already there, says Beverly Yates, N.D., a naturopathic physician and director of the Natural Health Care Group in Seattle.

She recommends taking two 70-milligram capsules with a meal prior to or while drinking. Look for a product that is standardized to 70 to 80 percent silymarin, the therapeutic factor in the herb.

## LIME AND SUGAR WATER: *An Ancient Ayurvedic Remedy*

Ayurveda, the ancient system of natural healing from India, says that the body is a combination of five elements: space, air, fire, water, and earth. When you have a hangover, the air element "pushes" the fire element, creating an excess of fire, which then "pushes" into the water and earth elements, creating mud. You feel clammy, dense, and sluggish, says DeAnna Batdorff, a clinical aromatherapist and Ayurvedic practitioner in Forestville, California.

Lime and sugar help "cut through the muck," she says. The sugar also helps stabilize blood sugar, which is typically low after heavy drinking. And she believes that the lime helps refresh and activate the liver, which is stressed from too much alcohol.

When you get up in the morning after a night of drinking, says Batdorff, add 2 teaspoons of fresh lime juice and ¼ teaspoon of sugar to an 8-ounce glass of water and drink it slowly.

## AROMATHERAPY: *For the Morning After*

Essential oils are a powerful way to relieve symptoms after a night of heavy drinking, Batdorff says. Here are her recommendations.

• If you're nauseated, smear a small drop of peppermint oil under your nose or dilute two to three drops in 1 ounce of olive oil and put a drop of the mixture on your belly, says Batdorff. "It will give you a refreshed feeling and help stop your stomach from churning."

• Coriander oil can also help with an upset stomach, says Batdorff. Put two drops, undiluted, on your belly button twice a day.

• Frankincense oil cools the body and can help stop the sweats, says Batdorff. Put one drop over your liver, which is on the upper right side of your abdomen.

• After a night of heavy drinking, you may feel heavy-hearted and full of remorse for your overindulgence. Grapefruit or orange essential oil can help lift your spirits, says Batdorff. Use it in a diffuser so your bedroom or house is filled with the smell.

Diffusing one or both of these essential oils in the house is also useful if cooking smells are nauseating you. "Grapefruit will cut through the smell and relieve the problem," says Batdorff.

• Feeling spaced-out? The essential oil vetiver is very grounding, says Batdorff. "It helps you find your center and regain focus after drinking," she says. Put two drops on the very top of your head.

• If you're not sure which essential oil to use, try marjoram, says Batdorff. "It is definitely for headaches, but it also balances the central nervous system," she says. Put one drop behind each ear.

# *Natural, Fast Relief from*
# **Headaches**

If you're one of the 45 to 50 million Americans who suffer from chronic headaches, let's start by relieving what may be your biggest "headache" of all: the never-get-better notion (still held by many doctors) that chronic headaches are psychological in origin.

"The majority of doctors do not understand that chronic headaches are *biological* in origin," says Fred D. Sheftell, M.D., director and cofounder of the New England Center for Headache in Stamford, Connecticut.

The biological or physical cause of headaches is a genetically based deficiency of the brain chemical serotonin. This deficiency alters the physiology of the blood vessels, pain receptors, and other elements in the brain to produce a headache, according to Lawrence Robbins, M.D., director of the Robbins Headache Clinic in Northbrook, Illinois. He says that 90 percent of the people in his practice with chronic headaches have a family history of them.

This single cause produces a variety of headaches. The two most common are migraines (throbbing or aching pain on one side of the head, often coupled with nausea, visual disturbances, and dizziness) and tension headaches (a throbbing forehead, dull pain on both sides of the head, and a sensation that the head is being squeezed, tightened, or pressed). There are many headache triggers, from foods to stress to hormones to weather changes, but you probably have to be genetically predisposed to chronic headaches for the triggers to affect you time and time again, Dr. Robbins says.

What do people typically do to stop the pain of a headache? Reach for a painkiller, of course. And these medications work, at least for a while.

# GUIDE TO
# PROFESSIONAL CARE

Chronic headaches can be symptoms of many different health problems; if you have severe or frequent headaches, see a medical doctor for an examination and diagnosis, says Lawrence Robbins, M.D., director of the Robbins Headache Clinic in Northbrook, Illinois.

Consult a doctor as soon as possible, Dr. Robbins says, if the headaches get progressively worse over days or weeks; if you've never had headaches, and they've started suddenly; if your headache began after coughing, straining, or exertion; if you have a headache accompanied by changes in memory, personality, or behavior; if you have a headache along with changes in vision, the ability to walk, or general weakness or numbness; if you have a headache with a stiff neck, fever and rash, or breathing problems; or if you have a headache after an injury or accident.

If you have a sudden, excruciating headache that's more painful than any you've had before, see a doctor immediately.

The best health professional to see for headache pain is a headache specialist, "who will not dismiss your problem as psychological and will be aware of the latest and most effective treatments, both conventional and alternative," Dr. Robbins says.

You may also want to consider seeing a psychotherapist after you've seen a medical doctor to learn how to improve your coping skills, he says. "People who have been through therapy typically use less medicine, have less severe headaches, and have less anxiety in general."

Unfortunately, chronic headache sufferers can quickly develop a tolerance to painkillers, causing them to need more medications to stop the pain. Eventually, it gets to a point where *not* taking medications can trigger headaches, as the body attempts to withdraw from the drug. This phenomenon, called rebound headache, affects millions of chronic headache sufferers, Dr. Robbins says.

Yes, there are many prescription and over-the-counter medications that, when used sensibly, can help control chronic headaches. According to Dr. Robbins, however, alternative remedies are often better choices, or they can be combined with medications so you need less painkiller.

"The treatment of chronic headache may not be successful with medications alone," says Dr. Sheftell. "The headache sufferer needs to include a variety of other strategies, such as proper diet, nutritional supplements, stress management, and many other factors."

In fact, after visiting your doctor to rule out a serious cause for your headaches such as a tumor or infection, there are many ways to achieve immediate headache relief that may be more effective than drugs. Start with the cold comfort of ice.

## ICE: *A Headache Sufferer's Best Friend*

"The majority of patients will find that during acute episodes, ice is the best form of pain relief," says Dr. Sheftell.

"Many of my headache patients say ice is their best friend," agrees Dr. Robbins. Ice cuts pain by reducing swollen blood vessels that are pressing on nerves, by overriding pain messages to the brain, and by lowering metabolism, which reduces muscle contraction.

A reusable ice pack, wrapped ice, or even a box or bag of frozen food will work. Cover the ice or cold object with a paper towel or a thin layer of cloth to protect your skin. Then place the ice on the painful area, but only for 20 minutes at a time to reduce the chance of skin damage.

The sooner you apply ice after the headache starts, the faster and more thorough the pain relief, says Dr. Robbins. He recommends trying Migraine Ice, a new product that provides cool relief without refrigeration.

## ACUPRESSURE: *Hand-to-Hand Pain Relief*

Pressing the acupressure point (called LI4) in the thick, meaty part of the web between your thumb and forefinger can help relieve headache pain, says Alexander Mauskop, M.D., director of the New York Headache Center in New York City. (For the exact location of the point, see An Illustrated Guide to Acupressure Points on page 700.)

Using your opposite hand, feel for the tender areas in the web and press and rub them, squeezing with your thumb on the back of your hand and one or more fingers hooked under your palm. Apply pressure with a rhythmic, pumping action.

The right amount of pressure, says Dr. Mauskop, will produce a twinge that isn't painful but isn't soothing, either. You can apply pressure for as long as necessary to reduce or eliminate your headache, working each hand for about a minute at a time.

One caution, however: Pregnant women should not use this point because it may cause premature contractions of the uterus.

## AROMATHERAPY: *As Effective as Ibuprofen*

Rubbing peppermint oil on your temples at the start of a tension headache can relieve pain just as effectively as taking ibuprofen, the popular over-the-counter pain reliever, says Dr. Robbins. Dilute one drop of peppermint essential oil in one to two drops of almond oil or other carrier oil to apply to your head, or add three drops to a warm bath.

Other essential oils, such as lavender or Roman chamomile, can also help relieve a tension headache, says Dr. Mauskop. Sprinkle one drop of the oil of your choice on a tissue and inhale deeply. Or take a bath in warm water to which you've added five to six drops of oil.

## VITAMIN $B_6$: *Stabilize Serotonin*

Vitamin $B_6$ may help stabilize the brain's serotonin levels, preventing headaches, says Dr. Sheftell. He recommends 50 milligrams a day for chronic headache sufferers.

## FEVERFEW: *Similar to Aspirin*

The herb feverfew may help reduce the frequency of migraines, says Dr. Mauskop. It contains compounds called sesquiterpene lactones, which may have anti-inflammatory properties similar to aspirin's.

Take 125 milligrams daily of prepared, dried feverfew, available in caplets, that's standardized for 0.2 percent parthenolide, says Dr. Mauskop. And check the botanical name on the label (*Tanacetum parthenium*) to be sure the product is authentic feverfew.

Or, he says, you can take one caplet twice a day of Migra-Lieve, a product that supplies magnesium, riboflavin, and feverfew, all of which have been shown to relieve migraines. It will take 1 to 3 months of regular use before relief occurs. If you plan to take it for more than 4 months, do so only with the approval and supervision of a physician experienced in the therapeutic use of herbs, says Dr. Mauskop.

## GINGER: *Perfect for "Vata" Headaches*

Your mind races, you start a lot of new things but never finish, you have irregular habits, and you need a lot of change in your life. If that description fits you, try the "grounding" herb ginger for your headaches, says neurologist David Simon, M.D., medical director of the Chopra Center for Well-Being in La Jolla, California.

Put 1 teaspoon of grated fresh ginger in a 16- to 24-ounce thermos of hot water and sip throughout the day, Dr. Simon suggests.

This remedy comes from Ayurveda, the ancient system of natural healing from India, which divides people into three constitutional types: vata, pitta, and kapha. Typical vata people have a lot of movement in their natures, says Dr. Simon.

### Uncovering the Truth About MSG and Migraines

It's an accepted scientific fact that the food additive monosodium glutamate, or MSG, can trigger migraines in people who are sensitive to it. But what isn't so well-known is that MSG can be an ingredient in a food but not be listed as MSG on the label.

Instead, it can masquerade as "hydrolyzed protein" or "yeast nutrient" or "natural flavoring" or any one of more than a dozen MSG-containing ingredients. In short, this so-called flavor enhancer, which makes every taste just a little bit tastier, is just about everywhere in packaged and processed foods.

And it's giving a lot of people migraines.

"I would say that 80 to 90 percent of my migraine patients can avoid headaches completely if they eliminate all sources of MSG from their diets," says Gerard L. Guillory, M.D., an internist in Aurora, Colorado.

If you have migraines, use the following list of MSG-containing ingredients when you shop, and don't buy foods with one or more of those ingredients on the label. If you eliminate all sources of MSG from your diet, and your migraines go away (it's quite likely that they will, according to Dr. Guillory), you'll know that you're probably sensitive to the additive and will need to avoid it in the future.

An important postscript: Aspartame (aspartic acid), the compound in NutraSweet, Equal, and other artificial sweeteners, has the same effect as MSG. So if you're sensitive to MSG and want to prevent migraines, you must avoid aspartame-based artificial sweeteners, too, says Dr. Guillory.

The following ingredients always contain MSG.

- Monosodium glutamate
- Hydrolyzed protein
- Sodium caseinate
- Yeast extract
- Yeast nutrient
- Maltodextrins
- Autolyzed yeast
- Textured protein
- Calcium caseinate
- Yeast food
- Hydrolyzed oat flour

The following ingredients often contain MSG.

- Malt extract
- Malt flavoring
- Bouillon
- Barley malt
- Broth
- Stock
- Flavoring(s)
- Natural flavoring(s)
- Natural beef flavoring
- Natural chicken flavoring
- Natural pork flavoring
- Food seasonings

## ALOE: *Great for "Pitta" Headaches*

Are you always fighting a deadline of one kind or another? Do you try to get a lot done in a short period of time? Are you irritable and critical? Have insomnia? Tend to suffer from heart-burn and skin rashes?

Try "cooling" aloe juice for your headaches, says Dr. Simon. Take 2 tablespoons twice a day. This remedy works for the typical pitta person in Ayurveda.

## FIBER AND WATER: *No Constipation, No Headaches*

"I've been surprised to see that a very high percentage of my patients with migraines are constipated and that improving their regularity helps reduce their headaches," says Dr. Simon.

To relieve constipation, Dr. Simon recommends a mostly vegetarian diet that includes at least five or six servings a day of fruits, vegetables, or grains plus legumes, nuts, seeds, and plenty of water, and minimizes animal fat. If you change your eating habits and are still constipated, says Dr. Simon, try a fiber supplement such as Metamucil; follow the directions on the label.

If that doesn't work, he recommends the herb triphala, a bowel tonic from Ayurvedic medicine. It's available as tablets; follow the dosage recommendations on the label.

### Trigger Foods:
### Discover the Headache Causers

Foods that contain a chemical called tyramine are strongly linked to chronic headaches in many people, according to Lawrence Robbins, M.D., director of the Robbins Headache Clinic in Northbrook, Illinois.

The only sure way to discover which of the following foods is giving you headaches is to eliminate all of them and then return one food at a time to your diet, noting if it gives you a headache, he says.

- Smoked and cured, aged and packaged meat
- Herring, caviar, and smoked fish
- Vinegar
- Pickled and fermented foods
- Aged cheese (such as Cheddar, Brie, and Gruyére)
- Products high in yeasts, including doughnuts, coffee cakes, and breads, especially hot, fresh bread

- Chocolate
- Sugar and all products made with processed sugar or corn syrup
- Citrus fruits in large quantities
- Figs
- Sour cream and yogurt
- The pods of lima beans, navy beans, and peas
- MSG
- Caffeine (more than 200 milligrams; small amounts actually help headaches)
- Alcoholic beverages, especially red wine

## FOOD: *Eat on Schedule*

Many people with chronic headaches believe that food sensitivities are the main cause of their problem. But food affects only one in three headache sufferers, says Dr. Robbins. In fact, he believes that to prevent a headache, when you eat is much more important than what you eat.

"Low blood sugar is a common headache trigger," he says. "Eating at least three meals a day, every day, will help keep blood sugar levels balanced."

### Mind-Body Healing Makes Stress
### Less of a Headache

While stress isn't the cause of chronic headaches, it can trigger episodes. And mind-body techniques, such as breathing, meditation, visualization, yoga, and the like, can help defuse stress and prevent headaches.

"Many of my patients who use mind-body techniques to reduce stress have far fewer headaches," says Dr. Robbins.

## MEDITATION: *Breathing a Sigh of Relief*

A woman with migraines for whom all other treatments had failed found relief by regularly doing the following breathing-awareness technique and drinking ginger tea, says Dr. Simon. The meditation is taken from his book, *The Wisdom of Healing*.

Close your eyes and gently focus awareness on your respiration. As you inhale and exhale, simply observe your breath.

Remain aware of your breathing without trying to alter it in any way.

As you observe your breath, it may vary in speed, rhythm, or depth. It may even seem to pause for a time. Without resisting, calmly observe these changes.

At times, your attention may drift to a thought passing through your mind, to a physical sensation in your body, or to some distraction in the environment. Whenever you notice that you are not observing your breath, gently bring your attention back to it. Relinquish any expectations that you may have during this technique. If you find yourself being drawn to a particular feeling, mood, or expectation, treat this as you would any other thought. Gently return your awareness to your breath.

When you're finished meditating, very slowly open your eyes and return your attention to the sights and sounds around you.

Do this meditation once a day for 20 minutes, says Dr. Simon. The first few times you do it, keep a clock nearby and peek at it every few minutes. After a few days, you'll be surprised at how adept your body becomes at knowing when the time is up.

## VISUALIZATION: *Help Yourself to See Straight*

This visualization exercise can help ease muscle tension in the forehead, thus relieving the pain of a tension headache, says Dr. Sheftell.

First, sit in a comfortable chair, loosen any restrictive clothing, and close your eyes. Inhale deeply and slowly to a count of three. Be sure that your abdomen moves more than your chest, since abdominal breathing increases your intake of oxygen. Hold for a second, then exhale to a count of three.

Continue deep breathing and begin to visualize the muscles in your forehead as scrunched-up lines. Imagine those lines slowly becoming straighter and more parallel. Continue the deep breathing and the visualization for 5 to 10 minutes.

## ENERGY HEALING: *Ground Your Body, Heal Your Headache*

You can relieve a simple headache (not a chronic tension headache or migraine) with a basic exercise that releases energy blockages in the lower half of the body, allowing energy to flow out of the head, says Catherine Karas, a physical therapist and energy healer in Tiburon, California. Here's how to do it.

Stand with your feet shoulder-width apart, your knees slightly bent, your eyes looking at the floor ahead of you, and your head straight, in alignment with your spine. Direct your thoughts to your pelvis and allow the energy there (you may feel a sense of blockage or stagnation) to travel down through your thighs, your knees, your calves, your ankles, and your feet, and then to drain into the ground. Next, let fresh energy flow into your body from the Earth, moving up your entire body into your head.

Whenever you feel a headache developing, do this exercise for 5 minutes. Repeat the first energy-out exercise, then follow with the energy-in exercises as many times as you like, says Karas. "It works particularly well for headaches caused by hours of computer work," she says.

## Relief for Menstrual Headaches

The right vitamins and minerals can ease headaches linked to your menstrual cycle. Here's what experts recommend.

### VITAMIN E: *Take It before Your Period*

Vitamin E can help stabilize estrogen levels and prevent migraines around the time of menstruation, says Dr. Sheftell. He recommends taking one dose of 400 international units daily, then increasing to two doses a day during menstruation, starting a few days before your period and stopping a day or two after it begins.

### MAGNESIUM: *Is a Deficiency Causing Your Migraine?*

According to Dr. Mauskop, 40 percent of women with migraines (particularly those caused by the hormonal changes of menstruation) have lowered blood levels of the mineral magnesium. And 85 percent of those women have fewer migraines when they take a magnesium supplement, he says.

He recommends 400 milligrams a day in the form of chelated magnesium or magnesium oxide for maximum absorption. To avoid diarrhea, a possible side effect of taking magnesium supplements, start with 200 milligrams a day and increase to 400 milligrams after 7 days.

**CALCIUM:** *Another Natural Medicine for Menstrual Migraines*

Calcium supplements can help decrease the frequency of menstruation-caused migraines, says Dr. Robbins. He recommends taking two Extra-Strength Tums daily, which supply 750 milligrams of calcium.

**RIBOFLAVIN:** *Fewer Migraines*

Taking 400 milligrams a day of riboflavin can help significantly reduce the frequency of menstrual and other types of migraines in 6 to 8 weeks, says Dr. Robbins.

While the possibility of side effects is very low, he recommends that someone using this dose of riboflavin, which is hundreds of times more than the government's Daily Value, do so only with the approval and supervision of a physician.

# *It May Be Possible to Reverse*
# **Hearing Loss**

There are many possible causes of hearing loss—a side effect from a medication, an infection, or even too much earwax—but the most common cause is aging.

Over time, the nerve cells in the cochlea, the organ of the inner ear that is responsible for hearing, are destroyed. And, like brain cells, they can't be "treated" or restored. When you lose hearing in this way, you never get any of it back, except with a hearing aid.

At least, that's what a conventional doctor will tell you. But Michael D. Seidman, M.D., isn't a conventional doctor. As an otolaryngologist (ear, nose, and throat specialist) and medical director of the tinnitus center at the Henry Ford Health System in West Bloomfield, Michigan, Dr. Seidman has a unique perspective on health, healing—and hearing.

Also, as a researcher who has conducted numerous studies

on nutrition and hearing, many sponsored by the government's National Institutes of Health, he has shown that age-related hearing loss can be slowed and even reversed in rats.

He says that those research results may be very promising for humans. "In scientific studies, we have treated aging rats with different types of nutrients and improved their hearing by 5 to 10 decibels," Dr. Seidman says. In one such study, he tracked the hearing of 18- to 20-month-old rats until they were 24 to 26 months old (the equivalent of an 80- to 90-year-old human). During that period, the rats had a decline in hearing of 7 to 10 decibels.

When a group of those rats was fed the nutrients for 6 weeks, however, their hearing improved by 5 to 10 decibels, while the hearing of the rats that weren't fed the compounds worsened by another 5 to 7 decibels over that time.

The secret of reversing age-related hearing loss, says Dr. Seidman, is in the mitochondria, the areas within cells that produce energy. As the mitochondria generate the body's fuel, they also produce pollutants called free radicals, which damage DNA—a process that may be the cause of all age-related degeneration.

The nutrients that Dr. Seidman gave to the rats "enhance the functioning" of the mitochondria, he says. In fact, they may actually repair mitochondrial DNA that has been damaged by free radicals.

Here are the four nutrients in the formula that Dr. Seidman used. While he says that there would have to be studies involving humans before these nutrients could be scientifically said to reverse hearing loss, he also says that he takes the nutrients himself to counteract the effects of age-related hearing loss.

So try this combination for 6 months to see if it might help improve your hearing, says Dr. Seidman. The supplements are safe to take long term.

## ACETYL-CARNITINE: *A Combination of Amino Acids*

This nutrient is made in the body from lysine and methionine, two amino acids. Without it, the mitochondria can't make energy from fat. Your regimen should include 150 milligrams of the nutrient daily.

---

## GUIDE TO
## PROFESSIONAL CARE

If your hearing is so impaired that you have trouble understanding what people say, or if you have sudden, unexplained hearing loss accompanied by ringing in your ears (especially on one side), you need to see an otologist (ear specialist) or otolaryngologist (ear, nose, and throat specialist). You should also see one of these specialists if you experience bleeding in, discharge from, or pain in the ear. These doctors can help rule out any underlying medical problems that could be causing your hearing difficulties.

Once a doctor has established that you have age-related hearing loss, you should see a clinical audiologist to be tested and fitted for a hearing aid, says Richard Carmen, a clinical audiologist in Sedona, Arizona.

---

### ALPHA-LIPOIC ACID: *A Powerful Antioxidant*

Antioxidants protect your body against free radicals, and alpha-lipoic acid may be one of the most powerful antioxidants of them all, Dr. Seidman says. It is essential in mitochondrial functioning. Take 150 milligrams daily.

### COENZYME Q$_{10}$: *Another Must for the Mitochondria*

This vitamin-like supplement carries fatty acids across the cellular membrane so they can be used by the mitochondria to make the body's energy. Take 60 milligrams a day.

### GLUTATHIONE: *Vitamins C and E Can't Work without It*

The enzyme glutathione is part of your body's antioxidant "dominoes"—without it, the antioxidant vitamins C and E can't do their jobs. Take 50 milligrams daily.

### You Don't Hear Only with Your Ears

"Hearing is not generated by just the nerve cells in the cochlea," says Mona Lisa Schultz, M.D., Ph.D., a neuropsychiatrist and neuroscientist in Yarmouth, Maine. Hearing, she says, also depends on how we focus and on our attitude about what we hear.

"If I had age-related hearing loss, I would try to augment my hearing by refining my attentional mechanisms and by changing my attitude," Dr. Schultz says. Here are two steps that you can take to do just that.

## FOCUS: *Your Internal Hearing Aid*

"What hearing you have left, you can augment because you have an 'internal hearing aid'—attention," says Dr. Schultz. She recommends that in situations where it's difficult to hear, such as in a crowded room, you very consciously and intentionally focus on what you want to hear and just tune out the rest.

## ATTITUDE: *You Can't Hear If You Don't Listen*

"Everyone knows that a man often loses his hearing in the range of his wife's voice," says Dr. Schultz. In other words, if there are things that you don't want to hear, you may find that you have more difficulty hearing them.

If you suspect that your attitude plays a role in your hearing loss, try not only to hear but also to listen—to be emotionally sensitive to what people in your closest relationships are saying to you. And try not to get verbally angry when other people communicate things that you may not like to hear.

In fact, says Dr. Schultz, ask your spouse or relatives or friends, "Do you think I have trouble listening to you?" If the answer is yes, slow down and pay more attention when they're speaking. You may find that when you listen better, you hear better, too.

# Better and Safer Ways
# to Cool Down
# **Heartburn**

Millions of Americans take antacids for heartburn. According to alternative practitioners, they're all making a big mistake.

"One of the worst things you can do for your health is take an antacid," says Pamela Sky Jeanne, N.D., a naturopathic doctor in Gresham, Oregon. "That's because, in order to break down proteins into amino acids that are usable by the body, you must have sufficient hydrochloric acid in your stomach.

"If you take antacids, you interfere with this natural digestive process. You also interfere with digestion in the small intestine and the entire length of the digestive tract.... In short, an antacid destroys your ability to absorb nutrients. And that can destroy your health."

It's not a mystery why Americans take antacids: Heartburn hurts. Doctors call this problem gastroesophageal reflux, and it occurs when a valve at the bottom of the esophagus, the tube that leads to the stomach, weakens. This allows stomach acid to reflux, or flow back into the esophagus, causing the intense burning of heartburn.

If you have gastroesophageal reflux disease, you may also have symptoms such as sore throat, hoarseness, a persistent cough, or difficulty swallowing. You may also have digestive symptoms such as queasiness, bloating, belching, and stomach pain.

Even though antacids make stomach acid less potent, they simply aren't healthy, says Richard Leigh, M.D., a retired physician in Fort Collins, Colorado. "Taking prescription or over-the-counter antacids for months on end for heartburn is crazy," he says.

A much better approach is to use natural—and safe—remedies,

---

# GUIDE TO
# PROFESSIONAL CARE

Since heartburn and gastroesophageal reflux disease respond well to home treatments, your symptoms will probably clear up fairly quickly. If they don't disappear after about a week, and your alternative practitioner has already ruled out food sensitivities or other common heartburn triggers, you'll want to see a medical doctor to be sure that there isn't a more serious problem.

In fact, you should see your doctor right away if the heartburn is accompanied by chest pain, especially pain that radiates to the jaw, neck, or arm, or is accompanied by other symptoms, such as cold sweats, nausea, or a squeezing sensation in the chest, says James Balch, M.D., a physician in Trophy Club, Texas. You could be having a heart attack, and you don't want to take any chances, he says.

---

Dr. Leigh says. In fact, he believes that in many cases, "acid indigestion" is really caused by not generating *enough* stomach acid to digest food properly.

## HYDROCHLORIC ACID: *More Can Be Better*

"Most often, people think heartburn is due to excess acid," Dr. Jeanne says. "That may not be the case. There may be a deficiency of acid, particularly in people over 50, since stomach acid decreases with age."

In fact, the discomfort of having too little stomach acid is nearly identical to the discomfort of having too much, adds Elizabeth Lipski, a certified clinical nutritionist in Kauai, Hawaii. Because stomach acid begins the digestion process, having too little of it interferes with proper digestion, causing nausea, bloating, belching, and other symptoms of heartburn.

Dr. Leigh recommends that people with heartburn try taking a supplement containing hydrochloric acid, such as Gas-X Extra Strength liquid, right before meals, following the label directions.

If your stomach is deficient in hydrochloric acid, you should get relief right away.

If, however, your stomach doesn't need the boost, you'll feel a mild (but not dangerous) burning sensation, which you can stop instantly by drinking either a glass of milk or a solution made by mixing ¼ to ⅓ teaspoon of baking soda in 1 cup of water, suggests Dr. Leigh.

## LICORICE: *A Natural Antacid*

If your symptoms continue after taking hydrochloric acid supplements, there's a good chance that the problem is too much acid.

Rita Elkins, a master herbalist in Orem, Utah, recommends using a form of licorice called deglycyrrhizinated licorice, or DGL, which is a chewable form of the herb. It protects the lining of the esophagus, which may be at risk in cases of chronic heartburn. This form of licorice is thought to be more effective than regular licorice and may not cause high blood pressure, which is a possible side effect of other forms.

"Licorice may also be used to protect against the possible formation of some ulcers by hyperacidity," Elkins says.

When using licorice for heartburn, take one or two chewable tablets three times daily on an empty stomach, says Mark Stengler, N.D., a naturopathic physician in San Diego.

## ALOE: *Stops Symptoms Fast*

"I suffer from acid indigestion, and drinking a cup of aloe gel whenever I develop symptoms stops them almost instantly," says James Balch, M.D., a physician in Trophy Club, Texas. The gel helps protect and heal the delicate lining of the esophagus, he explains. He says that you can dilute the gel or not, depending on your taste. Be sure to check the label to see that you're getting the form intended for internal use.

## SLIPPERY ELM: *Heals the Mucous Membranes*

"Slippery elm is a wonderful herb that helps relieve the symptoms of acid indigestion because it heals the mucous membranes that have been irritated or injured by acid reflux," Dr. Jeanne says. She recommends taking one capsule of the herb right before each meal.

## 12 Steps to Avoiding Heartburn

Natural remedies are very effective for treating heartburn, but it's often possible to prevent it entirely by avoiding the most common triggers, says David S. Utley, M.D., clinical instructor at Stanford University Medical Center. Here are 12 steps that he recommends.

**1.** Avoid high-fat foods. Dietary fat causes the body to produce a hormone that weakens the esophageal valve, thus letting acid into the esophagus.

**2.** Don't eat big meals. Eating a lot of food makes your body produce a lot of acid. Instead, eat five or six small meals a day.

**3.** Don't eat before bedtime. Lying down soon after eating makes it easier for stomach acid to flow into the esophagus. It's better to eat 3 to 4 hours before you go to bed, Dr. Utley says.

**4.** Cut out coffee and tea—both caffeinated and decaffeinated. It's not the caffeine that causes increased stomach acid but some other, unknown ingredient in these beverages.

**5.** Cut down on carbonated beverages (especially cola and beer), citrus fruits, and tomatoes. These foods can trigger your stomach to produce extra acid.

**6.** Watch out for spices. Spicy foods are common causes of excess acid.

**7.** Chuck the chocolate. The fat and other ingredients in chocolate can open the acid faucet, causing painful heartburn.

**8.** Loosen your belt after eating. Tight clothing, such as belts, pants, and support hose, can create additional pressure and make heartburn much worse.

**9.** Skip the spearmint and peppermint. These normally healthful herbs, often enjoyed in tea or as a flavoring in after-dinner mints, loosen the esophageal valve.

**10.** Nix the nightcaps. If you have acid indigestion, drinking alcohol in the evening almost guarantees a late-night episode of heartburn.

**11.** Lose weight. While losing may be easier said than done, being 10 to 20 percent over your ideal body weight puts you at risk for heartburn.

**12.** Stop smoking. Smoking weakens your esophageal muscle, thus allowing acid to pour into the esophagus.

## MSM: *Acid Protection*

The nutritional supplement MSM (methylsulfonylmethane) strengthens the lining of the esophagus, protecting it from stomach acid, says Teresa Rispoli, Ph.D., a licensed nutritionist and acupuncturist in Agoura Hills, California. She recommends taking one to three capsules twice a day with meals for as long as the symptoms continue.

## SLEEP: *The Right Way*

Sometimes, the best remedy is the simplest.

"Remember, your stomach is on your left side," said Dr. Leigh, "so if you sleep on your left side or on your back, this encourages stomach contents to flow up into the esophagus." So when you settle down to get your zzz's, lie on your right side, he suggests.

# *Natural Remedies to Stop or Even Reverse* **Heart Disease**

Your odds of dying of heart disease are one in four. Reading this chapter may help improve those odds in your favor.

Yes, one in four Americans dies of heart disease, often the result of years of eating a high-fat, low-fiber, overprocessed, nutrient-poor diet; of not exercising regularly; and of being battered by stress.

All of those factors (and many more) damage the arteries to the heart, allowing plaque to narrow the arterial passageways until they are so plugged that only a meager trickle of oxygen-carrying blood can squeeze through—and part or all of the heart muscle dies. In other words, you have a heart attack.

That scenario is as common as a sunset. In fact, it's a lot more common, since approximately 1,400 Americans die each day from heart disease. And most of those attacks are preventable.

"If you have heart disease, it's possible to reverse its progress and bring your arteries to healthier condition," says Julian Whitaker, M.D., founder and director of the Whitaker Wellness Center in Newport Beach, California.

Dr. Whitaker isn't talking about surgery or medications, the options that most conventional doctors recommend for controlling heart disease. He's talking about "simple, gentle, natural" alternative remedies, such as a healthier diet, taking the right nutritional supplements, exercising regularly, and learning how to deal with stress.

Remember, however, that you should use the remedies in this chapter only with the approval and supervision of a qualified health care practitioner.

---

## GUIDE TO
## PROFESSIONAL CARE

*Caution:* You should use the alternative remedies discussed in this chapter only as part of a treatment program that is guided and monitored by a qualified medical doctor in partnership with a qualified alternative practitioner, both of whom are experienced in caring for your condition. Check with your conventional doctor before changing or stopping any conventional medical treatments or medications, and keep all of your doctors and/or alternative practitioners informed of all treatments that you are receiving.

It should go without saying that if you have any type of chest pain, you need to see a physician for a diagnosis. Even if it subsides after a few minutes, chest pain can be a warning sign of an impending heart attack if it is accompanied by pain that spreads to the neck, shoulders, or arms; light-headedness; fainting; sweating; nausea; shortness of breath; stomach or abdominal pain; unexplained anxiety; weakness; fatigue; paleness; or palpitations. If you do have heart disease, you may need surgery, such as a coronary bypass operation, to extend or even save your life, says Seth Baum, M.D., an integrative cardiologist and founder of the Baum Center for Integrative Heart Care in Boca Raton, Florida. For many patients, however, alternative remedies can stop or even reverse heart disease, Dr. Baum says.

Who can help guide you in the use of those remedies? A doctor who actually uses them in his practice, says Julian Whitaker, M.D., founder and director of the Whitaker Wellness Center in Newport Beach, California.

"You can't expect a doctor who is not actively engaged in treating patients with nutritional and other natural modalities to know how they should be used, or to even agree that they should be used," Dr. Whitaker says. "Don't try to convert your doctor; just find a doctor who is more attuned to the direction you've taken in health care."

The best natural treatments for heart disease are not just nutrition and vitamin therapy but also exercise and stress control, says Glenn S. Rothfeld, M.D., regional director of American WholeHealth in Arlington, Massachusetts.

You may also want to explore chelation therapy, a series of intravenous treatments that can help reverse heart disease by cleaning your arteries of plaque, says Paul Beals, M.D., a naturally oriented physician in Laurel, Maryland.

## Getting to the Heart of Exercise

If your heart could plead, it would beg you to exercise. Regular exercise helps control weight, brings down high blood pressure, lowers blood sugar, increases HDL ("good") cholesterol, and reduces emotional stress. And all of these are important factors in preventing or reversing heart disease, says Stephen T. Sinatra, M.D., a cardiologist and director of the New England Heart Center in Manchester, Connecticut.

Just remember: Any level of increased activity can benefit the heart, says Dr. Sinatra. Whenever you're in a parking lot, for example, park your car farther away from the entrance so you have to do a little more walking. Use the stairs instead of the elevator. Stop using the remote control and walk across the room to change the TV channel.

If you're over 40 and want to start a more strenuous exercise program, see your physician for an exercise stress test. This will rule out any risk to your heart so that you can exercise without worry.

Here are some ways you can optimize the heart-healthy value of exercise.

• Be sure to do a brief warm-up (about 10 minutes) that includes deep breathing exercises, hamstring stretches, and lower back stretches to prepare your body for exercise to help you avoid injury.

• Choose the right exercise. Dancing and walking are good forms of aerobic exercise for strengthening the heart muscle and improving circulation, says Dr. Sinatra. Dancing is great because it uses the whole body, he says, and since walking is so enjoyable, it's easy to exercise regularly. Swimming, bicycling, rowing, cross-country skiing, jumping rope, and hiking are other good options for aerobic exercise.

• Plan your exercise sessions for 15 to 30 minutes.

• Exercise three to five times a week for the greatest benefits.

• Monitor your intensity. After your stress test, your doctor will tell you your maximum heart rate—for example, 150 beats per minute. Exercise at no more than 70 percent of that maximum; in this example, that's about 105 beats per minute.

• Go slowly. Perhaps you've been walking for 15 minutes a day a couple of times a week. Now you're feeling fitter and want to walk longer. Don't rush! Increase your time by no more than 10 percent a month, says Dr. Sinatra.

## FOOD: *Nature's Best Cure*

One of the simplest and best dietary remedies for healing heart disease is to eat only foods that grow out of the ground, in their whole, unprocessed form.

"Preventing and healing heart disease is truly that simple," says Kitty Gurkin Rosati, R.D., a registered dietitian and nutrition director of the Rice Diet Program at Duke University in Durham, North Carolina. "If we would eat only foods that were just picked, I would need to find another profession!"

That's because those foods—vegetables, fruits, grains, and beans—are low in the heart-hurting saturated fat found in meat and dairy products, high in heart-healing fiber, and loaded with heart-nourishing vitamins and minerals.

Rosati adds to that dietary advice a recommendation for no more than a cup of nonfat dairy products daily for bone-protecting calcium, and 3 to 6 ounces of fish a couple of times a week for artery-clearing fatty acids.

## FLAXSEED OIL: *To Prevent Artery-Clogging Clots*

If eating fish twice a week isn't your cup of chowder, be sure to get a tablespoon or two of flaxseed oil every day. This oil is rich in both omega-3 and omega-6 fatty acids, which help reduce the stickiness of platelets, blood components that can bunch together and form the kind of clot that lodges in an artery and causes a heart attack.

You can take the oil straight or use it on salads or as a butter substitute on bread, says Paul Beals, M.D., a naturally oriented physician in Laurel, Maryland.

## APPLE-CIDER VINEGAR: *May Erode Arterial Plaque*

Using apple-cider vinegar on salads seems to help dissolve arterial plaque, says Patrick Quillin, R.D., Ph.D., director of the Rational Healing Institute in Tulsa, Oklahoma. It appears to do this by enhancing the number of friendly bacteria, which improves cholesterol reduction and immune functions. Or you can add a teaspoon of the vinegar to a cup of regular apple cider and drink it three times a day, he says.

## B-COMPLEX VITAMINS: *The Homocysteine Defense*

As your body metabolizes protein, it converts the amino acid methionine into another amino acid, cystine, making the chemical homocysteine in the process. High levels of homocysteine can have a direct, toxic effect on the coronary arteries, damaging them in such a way that arterial plaque can get a foothold, says Seth Baum, M.D., an integrative cardiologist and founder of the Baum Center for Integrative Heart Care in Boca Raton, Florida.

Perhaps as much as 30 percent of all heart disease is directly caused by high homocysteine levels, he says. That's the bad news. The good news is that three B vitamins—folic acid, $B_6$, and $B_{12}$—can help convert homocysteine to methionine or cystine, thus protecting your heart.

Dr. Baum recommends taking 800 to 1,000 micrograms of folic acid, 400 micrograms of vitamin $B_{12}$, and 50 milligrams of vitamin $B_6$ daily.

## CoQ$_{10}$—Extra Energy for Damaged Hearts

When you have a heart attack, a big chunk of heart muscle is destroyed, and the muscle that's left tries to take over the entire job of keeping the heart pumping. The remaining heart cells eventually become exhausted from the extra effort, and the heart starts to do a poor job of pumping blood to the rest of the body, leading to swollen ankles, fatigue, and shortness of breath when you exert yourself.

In medical terms, you have congestive heart failure. In practical terms, your heart cells need more energy. The supplement coenzyme Q$_{10}$ (coQ$_{10}$) can give it to them, says Stephen T. Sinatra, M.D., a cardiologist and director of the New England Heart Center in Manchester, Connecticut.

The vitamin-like coQ$_{10}$ stimulates the body to form ATP, a key chemical for producing energy in every cell. When the myocardial cells are energized, they contract with more force, and the entire heart pumps with greater vigor. The result: congestive heart failure frequently improves.

"I personally use it in every one of my patients with congestive heart failure if they are willing to take it," says Dr. Sinatra. "It has a considerable impact on their quality of life."

Different patients need different levels of coQ$_{10}$, ranging from 90 to 400 milligrams daily. Because there's such a wide range of effective doses, Dr. Sinatra says to use it only under the care and supervision of a nutritionally oriented physician.

At whatever level you take it, look for yellow, soft-gel capsules, which Dr. Sinatra says are the best absorbed of the coQ$_{10}$ products.

## VITAMIN E: *Stops Free Radicals*

Vitamin E is an antioxidant that can help stop free radicals (unstable molecules that harm cells by oxidizing the fats in cell membranes) from damaging the lining of your arteries and contributing to heart disease, says Michael Janson, M.D., consultant physician at Path to Health in Burlington, Massachusetts. He recommends taking 400 to 800 international units of vitamin E a day to protect your arteries.

## MAGNESIUM: *Helps Reverse Heart Disease*

This mineral is critically important in helping to reverse heart disease, says Dr. Janson. It can relax blood vessels, improve circulation, reduce angina, and help lower blood pressure. He recommends 500 to 1,000 milligrams of supplemental magnesium daily, half with breakfast and half with dinner.

## COENZYME Q$_{10}$: *Helps Prevent Heart Disease*

The vitamin-like supplement coenzyme Q$_{10}$ can help stop the oxidation of LDL cholesterol—"the pivotal step in the process of atherosclerosis," or hardening of the arteries, says Stephen T. Sinatra, M.D., a cardiologist and director of the New England Heart Center in Manchester, Connecticut.

To help prevent heart disease, he recommends taking 90 to 180 milligrams of coenzyme Q$_{10}$ a day in three divided doses.

## QIGONG: *Brings Healing Energy to Your Heart*

The qigong exercises of Traditional Chinese Medicine can suffuse your heart with more life force, or chi, says Glenn S. Rothfeld, M.D., regional director of American WholeHealth in Arlington, Massachusetts. The following exercise is particularly good for releasing blocked chi in the heart area, he says.

Put your right palm on the left side of your chest and massage slowly in a clockwise circle while silently repeating the word *ho*. Do this exercise for as long as you like, at least once a day.

## YOGA: *Expand Your Horizons*

The yoga exercise known as the chest expansion pose can help improve circulation. Here's how Dr. Rothfeld says to do it.

Hold your arms out to the sides, then bend your elbows and slowly move your arms back until you can clasp your hands behind your head at about shoulder level (*a*).

Keeping your hands clasped, slowly stretch your arms up without straining, holding your trunk straight (*b*).

Stretch your arms backward, with your hands still clasped, and gently arch your back, holding the stretch for about 5 seconds (*c*).

Slowly bend forward, dropping your head and stretching your clasped hands downward, for about 10 seconds (*d*).

Finally, stand up, drop your arms to your sides, and relax. Do this pose once or twice each day on an ongoing basis, says Dr. Rothfeld.

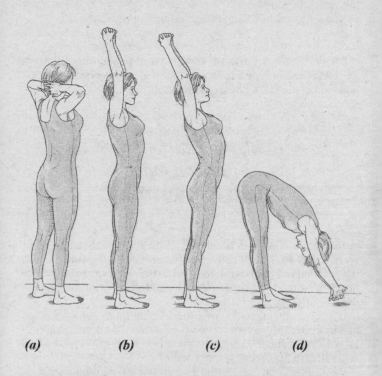

*(a)*              *(b)*              *(c)*              *(d)*

## AROMATHERAPY: *Calm Your Heart*

Essential oils can relieve some of the anxiety of having heart disease, says Jane Buckle, R.N., a nurse and aromatherapist in Albany, New York.

If you have heart disease, she recommends using one of the following: sweet marjoram, lavender, neroli, or damask rose. She believes that damask rose has been particularly useful in helping people recover from heart attacks. To use an essential oil, try the following techniques.

• Put a few drops in a warm bath before soaking for 10 to 15 minutes.

• Put a few drops on a cotton ball and place it next to your pillow while you sleep.
• Add a few drops to a massage oil before receiving a massage.

People with heart disease should avoid peppermint oil, says Buckle. Some research indicates that it can cause heart palpitations in people taking heart medication.

## *Cool, Alternative Ways to Head Off*
# Heat Exhaustion

Talk about hot and bothered! With heat exhaustion, your body is way too hot, because you haven't been drinking enough fluids to keep it cool. And you feel extremely bothered. You're likely to be pale, dizzy, nauseated, and thirsty, with a headache the size of the sun.

If you're outside and start experiencing those symptoms, go inside, preferably where it's air-conditioned. And start drinking lots of fluids, either water or a sports beverage. If you don't feel any better in 30 minutes, see a doctor.

Preventing heat exhaustion is a matter of common sense— drinking plenty of fluids, exercising during the coolest parts of the day, and wearing loose-fitting clothes that help keep you cool, including a hat. Plus, alternative healers have a few extra tricks, for both prevention and treatment, up their loose-fitting sleeves.

**LIQUID MINERAL:** *For Prevention*
One reason for heat exhaustion is that the body runs out of electrolytes, the minerals that help prevent muscle cramps, says Beverly Yates, N.D., a naturopathic physician and director of the Natural Health Care Group in Seattle. To avoid the problem, especially if you're planning to be physically active in sunny,

---

# GUIDE TO
# PROFESSIONAL CARE

Heat exhaustion means that your vital organs aren't getting enough blood. With less blood available, you will feel light-headed and weak. Other symptoms include cool, pale, clammy skin; thirst; headache; nausea; a fast, weak pulse; fatigue; confusion; and anxiety. If you've taken steps to relieve heat exhaustion but your symptoms get worse or don't improve after 30 minutes, get medical help without delay.

Heat exhaustion may lead to heatstroke, a condition in which your body temperature rises to dangerous, potentially fatal levels. The signs of heatstroke are an altered mental state, which can range from confusion to unconsciousness; slurred speech; very hot, flushed skin; a rapid pulse; headache; dilated pupils; and muscle spasms. Heatstroke is a medical emergency.

---

hot weather, take liquid mineral supplements during the hotter times of the year.

Dr. Yates says to look for supplements that include magnesium, calcium, and manganese and recommends those that are water-based to help with rehydration. She favors the liquid variety because she says that they're better absorbed. The dosage is ½ teaspoon in 4 ounces of water three times a day.

### LEMON BALM: *Keep Your Internal Temperature Down*

Some people are more sensitive to hot weather than others, says Pamela Fischer, founder and director of the Ohlone Center for Herbal Studies in Concord, California. If summer weather makes you feel as gritty, sweaty, and crumpled as a used beach towel, try drinking a few glasses a day of herbal iced tea made from lemon balm (also known as melissa), which is cooling to the body.

To make the tea, add ¼ cup of the dried herb to 1 quart of boiled water. Steep for 30 minutes to an hour, strain, and refrigerate until chilled.

## FLOWER ESSENCES: *Be Sensitive to St. John's Wort*

Take four drops of St. John's wort flower essence a day for at least a month if you seem to be extra-sensitive to the sun or prone to symptoms of heat exhaustion. This flower essence, from the herb that is used to treat depression, can treat all maladies related to darkness and light, says Patricia Kaminski, director of the Flower Essence Society in Nevada City, California. You can take this for up to several months until your sensitivity improves.

## FOOD: *Eat As If You're on Vacation*

If you travel to tropical climes during the summer, heat exhaustion is more likely because your body will face a number of significant stressors besides a hotter climate, including changes in time zones, language, and foods. To minimize the stress, Dr. Yates suggests that you change your diet before your trip, emphasizing foods that are eaten in that climate.

"A lot of tropical fruits are very tasty and full of electrolytes and water," she says. They include mangoes, papayas, guavas, bananas, and pineapple.

## HOMEOPATHY: *Cool Your Symptoms with Glonoinum*

This cooling remedy is for people with heat exhaustion who have a "throbbing, bursting headache" and a "glowing red face," says Dr. Yates. She recommends dissolving two pellets of 12C potency Glonoinum under your tongue every 15 minutes. If you don't feel better after two doses, see a doctor. If you do improve, take two pellets every 3 to 4 hours for the rest of the day.

# *Relieve the Itch and Speed the Healing of* **Heat Rash**

Heat rash is a discomfort, not a disease. It occurs when sweat becomes stuck in the pores and spreads into surrounding tissue, irritating it.

As a result, you're not only overheated and sweaty, you also have tiny red or pink, blisterlike bumps that are extremely itchy on your chest, back, and even your armpits or the creases of your elbows or groin.

This "prickly heat" should go away in 3 to 4 days without you having to do anything at all, short of staying cool and dry, wearing light cotton clothing, and exposing the affected area to the air. If you want to speed its exit, however, or relieve the itching, alternative healers suggest these remedies.

## HYDROTHERAPY: *Minty Itch Relief*

Taking a cool bath with peppermint added to the water is great for relieving the itch of a heat rash, says Bradley Bongiovanni, N.D., a naturopathic physician in Cambridge, Massachusetts.

Wrap a cup or two of fresh peppermint leaves in cheesecloth, fill the tub with cool water, immerse the mint in the water for 3 to 5 minutes, then soak for 5 to 10 minutes. Do this as often as necessary to relieve the itching.

## CUMIN AND CORIANDER: *Ayurvedic Relief*

In Ayurveda, the ancient healing system from India, a heat rash is seen as an imbalance of the "pitta," or fire element, in the body.

You can help cool pitta with coriander and cumin seeds, says Pratima Raichur, an Ayurvedic practitioner in New York City. Soak 1 teaspoon of cumin seeds and 1 teaspoon of coriander seeds in 12 ounces of water overnight. "In the morning, strain and drink the liquid," Dr. Raichur says. Do this daily until the rash goes away.

### CALENDULA: *Soothing and Healing*

Using a water-based gel of the herb calendula on the rash can speed healing, Dr. Bongiovanni says. But avoid calendula ointment or cream; it cuts off the flow of air to the rash, which could make it worse. Use this remedy as needed.

### LAVENDER ESSENTIAL OIL: *Alone or with Calendula*

Essential oil of lavender helps normalize and regenerate skin cells and is very healing for any kind of skin problem, says Therese Francis, Ph.D., an herbalist in Santa Fe, New Mexico. You can use a drop or two of lavender oil directly on the rash three or four times a day.

You can also add a drop or two of lavender oil to calendula gel to give it even more healing power, Dr. Francis says.

# *Natural Relief for*
# **Heel Pain**

A heel, as you probably know all too well, is someone who has betrayed you—in dictionary terms, an "untrustworthy person."

When it comes to feet, a lot of heels *are* heels: You depend on them for constant support, and suddenly, they cause you pain.

How can you make a treacherous heel behave in a more trustworthy manner? In most cases, you'll need to seek medical help, but alternative foot specialists suggest a few home remedies to lessen the pain while your heel is healing or while you're waiting for your custom-made orthotic.

### TURMERIC: *For Herbal Relief*

Turmeric can help relieve the stiffness and aching of heel pain, says Steven Subotnick, D.P.M., N.D., a podiatrist in

Berkeley and San Leandro, California. Take the capsules according to the dosage recommendations on the label, he says.

## BOSWELLIA: *An Ayurvedic Cure*

This herb from Ayurveda, the ancient system of natural healing from India, can help relieve inflammation and pain, Dr. Subotnick says.

He recommends a product called Inflavonoid Intensive Care, manufactured by Metagenics, that contains boswellia, turmeric, and other anti-inflammatory nutrients and herbs. Or look for any other product that contains turmeric and boswellia and is meant to lessen pain in the joints, he says. Follow the directions on the label for the correct dosage.

## HOMEOPATHY: *Putting Your Best Foot Forward*

Homeopathic remedies can provide pain relief and speed healing of plantar fasciitis, the most common cause of heel pain, says Dr. Subotnick. Here are his recommendations for choosing the best remedy for you.

• If the bottom of your foot is very stiff after rest in the morning, if it's better with continued movement and worse when you're sitting, and if you feel restless, try Rhus toxicodendron or Valerian.
• If movement makes you tired and cranky, if you're depressed, and if the pain is worse when you take a step, try Ruta graveolens.
• If you feel better sitting with your foot up and worse when your foot is hanging down, if the pain feels like an electric shock, and if it feels better when you're warm and resting and when you move, try Phytolacca decandra.
• If it's hard to tell whether your pain is better or worse when you move, if the pain is shooting and darting, and if your foot feels better when it's warm and worse when it's cold, try Stellaria media.
• If an approaching storm makes the pain worse, try Rhododendron chrysanthum.
• If the pain is worse during a storm, try Phosphorus.
• If the pain on the bottoms of your feet is pulsating, try Natrum carbonicum.
• If the pain is better on a rainy day, and you're "a rebellious type of person," try Causticum.

# GUIDE TO
# PROFESSIONAL CARE

If your heel pain was caused by an injury or doesn't clear up within a few days, see a podiatrist. Orthopedic surgeons treat bones and joints, so they can also diagnose the cause of heel pain.

Using self-care to resolve heel pain completely may not work for two reasons. First, the problem can be complex. There are many types of heel pain, and it takes a professional to figure out the cause. Second, the best treatment is usually a custom-made shoe insert (an orthotic) tailored by a podiatrist to your foot shape, gait, and the exact cause and site of your pain.

Among the many types of heel pain that a podiatrist may diagnose, the most common are caused by athletic overuse or exercising or by standing or walking on hard surfaces. Here are some of them, as explained by Steven Subotnick, D.P.M., a podiatrist in Berkeley and San Leandro, California.

• The most common type of heel pain is plantar fasciitis, an inflammation of the band of tissue (fascia) that runs from the heel bone to the metatarsal bones at the base of the toes. It causes pain on the bottom of the foot near the heel that's worse when you wake up and lessens during the day.

• Heel spurs, which are bony and sometimes painful growths on the heel, occur when the plantar fascia is pulled slightly off the heel bone.

• Painful bumps on the back of the heel, called pump bumps, are caused by irritation from the back of a shoe.

• Stress fractures, or microscopic cracks in the bone, hurt in the morning and worsen during the day.

• If your heel hurts only when you push down on it or press it with your fingers, it may be bruised.

• Arthritis, gout, an infection, or, rarely, a benign tumor, can also cause heel pain.

For each of the remedies, take two tablets a day of the 6X or 12X potency, Dr. Subotnick suggests. Take only one homeopathic remedy at a time unless directed otherwise by your homeopath, and take it only for as long as you have the pain.

## STRETCHING: *To Prevent Pain*

Tight calf muscles can be a hidden cause of heel pain. If the muscles can't absorb the constant pounding of running or other types of impact exercises, the shock goes to the heels.

Here's an easy exercise that can keep your calf muscles stretched and help prevent—even cure—heel pain, says Stephanie L. Tourles, a licensed esthetician, reflexologist, and herbalist in West Hyannisport, Massachusetts. It's best to do this exercise after taking a short walk or a warm bath or after doing a bit of gardening. The calf muscles need to be warmed up before stretching to prevent injury.

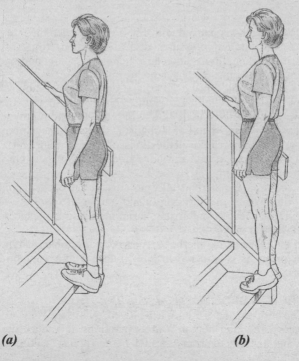

*(a)*                                                    *(b)*

Stand on a bottom stair step or an exercise bench step and hold on to the railing or another stationary object for support. Step back and lower your heels over the edge of the step as far as you comfortably can to give your calves (and heels) a good stretch (*a*). Next, rise up onto your toes (*b*), then lower your heels again; repeat 20 or 30 times.

Do this exercise once a day. If you have weak calf muscles, start with 5 repetitions and gradually build up to 10, 20, and 30.

# *All-Natural Relief from Painful* **Hemorrhoids**

The anal canal is packed with small veins. When these veins, because of internal pressures or just irritation from sitting, swell like little balloons and cause itching, burning, and sometimes even bleeding, you have hemorrhoids.

If you want relief, just use Preparation H—Preparation *Herb*, that is. "You will get quicker results with over-the-counter hemorrhoid preparations than you will with herbal ointments," admits Rita Elkins, a master herbalist in Orem, Utah. "But over-the-counter hemorrhoid medications offer only temporary relief from symptoms and can have side effects such as chronic irritation of surrounding tissue."

In addition, the hemorrhoids usually come back, meaning that you have to use the drug again and again. Worse, some hemorrhoid medications irritate surrounding tissue, especially vaginal tissue in women.

On the other hand, "herbal preparations don't have anything in them that is considered unsafe to absorb into your body," Elkins says.

## BUTCHER'S BROOM: *Shrinks Swollen Tissues*

"The herb butcher's broom is believed to have the same effect as over-the-counter hemorrhoid preparations. It's an astringent herb, and it works to shrink swollen hemorrhoids," Elkins says.

She recommends using butcher's broom tincture or powder to make an ointment. Using a spoon, mix 10 to 15 drops of tincture or the powder from five capsules (which usually contain 100 to 200 milligrams of butcher's broom) into a small container of beeswax (about ¼ cup). You can apply the ointment generously directly to the area of discomfort. You can also add a few drops each of vitamin E and aloe gel to the ointment to help reduce inflammation and speed healing, Elkins says. You can use the ointment as often as necessary.

At the same time you're using butcher's broom ointment, Elkins recommends drinking butcher's broom tea or taking capsules. Make the tea by pouring 1 cup of boiling water over 1 to 2 grams, or about ½ teaspoon, of the herb and steeping for 10 minutes. She advises straining the tea and drinking up to four cups a day. For capsules, the dosage is two 200-milligram capsules three times a day. When using capsules, look for a product that's standardized for 9 to 11 percent ruscogenin, the herb's active ingredient.

## FLAVONOIDS: *Strengthen the Veins*

Alternative practitioners believe that supplements that contain flavonoids—natural healing compounds that are also found in fresh fruits and vegetables—can help strengthen the anal veins so that hemorrhoids are less likely to occur.

They can also reduce inflammation and help hemorrhoids heal, says Teresa Rispoli, Ph.D., a licensed nutritionist and acupuncturist in Agoura Hills, California. Supplements that contain hydroxyethylrutosides, rutin, and citrus bioflavonoids are most effective for treating hemorrhoids, she says. Just follow the directions on the label.

## GLYCOSAMINOGLYCANS: *Repair Damaged Cells*

For hemorrhoids that are extruded, or prolapsed, Dr. Rispoli recommends taking supplements that contain glycosaminoglycans. These are the purified structural components of blood vessels, and they can help repair damaged cells, she says. Follow the directions on the label, she advises.

## HYDROTHERAPY: *Sitz Baths for Instant Relief*

Sitting in a tub of warm water, or sitz bath, for 10 minutes several times a day is one of the fastest ways to help relieve the

# GUIDE TO
# PROFESSIONAL CARE

Hemorrhoids, commonly located inside the anal canal, around the anus and lower rectum, are usually little more than an annoyance. (If you notice blood covering the stool, in the toilet bowl, or on the toilet paper, which can be common with internal hemorrhoids, be sure to call a doctor, since it could indicate something more serious.)

Sometimes, hemorrhoids protrude outside the anal canal and may involve painful swelling or a hard lump around the anus that occurs when a blood clot forms. If irritated, they can itch and bleed. This type of hemorrhoid can be intensely painful and needs to be surgically removed, says Steve L. Gardner, N.D., a naturopathic doctor in Milwaukie, Oregon.

Conventional doctors usually remove hemorrhoids with ligation (wrapping a rubber band around the hemorrhoid and depriving it of circulation until it falls off), with a laser (destroying the hemorrhoid), or with surgery (cutting it off). All of these methods can cause a great deal of pain and may require days and even weeks of recovery.

Another method, invented in the 1950s by a medical doctor but little used today, involves applying negative galvanic electricity directly to the hemorrhoid. This method causes the tissues to shrink instantly, nearly without pain.

"This method has been adopted by alternative care practitioners as a more patient-friendly way to remove hemorrhoids," Dr. Gardner says. "A patient can be treated and go right back to work. I've had long-haul truckers, who are prone to hemorrhoids, come to see me, be treated, and get right back in their trucks. That would be impossible with any of the conventional treatments."

discomfort of hemorrhoids, says Mark Stengler, N.D., a naturopathic physician in San Diego.

## PSYLLIUM: *Soften the Stools*

One of the most common causes of hemorrhoids is a low-fiber diet, which produces small, hard stools that are difficult to pass. The resulting straining damages the anal veins, says Elizabeth Lipski, a certified clinical nutritionist in Kauai, Hawaii.

Psyllium seeds, either in bulk form or as an ingredient in fiber supplements such as Metamucil, help make stools softer and easier to pass. This not only helps prevent hemorrhoids, it also makes bowel movements less painful, Lipski says.

She recommends making psyllium seeds part of your regular diet. For one week, take a teaspoon of seeds at breakfast by adding them to an 8-ounce glass of water. Starting the second week, take the seeds at breakfast and lunch. During the third week, take them at breakfast, lunch, and dinner, then stay at that level. Once you reach this point, you can stop taking any other fiber supplements if you no longer have discomfort. Adding psyllium to your diet gradually will help control the gas that sometimes accompanies a sudden increase in fiber, she says.

Fiber creates large, soft stools by absorbing water, Lipski adds, so when you're taking psyllium or any other form of fiber, you need to drink up. She recommends drinking ½ ounce of water for each pound you weigh. Thus, if you weigh 130 pounds, you should drink 65 ounces of water; if you weigh 160, you need 80 ounces.

## HIGH-FIBER FOODS: *Natural Healers*

There's nothing wrong with using psyllium seeds or other fiber supplements, but you can get the same effect by eating lots of high-fiber foods, says Lipski. "Increase your intake of fruits, whole grains, and vegetables, especially those containing good amounts of fiber, such as asparagus, brussels sprouts, cabbage, carrots, cauliflower, corn, peas, kale, and parsnips," she says.

Eating a high-fiber breakfast cereal (one that supplies 5 grams or more per serving) will also significantly increase your fiber intake, she adds.

# Avoid Standard Treatments That May Worsen
# Hepatitis C

Some 4 million Americans have an extremely serious liver disorder called hepatitis C. Caused by a viral infection, it damages the liver and greatly increases the risk of liver failure as well as cancer.

The standard treatment for hepatitis C is a powerful antiviral drug called interferon, along with other medications. The treatment lasts a year, and it causes fever, muscle aches, and other flulike symptoms in about 60 percent of people who take it.

What's worse, the treatment doesn't always work. Even when it banishes the virus for a while, there's no scientific evidence that it prevents liver failure.

Alternative practitioners believe that, in many cases, there is a better way to treat this disease. "Interferon and other pharmaceuticals can actually delay the healing process by toxifying the body," says Christopher Hobbs, an herbalist and expert in Traditional Chinese Medicine in Santa Cruz, California.

Probably the best way to strengthen the body against hepatitis C is with liver-protecting herbs, says Hobbs. Along with nutritional therapies, herbal treatments can help your body recover from this dangerous viral assault. If you think you have hepatitis C or have been diagnosed as having it, seek medical care. Talk to your doctor or your alternative practitioner before trying these or other alternative remedies.

**MILK THISTLE:** *Rebuilds Damaged Cells*
The herb milk thistle contains a group of chemicals called silymarin, which stimulate the synthesis of protein in liver cells and actually help the liver regenerate itself. Hobbs recommends taking two 150-milligram tablets or capsules of milk thistle extract, standardized to contain 70 to 80 percent silymarin, three or four times a day.

## GUIDE TO PROFESSIONAL CARE

*Caution: You should use the alternative remedies discussed in this chapter only as part of a treatment program that is guided and monitored by a qualified medical doctor in partnership with a qualified alternative practitioner, both of whom are experienced in caring for your condition. Check with your conventional doctor before changing or stopping any conventional medical treatments or medications, and keep all of your doctors and/or alternative practitioners informed of all treatments that you are receiving.*

Since hepatitis C is a potentially life-threatening condition, it's essential to see a medical doctor at the first sign of symptoms. These include jaundice (yellowing of the skin or the whites of the eyes), pain in the lower right abdomen, loss of appetite, dark urine, nausea, chills, or fever, says Elizabeth Sander, M.D., an internist in Los Angeles.

Since people with hepatitis C also have an increased risk for hepatitis A and hepatitis B infections, it's a good idea to talk to your doctor about being vaccinated. Vaccines that protect against these illnesses are readily available and are very effective.

Another option is to take a multiherb supplement. Look for one with a standardized silymarin extract of 10 to 50 percent that's blended with other liver-protecting herbs such as turmeric, artichoke leaf, gentian, and ginger. Follow the dosage recommendations on the label.

**HERBS:** *Kill the Virus and Build Immunity*
There are many herbs that help protect the liver from hepatitis C, says Hobbs, including lemon balm, St. John's wort, shitake mushrooms, schisandra, and garlic. Each of these herbs is taken in a different way, according to Hobbs.

• Lemon balm: Make a tea by adding 1 teaspoon of dried or fresh herb to 1 cup of boiling water. Steep for 15 minutes, strain, and drink two to three cups a day.

• St. John's wort: Take one 300-milligram capsule twice a day. Look for an extract standardized for 0.3 percent hypericin, Hobbs advises.
• Shiitake: Take 1,500 to 2,000 milligrams in capsule or tablet form twice a day with meals.
• Schisandra: Take a 100-milligram capsule standardized to contain 9 percent schisandris twice a day.
• Garlic: All forms are effective. You may want to eat a few cloves a day of fresh or cooked garlic or take a daily dose of two or three capsules containing 3,000 to 4,000 micrograms of allicin each.

## The Anti-Hepatitis C Diet

Ramona Jones is a certified nutritional consultant in Shawnee, Oklahoma. She also has hepatitis C.

By using natural methods—herbal remedies and nutritional supplements along with a body-strengthening diet—she has managed to remain symptom-free and healthy.

Jones has found that a healthful diet is essential for people with hepatitis C because it's the liver's job to filter and detoxify all of the potentially harmful substances in your body. Your goal should be to avoid taxing your liver with foods such as the following, which are hard for the body to detoxify.

• Animal products, especially red meats, which are loaded with antibiotics, growth hormones, and steroids. Meat complicates the digestive process, stressing the liver, gallbladder, and pancreas, Jones explains. It is one of the hardest foods to digest, she adds.
• Dairy foods, which put added strain on the liver.
• Alcohol, which is notorious for its liver-harming effects.
• Caffeine, which stimulates and stresses the liver. Look for it not only in coffee, tea, and colas but also in many over-the-counter medications.
• Tap water, which often contains much more than you bargained for, including chlorine, fluoride, inorganic chemicals, and compounds that the liver is unable to process. Drink distilled water only, Jones suggests.
• Junk food, which is not only a poor source of nutrition but is also chock-full of the things we should avoid to minimize

stress to the liver—sugars, fats, hydrogenated oils, chemical additives, and preservatives.
• Fruit juices, which are high in concentrated sugar. Sugar is a shock to the liver, it stresses the digestive process and the pancreas, and it may "feed" the hepatitis C virus, Jones says.
• Artificial sweeteners, which are extremely hard for the liver to process. Your poor liver doesn't even recognize what these substances are, Jones says. Use liquid stevia, derived from an herb, instead.

## Acupressure for Acute Attacks

Hepatitis C is a chronic, or long-term, illness. As with other long-term conditions, it may cause acute episodes—in this case, periods when the liver is particularly inflamed. During these episodes, you're likely to experience symptoms such as fatigue, nausea, and diarrhea.

You can relieve many of the acute symptoms of hepatitis C with acupressure, says Misha Cohen, O.M.D., a doctor of Oriental medicine and an acupuncturist in San Francisco.

Here's what she recommends. (For the precise locations of the points, see An Illustrated Guide to Acupressure Points on page 700.)

• For nausea, press the PE6 point, located on the inside of the wrist three finger-widths above the wrist crease, between the two bones.
• For fatigue, massage ST36, located four finger-widths from the hollow of the knee on the outside of the leg and one finger-width from the crest of the shinbone. You may also want to massage SP4, on the inside of the foot in the hollow behind the bone of the big toe.
• For diarrhea and abdominal cramps, massage ST37, which you'll find six finger-widths below the kneecap, on the outside of the leg next to the shinbone. Or try the ST25 points, located on the abdomen three finger-widths to the right and left of the navel.

As for foods that you *should* eat, Hobbs recommends easy-to-process sources of protein such as fish, organic chicken and turkey, and soy products. And don't forget beans, he says.

Lentils, chickpeas, and adzuki, navy, pinto, and mung beans are all great choices.

In addition, he recommends eating lightly steamed green vegetables, along with squash. Summer squash and zucchini are especially good. "They're the easiest on digestion," he says.

Fresh fruit is always good, although Jones advises not having more than three servings a day. "Too much sugar in any form stresses the liver," she says.

Finally, be sure to eat plenty of whole grains, which are loaded with liver-strengthening B vitamins.

## *Nutrition Is Better Than Drugs for* **High Blood Pressure**

There are literally dozens of powerful medications for lowering high blood pressure. According to the nation's top alternative physicians and other experts, however, most people can lower their blood pressures into the safety zone without resorting to drugs.

"Volumes of scientific research show that dietary changes can eliminate high blood pressure—or hypertension—in most patients," says Julian Whitaker, M.D., founder and director of the Whitaker Wellness Institute in Newport Beach, California. "In spite of that, the routine approach of most doctors is to immediately start a patient on drugs—and usually without any recommendation for dietary change. The dangerous side effects of high blood pressure drugs often make this approach, in my opinion, more harmful to the patient than beneficial."

Eric Braverman, M.D., director of the Place for Achieving Total Health in New York City, agrees that medications can cause problems without getting to the root of the condition.

"Drugs treat the symptoms of high blood pressure, which can be necessary in some cases, but curing the problem requires nutritional supplements and dietary and lifestyle changes," he says.

So, if you have been diagnosed with high blood pressure (this usually means that your reading is higher than 140/90), here are the remedies that alternative healers say can bring your pressure down to a healthier level. It's worth doing, because high blood pressure can lead to a host of other problems, including heart disease, he says.

## WATER: *The Remedy That's Too Good to Be True*

Dr. Whitaker's number one recommendation for lowering high blood pressure is to drink 15 glasses of water a day. "Almost all of the blood pressure medications mimic the effects of increased water intake," he says.

Water, he explains, relaxes your entire system, including your arteries—and tight, constricted arteries are the main cause of high blood pressure. "This remedy is so easy and simple, it seems too good to be true," he says. Yes, 15 glasses is a lot of water. He recommends drinking one 8-ounce glass every hour that you're awake.

## POTASSIUM-RICH FOODS: *Bounce Salt from the Body*

Lowering sodium is important because this mineral can raise blood pressure in those who are sensitive to it. Unlike many physicians, though, Dr. Whitaker doesn't tell patients to go on low-sodium diets.

"I tell them to increase their intake of the mineral potassium," he says. Potassium and sodium act like a seesaw in your body. The higher your intake of potassium, the lower your level of sodium.

Dr. Whitaker cites scientific studies in which people who were taking blood pressure medications were able to get off the drugs just by eating a lot more fruits and vegetables, which are excellent sources of potassium.

He recommends eating at least two bananas a day (they're loaded with potassium) along with at least five servings of other high-potassium fruits and vegetables. (Fruits and vegetables also supply plenty of fiber, which is another food factor that can help lower blood pressure.)

"A high potassium intake can prevent high blood pressure and lower existing high blood pressure," agrees Kitty Gurkin Rosati, R.D., a registered dietitian and nutrition director of the Rice Diet Program at Duke University in Durham, North Carolina.

# GUIDE TO
# PROFESSIONAL CARE

*Caution: You should use the alternative remedies discussed in this chapter only as part of a treatment program that is guided and monitored by a qualified medical doctor in partnership with a qualified alternative practitioner, both of whom are experienced in caring for your condition. Check with your conventional doctor before changing or stopping any conventional medical treatments or medications, and keep all of your doctors and/or alternative practitioners informed of all treatments that you are receiving.*

Since dietary changes, nutritional supplements, exercise, and stress control can be so helpful for controlling high blood pressure, the best professional to treat your blood pressure problem may be a naturally oriented physician, says Julian Whitaker, M.D., founder and director of the Whitaker Wellness Institute in Newport Beach, California.

If your blood pressure is 160/100 or higher, however, you may need pressure-lowering drugs as well as natural remedies, he cautions. Have your blood pressure checked annually, especially if you have a family history of hypertension. Because there are often no physical symptoms to alert you, regular checks are the only way to tell if you have the condition.

---

Besides bananas, some of the fruits highest in potassium include apricots, cantaloupe, dates, honeydew melons, kiwifruit, mangoes, nectarines, watermelon, avocados, grapefruit juice, oranges, papayas, pomegranates, prune juice, and raisins.

Some of the richest vegetable sources of potassium are Swiss chard, celery, spinach, parsley, watercress, endive, kohlrabi, broccoli, tomato juice, cucumbers, cauliflower, asparagus, artichokes, potatoes, sweet potatoes, and winter squash.

If you have kidney disease, high levels of potassium can be harmful. You should talk to your doctor before increasing your intake of potassium-rich foods.

### FISH: *For Oils Your Arteries Need*
Lowering your intake of artery-hurting saturated fat—the kind found in red meats and dairy foods—should be part of any

plan to lower high blood pressure. But omega-3 fatty acids, a type of fat found in cold-water fish, can actually help lower blood pressure, Dr. Braverman says.

"Eat fish daily, or even twice daily, if you can," he says. Some of the fish highest in omega-3's include mackerel, sardines, bluefish, salmon, mullet, herring, and lake trout.

If fish isn't your favorite food, you can still get your daily omega-3's by taking a fish-oil supplement, Dr. Braverman says. He recommends taking seven capsules daily of a high-potency fish oil, with a minimum of 1,000 milligrams per capsule. Or you can take 3 tablespoons daily of EPA-emulsified fish oil.

## MAGNESIUM GLUCONATE: *Less Arterial Tension*

Magnesium relaxes arteries, thus helping to lower blood pressure, Dr. Whitaker says. He recommends taking 500 to 1,000 milligrams of magnesium gluconate a day, divided into three doses. Since amounts this high may pose problems for people with existing heart conditions, check with your doctor before supplementing.

## COENZYME $Q_{10}$: *Like Exercise for the Arteries*

"The use of coenzyme $Q_{10}$ is a pivotal component of my core protocol to lower blood pressure," says Stephen Sinatra, M.D., a cardiologist and director of the New England Heart Center in Manchester, Connecticut.

Research indicates that many people with high blood pressure are deficient in this important nutrient. Coenzyme $Q_{10}$ helps generate energy in every cell in your body, and it may help improve the "tone" of the arteries, reducing blood pressure, says Dr. Sinatra. He recommends taking 60 to 90 milligrams of coenzyme $Q_{10}$ three times a day after a meal, for a daily total of 180 to 270 milligrams.

### Hidden Emotions: A Common Cause of High Blood Pressure

Did you develop high blood pressure suddenly—almost overnight?

Do you have high blood pressure but no obvious risk factors, such as being overweight or having a family history of hypertension?

Did your high blood pressure begin at a very early age?

Do you have uncontrollably high blood pressure?

Do you have recurrent episodes of high blood pressure, even though, outwardly, there have been no great or stressful changes in your life?

If you answered yes to any of these questions, the cause of your high blood pressure may be hidden emotions. These are not the emotions that you feel but the ones that you *don't* feel, the ones that you may be subconsciously hiding from yourself.

Hidden emotions may cause as many as half of all cases of high blood pressure, says Samuel J. Mann, M.D., associate professor of clinical medicine at the hypertension center of New York Presbyterian Hospital–Cornell Medical Center in New York City. After treating thousands of people with high blood pressure, Dr. Mann has discovered that unwanted, unacknowledged, repressed feelings (such as from a childhood trauma, for example) may "eat away" at the body, causing many cases of hypertension. When the emotions are acknowledged and experienced, the hypertension may be cured.

People who aren't aware of their negative feelings are often described by others as Mr. Nice Guys, Dr. Mann says. They may be even-tempered, emotionally self-reliant, emotionally unavailable, model citizens, inflexible know-it-alls, or workaholics—in short, supermen or superwomen. Or they may be people who insist that they aren't as tense or angry as they look.

If you're having trouble controlling hypertension, and one of the previous descriptions seems to fit you, consider taking the following actions, which will help you begin to feel your emotions.

• Listen to music regularly to help bring up emotions.
• When you're feeling upset or under stress, talk about it with a friend. You don't have to solve the problem; just acknowledge your feelings.
• Keep a journal and write down your thoughts and feelings.
• Put time aside for introspection and reflect on your past. Embrace the emotions that come up. Allow yourself to just sit quietly for 15 to 30 minutes a day.
• Look for a psychotherapist or spiritual resource that can help you heal.

If you try this strategy, however, and your blood pressure remains high, you may need medication to lower it.

**EXERCISE:** *Walk to Better Health*

Eating the right foods is crucial for lowering and preventing high blood pressure. But so is regular exercise.

"I recommend 30 minutes of aerobic exercise four times a week for my patients with high blood pressure," says Mark Stengler, N.D., a naturopathic physician in San Diego. "Regular exercise relaxes artery walls and decreases stress. It can also help a person lose weight, and being overweight is a major risk factor for high blood pressure."

"Walking is the best exercise for people with high blood pressure," adds Donald Carrow, M.D., founder and director of the Florida Institute of Health in Tampa. "It's the easiest exercise. People can slowly build up the time they exercise, starting with as little as 5 minutes and increasing as they get stronger. And for someone with high blood pressure, it's the least traumatic exercise. High-intensity exercise like running or racquetball can be too stressful for those with hypertension."

**HAWTHORN:** *Good for the Heart and Arteries*

Plan on taking 250 milligrams of a standardized extract of the herb hawthorn daily until your blood pressure reaches normal levels, at which point, you can reduce or eliminate it. This herb can help lower blood pressure by relaxing arteries and strengthening the heart, says Michael Janson, M.D., consultant physician at Path to Health in Burlington, Massachusetts.

**GARLIC:** *Lowers Blood Pressure Naturally*

Scientific studies have shown that garlic, either fresh or in supplement form, can help lower blood pressure, Dr. Braverman says.

"Eat as much garlic as possible—two or three cloves a day, minimum," adds Dr. Sinatra. (You can counteract garlic breath by chewing on fresh parsley.)

Even people who like garlic may have trouble eating this much, however. That's why doctors often recommend using garlic supplements, following the directions on the label, Dr. Stengler says.

# *Antioxidants Can Win the War Against* **High Cholesterol**

Maybe you think of cholesterol as a kind of evil plug. The usual story goes like this: You eat too much cholesterol or animal fat, which is converted to cholesterol in your body, the cholesterol clogs your coronary arteries, and blood and oxygen can't get through to your heart, causing a heart attack. The idea is that if you lower your cholesterol, all will be well.

But, if cholesterol is so bad, why does your body synthesize up to 1,500 milligrams (almost the amount in 10 eggs) a day, using it for all kinds of crucial functions, such as the manufacture of hormones?

Why do Eskimos, who typically eat a diet loaded with animal fat, have very low rates of heart disease?

The answer is that high cholesterol isn't the cause of heart disease; *oxidized* cholesterol is.

That's the opinion of many alternative physicians, including Philip Lee Miller, M.D., founder and director of the Los Gatos Longevity Institute in California. "I'm one of those people who have been saying for 30 years that cholesterol does not cause heart disease," he says. "It's a recruit in the process, like a soldier is a recruit in a war, but it doesn't cause the war."

Dr. Miller believes that lowering LDL (low-density lipoprotein) cholesterol plays a critical role in preventing hardening of the arteries. LDL cholesterol is manufactured and secreted by the liver and is carried to the arteries in the heart in the same way furniture is carried in a moving van. Once there, the cholesterol may be oxidized by the same oxygen-sparked, cell-destroying process that rusts iron or turns an apple brown after it's been cut.

The destructive process of oxidation is literally inflammatory—it's like a fire in the body. The immune system, your body's fire department, rushes "foam cells" to the area to

### GUIDE TO
### PROFESSIONAL CARE

Since uncontrolled high cholesterol can be a serious health threat, it's important to have your level tested every 6 months. If your total cholesterol reading is 200 or higher, your doctor will likely want to test you every 3 months and work aggressively to get it under control. In most cases, you'll have success with a combination of diet, nutritional supplements, and lifestyle changes. Your doctor will decide the best treatment for you, based primarily on your LDL levels, and may recommend using cholesterol-lowering drugs to bring the numbers into a healthier range.

You'll also certainly want to talk to an alternative physician about various factors that may be contributing to the problem, such as dietary and mineral deficiencies, hormone imbalances, or even heavy metal poisoning with mercury, adds Sandra Denton, M.D., a naturally oriented physician in Anchorage.

douse the blaze. But just as firemen sometimes have to ax down a door to get into a burning building, the anti-inflammatory process can damage the lining of the artery. This roughened, injured area is a perfect foundation for the buildup of plaque, the truly evil plug that clogs arteries and triggers heart attacks.

"Oxidized LDL starts an inflammatory reaction that the body tries to heal, but the healing causes more problems than it resolves," says Dr. Miller. The best way to prevent this heart-hurting process, he says, is to prevent the oxidation of LDL cholesterol. And the best way to do that, says Dr. Miller, is to make sure you get enough of the antioxidants vitamin E, vitamin C, and glutathione.

Antioxidants work by calming unstable oxygen molecules called free radicals, which are responsible for oxidizing cells. When antioxidants neutralize free radicals, they're on a type of suicide mission. The antioxidants themselves are oxidized, or, in chemical terms, reduced.

Fortunately, the body has a system to help ensure that there are always plenty of antioxidants available, Dr. Miller says. When vitamin C is oxidized, vitamin E comes to the rescue, donating some of its molecules to restore the vitamin C to its full antioxidant status. In the process, the vitamin E is reduced, but the glutathione replenishes it. That's why you need all three nutrients, says Dr. Miller.

## VITAMIN C: *The First Line of Defense Against Heart Disease*

Vitamin C is a very powerful antioxidant. Dr. Miller recommends taking anywhere from 1,000 to 4,000 milligrams a day to reduce the oxidation of LDL and prevent heart disease. Any type of vitamin C is effective, but his favorite is a form called ester-C, which is nonacidic and perhaps a little less irritating to the digestive tract than other forms.

## VITAMIN E: *A Mixed Bag of Protection*

Like vitamin C, vitamin E is a powerful antioxidant. Dr. Miller says that 800 international units daily is the ideal dose to prevent cholesterol from oxidizing. He recommends using vitamin E supplements that are natural, not synthetic. For maximum potency, they should also contain mixed tocopherols; the label will specify the ingredients alpha-, beta-, and gamma-tocopherol.

"A mix of tocopherols, not just one, is the way vitamin E is found in nature," he explains.

## NAC: *To Create Glutathione*

Vitamins C and E are most effective when your body has high levels of glutathione, says Dr. Miller. A doctor can measure your glutathione levels, and if they are low, Dr. Miller recommends taking a supplement called n-acetylcysteine (NAC), which helps build and conserve your body's store of glutathione.

The body doesn't do a good job of absorbing most glutathione supplements, Dr. Miller says. But NAC, a form of the amino acid cysteine, he says, provides the right chemical precursors for your body to create glutathione. He recommends taking 3,000 milligrams a day.

## Improving Your Cholesterol Balance

Stopping the oxidation of LDL cholesterol is crucial to preventing heart disease, says Dr. Miller. But if there's less LDL cholesterol in your body, there's less to oxidize, so reducing LDL is important.

It's also important to increase HDL (high-density lipoprotein) cholesterol, which hauls the LDL away from your arteries and back to your liver. There are a variety of supplements and herbs that help lower LDL, raise HDL, or do both at the same time.

### NIACIN: *Strong Natural Medicine*

Niacin is a B vitamin that works powerfully to lower LDL cholesterol, says Mark Stengler, N.D., a naturopathic physician in San Diego.

He recommends taking 1,500 milligrams of niacin a day in the form of inositol hexanicotinate. This form doesn't cause the tingling, itchy, hot rush of blood into the face and upper body, called flushing, that may occur with other forms.

"In my experience, this vitamin is as effective as any cholesterol-lowering drug on the market," says Dr. Stengler. He recommends starting with 500 milligrams and increasing the dose by 500 milligrams a week until you reach the full amount. Since high levels of niacin may cause liver problems, you should take inositol hexanicotinate, or any other form, only with the approval and supervision of your doctor.

### SELENIUM: *Helps in Three Ways*

The trace mineral selenium is very helpful for controlling cholesterol. First, it boosts levels of glutathione. Second, it works on its own to lower LDL. Third, it increases healthful HDL, says Dr. Miller. "Selenium is absolutely critical to any cholesterol-lowering program," he says. He recommends long-term use of a daily multivitamin that contains at least 200 micrograms of selenium.

### ZINC AND COPPER: *More Minerals to the Rescue*

Zinc and copper increase HDL and reduce LDL, says Amy Rothenberg, N.D., a naturopathic physician in Enfield, Connecticut. She recommends taking 30 milligrams of zinc and 1 to

2 milligrams of copper daily, preferably as part of a multivitamin/mineral supplement.

## GUGGUL: *A Cholesterol-Lowering Herb*

"I have dramatically reduced LDL cholesterol and increased HDL cholesterol with just this one herb," says Virender Sodhi, M.D. (Ayurved), N.D., an Ayurvedic and naturopathic physician and director of the American School of Ayurvedic Sciences in Bellevue, Washington.

Dr. Sodhi recommends using a product standardized for 10 percent guggulsterones, the active ingredients in the herb. Take three doses totaling 900 milligrams a day, he advises, but only under the supervision of an Ayurvedic physician. Once your cholesterol levels are back to normal, Dr. Sodhi recommends reducing the dosage to 300 milligrams a day.

### Foods for Cholesterol Control

Many different types of foods, and components of foods, can help lower LDL and boost HDL. Here are the ones that alternative practitioners recommend most.

## OAT BRAN: *Locks Up Cholesterol*

Oat bran is rich in soluble fiber, a substance that binds with cholesterol in the intestine and ushers it out of the body. "Eating ¾ cup of cooked oat bran cereal a day can lower cholesterol by 10 percent," says Dr. Rothenberg. "However, if you're more likely to eat an oat bran muffin, that works, too."

## ONIONS AND GARLIC: *Pungent Protection*

"Cook with garlic and onions whenever possible," says Dr. Stengler. Both have been shown to cut cholesterol. Or, he says, you can take garlic supplements, following the dosage recommendations on the label.

## WALNUTS: *The Healthiest Nuts Around*

Walnuts contain alpha-linolenic acid, which can help lower cholesterol, says Kitty Gurkin Rosati, R.D., a registered dietitian and nutrition director of the Rice Diet Program at Duke University in Durham, North Carolina. Other good sources of this good-for-you fat include olive oil, flaxseed oil, linseed oil, canola oil, soybean oil, and purslane, a salad green. To get a double dose, sauté purslane in a teaspoon of olive oil, says Rosati.

### LECITHIN: *Dissolves Cholesterol*

Lecithin granules contain phosphatidylcholine, which helps liquefy cholesterol in your body so it doesn't end up frozen in arterial plaques, says Dr. Rothenberg. She recommends sprinkling 1 tablespoon of granules on your cereal each day. Or toss some in a blender with fruit and nonfat yogurt.

### SOY: *Any Form Will Do*

Tofu, tempeh, and other soy foods contain compounds called isoflavones, which can help lower cholesterol, says Dr. Stengler. An easy way to incorporate isoflavones into your diet is to add soy protein powder to a shake. Or eat more tofu and miso, two popular soy foods that are versatile and easy to cook with.

## *Boost Your Defenses Against* HIV and AIDS

HIV is the virus that causes AIDS, a disease that destroys the immune system and ravages the body. There is no cure for AIDS, no way to eradicate HIV (the human immunodeficiency virus) from the body.

Yet, according to Jon Kaiser, M.D., director of the Jon Kaiser Wellness Center in San Francisco, "the progression of HIV disease in my practice is an extremely rare event."

So far, conventional doctors have been unable to find long-term solutions to control this dreadful virus. Yet, Dr. Kaiser has devised an immune-strengthening, alternative treatment program that he says has stopped the progression of HIV infection in more than 1,000 of his patients. The program consists of whole foods, nutritional supplements, herbs, exercise, stress reduction, and techniques for emotional and spiritual growth.

It's not that Dr. Kaiser doesn't use the new array of antiviral drugs (like protease inhibitors) that help slow the progression of HIV infection, but he uses them only when they're absolutely necessary. These drugs have a daunting variety of body-punishing side effects, he explains, from headaches to heart disease. And because people with HIV can quickly become resistant to antiviral drugs, he prefers to use them as a last resort.

"I am able to keep a high percentage of my HIV-positive patients off antiviral drugs completely for a significant period of time," he says. "And if they must take antiviral medications, I believe that combining them with natural therapies helps the drugs work better and longer, with fewer side effects."

## AFFIRMATIONS: *Health from Within*

One of the cornerstones of Dr. Kaiser's program is providing emotional and spiritual uplift, using techniques such as meditation, prayer, or yoga. Relaxing the body, decreasing stress, and helping people connect with their spiritual sides can be powerful healing forces, he says. "Healing does not come from little bottles," he explains. "It comes from within."

Long-held negative beliefs or fears, such as "I'm not good enough to succeed in life," or "I can't heal," cause changes in the body that can weaken the immune system, says Dr. Kaiser. You can change your beliefs from negative to positive by using affirmations—positive statements that are written or spoken aloud many times during the day.

First, write out a few of your fears, such as "I am afraid of becoming sick." Then write out a new belief, such as "I am a healthy human being, and my healthy emotions and thoughts will manifest a healthy body." Here are some other examples.

• I breathe in love and light and exhale fear and darkness.
• I am confident and powerful.
• I am at peace with myself.
• I will listen to my body's guidance through my healing journey.

"I believe that using affirmations can literally change the ways the body works, and this in turn can help with healing," Dr. Kaiser explains.

# GUIDE TO
# PROFESSIONAL CARE

*Caution: You should use the alternative remedies discussed in this chapter only as part of a treatment program that is guided and monitored by a qualified medical doctor in partnership with a qualified alternative practitioner, both of whom are experienced in caring for your condition. Check with your conventional doctor before changing or stopping any conventional medical treatments or medications, and keep all of your doctors and/or alternative practitioners informed of all treatments that you are receiving.*

HIV infection is extremely complicated to treat. People who have HIV need to see someone who specializes in this condition and sees a lot of HIV patients, says Jon Kaiser, M.D., director of the Jon Kaiser Wellness Center in San Francisco.

"A doctor who is an HIV specialist will give you better care," he says. Many HIV specialists are also open-minded about alternative medicine, he adds. This means that they'll be willing to work with you as a partner, which is essential in any long-term treatment plan.

## ESSENTIAL FATTY ACIDS: *Good for the Skin*

Infections and other skin problems are common in people with HIV, says Allen Green, M.D., director of the Center for Optimum Health in Fountain Valley, California. Essential fatty acids (EFA), which are abundant in cold-water fish, flaxseed oil, and borage oil, help keep the skin healthy.

Dr. Green suggests taking a daily EFA supplement, following the directions on the label. For vegetarians, he recommends supplements containing 4,000 to 6,000 milligrams of flaxseed oil. For nonvegetarians, supplements of both fish oil in 2,000- to 4,000-milligram doses and borage oil in 240- to 480-milligram doses may be helpful. Take these doses daily.

## The Need for Protein

Protein feeds the immune system. Since HIV attacks the immune system, people with the virus need all the protein they can get.

"I believe that adequate consumption of protein can make the difference between a healthy immune system and one that is in a progressive state of decline," says Dr. Kaiser. He recommends that people with HIV get 0.6 gram of protein for every pound of body weight. For someone who weighs 150 pounds, for example, that would mean at least 90 grams of protein a day. Here are a few ways to ensure that you get enough.

### THE 20-GRAM RULE: *A Guideline for Every Meal*

An easy way to keep track of your protein intake is to make it a point to eat at least 20 grams at every meal. High-protein animal foods recommended by Dr. Kaiser include beef (just 4 ounces supplies about 28 grams of protein), ham, turkey, chicken, shrimp, halibut, salmon, and tuna.

High-protein plant and dairy foods include tofu (½ cup supplies 10 grams of protein), barley, peanut butter, beans, nuts, pasta, and eggs (one egg has 7 grams).

### PROTEIN SNACKS: *Eat Them Between Meals*

Look for protein bars that provide 5 to 10 grams of protein, and eat no more than two or three bars a day, says Dr. Kaiser. Be sure to choose bars that have a minimum of sweeteners, which can depress immune function, he adds.

### PROTEIN POWDER: *Truly Great Shakes*

A convenient way to get a lot of protein is to make a daily shake with protein powder that provides at least 25 grams of protein per serving. Avoid any powder that lists sugar, sucrose, dextrose, corn syrup, or fructose as one of its first two ingredients, says Dr. Kaiser. Also avoid powders with artificial flavors or colors.

If you have chronic diarrhea (a common symptom of HIV), try a powder with hydrolyzed protein, which is easily absorbed. "Mixing hydrolyzed protein supplements with rice or soy milk makes a good-tasting, easy-to-digest source of protein," says Dr. Kaiser.

## Healing Foods

A number of foods are thought to help people with HIV, both by controlling various symptoms and by bolstering immunity.

Here are the foods that many alternative practitioners recommend.

## GARLIC: *Good for Protection*

Garlic contains allicin, a powerful compound that can help kill bacteria, fungi, and viruses. This is important for people with HIV because the virus damages the immune system, giving many different types of organisms the opportunity to flourish.

Tai Lahans, an acupuncturist and practitioner of Traditional Chinese Medicine in Seattle who specializes in treating people with HIV, advises HIV-positive patients to take at least 9 grams of raw garlic a day in juiced form, or about three medium cloves. The garlic can be taken in three doses of 3 grams each at morning, noon, and evening. The juiced form is very active and can be added to other fresh juices.

You can also take garlic supplements. Dr. Kaiser recommends two to eight capsules a day.

Garlic may do more than protect against random infections. It also may slow the progression of the disease itself. "HIV spreads through clumps of white blood cells called aggregated lymphocytes," says Lahans. "Garlic helps dissolve those clumps, slowing the infection."

## Dr. Kaiser's Anti-HIV Nutrient Program

People with HIV should take several types of nutritional supplements, says Jon Kaiser, M.D., director of the Jon Kaiser Wellness Center in San Francisco. He recommends a multivitamin/mineral supplement, a separate multimineral supplement, and individual vitamins as well as other supplements that can help stall HIV and keep it from progressing to AIDS. (Dr. Kaiser notes, however, that these doses are much higher than normal, and people with HIV should take them only with the supervision of a health care professional.) Here's what to look for.

### Multivitamin/Mineral Supplement

- Vitamin A/beta-carotene: 10,000 to 20,000 international units
- B vitamins (thiamin, riboflavin, pantothenic acid, and $B_6$): 50 to 100 milligrams
- Vitamin $B_{12}$: 500 to 1,000 micrograms

- Vitamin C: 250 to 1,000 milligrams
- Vitamin E: 150 to 400 international units
- Iron: 9 to 18 milligrams
- Zinc: 10 to 25 milligrams
- Calcium: 50 to 250 milligrams
- Magnesium: 25 to 125 milligrams
- Selenium: 100 to 200 micrograms

**Multimineral Supplement**
- Iron: 9 to 18 milligrams
- Zinc: 25 to 50 milligrams
- Copper: 1 to 2 milligrams
- Calcium: 1,000 milligrams
- Magnesium: 500 milligrams
- Selenium: 100 to 200 micrograms

**Individual Vitamins**
- Vitamin C: 1,000 milligrams twice a day
- Vitamin E: 400 international units twice a day
- Vitamin $B_6$: 100 milligrams twice a day

**Other Supplements**
- N-acetylcysteine (NAC): 500 milligrams twice a day. NAC can help boost levels of the antioxidant glutathione. Studies show that people with HIV who have low glutathione levels move more quickly into AIDS.
- Coenzyme $Q_{10}$: 30 milligrams twice a day. This supplement is thought to provide cells with additional energy, boost immunity, and help relieve fatigue.
- Acidophilus: Daily, according to label directions. Acidophilus can help people with HIV avoid digestive problems that result from taking antibiotics and other drugs, which can destroy beneficial bacteria in the digestive tract.

**CONGEE:** *Calms Diarrhea*

Severe, chronic diarrhea affects most people with HIV, says Misha Cohen, O.M.D., a doctor of Oriental medicine and licensed acupuncturist in San Francisco. You can help control it by eating congee, or boiled rice pudding, she says.

"Chronic diarrhea produces extreme discomfort, makes it

difficult to have a normal social life, destroys the appetite, robs the person of nutritional support, and causes severe weight loss and wasting," Dr. Cohen explains. According to practitioners of Traditional Chinese Medicine, a daily meal of congee is said to provide warmth (yang) to the abdominal area. This is important because HIV and the drugs used to treat it tend to make this area very cold (yin), Dr. Cohen says.

To make congee, combine 1 cup of white rice with 7 to 9 cups of filtered water in a pot, cover, and cook on low heat for 6 to 8 hours. You may need to add more water during cooking to keep it from drying out. You can also make it in a slow cooker, says Dr. Cohen.

People with severe diarrhea may need to eat congee as a meal three times a day if that's all they can tolerate. In that case, you can add soup stock to the base. Otherwise, eat 1 to 3 cups a day.

## CHINESE HERBS: *For More Potent Congee*

Many alternative practitioners recommend adding healing foods or herbs to congee while it's cooking, Dr. Cohen says. For treating diarrhea, for example, she recommends adding 6 grams of lotus seeds (*lian zi*), 3 grams of euryale (*qian shi*), 3 grams of dried ginger (*gan jiang*), 6 grams of dioscorea (*shan yao*), 9 grams of poria (*fu ling*), 3 grams of codonopsis (*dang shen*), and 2 pieces of red dates (*hong zao*), plus fresh dates and cinnamon to taste. These herbs can be obtained from a Chinese herbal pharmacy or a practitioner of Traditional Chinese Medicine.

# Skip the Side Effects with Drug-Free Help for
# Hives

Hives are red bumps on your skin that are so maddeningly itchy that you'd do just about anything to prevent another attack.

Prescription medications such as antihistamines and cortisone are very effective at controlling hives, but they also can cause side effects. Antihistamines can make you drowsy, and cortisone can cause a wide range of body-damaging reactions. Cortisone is particularly damaging if you have chronic hives (episodes that last more than 6 weeks) and need to take the drug on a regular basis.

"I believe you need symptomatic relief for hives that is natural and free of side effects," says Jacqueline Krohn, M.D., a physician in New Mexico. "And, what's more important, you need to discover the cause of the hives so you can eliminate the problem."

Discovering the cause of hives can be difficult, and your best

## GUIDE TO PROFESSIONAL CARE

If you've had hives for more than 6 weeks, you have chronic hives as opposed to the acute variety, which may happen only once in a while. It's likely that chronic hives have multiple triggers, and you will need the help of an allergist or dermatologist to discover the causes, which could be food, chemicals, medications, molds, animal dander, the sun, cold, or many other possible factors.

In some cases, hives can be the first sign of a life-threatening allergic emergency called anaphylactic shock, particularly if they are inside your mouth, on your palms and the soles of your feet, on the top of your scalp, or near your genitals. The only way to counter this emergency is with an immediate injection of adrenaline (epinephrine), says Jacqueline Krohn, M.D., a physician in New Mexico. If you feel your throat closing up and you have trouble breathing, call 911 immediately or have someone drive you to the emergency room.

Carrying an injection device is advisable for people who are allergic to bee stings or common foods such as nuts or shellfish. For people who are allergic to foods, accidental exposure in restaurants can bring on acute hives and itching and may cause breathing problems. Talk to your doctor about getting a prescription for an injection device, then keep it handy.

bet is to work with an allergist who can help you pinpoint the possible trigger. Even so, there's plenty that you can do on your own to relieve the symptoms. Here's what alternative experts suggest.

## HYDROTHERAPY: *Stop a Hive Attack*

When triggered by an allergen, mast cells in your immune system release a chemical called histamine, which causes hives. Taking a very warm shower (as warm as you can tolerate without it being painful) also triggers the release of histamine. Once it has all been released, the itching stops, and it takes several hours for the body to make more histamine—which means no more hives.

"Taking this kind of shower for 10 to 15 minutes 'degranulates' all the mast cells, which means there's no more histamine, and your itching will be relieved," says Bradley Bongiovanni, N.D., a naturopathic physician in Cambridge, Massachusetts. "This remedy doesn't correct the problem, but it is helpful for managing it."

## QUERCETIN: *A Natural Antihistamine*

Quercetin is a plant pigment found in onions, apples, leafy green vegetables, and other foods. It's a natural antihistamine, and a quercetin supplement can help reduce or eliminate hives, Dr. Krohn says.

A secretary in the doctor's office who had chronic hives that made her face swell was able to clear up the problem by taking 500 milligrams of quercetin twice a day, she says. "This is an excellent supplement for anyone with the problem."

## HOMEOPATHY: *Customized Relief*

Homeopathic remedies can be effective for relieving acute hives or controlling chronic hives, Dr. Krohn says. She recommends using a 200C potency for acute hives. (While you may not be able to find more than a 30C potency in most health food stores, don't worry; it will still be effective.)

Follow the dosage recommendations on the label, which are likely to instruct you to take three or four pellets a day. Alternatively, says Dr. Krohn, you can dissolve one pellet in 4 ounces of water and take 1 teaspoon four to six times a day. "Taking the remedy this way has a more gradual but deeper effectiveness," she says. Here are the homeopathic remedies she says work best.

• Apis is good if the hives are hot, red, and very itchy or burning, and if they are worse when you're overheated and better when you're cold or cold is applied to them.
• Natrum muriaticum is for chronic hives, especially when they are white; appear on the joints, ankles, or hands; and are worse when you're overheated or under emotional stress.
• Rhus toxicodendron is for very red, large hives, with prickling itching, that appear on your forearms and hands, are worse when they get wet or are in cold air, and are accompanied by a recurring fever.
• Urtica urens is for hives on the scalp, hands, or fingers that sting, burn, and itch violently (making you want to rub constantly), and are worse in the heat and better when you're lying down and rubbing them.
• Arsenicum album is good if the hives burn and you have chills, and if they're worse at night and in cold air and better when you're warm and exerting yourself.

## SANDALWOOD ESSENTIAL OIL: *Soothe the Itch*

In Ayurveda, the ancient natural healing system from India, hives are said to be a "pitta," or fiery, condition. A classic remedy for fiery, itchy skin is sandalwood essential oil, says Pratima Raichur, an Ayurvedic practitioner in New York City.

"Sandalwood oil is cooling and calming—almost like a sedative for the skin," she says. To use it, add 20 drops of sandalwood essential oil to 1 ounce of a carrier oil such as coconut or almond. Apply it to the hives every 3 to 4 hours.

## MINT: *Cooling Cubes for Hives*

Putting ice directly on the hives can cool the itching, says Norma Pasekoff Weinberg, an herbal educator in Cape Cod, Massachusetts. Adding fresh mint to the cubes makes it even more effective.

To make the mint ice cubes, you'll need 2 teaspoons of crushed fresh mint leaves (such as peppermint) or 1 teaspoon of dried leaves. Pour boiling water over the leaves, cover, and steep for 5 minutes. Strain the tea, pour it into ice cube trays, and freeze. When the cubes are frozen, put them in a plastic freezer bag and label them. Then, when you have hives, rub a cube across the area to cool the itchy, irritated skin, Weinberg says.

**FLOWER ESSENCES:** *To the Rescue*

Flower essences are specially prepared distillations of flowers that can positively affect the body, mind, and emotions. The flower remedy called Rescue Remedy can help turn off an allergic reaction and reduce the emotional stress of having hives, says Dr. Krohn. Follow the dosage instructions on the label or add 3 to 5 drops to a glass of water and drink once a day until symptoms subside.

## *Boosting Chi Beats* **Hypoglycemia**

You're tired. You can't concentrate. You feel anxious. You're shaky, pale, and dizzy. Maybe you've broken out in a cold sweat.

Those symptoms are hallmarks of hypoglycemia, or low blood sugar, says Maoshing Ni, O.M.D., Ph.D., a doctor of Oriental medicine and director of the Tao of Wellness Center in Santa Monica, California.

And, just like a fuel gauge, those symptoms are pointing to a very obvious fact: Your body's energy is low, and you need to increase it. Practitioners of Traditional Chinese Medicine (TCM) call that energy chi.

In the case of hypoglycemia, TCM says that the chi in your body, particularly in your pancreas and spleen, is deficient and that restoring chi to those organs will help remedy the problem. The healing can start once you get the point—the acupressure point, that is.

## ACUPRESSURE: *Cure Yourself in 10 Days*

Chi, according to TCM, circulates in your body along energy tracks called meridians. Pressing certain acupressure points on those meridians can help send more chi to specific organs. In every case except for the CV point, you'll press the same acupressure points on both sides of your body symmetrically, first on one side, then on the other. Here are the four points that restore energy to the pancreas and spleen, says Dr. Ni. (For the exact locations, see An Illustrated Guide to Acupressure Points on page 700.)

• ST36 is four finger-widths below the lower ridge of your kneecap, in the hollow or indentation at the front of your shinbone.
• SP4 is at the beginning of the arch on the inside of your foot, right behind the bone of the big toe.
• CV6 is two finger-widths below your navel, on an imaginary vertical line running down the middle of your body and directly through your navel.
• BL20 is two finger-widths from your spine, level with what doctors call the 11th thoracic vertebra, which is between your waist and the middle of your shoulder blades.

Use your thumb or finger to press each point with very steady pressure for 2 minutes, says Dr. Ni. You can press all

---

## GUIDE TO
## PROFESSIONAL CARE

Hypoglycemia, or low blood sugar, can cause a wide array of symptoms, including cravings for sweets, irritability, fatigue, dizziness, headaches, poor memory, heart palpitations, shakiness, blurry vision, depression or mood swings, and frequent anxiety or nervousness.

If you have several of these symptoms or any of them in a severe form, see a nutritionally oriented physician for diagnosis and treatment, says Michael Janson, M.D., consultant physician at Path to Health in Burlington, Massachusetts.

of the points consecutively for quick, symptomatic relief whenever you're experiencing the symptoms of hypoglycemia, he says. For long-term relief, alternate the points every other day; for example, press ST36 and SP4 on Monday, CV6 and BL20 on Tuesday, ST36 and SP4 on Wednesday, and so on.

After 10 days, your condition should be stabilized, says Dr. Ni. As with the alignment of a car, however, he notes that your body's internal balance may go out of alignment again after a period of stress, poor diet, or other negative situations.

### PROTEIN: *Be Proactive with Your Diet*

A diet that includes more protein sources and fewer simple carbohydrates such as white sugar and flour strengthens your spleen and pancreas, says Dr. Ni. Eat more tofu and other soy products as well as more chicken, turkey, fish, and beans.

### GINSENG: *Use the Right Kind*

If acupressure and diet don't remedy the problem, "a person should use Chinese herbs," says Dr. Ni. He says that ginseng promotes more energy in the spleen/pancreas system, but you need to take the right type: either Chinese or Korean, not American or Siberian. American and Siberian ginseng don't have as potent an effect, according to Dr. Ni.

Chinese and Korean ginseng help the liver convert the substance glycogen to glucose, or blood sugar. Follow the dosage instructions on the label, Dr. Ni says. You will need to take it for 2 to 4 weeks before you see results. Once you have experienced no symptoms for a few days, or if you don't notice any results after several weeks, stop taking it.

### Vitamins and Minerals: The Best Kinds of "Sugar Pills"

With hypoglycemia, blood sugar levels fluctuate wildly up and down—"sometimes way too low, sometimes way too high," says Michael Janson, M.D., consultant physician at Path to Health in Burlington, Massachusetts.

The following vitamins and minerals, he says, can help normalize your blood sugar levels and protect your body against some of the damage that can result from levels that are sometimes too high and sometimes too low.

The first nutritional supplement that Dr. Janson recommends is a high-potency multivitamin/mineral supplement. To make sure it's high-potency, look for a supplement with at least 400 to 500 milligrams of magnesium, 100 to 200 micrograms of selenium, 20 to 30 milligrams of zinc, 500 to 1,000 milligrams of vitamin C, 200 to 400 micrograms of chromium, and 400 international units of vitamin E.

"Those levels of nutrients should guarantee that the entire spectrum of vitamins and minerals in the supplement is high enough to help remedy hypoglycemia," says Dr. Janson.

In addition to your daily vitamin/mineral supplement, he recommends that you take the following individual supplements (but only with the approval and supervision of your physician).

- Vitamin C: 1,000 milligrams
- Bioflavonoids: 1,000 milligrams
- Magnesium: 200 milligrams
- Vitamin E: 400 international units
- Chromium: 200 to 400 micrograms
- Coenzyme $Q_{10}$: 100 to 200 milligrams
- Standardized milk thistle extract containing silymarin: 250 to 500 milligrams

## CODONOPSIS : *The "Poor Man's Ginseng"*

If ginseng is too expensive, try the herb codonopsis, says Dr. Ni. You may also find it under the name dang shen or bellflower. It works like ginseng, only more slowly, he says, and at about one-tenth the price. He suggests taking five 300-milligram capsules three times a day.

## FOOD: *Beating the Blues*

The American diet is red, white, and blues: Too much fatty, fiber-free red meat and too many refined carbohydrates like white sugar and white bread can result in the brain-numbing blues of hypoglycemia.

The remedy? Michael Janson, M.D., consultant physician at Path to Health in Burlington, Massachusetts, advocates a low-fat, mostly vegetarian diet that includes fish and emphasizes natural, high-fiber (or slowly digested complex car-bohydrate) foods such as grains, vegetables, fresh fruits, legumes, seeds, and nuts. And he says that snacking on those foods between meals can also help balance blood sugar levels.

## *Drug-Free Help for*
# Impotence

With all of the hype surrounding sildenafil citrate, better known as Viagra, you might think that the erection-bestowing prescription drug is the only option for men with impotence.

It's not, say alternative physicians.

"I believe that there are natural treatments that appear to be just as effective in restoring erectile ability, are probably a lot safer, and are certainly less expensive than Viagra," says Jonathan Wright, M.D., a nutritionally oriented physician and director of the Tahoma Clinic in Kent, Washington. "Before a man tries Viagra, I strongly suggest that he give these remedies a try."

In particular, men who are taking medication for heart problems should explore alternatives to Viagra. It's known that taking nitrate drugs such as nitroglycerin with Viagra can cause a deadly drop in blood pressure, says Gerald Melchiode, M.D., professor of psychiatry and lecturer at the University of Texas Southwestern Medical Center in Dallas.

Here are some effective, nondrug erection enhancers.

### ARGININE: *Natural Viagra*

Viagra works by blocking an enzyme called PDE5 that destroys nitric oxide, the chemical in your body that's responsible for allowing the penis to fill with blood during an erection. Well, the amino acid arginine is the body's main source of nitric oxide, says Dr. Wright. So does that mean that increasing your intake of arginine can help you defeat impotence?

"Yes," says Dr. Wright, "taking arginine supplements can improve a man's ability to have an erection."

In fact, you should consider using arginine before you try Viagra, he says. It's a natural, safe substance, he points out, while Viagra is a drug with side effects that can include common problems such as headaches, facial flushing, digestive upset, and abnormal vision.

If you decide to take arginine to enhance sexual function, Dr. Wright recommends 3,000 milligrams a day. It will take about 3 to 4 weeks to take effect. If you feel that extra help is necessary, you may take an additional dose of 3,000 milligrams about an hour prior to having sex.

You should take this supplement only under the supervision of a knowledgeable medical doctor. Do not take it if you have genital herpes or if you are also using lysine supplements.

**GINKGO:** *For Circulatory Problems*

Ginkgo, which is well-known for boosting memory by improving circulation to the brain, also boosts circulation to the penis, thus helping to reverse erectile dysfunction, says Dr. Wright. He recommends 60 milligrams daily, but he also counsels patience, since the herb typically takes 2 to 6 months to work.

## GUIDE TO
## PROFESSIONAL CARE

If you're having difficulties such as a total inability to have an erection or an inconsistent ability to have or maintain one, see a urologist to rule out a physical problem, such as circulatory disease. Tell the urologist about your current medications, since many common prescription drugs, such as drugs for high blood pressure and antidepressants, can cause sexual dysfunction.

The next step is for you and your partner to see a mental health professional such as a psychiatrist, who can recommend a medical treatment (such as Viagra) as well as address any relationship issues that may underlie the problem.

### The Tantric Way

The branch of yoga known as Tantra teaches techniques for improving sexual performance with the goal of generating extra energy for spiritual practice, says Charles Muir, director of the Source School of Tantra Yoga in Wailuku, Hawaii.

Some of the techniques show a man how to make love without an erection and become erect in the process. "Most men think that if they don't have an erection, they can't do anything," says Muir. "But these techniques can bring circulation and energy to the penis, causing an erection."

Don't worry, however, if you don't get an erection while doing these techniques. Just have fun and see what happens. Here are two that Muir teaches.

**YOGA:** *Holding the Wand*

"In this technique, either partner grasps the penis with the fingers or hand and manipulates it as if it were a wand, gently rubbing the head across the outside of the vagina, especially over and around the clitoris," says Muir. "The stimulation and contact with your lover's vagina will usually inspire an erection pretty quickly, but a soft penis can provide a woman great pleasure. A lubricant is necessary in this technique to eliminate friction and enhance enjoyment."

He adds that a woman can derive great sexual pleasure from assuming the active role in this technique by holding the penis and moving it in ways that she finds stimulating.

**YOGA:** *Tapping into Pleasure*

"Another hand-assisted technique is to tap the penis against the lips of the vagina and the clitoris," says Muir. "Again, either the man or the woman can perform this move, holding the penis as if it were a conductor's baton, tapping it to a slow tempo that builds faster and faster, using it to contact the woman with a touch that varies from gentle to firm, then back to gentle." This technique can be used whether the penis is soft or hard, he says.

# *Put Yourself in Control of* **Incontinence**

Take a drug. Have an operation. Wear an adult diaper.

Those are the three options offered by most doctors when they treat someone for urinary incontinence, the involuntary leaking of urine. But some alternative-minded experts say that those therapies should be last resorts, not standard recommendations. They estimate that between 80 and 90 percent of people with urinary incontinence, most of whom are women, can find relief with safer and less bothersome therapies.

Medication can have side effects. Surgery has its risks. An absorbent pad isn't a solution.

Before resorting to such drastic measures, most people should try behavioral and dietary methods to solve the problem, says Genevieve M. Messick, M.D., a physician in Columbus, Ohio, who specializes in urinary incontinence and pelvic floor dysfunction. Only when natural treatments fail should people resort to the others.

## CAFFEINE: *Cut Down to Reduce Irritation*

"Caffeine is an irritant that causes the bladder to be more spastic," explains Dr. Messick. It's also a diuretic, which means that it makes your body produce more urine. "These two factors can make incontinence worse," she says.

Caffeine isn't found only in cola, tea, and coffee, adds Diane Kaschak Newman, a nurse practitioner who works with adults in Philadelphia. It's also present in chocolate and some over-the-counter drugs, such as Excedrin, Anacin, and Midol.

"If you suspect that caffeine intake is causing your bladder problems, gradually decrease the level of caffeine you're getting and see if there's an improvement in symptoms," Newman advises.

# GUIDE TO
# PROFESSIONAL CARE

Only about half of the people with urinary incontinence seek medical care, says Genevieve M. Messick, M.D., a physician in Columbus, Ohio, who specializes in urinary incontinence and pelvic floor dysfunction. Many of these people resort to using absorbent pads because they've been convinced by television advertising that incontinence is a normal part of aging and that wearing pads is a reasonable way to control the problem.

In many cases, however, with the proper treatment, incontinence can be controlled or eliminated, making pads unnecessary, says Dr. Messick. The best place for that treatment, she says, is a center dedicated to continence care.

First, a surgeon, gynecologist, or urologist at the center will rule out any kind of problem that would require surgery. Then you'll be taught about diet. You'll receive instructions for behavioral techniques such as those discussed in this chapter. And you'll receive counseling to help you deal with the emotional and lifestyle challenges of incontinence. Most important, your continence program will be designed specifically for you; there is no one-size-fits-all answer to the problem, says Dr. Messick.

The National Association for Continence can provide a recommendation for a continence center in your area, says Dr. Messick. Write to NAFC-CRS, PO Box 8310, Spartanburg, SC 29305-8306.

---

**ALCOHOL:** *Abstinence Can Counter Incontinence*

The muscles of the pelvic floor control the opening and closing of the urethra, the tube through which urine leaves the bladder. Weak pelvic floor muscles are one of the main causes of urinary incontinence in women. Alcohol causes these muscles to weaken further, and since alcohol also has a diuretic effect, the weak muscles are forced to hold back extra urine. Thus, the wisest course is to cut back on—or cut out—alcohol and see if your symptoms improve, Dr. Messick advises. If they do, you know you have to curtail your alcohol consumption.

## ASPARTAME: *Bitter for Your Bladder*

"Artificial sweeteners containing aspartame can irritate the bladder. From my experience, they appear to be a common cause of bladder dysfunction, urinary urgency or frequency, and incontinence," says Newman.

"I had a patient who had been through surgery and had taken medications, all without relief," she says. "But when she abstained from using aspartame, her incontinence cleared up."

## WATER: *More Is Better*

People with urinary incontinence sometimes try to gain control by drinking less water. After all, less water means less urine, which means less chance of an accident, right? Not so, says Newman. Drinking less produces more concentrated urine, which irritates the bladder. This in turn may increase the frequency of urination and the chance of an accident.

She recommends drinking eight 8-ounce glasses of water a day, but sip it throughout the day rather than drinking a lot at one time. This will help prevent those overwhelming sensations of urgency, says Newman.

The one time that you want to drink less is in the evening, she adds. She suggests that you not drink any liquids for at least 3 hours before you go to bed. That way, you'll be less likely to wake up during the night with the urge to urinate.

## KEGELS: *Do Them Right*

The muscles of the pelvic floor are like a sling supporting the bladder and urethra. Strengthening those muscles allows women with incontinence (or men who are incontinent following prostate surgery) to keep urine in the bladder until they decide to let it out.

"Some health professionals will tell you that exercises to strengthen the muscles of the pelvic floor (called Kegels, after the gynecologist who invented them in the 1940s) don't work," says Kathryn Burgio, Ph.D., director of the continence program at the University of Alabama at Birmingham. But, she says, that's because Kegels usually aren't taught properly. Done correctly, the exercises work for most people who do them.

In fact, you may see significant improvement after 8 weeks, says Dr. Burgio. Here's how to do them right.

First, you need to know where the muscles are. You can locate them by stopping or slowing the stream of urine the next time you go to the bathroom, says Dr. Burgio. The muscles that you use to do that are the pelvic floor muscles. Another way to identify them is to tighten the same muscles that you use to stop yourself from passing gas in public. Women can also find them by tightening the vaginal muscles.

Several times a day, squeeze the muscles and hold the contraction for 10 seconds, says Dr. Burgio. At first, you may not be able to hold for that long, but don't worry. Start by holding for a count of 3 (1, Mississippi; 2, Mississippi; 3, Mississippi), then let go. Over time, build up to a count of 10.

Some people have a tendency to contract their abdominal muscles by mistake. Breathing normally and regularly while doing the Kegels will help keep your abdomen relaxed, says Dr. Burgio. Also, you can put one hand over your abdomen to double-check that you're not tightening the muscles there, she adds.

When you're doing Kegels correctly, you'll feel a lifting sensation in the area of your vagina or a pulling sensation in your rectum, says Newman.

To build up the muscles, you need to do 45 Kegels a day. It's best to do them 15 times in a row three times a day.

"The most common error is that people simply forget to do them," says Dr. Burgio. The best way to remember to do your Kegels is to pick a few activities that you do every day, such as taking a shower, brushing your teeth, or eating a meal, and do the exercises during those activities.

Does that sound like too much distraction? Just stay with it. "At first, you'll have to concentrate quite a bit," says Dr. Burgio. "But after they become a habit, you'll start doing them automatically."

## URGE STRATEGY: *To Gain Control*

Imagine that you have a powerful urge to urinate. It's a sensation that you can't ignore. The moment you feel the urge, you rush to the bathroom because you're afraid that if you don't, you'll have an episode of urge incontinence, which simply means losing urine before you make it to the bathroom.

People with this type of incontinence often find that urges come more and more frequently, and pretty soon, their bladders seem to have taken over their lives. What's worse, all of that rushing just jiggles the bladder and increases abdominal pressure, which can push urine out.

Well, it's time to regain control—with an "urge strategy." Here's what Dr. Burgio recommends.

**1.** When you get the urge, stop what you're doing and stay put. Sit down when possible, or stand quietly.
**2.** Remain very still. When you are still, it's easier to control your urge.
**3.** Squeeze your pelvic floor muscles quickly several times, but don't relax fully between contractions.
**4.** Relax the rest of your body. Take a few deep breaths and let go of your tension. Concentrate on suppressing that urgency.
**5.** Wait until the urge subsides.
**6.** Walk to the bathroom at a normal pace. Do not rush. Continue squeezing your pelvic floor muscles quickly while you walk.

If you do this each time the urge strikes, "you will have a much better chance of staying dry on your way to the toilet," says Dr. Burgio.

# Alternative and Modern Medicine Can Treat
# **Infertility**

Couples who are having trouble conceiving should see an infertility specialist. But even before and while you're working with the specialist, consider using alternative remedies to improve your chances of having a baby.

"Combined conventional and alternative medical approaches are the best ways to treat infertility," says Roger C. Hirsh, O.M.D., a doctor of Oriental medicine and specialist in herbal medicine in Beverly Hills. And, he says, some of the most powerful alternative methods are from the ancient healing system of Traditional Chinese Medicine (TCM).

## Using TCM to Enhance Fertility

The first and most important step is to restore general health to the man and woman through a dietary regimen, herbal decoctions, and acupuncture. Even if you and your spouse can't see a TCM practitioner to help boost your fertility by restoring health, the following home remedies can be extremely helpful.

### ACUPRESSURE: *Stimulate the Conception Vessel*

Acupuncture points can be stimulated with finger or palm pressure to regulate the chi, or life-energy, as it circulates throughout the body in currents along pathways called meridians.

In men, the best acupressure area for increasing fertility is called CV4, located four finger-widths directly below the navel. It balances and enhances the kidney meridian and reproductive essence in the pelvic cavity. This area is most important to the health of the reproductive organs. To stimulate the point, cover it with the palm of your right hand, then, with your left hand on top of the right, press and rub 100 times in a clockwise direction. Use about 5 to 7 pounds of pressure (to determine how much pressure that is, press on your bathroom scale with your hand).

Women also can benefit from acupressure on this point. Stimulating the liver meridian, however, which spreads the energy in the chest, helps the emotional awareness that plays such a major role in conceiving a baby. Dr. Hirsh recommends using the same palm-rubbing technique on CV17, which is in the center of the chest directly between the nipples. (For the exact locations of both points, see An Illustrated Guide to Acupressure Points on page 700.)

### FOOD: *Make the Abdomen Happy*

"A woman needs a nice, warm, cushy environment in the uterus for the egg to implant," Dr. Hirsh says. The way to produce this environment is to emphasize "warming" foods rather than "cooling" foods such as salads.

Dr. Hirsh recommends a protein-rich diet of cooked foods in which small portions of meat, such as lamb (which, in TCM, is said to warm the uterus) and other lean meats, are used as condiments with tofu, grains, beans, cooked vegetables, and other

# GUIDE TO
# PROFESSIONAL CARE

A woman under 35 who has not become pregnant after a year of unprotected intercourse, or a woman over 35 who has not become pregnant after 6 months, should "go straight with her husband to an infertility specialist," says Alice Domar, Ph.D., director of the Behavioral Medicine Program for Infertility at Beth Israel Deaconess Medical Center in Boston.

A reproductive endocrinologist will test the man for sperm abnormalities and the woman for ovulatory dysfunction, the two biggest causes of infertility. The woman will also receive tests to see if her fallopian tubes are open and healthy and if her reproductive hormones are normal. Checking thyroid function is also very important, and there are other tests as well. Once a diagnosis is made, treatment begins, often with fertility-enhancing drugs. More than half of all couples who are treated for infertility will be successful.

During treatment, which could take several years, Dr. Domar strongly advises couples to attend a support group sponsored by RESOLVE, a national network for infertile couples. Or call your local hospital or academic medical center to see if it has a mind-body infertility program.

whole foods. Other high-protein items include fish, seafood, milk, and eggs.

Although fruit is cooling, it's good for sperm production, since too much heat damages sperm. Sperm count and motility (movement) are generally enhanced by a cool environment. Therefore, for men, whole fruit and fruit nectars are useful for increasing sperm count and the amount of ejaculate.

Herbs can also be helpful. For recommendations, it's best to see a qualified herbal practitioner. To find out who is licensed, contact your state medical board, says Dr. Hirsh.

## SEXUAL TECHNIQUE: *Yin and Yang Unite in Conception*

TCM suggests that both partners should achieve orgasm together to create the ideal opportunity for conception, Dr. Hirsh says. When the man ejaculates, he should use his consciousness to direct the ejaculate to the center of his partner's brain to effect hormone stimulation. During her orgasm, the woman should "embrace the Earth with her being."

For the man, "aiming" helps encourage the sperm to be deposited high in the uterus, where it has the greatest chance of traveling up the fallopian tube for conception, Dr. Hirsh says. For the woman, bearing down during orgasm and relaxing afterward helps the cervix draw more sperm into the uterus.

## Mini-Relaxation: The Mind-Body Conception Connection

What with endless visits to clinics and hospitals, "advice" from well-intentioned relatives, a marriage strained by calendar-determined sex, and month after month of disappointment, infertility can be stressful. Moreover, the emotions associated with that stress, such as depression, anxiety, and anger, can actually decrease your chances of conception.

That's why mind-body strategies that calm emotions and release stress not only improve the quality of life for infertile couples but also increase their chances of conception, says Alice Domar, Ph.D., director of the Behavioral Medicine Program for Infertility at Beth Israel Deaconess Medical Center in Boston.

Dr. Domar advises women in her program to spend 20 minutes a day practicing one of the various mind-body techniques—meditation, visualization, yoga, or diaphragmatic breathing, to name a few. But anyone can quickly learn a simple stress-beating technique called mini-relaxation that she teaches as part of her program. Here's how.

Take slow, deep breaths—not from your chest but from your diaphragm, the flat strip of muscle above your abdomen that controls your breathing. To identify the area, put one hand over your abdomen just above your belly button. When you breathe from your diaphragm, your hand will rise and fall about an inch.

Next, mentally count down from 10 to zero with each breath, saying "10" with your first inhalation and exhalation, "9" with your second, and so on.

"When you get to zero, see how you are feeling," Dr. Domar says. "If you're feeling better, great. If not, try doing it again."

### KEGELS: *Build Your Prostate Health*

"In men, good prostate health is important for fertility because the sperm travel as ejaculate on prostatic fluid," Dr. Hirsh says. One way to tone and encourage your prostate health is with Kegel exercises, in which you repeatedly pull up and tighten the root of the penis in the same way you would to stop the flow of urine in midstream. This will strengthen ejaculate power.

Dr. Hirsh recommends doing 30 Kegels three times a day. For each Kegel, inhale and pull up for three counts, hold for one count, then exhale for three counts while you relax.

## Nutrition Advice for Women

The most important alternative approaches for conception are nutritional, says Jacob Teitelbaum, M.D., a physician in Annapolis, Maryland. Here's his advice for women.

### BEVERAGES: *Avoid Your Enemies*

Some common drinks might be considered birth control in a glass. If you're trying to get pregnant, Dr. Teitelbaum recommends that you stay away from the following beverages.

• Coffee. Drinking more than four cups a day—and possibly consuming any amount—can decrease fertility.
• Caffeinated soda. Just one drink of caffeinated soda a day can decrease your chances of becoming pregnant.
• Alcohol. If your infertility is caused by problems with ovulation, one drink a day can increase the difficulty of becoming pregnant by 30 percent. Having two drinks a day more than doubles the difficulty.

### IRON: *A Deficiency Could Be the Problem*

The typical blood test for iron includes a measurement of ferritin, a protein in the body that stores iron. While a woman may have ferritin levels that are high enough to prevent anemia, her levels may still be low enough to cause infertility, Dr. Teitelbaum says. He cites a study in which half of the women with low ferritin levels quickly became pregnant when they began taking iron.

If for some reason you can't have your ferritin levels checked, Dr. Teitelbaum says to take iron supplements for at least 4 months while trying to get pregnant. He recommends taking one tablet, or 50 milligrams, a day of the product Ferro-Sequels. You should take iron on an empty stomach, and don't take it within 6 hours of taking thyroid hormone, says Dr. Teitelbaum.

### VITAMIN C: *Women Should Cut Back*

One study found that doses higher than 1,000 milligrams of vitamin C a day can cause infertility in women, says Dr. Teitelbaum. He recommends that you take no more than 500 milligrams a day.

### VITAMIN B$_6$: *If You Have Irregular Periods*

In women who have irregular or absent periods, extra vitamin B$_6$ can boost fertility, Dr. Teitelbaum says. He recommends 50 milligrams a day.

### MULTIVITAMIN/MINERAL SUPPLEMENT: *A Must for Both Sexes*

Taking a multivitamin/mineral supplement is essential for optimum fertility, Dr. Teitelbaum says. He recommends My Favorite Multiple, manufactured by Natrol.

### Nutrition Advice for Men

Men can cause or contribute to infertility due to a low sperm count or poor sperm motility—that is, slow, sluggish sperm that are less likely to fertilize an egg. Here are Dr. Teitelbaum's nutritional suggestions for correcting those problems.

### VITAMIN C: *For a Better Sperm Count*

Supplementing the diet with vitamin C is thought to increase the number and speed of the sperm. Take 500 milligrams twice a day, Dr. Teitelbaum says.

### ARGININE: *For Healthier Sperm*

This amino acid can improve sperm count and motility, says Dr. Teitelbaum. If the problem is low sperm count, he recommends taking 4,000 milligrams a day. If the problem is poor motility, take 8,000 milligrams. Either l-arginine or free-form arginine is effective, he says.

Do not take arginine unless under the supervision of a knowledgeable medical doctor. Do not take it if you have genital herpes or if you are also using lysine supplements.

**ZINC:** *Another Way to Boost the Count*

Low sperm count can also be improved with the trace mineral zinc, Dr. Teitelbaum says. He recommends 30 milligrams a day for 4 months.

**ASTRAGALUS:** *More Motility*

The Chinese herb astragalus can improve sperm motility, says Dr. Teitelbaum. Follow the dosage recommendations on the label.

# *Drugs Aren't Enough for* **Inflammatory Bowel Disease**

The walls of a healthy colon are evenly coated with a protective layer called the mucosa. Viewed from the inside, this lining has a smooth surface that's a healthy shade of pink. In people with inflammatory bowel disease, however, the tissue becomes inflamed and irritated. Sometimes, it bleeds, causing bloody diarrhea.

The conventional treatment for inflammatory bowel disease, which is thought to occur when the body's immune system mistakenly attacks the intestine, is to give people powerful anti-inflammatory drugs. If those drugs don't help, they may be given even stronger ones with more serious side effects. And when that doesn't work, the only recourse may be to surgically remove the diseased part of the intestine.

"People may need prednisone and other anti-inflammatory drugs if a flare, or episode, of the disease is serious enough," says Patrick Donovan, N.D., a naturopathic physician in Seattle. "But once people are stable, there are more natural treatments that can reduce the inflammatory process without the side effects of drugs."

Inflammatory bowel disease, which actually includes two conditions, Crohn's disease and ulcerative colitis, is a serious condition that always requires professional care, Dr. Donovan says. Still, he believes that there are a number of natural home treatments that, when used under the supervision of a physician, can help reduce discomfort and limit damage to the intestinal wall. Dr. Donovan suggests that you check with your doctor for specific information, such as dosage guidelines, before trying any of these remedies.

### GLUTAMINE: *Nourishing the Small Intestine*

This amino acid is thought to "feed" the cells lining the small intestine. It can help correct the malabsorption of nutrients that can occur with Crohn's disease and also relieve symptoms, says Dr. Donovan.

### BUTYRATE: *Good for the Colon*

This supplement contains cal-butyric acid, a compound that is believed to help cells in the colon "regenerate and stay healthy," says Dr. Donovan. He recommends it for people who have colitis (inflammation of the colon). For maximum absorption, Dr. Donovan suggests a product called Cal-Mag Butyrate.

### BOSWELLIA AND TURMERIC: *More Help for Inflammation*

Another way to reduce inflammation in the intestine is with the herbs boswellia and turmeric (which contains the active ingredient curcumin). "These are very strong anti-inflammatory herbs with minimal side effects," Dr. Donovan says. He usually recommends a product called Marinecare, which also supplies extracts of sea cucumber.

### VITAMIN E: *Reining In Free Radicals*

Inflammatory bowel disease unleashes torrents of free radicals, unstable oxygen molecules that cause additional damage to intestinal cells. Vitamin E helps neutralize free radicals and can help minimize the damage, says Dr. Donovan.

# GUIDE TO
# PROFESSIONAL CARE

*Caution: You should use the alternative remedies discussed in this chapter only as part of a treatment program that is guided and monitored by a qualified medical doctor in partnership with a qualified alternative practitioner, both of whom are experienced in caring for your condition. Check with your conventional doctor before changing or stopping any conventional medical treatments or medications, and keep all of your doctors and/or alternative practitioners informed of all treatments that you are receiving.*

Inflammatory bowel disease is a complex condition that occurs in a variety of locations within the digestive tract and has several possible causes. When you're first having symptoms, which include frequent diarrhea, rectal bleeding, and painful cramping, there are a number of medical tests that should be performed to ensure an accurate diagnosis, says Patrick Donovan, N.D., a naturopathic physician in Seattle. These include stool tests to check for bacterial infections or parasites, a full blood count to evaluate the nutritional condition of the patient, an evaluation of the level of inflammation in the bowel, and a test to check for the presence of blood and other disease indicators in the stool.

Your physician may order a colonoscopy, which allows the doctor to visually inspect the colon and part of the small intestine. If he suspects Crohn's disease, he may want to use a procedure called endoscopy to look at the upper part of your intestinal tract. Finally, Dr. Donovan recommends simple blood tests to detect whether celiac disease or food allergies are aggravating the inflammation.

For the best care, Dr. Donovan says, people with inflammatory bowel disease should work with two practitioners, a gastroenterologist and a naturally oriented practitioner who understands nutritional treatments.

## VITAMINS AND MINERALS: *Prevent Malnutrition*

One reason that inflammatory bowel disease, specifically Crohn's disease, is so serious is that the small intestine may lose its ability to absorb essential nutrients. Dr. Donovan believes that everyone with this condition should take a high-potency multivitamin/mineral supplement daily.

Individual supplements may be necessary in addition to the multivitamin, Dr. Donovan adds. Vitamin A is thought to help regenerate the damaged lining of the gut. The same is true of folic acid, and a supplement is doubly important since some of the drugs used to treat this condition can reduce folic acid absorption. Zinc can help repair gut cells, and many people with inflammatory bowel disease are deficient in this mineral. Finally, since this disease may damage the area of the gut where vitamin $B_{12}$ is absorbed, a supplement is a must for many people.

## IRON: *Battling Anemia*

In his practice, Dr. Donovan finds that some people with Crohn's disease and most people with colitis have iron-deficiency anemia. The type of iron (ferrous sulfate) usually recommended for treating anemia, however, may worsen inflammation in people with inflammatory bowel disease, he says.

For his patients with anemia, Dr. Donovan recommends a supplement of ferritin, a nonirritating form of iron, as well as weekly injections of a liver compound that contains 40 milligrams of organic iron. (Ferritin supplements are available over the counter, but injections can be obtained only from your physician.)

## LIQUID DIETS: *Best for Flare-Ups*

Inflammatory bowel disease typically has both quiet and active periods. When the symptoms are flaring, Dr. Donovan recommends a liquid diet of herbal tea, high-protein broth (such as fish, chicken, or meat broth), and fresh vegetable juices. This allows the body to absorb essential nutrients without having to do the extra work of digesting solid foods, he says. You should use a liquid diet only under the supervision of your doctor, he adds.

**FATTY ACIDS:** *Reduce Inflammation and the Risk of Cancer*

People with inflammatory bowel disease may have a higher risk of colon cancer than those without the disease. The fatty acids in fish oils, which are found in supplements labeled EPA (eicosapentaenoic acid) and DHA (docosahexaenoic acid), are thought to help inhibit chemical reactions in the body that produce inflammation, and they may reduce the risk of colon cancer as well.

# *Heart-to-Heart Exercises for Couples Can Boost* Inhibited Sexual Desire

There are a lot of reasons that interest in sex diminishes in a relationship.

"It could be stress, overwork, or child-rearing responsibilities, all of which create barriers to a regular and satisfying sex life," says Seth Prosterman, Ph.D., a sex therapist and licensed marriage and family therapist in San Francisco.

The biggest reason, however, according to Dr. Prosterman, is the same one that often leads partners to divorce: Lack of communication. When thoughts and feelings aren't shared, intimacy withers, and so does sexuality.

To make the relationship—and the sex—fresh and exciting again, both partners first have to decide that they truly want to be intimate. Even then, there's no quick fix, but there are steps recommended by alternative practitioners that can help in the delicate process of increasing intimacy and restoring your sexual connection.

**YOGA:** *Two Hearts Beat As One*

Paul and Marilena Silbey of American Tantra in Fairfax, California, creators of the video "Intimate Secrets of Sex and Spirit," recommend a yoga exercise that brings more energy to the "heart chakra," the area in the chest that, according to yoga teaching, is the energetic center of love and intimacy.

Sit cross-legged on the bed facing each other, perhaps with the woman sitting in the man's lap with her legs around him and his around her, as if making love sitting up. If that isn't comfortable, you can stand and face each other. Then each of you should put your left hand over the other's heart and your right hand palm-down over the other's left hand.

Next, look into each other's eyes and synchronize your breathing, inhaling and exhaling together. Feel that all of the energy coming out of your eyes is flowing into the other person and that this energy then comes out of their hands and arms into you. Also feel that your energy is flowing into your hands and into the other person.

Do this as often and for as long as you find pleasurable, say the Silbeys. "This exercise creates a circular flow of energy between the two partners, uniting them at the heart chakra," says Paul Silbey.

You should do the exercise, either clothed or unclothed, in a private environment that fosters intimacy. If it leads you to express your intimacy in a sexual way, that's great, say the Silbeys.

### BREATHING: *Feeding the Heart*

"Face each other and look into each other's eyes," says Paul Silbey. "Not at the newspaper, not at the bills, not out the window, but really focusing on the eyes."

Next, begin to breathe together slowly and deeply. On each exhalation, each of you should sigh audibly, making the sound "a...a...h...h."

"This sound feeds the heart just as water feeds a plant," says Marilena Silbey. It also creates a field of energy around the couple, increasing intimacy, she says. Do this exercise in any private environment that promotes intimacy for 1, 5, or 10 minutes, or however long you want to stay in the pleasurable field of energy that you're creating with your partner.

### TOUCHING: *Do an Erogenous Zone Search*

If it's been a long time since you've had enjoyable sex with your partner, or if sex has been infrequent for many months, it

---

# GUIDE TO
# PROFESSIONAL CARE

Inhibited sexual desire can be a complex problem that requires professional help. If sexual frequency has become a troubling issue in your relationship, both partners should see a sex therapist together.

If your own level of desire has suddenly plummeted, particularly if you're over 40, see a medical doctor who understands and treats hormone imbalances, which may be the cause of the problem, says Eugene Shippen, M.D., a physician in Shillington, Pennsylvania.

Dr. Shippen also counsels women and men to have both their primary care physicians and their pharmacists evaluate their medications, since many drugs (particularly those for high blood pressure) can decrease sex drive.

---

may be time for an exercise called the erogenous zone search, says Dr. Prosterman.

"The point of this exercise isn't to 'get sexy' with your partner but to discover new things about each other's sensuality so you can bring that newness into your sex," he says.

Touch all the areas of your partner's body—feet, legs, buttocks, hips, belly, chest, back, arms, hands, neck, face, and ears—with light, short strokes. When one partner is finished, the other starts. As you do the exercise, the partner being touched rates the pleasurable level of each area that's stroked on a scale of plus 3 to minus 3, with 0 being neutral.

You may also want to do a similar exercise called guided touching, in which you tell your partner what kind of genital touch you find sexually stimulating.

"Be very specific," says Dr. Prosterman. For example, the woman might say, "I like it when you touch my clitoris on the left side," or the man might say, "The head of my penis is too sensitive for that firm a stroke."

Keep in mind that this type of communication during a sexual encounter often leads to frustration. "It's much better to take the time outside of sex to discover how your partner likes to be touched, " says Dr. Prosterman.

## TRADITIONAL CHINESE MEDICINE: *Herbs That Heighten Desire*

A number of Chinese herbs are thought to help stimulate sexual desire, says Christopher Hobbs, an herbalist and expert in Traditional Chinese Medicine in Santa Cruz, California.

He recommends taking a supplement of one or more of the following Chinese herbs and herbal formulas: Asian (panax) ginseng, ligustrum, denodrobium, or the Chinese formula called 8-Flavor Tea Pills. Follow the dosage recommendations on the product label.

## FLOWER ESSENCES: *Increase Your Motivation*

Bach flower remedies—flower-derived tinctures that help balance emotions—can energize a woman's sexual desire, says Judy Howard, a nurse and director of training at the Bach Centre in Sotwell, England.

If you feel a complete lack of interest each time your partner approaches you, try the remedy hornbean, she says.

If you feel that your sex life is in a rut, and you want to focus on bringing more excitement into your sexual play, try wild rose. "This remedy will help you feel motivated to bring your sex life back to life," she says.

If your lack of sexual desire is caused by fatigue, try olive, Howard suggests.

# *Meditation, Not Medication,*
# *Is One Way to Beat*
# **Insomnia**

What's the best treatment for insomnia?

Ask most doctors that question, and they'll have a ready answer (and a ready prescription): Sleeping pills.

"The majority of physicians consider sleeping pills to be the most effective treatment for insomnia—which they are not—and continue to overprescribe them," says Gregg Jacobs, Ph.D., an insomnia specialist at the sleep disorders center of Beth Israel Deaconess Medical Center in Boston.

Dr. Jacobs considers sleeping pills to be overprescribed because he says they don't address the cause of insomnia, are potentially addictive, and can actually make insomnia worse.

"Sleeping pills can be effective for the treatment of short-term insomnia," Dr. Jacobs says. "But they can become increasingly ineffective with regular use, and they can cause many side effects that far outweigh their moderate benefits."

Another reason that Dr. Jacobs considers sleeping pills to be overprescribed is that most people with insomnia can reduce or eliminate their sleep problems without drugs, using natural self-help methods.

## THE RELAXATION RESPONSE: *Put Stress to Sleep*

Stress is everywhere, from time pressures to noise pollution and family problems, from information overload to money worries. And too much stress can ruin sleep.

"Stressful life events are the most common precipitators of chronic insomnia," says Dr. Jacobs. You can learn a technique to help your mind and body defuse the negative effects of stress; it's called the relaxation response.

Research has shown that the relaxation response is an effective treatment for insomnia, says Dr. Jacobs. To help beat insomnia, practice the relaxation response for 10 to 20 minutes a

# GUIDE TO PROFESSIONAL CARE

Nondrug remedies are fine to use as an initial treatment approach to chronic insomnia, says Gregg Jacobs, Ph.D., an insomnia specialist at the sleep disorders center of Beth Israel Deaconess Medical Center in Boston.

If nondrug techniques don't work, however, you should contact the sleep disorders center nearest you and ask for an appointment with a psychologist or physician who specializes in behavioral techniques for insomnia.

While Dr. Jacobs says that the majority of people with chronic insomnia don't have underlying physical or mental problems, he recommends a complete medical exam to rule out possible causes such as sleep apnea or depression.

day, he says. Find the time of day that works best for you, then reserve that time every day to de-stress your life. Here's how to do it.

**1.** Choose a quiet place where you won't be disturbed by noise, people, or pets. Sit or lie in a comfortable position and close your eyes. If you fall asleep during the relaxation response, that's fine, but set an alarm for 20 minutes in case you do doze off, and don't do the exercise within an hour or two of bedtime because you might have a harder time falling asleep when you go to bed.

**2.** Focus your attention on each body part and feel relaxation spreading through them: your feet, calves, thighs, stomach, chest, back, hands, forearms, upper arms, shoulders, neck, jaw, cheeks, eyes, and forehead. You may notice warmth, tingling, or heaviness, or you may just feel the body part. "At the end of this exercise, take a few moments to concentrate on how your entire body is relaxed," says Dr. Jacobs.

**3.** To monitor your breathing, place one hand on your stomach and the other hand on your chest. "If you are breathing abdominally, only the hand on your stomach will move," he says. "As you breathe abdominally, respiration will

slow and deepen naturally." Deep, abdominal breathing is more relaxing than shallow chest breathing, says Dr. Jacobs.
**4.** Your muscles are relaxed. You're breathing deeply. Then, says Dr. Jacobs, "direct your attention from everyday thoughts by using a mental focusing device that is neutral and repetitive." He recommends a word such as *one*, *relax*, *peace*, or *heavy*. "For many people, it is helpful to repeat the word silently with each exhalation," he says.

You can also focus on a visual image of an enjoyable, relaxing place, says Dr. Jacobs. Imagine a vacation spot; a beach, meadow, or mountain; a place in a book, magazine, or movie; or floating on a cloud.

## Escape the Sleeping Pill Trap

Sleeping pills are a nightmare.

Consider benzodiazepines, or BZs, tranquilizers that are commonly prescribed for insomnia. According to Gregg Jacobs, Ph.D., an insomnia specialist at the sleep disorders center of Beth Israel Deaconess Medical Center in Boston, people who use them still take an average of 46 minutes to fall asleep. Because the drugs cloud thinking and memory, however, they make insomniacs forget that they were awake during the night.

These medications can interfere with normal brain functioning, causing light, poor-quality sleep. They can also cause a hangover, making you even less effective at the day's tasks than you would be if you didn't sleep well. And, to add insult to insomnia, the brain quickly becomes accustomed to the drugs. After 4 to 6 weeks of nightly use, they're no longer effective. "Yet, surprisingly, BZs are routinely prescribed by physicians for months or even years," says Dr. Jacobs.

And, he says, longtime users who stop taking the drugs can experience rebound insomnia, which is worse than the original problem and can make people start taking the drug again. In other words, BZs are addictive.

"Ultimately, this trap results in chronic use of sleeping pills that persists for years and causes psychological dependency and feelings of loss of control," says Dr. Jacobs. Other types of sleeping pills, such as antidepressants and over-the-counter products, are no better, he says.

You can escape the sleeping pill trap by gradually reducing your medication, says Dr. Jacobs. He recommends not starting to reduce your medication when your life is exceptionally hectic or stressful, however. He also advises telling someone close to you (along with your doctor) that you are implementing these techniques so that you'll have social support. Here's how to sleep drug-free.

First, start using the alternative home remedies offered by Dr. Jacobs in this chapter. Next, on one of the nights that you take medication, cut your dose in half. The best time is a weekend night, when the following day offers few pressures.

Once you're sleeping well on this reduced-dosage night, which may happen right away or may take a few weeks, cut your dose in half on another of the nights that you take medication. Space the two reduction nights far enough apart, Dr. Jacobs says, "so that if you don't sleep well, you won't experience disturbed sleep for two nights in a row."

Continue with this night-by-night process until you have cut the dose in half on all the nights that you take sleep medication. "At all costs, avoid going back to the original dose," says Dr. Jacobs.

Next, eliminate the remaining half-dose in the same gradual fashion, first on one night a week, then on two, and so on, until you're medication-free. "If you are taking multiple medications for sleep, use these techniques to get off one first, then work on reducing the second medication," he says.

If you've been on medications for a long time, you may need the help of a behavioral psychologist or a sleep disorders center to reduce your medication, says Dr. Jacobs. But you can do it, no matter how long you've been on sleeping pills. "If you follow these medication-reduction guidelines, you can overcome your dependency on sleeping pills as many of my patients have," he says.

## SUNLIGHT: *Rays Yourself from the Dead Tired*

Sunlight regulates melatonin, a brain chemical that controls body temperature. Normal rhythms in body temperature create normal sleep, which is why too little exposure to sunlight can cause insomnia, says Dr. Jacobs.

If you have trouble falling asleep, you need more early-morning sunlight, says Dr. Jacobs. Open the drapes or shades immediately upon awakening, eat breakfast near a sun-exposed window, avoid dark sunglasses in the morning, and take an early-morning walk.

If you wake up too early in the morning, you need more late-day sunlight, he says. Avoid dark sunglasses late in the day, take a late-afternoon walk, sit near a sun-exposed window the hour before sunset, and leave the drapes open until dark.

## CARBOHYDRATES: *The Best Bedtime Snack*

A high-carbohydrate snack such as bread, bagels, or crackers eaten immediately before bedtime can increase serotonin, a brain chemical that promotes sleep, says Dr. Jacobs.

## POSITIVE THINKING: *Change Your Thoughts, Change Your Sleep*

Negative sleep thoughts can keep you awake, says Dr. Jacobs. "When they occur at bedtime or while you are awake in the middle of the night, negative sleep thoughts have a forceful effect on making you feel anxious and frustrated, creating another night of insomnia." These troubling thoughts include phrases such as the following.

- I don't think I can fall back to sleep.
- I can't fall asleep without a sleeping pill.
- This is going to be another night of insomnia.
- My insomnia is getting worse.
- I need more sleep.

If you recognize negative thoughts and replace them with positive ones, you will be less anxious and frustrated about insomnia, says Dr. Jacobs. "As a result, you will relax and sleep better."

In the morning, says Dr. Jacobs, "write down any negative sleep thoughts that you experienced at bedtime, while awake during the night, or upon rising from bed in the morning." Then, write a positive thought below that list. For example, positive thoughts to counter the negative ones above could include:

- I always fall back to sleep sooner or later.
- I need less sleep than I thought.
- My sleep is getting better and better.
- My sleep will improve as I use positive sleep thoughts rather than negative sleep thoughts.

Each morning, write down one or more positive sleep thoughts. "By practicing this every day, you will start to think more positively and confidently about sleep, you'll gain more control over sleep, and you'll soon start to sleep better," Dr. Jacobs says.

## TRADITIONAL CHINESE MEDICINE: *Massage for Restful Sleep*

Self-massage from Traditional Chinese Medicine is an effective alternative home remedy for insomnia, says Bob Flaws, a licensed acupuncturist and expert in Chinese medicine in Boulder, Colorado.

Massage balances the chi, or life-energy, in your body, allowing you to fall asleep more easily. Flaws recommends doing this massage right before you lie down and turn off the light. The best results come with daily practice over a period of weeks and months.

"As you massage, calmly focus on the physical sensations under your hands, and don't let your mind wander to your worries about today or tomorrow," he says. The entire massage should take 20 to 30 minutes. (For the locations of the acupressure points, see An Illustrated Guide to Acupressure Points on page 700.)

1. Start by pressing and kneading the center and top of your skull, which helps calm the entire body. Do this about 100 times. This massage also works acupressure points on your head.
2. Use the fingertips of both hands to knead the ends of your eyebrows closest to the bridge of your nose, which stimulates acupressure point BL2. Do this about 30 times.
3. With your index fingers and thumbs, massage the upper edges of the bones in your eye sockets, then do the lower edges. Work from the inner corners of the eyes to the outer corners 20 to 30 times.
4. Rub the palms of your hands together vigorously until they feel warm. Place your warm palms over both eyes and keep them there for 30 to 60 seconds. Very lightly rub your closed eyes 10 times.
5. Find the depressions just below the base of your skull on the back of your neck, midway between the bones behind your ears and the muscles on either side of your spine. These points are known as GB20. "It's where most people instinctively massage

when they have a tension headache or stiff neck," says Flaws. With both hands, press and knead both points 30 to 50 times.

**6.** Using the palm of your hand, rub circles around the center of your upper abdomen, then do the same on your lower abdomen. On each area, rub first clockwise and then counterclockwise, about 100 times in each direction.

**7.** Find the point on the inside of your forearm between the two tendons, approximately 1½ inches above the wrist. This point is known as PE6 in acupressure. With your thumb, press and knead the point on your left arm, then do the right arm, 30 to 50 times on each side.

**8.** Find acupressure point HE7 at the crease of your wrist right below the base of your pinky finger. Massage the point on each wrist 30 to 50 times.

**9.** Find the point located 3 inches below the lower outside edge of your kneecap when your leg is bent; it's in a depression between the muscles of the lower leg. Massage the point on each leg 30 to 50 times. This is acupressure point ST36.

**10.** Find the point 3 inches above the tip of your inner anklebone on the back of your lower leg. In acupressure, this point is known as SP6. Massage 30 to 50 times on each ankle.

**11.** Stimulate the acupressure point KI1, located in the depression just behind the ball of your foot toward the heel. Use the palm of the opposite hand until the palm feels hot. Repeat on the other foot.

## Three Homeopathic Remedies
## for Three Types of Insomnia

The simple remedies of homeopathy can help almost anyone sleep better, says Steve Nenninger, N.D., a naturopathic physician in New York City. For each of these remedies, take the 30C potency, letting three pellets dissolve under your tongue three times a day, for as long as symptoms persist, he says. Here are his recommendations.

### IGNATIA AMARA: *If You Can't Fall Asleep*
This remedy works best for people who have trouble falling asleep and who have a past history of grief, says Dr. Nenninger.

**ARSENICUM ALBUM:** *If You Wake Up in the Middle of the Night*

This is the right remedy if you wake up in the middle of the night feeling anxious or restless and take a long time to fall back to sleep, says Dr. Nenninger.

**NUX VOMICA:** *If You Wake Up Early in the Morning*

If you wake up early in the morning worrying about business or stressful events, and you can't fall back to sleep, use Nux vomica, says Dr. Nenninger.

# *Walk Away From the Pain of* **Intermittent Claudication**

When you have intermittent claudication, the arteries that feed the muscles of your legs are blocked. The resulting calf discomfort can range from painful to debilitating.

The typical drug treatment for intermittent claudication consists of two medications that improve circulation by "thinning" the blood: pentoxifylline (Trental) and aspirin.

Some patients with the problem end up having surgery that's similar to a heart bypass. Arteries are "stripped" from another part of the body and implanted in the legs. Or patients undergo angioplasty, in which a balloon-like device is inserted into the artery and inflated, clearing the blockage. Another alternative is stenting, which uses a balloon-like device along with wire mesh, which is left within the artery to keep it open.

But Seth Baum, M.D., an integrative cardiologist and founder of the Baum Center for Integrative Heart Care in Boca Raton, Florida, has found that unless symptoms are extremely debilitating or a patient may be facing amputation, natural approaches for intermittent claudication are actually superior to conventional approaches.

## CARNITINE: *Alternative Fuel for Muscles*

This supplement is similar to an amino acid, a component of protein. Many practitioners believe that it helps muscle cells work even when they're not getting enough oxygen by supplying them with higher levels of fatty acids, a nutritional fuel.

For someone with intermittent claudication—someone whose leg muscle cells can't get enough oxygen and are desperately in need of another type of fuel—carnitine may be a godsend.

# GUIDE TO PROFESSIONAL CARE

Intermittent claudication can be a real pain—usually a burning, cramplike sensation that typically hits after you've walked short distances. If you have intermittent claudication, it's almost certain that you have severe arterial disease in other parts of your body and are at risk for heart attack and stroke. Thus, you must be under the supervision of a medical doctor, who will treat you for clogged arteries, says Glenn S. Rothfeld, M.D., regional medical director of American WholeHealth in Arlington, Massachusetts.

But, according to Julian Whitaker, M.D., founder and director of the Whitaker Wellness Institute in Newport Beach, California, you should consider choosing an alternative physician who uses EDTA chelation, a series of intravenous treatments that Dr. Whitaker believes can clear clogged arteries.

"This is a highly controversial therapy among conventional doctors, but I think it's one of the best therapies for intermittent claudication," he says. "Every cardiologist and internist has had intermittent claudication patients who have been scheduled for amputation. Well, I have seen many such patients who were going to have their lower limbs removed and who were saved from this procedure by chelation therapy."

To control the painful symptoms of intermittent claudication, you may also want to try acupuncture. "Acupuncture is based on the circulation of life-energy, called chi. The improved circulation can lessen pain and improve function," Dr. Rothfeld says.

"Eighty percent of my patients with intermittent claudication who take carnitine either have a complete resolution of symptoms or can walk significantly farther without pain," says Dr. Baum.

The key factor in using this nutrient is making sure that you get enough. Dr. Baum has found that the best level is 2,000 milligrams twice a day. Carnitine has no significant side effects, he says, and it's safe to use indefinitely.

## GINKGO: *Outperforms Prescription Drugs*

Several studies show that the herb ginkgo lets people with intermittent claudication walk farther without pain, says Glenn S. Rothfeld, M.D., regional medical director of American Whole-Health in Arlington, Massachusetts.

In fact, numerous studies tested the herb against placebos (inactive substances) or pharmaceutical drugs commonly used to treat the disease. The studies confirmed ginkgo's ability to increase walking capacity, and many of them have shown that ginkgo improves circulation.

Dr. Rothfeld gives his patients a 24 percent extract of 40 milligrams of ginkgo three times a day. It's safe to take this dosage for 3 months, then take a month off. If you are taking a blood-thinning medication such as warfarin (Coumadin), however, do not use ginkgo.

## VITAMIN E: *Improves Circulation*

Dr. Rothfeld has all of his intermittent claudication patients take 400 international units of vitamin E daily. He says that studies have shown that people with intermittent claudication who took that level of vitamin E every day could walk farther without pain. "It probably works by making blood less 'sticky,' improving circulation," he says. It's safe to take this longterm.

## NIACIN: *For Your Arteries*

The B vitamin niacin is thought to help widen arteries, bringing more oxygen to the leg muscles. Studies show that niacin can help people with intermittent claudication increase the distance that they can walk, says Dr. Rothfeld.

He recommends a special form of niacin called inositol hexaniacinate (or inositol hexanicotinate), which he believes is the most effective form for people with intermittent claudication.

It's also the safest. It doesn't cause liver problems, a possible side effect of niacin, nor does it trigger a "niacin flush," the overheated, itchy, red-faced reaction that some people develop after taking the niacin, he says.

He suggests taking 500 milligrams twice daily. Try it for 3 months, then take a month off.

## OMEGA-3 FATTY ACIDS: *For Efficient Oxygen Delivery*

The type of fats found in fish oil, known as omega-3 fatty acids, are thought to soften the membranes of red blood cells so that they can more easily deliver their oxygen to muscle cells.

Jill Stansbury, N.D., chair of the botanical medicine department at the National College of Naturopathic Medicine in Portland, Oregon, recommends that people with intermittent claudication take a 500- to 1,000-milligram omega-3 supplement daily, following the dosage recommendations on the label. It's safe to take this longterm.

There's one caution, however. Since fish oils can possibly contribute to nosebleeds and easy bruising, and may cause upset stomach, do not take them if you take blood thinners or use aspirin regularly.

## YOGA: *Make a Shoulder Stand*

The shoulder stand is a yoga posture that can help improve leg circulation in people with intermittent claudication, says Dr. Rothfeld. Here's how to do the pose.

Lie on your back with your knees bent, your feet flat on the floor, and your arms at your sides with your palms down. As you exhale, push your palms down and draw your knees in and up. Then straighten your legs as you raise your hips (*a*).

Bend your elbows, place your hands on the back of your pelvis, and slide your hands up to your lower back as you continue to raise your hips. Keep your legs straight, but don't lock your knees. Your feet should be directly over your head (*b*). Stay in this position for as long as you feel comfortable, up to 5 minutes.

Next, ease your hips to the floor, using your hands for support, then bend your knees and lower your feet to the floor. Dr. Rothfeld says to do the pose once or twice a day.

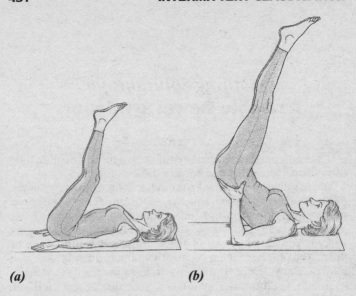

*(a)*                                        *(b)*

## HYDROTHERAPY: *Get Back in Circulation with Foot Baths*

A hot-and-cold foot bath first expands and then constricts the arteries in your legs, creating a pumping action that stimulates circulation, says Mark Stengler, N.D., a naturopathic physician in San Diego.

You'll need two basins large enough to hold both feet. Fill one with cold water and the other with hot water (be sure that it's not painfully hot). Put your feet in the hot water for 1 minute, then put them in the cold water for 20 seconds. Repeat this sequence three times. For best results, use these foot baths three or four times a day, says Dr. Stengler.

## *Soothing Solutions for*
# Irritable Bowel Syndrome

It's the mongrel of digestive disorders, a motley combination of intestinal woes that can be very difficult to tame.

You may have abdominal pain in the form of cramps, aches, or sharp, burning stabs. You may have problems with bowel movements, either constipation or diarrhea or a seesaw of both. You may have raging indigestion—gas, bloating, belching, or nausea. You may have all of these symptoms or just some of them. You may have them constantly or intermittently. And you may have any degree of discomfort, from miserable to mild.

To add insult to intestinal injury, your doctor can't tell you what causes your irritable bowel syndrome (IBS). Medical science hasn't figured out what triggers it, which is why physicians call it a functional disorder, meaning a problem with no obvious cause.

About all they can do is treat the symptoms. Your doctor may give you a prescription for abdominal cramps, another for diarrhea, and maybe even a tranquilizer for your nerves, since stress can worsen the symptoms.

What most doctors don't know is that it may be possible to eliminate the symptoms of IBS—in effect, curing the problem—without drugs, says Tammy Born, D.O., an osteopathic physician and director of the Born Preventive Health Care Clinic in Grand Rapids, Michigan.

"Doctors are not taught in medical school that there are effective treatments for irritable bowel syndrome," Dr. Born says. "But you can solve this problem." Here are some natural ways to reduce symptoms and restore the health of your intestinal tract.

### PEPPERMINT: *It's Strong Medicine*

"This is my number one recommendation for reducing the symptoms of irritable bowel syndrome," says Andrew Gaed-

# GUIDE TO
# PROFESSIONAL CARE

If you're having one or more symptoms of irritable bowel syndrome, such as diarrhea or bloating, that don't go away within 2 to 4 weeks, you'll want to consider seeing a gastroenterologist, a specialist in digestive conditions. It's important to be sure that you don't have a serious digestive problem, such as intestinal cancer or inflammatory bowel disease, that has similar symptoms, says William B. Salt II, M.D., clinical associate professor of medicine at Ohio State University College of Medicine and Public Health in Columbus.

It's important, however, to find a gastroenterologist who's willing to begin by putting you on a self-help program and then examine you after 6 to 8 weeks to see how you're doing. If there has been no progress in reducing symptoms, you should be tested for more serious problems, says Dr. Salt. If you have additional symptoms such as fever, involuntary weight loss, blood in the stool, or a mass that's detected on abdominal examination, you will need immediate medical treatment rather than a self-help program.

Anyone who has symptoms of irritable bowel syndrome should be tested for food allergies, adds Tammy Born, D.O., an osteopathic physician and director of the Born Preventive Health Care Clinic in Grand Rapids, Michigan.

"Allergies to dairy products are particularly likely to cause bowel symptoms," Dr. Born says. You should also have a test called a comprehensive digestive stool analysis, which will detect other bowel abnormalities, such as unhealthy bacteria or a yeast infection. Only physicians who are experienced in alternative medicine are likely to order these additional tests, she says.

dert, a professional member of the American Herbalists Guild and director of the Get Well Clinic in Oakland, California.

Peppermint is thought to soothe the entire digestive tract, he explains. He recommends three or more cups of peppermint tea a day. Follow the directions on the package.

**MAGNESIUM GLYCINATE:** *Prevents Intestinal Spasms*

This mineral is believed to tone and relax the muscles of the intestinal tract, helping to prevent painful spasms, says Teresa Rispoli, Ph.D., a licensed nutritionist and acupuncturist in Agoura Hills, California. Follow the directions on the label.

**HYDROLIZED FISH PROTEIN:** *Repairs Intestinal Walls*

"This supplement has been exceptional in healing my patients with irritable bowel syndrome," says Dr. Born. Repairing the intestinal tract, which may have been damaged by medications, chemicals in foods, food allergies, stress, and other hazards of modern life, is the key to healing this condition, she explains.

She recommends a product called Seacure. "Taking two capsules before each meal can be an important part of the IBS puzzle," she says.

**DEEP BREATHING:** *Helps Neutralize Stress*

Breathing slowly and deeply helps to relieve stress in a hurry—and stress can play a major role in IBS, says Gerard L. Guillory, M.D., an internist in Aurora, Colorado.

If you begin to feel tense, place your hands over your abdomen and feel your stomach expand as you inhale. Inhale slowly and deeply through your nose, hold your breath for a second or two, then slowly exhale through your mouth. Do this several times until you feel relaxed, he advises.

## Dietary Keys to Healing

Changing the way you eat can bring permanent relief from the pain and discomfort of IBS, alternative practitioners say. Here is their best nutritional advice.

**INSOLUBLE FIBER:** *The Best Solution*

Adding more insoluble fiber (the kind found in whole grains) to your diet helps create firm, bulky stools. It normalizes digestion and may help relieve many of the symptoms of IBS, such as constipation, diarrhea, abdominal pain, and bloating, says Dawn Burstall, R.D., a registered dietitian in Halifax, Nova Scotia.

"Everyone with an irritable bowel needs between 20 and 35 grams of fiber daily," she says. Every day, says Burstall, eat three to five servings of wheat-based, whole-grain products, such as whole-wheat bread, wheat bran bread, whole-wheat crackers, wheat bran muffins, and whole-wheat cereal.

You should also eat one serving of a concentrated fiber source every day, such as a high-fiber cereal like All Bran, Fiber One, or Bran Buds with Psyllium. Or take a high-fiber bulking agent, such as Metamucil, Prodiem Plain, Normacol, or Citrucel. These sources supply 10 or more grams of fiber a day, says Burstall.

One caution, though. You should introduce high-fiber foods into your diet gradually, says Burstall. For the first 7 to 10 days, for example, eat only ¼ cup of very high fiber cereal, increasing the amount to ½ cup after 10 days. That will reduce some of the flatulence that can occur as your bowels adapt to more fiber.

Even if you experience a little discomfort, though, stick with your high-fiber diet, says Burstall. After 2 to 3 weeks, your bowels will adjust to the change, and your symptoms should start to go away.

## The Write Solution

Digestive tracts are as individual as fingerprints, which means that a food that is fine for one person with irritable bowel syndrome could be devastating for you. How can you discover and eliminate your unique trigger foods? By using a diet diary, says Gerard Guillory, M.D., an internist in Aurora, Colorado. "All you need is commitment, a pen or pencil, and a notebook," he says. Here's how to do it.

• Write down everything you eat and when you eat it. Details are crucial, says Dr. Guillory. Include brand names and the exact amount you ate, and don't forget about extras like salad dressings and beverages.
• Each time you record a food, write down the type of day you're having, such as "Rushing," "Late for work," or "Relaxing day at the beach." Also record your level of stress at the time of the meal, rating it from 1 to 5, with 1 being the lowest level and 5 being the highest.
• Record your symptoms. Anytime you have a symptom—abdominal pain, diarrhea, gas, belching, or any other kind of digestive discomfort—write down what happened and when.

Keep your diary for at least 2 weeks, says Dr. Guillory (a month is even better). Then examine the diary, looking for patterns such as the connection between foods, food groups, and symptoms.

"Many people are able to determine the specific food groups or circumstances that worsen their symptoms," he says. You might find, for example, that when you skip breakfast, eat a skimpy lunch, and have a large dinner late at night, your symptoms are particularly bad the next day. Or you might find that Chinese food always makes you feel worse. You might also discover that your symptoms are more related to factors that increase stress than to specific foods.

"Your diary can help you track down and eliminate any foods or lifestyle factors that are contributing to your symptoms," says Dr. Guillory.

## WATER: *The Key to Making High-Fiber Diets Work*

Eating a lot of dietary fiber won't do any good unless you drink eight 8-ounce glasses of water every day.

"Skip this, and the high-fiber diet will not work," says Burstall. That's because fiber is hydrophilic, meaning that it forms firm, bulky stools by attracting water. No water, no bulking—and no digestive benefits.

## LOW-FAT FOODS: *Good for the Gut*

Saturated fat (found in animal and dairy foods) is a common trigger for the symptoms of IBS, says William B. Salt II, M.D., clinical associate professor of medicine at Ohio State University College of Medicine and Public Health in Columbus. "It stimulates contractions in the gastrointestinal tract, causing cramping and diarrhea," he explains. He recommends following a low-fat diet.

## BUTTER: *Try a Teaspoon a Day*

Even though most saturated fats can worsen IBS, butter in small amounts may be an exception, according to some alternative practitioners. It's rich in butyric acid, which is believed to nourish the cells of the intestinal walls, says Dr. Rispoli.

## GAS-PRODUCING FOODS: *Take Precautions*

Eating a high-fiber diet and avoiding gas-producing foods is often the best combination for easing IBS, says Burstall. The worst gas offenders tend to be beans, cabbage, brussels sprouts, broccoli, and asparagus.

If those are among your favorite foods, try Beano, advises Dr. Guillory. It contains an enzyme that breaks down the indigestible carbohydrates in those foods that produce the gas. You can put a few drops of Beano on food before you eat it, or you can take Beano tablets before a meal. Cooking with Beano or putting it on piping-hot food may destroy the gas-preventing enzyme, says Dr. Guillory.

## CAFFEINE: *A Must to Avoid*

Eliminating caffeine is a must, says Dr. Salt. "It is a direct stimulant of the GI tract, and it can trigger or aggravate irritable bowel syndrome," he explains. So whether the caffeine is in coffee, tea, cola, or chocolate, your best bet is to stay away from it.

## ALCOHOL: *Beer Is the Worst*

Any alcoholic beverage can make IBS symptoms worse, but beer seems to be the major offender, says Dr. Guillory. In addition to alcohol's irritating effects, the carbonation can cause bloating and other discomfort.

# *Fly Naturally to Avoid*
# Jet Lag

You've just flown across four time zones, and now you only wish you could crash (fall asleep, that is). But your body doesn't believe the luminescent "11:45 P.M." on the digital clock in your hotel room. It's convinced that the correct time is 7:45 P.M.

Not only that, but you're beginning to realize that tomorrow, after the stress of travel and a major bout of sleep deprivation, you'll probably feel headachy, exhausted, and cranky and have the attention span of a 2-year-old.

In short, you'll have jet lag.

---

# GUIDE TO
## PROFESSIONAL CARE

Almost everyone can self-treat the symptoms of jet lag, says Martin Moore-Ede, M.D., Ph.D., former professor of physiology at Harvard University and president of Circadian Technologies in Cambridge, Massachusetts. The rare exceptions are people with conditions such as manic-depressive disorder, who are prone to psychotic events and for whom travel across time zones can trigger an episode of the disease that would require professional care.

---

Better take a sleeping pill while there's still time, right? Maybe not, says Martin Moore-Ede, M.D., Ph.D., former professor of physiology at Harvard University and president of Circadian Technologies in Cambridge, Massachusetts. "You'll probably only make things worse for yourself," he says.

That's because sleeping pills can cause a hangover, a leftover dose of daytime grogginess from the sedating medication. Since you haven't dealt with one of the main causes of jet lag—a disruption of your body's internal clock, which regulates your sleep-wake cycle—taking a sleeping pill might make it even harder for you to fall asleep tomorrow night. Instead of a sleeping pill, says Dr. Moore-Ede, you might want to consider nondrug methods to prevent or clear up the symptoms of jet lag.

### LIGHT: *Let the Sun Reset Your Internal Clock*
The "clock" in your brain is a tiny group of cells called the suprachiasmatic nuclei, or SCN. It's set by being exposed to bright light, Dr. Moore-Ede says. Thus, if you travel from east to west, try to get a dose of bright light in the evening. Taking a walk outside for about an hour is the simplest way. That will help delay your sleep-wake cycle, allowing you to go to bed and wake up later.

If you travel from west to east, go for that walk for an hour or two in the morning, which will help shift your body to an earlier bedtime.

**MELATONIN:** *Take a Small Amount at Bedtime*

The natural hormone melatonin can also help reset the sleep-wake cycle, says Beverly Yates, N.D., a naturopathic physician and director of the Natural Health Care Group in Seattle.

But the typical per-pill dose of most products—3 to 5 milligrams—is way too much, she says. She recommends looking for a 500-microgram (0.5 milligram) supplement, and starting to take it the day before your trip.

"When you're traveling, melatonin can help you fall asleep faster and sleep more deeply," Dr. Yates says. Take this supplement only under the supervision of a knowledgeable medical doctor.

**FOOD:** *Try the "Destination Diet"*

"A week to 3 days before they travel from a cold to a warm climate, I advise my patients to start eating more of the foods that they'll find at their destination, such as mangoes and papayas," says Dr. Yates.

Eating in this way helps the body adapt more quickly to the new climate and reduces the symptoms of jet lag, she says.

"Changing your diet to that of your destination tells your body that it is about to experience a change. By taking the changes in pieces rather than all at once, you can ease the shock of significant shifts in eating, sleeping, and general well-being. This technique helps smooth the transitions and stresses that travel can introduce," says Dr. Yates.

You'll also want to prepare for your return trip. "A day or two before you're about to return, start eating as you will when you get home," says Dr. Yates.

**WATER:** *Stay Hydrated*

Many of the symptoms of jet lag are really "wet lag," or dehydration. "The air in airplanes is extremely dry, so you should drink plenty of water to avoid dehydration," says Dr. Moore-Ede. He recommends 1 liter (about 34 ounces) of water for every 6 hours of flying.

Also, don't drink coffee or alcohol en route, he says. They're diuretics, which flush water out of your body.

**HOMEOPATHY:** *Arnica Softens Those Bruising Seats*

Sitting for hours in the cramped space of an airplane seat can beat up your body. To feel less achy, stiff, and bruised after a long flight, take the homeopathic remedy Arnica, says Dr. Yates. Take three tablets of the 30C potency three times a day, beginning the day before your flight and continuing on the day you fly and the day after.

# Nutritional Remedies
# Can Ward Off
# Kidney Stones

If you have had a kidney stone, ask your doctor if there are nutritional remedies that will prevent a recurrence. If your doctor says no, find another doctor.

That's the advice of Wynne A. Steinsnyder, D.O., an osteopathic physician and urologist in North Miami Beach. "There are readily available and effective forms of alternative therapies for preventing the recurrence of kidney stones," he says.

Once you've had that excruciatingly painful experience with a kidney stone—a dense collection of tiny, sharp-edged crystals that can tear the delicate tissues of your urinary tract as they exit from your body—you know that you don't want it to happen ever again.

Approximately 70 to 80 percent of kidney stones are composed of calcium oxalate crystals, while another 10 percent or so are made of uric acid crystals. (There are also a few other, relatively rare types.) You need to know the type of stone you had, because each type requires a slightly different preventive approach, Dr. Steinsnyder says.

If your first stone was recovered, your doctor may have analyzed its content. Another way to find out is for your doctor to analyze the sediment in your urine to see whether it contains traces of either calcium oxalate or uric acid crystals. Once you

## GUIDE TO
## PROFESSIONAL CARE

*Caution:* You should use the alternative remedies discussed in this chapter only as part of a treatment program that is guided and monitored by a qualified medical doctor in partnership with a qualified alternative practitioner, both of whom are experienced in caring for your condition. Check with your conventional doctor before changing or stopping any conventional medical treatments or medications, and keep all of your doctors and/or alternative practitioners informed of all treatments that you are receiving.

Kidney stones can be caused by a number of serious diseases, so if you've had an attack, see a doctor for a thorough evaluation, says Wynne A. Steinsnyder, D.O., an osteopathic physician and urologist in North Miami Beach.

Also, you should see a doctor immediately if you have an attack of kidney stones, especially if it is accompanied by pain that isn't relieved by drinking large amounts of fluids and taking over-the-counter painkillers, or blood in your urine or the inability to pass urine, or a fever, or pain near the kidneys (located in your lower back near the end of the rib cage).

know the composition of your stone, you can choose the remedies that are right for you.

## Calcium-Containing Stones

"There is no question that a typical high-fat, low-fiber Western diet causes calcium stones," Dr. Steinsnyder says. That type of diet increases both the calcium oxalate crystals in your urine and the factors that cause them to form a stone. Here are the nutritional remedies that he suggests.

### FOOD: *A High-Fat Chance of Getting Stones*

Lots of fat. Not much fiber. Plenty of white sugar and white flour. Heavy on the red meat. That's the recipe for many degenerative diseases, including heart problems and cancer. It's also the way to set yourself up for kidney stones, Dr. Steinsnyder says. The opposite type of diet—high in fiber, low in fat, easy on refined carbohydrates, and light on red meat—is the way to go, he says.

There are also some healthy foods that you should avoid with calcium stones. Certain leafy green vegetables, including spinach, Swiss chard, and beet greens, are high in oxalates, acids that the body cannot process and that are passed through the urine. For people who are sensitive to oxalates, eating too many of these greens can cause kidney stones.

## WATER: *Drink a Lot*

While you're eating all that healthy food, drink a lot of water, too. "Inadequate fluid intake is a major factor in allowing crystals to accumulate in the urine," Dr. Steinsnyder says. He tells his patients to drink six 8-ounce glasses of water a day.

## VITAMINS AND MINERALS: *An Anti-Stone Supplement Program*

The following vitamins and minerals can help prevent calcium stones, says Dr. Steinsnyder.

• Calcium: Surprisingly, this is the first and most important of the supplements. By binding to the oxalate in your body, calcium can help keep stones from forming. Take 600 milligrams a day.
• Magnesium and vitamin D: Use a calcium supplement that also supplies 300 milligrams of magnesium and 400 international units of vitamin D. These two nutrients aid in the absorption of calcium, and magnesium by itself can help block stone formation.
• Vitamin $B_6$: This vitamin can reduce the production and excretion of oxalates. Dr. Steinsnyder recommends 100 milligrams a day taken as part of a high-potency B-complex supplement.

## TRIBULUS TERRESTRIS: *Blocks Stone Formation*

This Ayurvedic herb, also known as gokshura, reduces the body's production of calcium oxalate and can help prevent calcium stones, Dr. Steinsnyder says. Follow the dosage recommendations on the label.

**EXERCISE:** *No Sweat*

Exercise helps keep calcium from draining out of the bones and ending up in the urine, where it could contribute to the formation of stones, Dr. Steinsnyder says. His recommendation is to walk briskly for 20 to 30 minutes a couple of times a week.

He also tells his patients with kidney stones not to go out to a gym and dehydrate themselves with a lot of sweaty exercise, however, since dehydration is a major risk factor for developing new stones.

## A Ginger Compress:
## Just What the Doctor Ordered

When Guillermo Asis, M.D., director of the Path to Health clinic in Burlington, Massachusetts, had an excruciating bout of kidney stones, he knew just what to do to relieve his pain. He made a compress, a soothing topical application of warm water and the herb ginger. Here are his instructions so that you can do the same if you need pain relief.

You'll need someone to help you with the procedure, and you'll also need to be careful that neither of you is burned while preparing the compress.

• Fill an 8-quart or larger pot with water and bring it to a boil.
• Use a piece of fresh ginger about the size of your palm. Wrap it in a piece of cheesecloth and attach a string so that it resembles a large tea bag, then put it into the boiling water for 2 to 3 minutes.
• Reduce the heat somewhat so that the water is hot but not boiling. Use the string to remove the cheesecloth bag, squeeze it over the pot so the juice from the softened ginger runs into the water, then replace the bag in the bottom of the pot.
• Next, remove the pot from the heat and soak a washcloth in the hot ginger water. Remove it and wring it out thoroughly so that it is wet but not dripping, and check the temperature. It should be hot but not scalding.
• Place the cloth on your lower back over the area of the affected kidney, put a piece of plastic (such as a small trash bag) directly on top of the compress, then put a dry towel on top of the plastic.

• Repeat the application of these three layers every 5 to 10 minutes for 30 to 45 minutes so that the area stays warm. If it's still painful in 12 hours, try a second application.

"When I had my attack and did this, I didn't need to take any painkillers, and my stone passed without strain," Dr. Asis says. The heat and moisture open the urinary duct, which is connected to the kidney, and allow maximum penetration of the pain-relieving ginger, he says.

## Uric Acid Stones

There are two keys to preventing a recurrence of uric acid stones, Dr. Steinsnyder says. One is to balance the chemistry, or pH, of your urine, keeping it as alkaline (as opposed to acid) as possible. Another is to limit your intake of purines, food components that increase uric acid. Here's the dietary advice to fulfill both goals.

### FOOD: *Dietary Do's and Don'ts*

Drink more orange, grapefruit, and tomato juice to keep the right pH balance. Aim for two to three glasses a day.

To reduce purines in your diet, avoid anchovies, sardines, meat extracts, gravies, liver, kidney, sweetbreads, and fried foods; don't eat more than 3 ounces of lean meat or one serving of oatmeal, oysters, crabs, tuna, ham, lima beans, asparagus, cauliflower, mushrooms, peas, or spinach daily.

Don't worry, however, if you occasionally violate any of these restrictions, Dr. Steinsnyder says. "Just drink more water than usual and take Alka-Seltzer, which alkalinizes your urine," he says. Follow the directions on the package.

### WATER: *Keep Drinking*

Aim for at least eight 8-ounce glasses of water a day to prevent uric acid stones, says Dr. Steinsnyder.

### Passing a Stone

If you're having a kidney stone attack, you should see a doctor immediately. In addition, there is an herb that helps stones pass more easily and therefore dramatically reduces the pain.

**CORN SILK:** *Reduces Friction*

Corn silk reduces friction as the stone moves along, says Dr. Steinsnyder. You can use capsules, liquid, or tea bags, following the dosage recommendations on the label.

# *Walking Away from*
# Knee Pain

The knee is composed of two bones (the femur and the tibia) balancing on one another and lashed in place on all sides by muscles and connective tissue. It is the only weight-bearing joint in the body with this design. And that makes the knee prone to arthritis, injuries, and pain.

While it is important to check with your doctor about any suspected knee injury or long-lasting pain to rule out serious damage to the knee, effective treatment may not necessarily need to focus on the knee joint.

"Often, the conventional medical approach to treating knee pain is to focus attention solely on the area that hurts—the knee itself," says Sharon Butler, a certified practitioner of Hellerwork (a structural bodywork and movement therapy) in Paoli, Pennsylvania. "Proper pain-free function of the knee relies on the balance of all muscles, tendons, and ligaments that wrap the knee joint. When one or more of these elements is tighter or more restricted than the others, knee pain is often the result."

Butler first evaluates the alignment and balance of the ankle joints. "If the ankle joints do not support the weight of the body evenly, by rolling either inward (pronation) or outward (supination), the bone of the lower leg becomes twisted, leading to

# GUIDE TO
# PROFESSIONAL CARE

According to Rosemary Agostini, M.D., a physician at the Virginia Mason Sports Medicine Center and clinical associate professor of orthopedics at the University of Washington, both in Seattle, you should see an orthopedist or medical doctor for diagnosis and treatment if you have stiffness and pain in one or both knees, especially if it lasts for more than 6 weeks; knee pain, swelling, or tenderness, especially swelling that occurs within 24 hours of an injury; or any other pain than interferes with mobility or daily activities.

One particularly effective alternative medical treatment for knee pain is reconstructive or neural-fascial therapy, says William Faber, D.O., an osteopathic physician and director of the Milwaukee Pain Clinic. The therapy consists of a series of injections of anesthetic into the joint, which helps stabilize tissue and strengthens the joint, cartilage, ligaments, and tendons.

"With each treatment, pain becomes less and less and disappears in almost all cases," says Dr. Faber.

---

strain in the soft tissues at the knee joint. This leaves the knee at particular risk for injury, especially in sports activities that put unusual strain on the knees, such as tennis, basketball, and jogging."

When ankle alignment problems are evident, Butler often chooses the following exercise to teach her patients how to walk properly and to help restore balance to the soft tissues of the knee.

**EXERCISE:** *Walk a Tightrope—on the Floor*

"This exercise helps align the ankle over the foot and the knee over the ankle, eliminating the type of structural misalignment that can cause knee pain," says Butler.

Find a place in your home that has a long, unobstructed area without any turns, such as a long hallway or a large room. Put two parallel lines of masking tape 6 inches apart on the floor.

In your bare feet, walk on the lines of tape. As you take each step, align the center of each heel and the second toe of each

foot with the inner edge of the tape. Just walk back and forth
for 5 minutes two or three times a day, recommends Butler.

"This gently corrects knee pain by educating you in a walking
style that transfers weight more appropriately through the knee
joint," she says.

## WALKING: *Watch Your Step*

When you're out for a walk, look down every once in a while
to see how your feet are "tracking," says Butler. Are your toes
pointing outward (a common habit)? Consciously use the foot
position that you use when you "walk the tightrope," she says.

## REFLEXOLOGY: *Treat the Knee Reflex Point*

Your feet have many reflex points, each of which corresponds to a particular part of the body. "Stimulating a reflex
point with a therapeutic-grade essential oil can relieve pain in
the corresponding body part," says Terri Moon, a certified massage technician and director of Touched by the Moon holistic
health center in Santa Rosa, California.

To find the knee reflex point, run a finger down the outside
edge of your foot. You'll encounter a protruding bony area midway between your heel and little toe; the reflex point is right below that spot on the bottom of the foot.

For ligament pain, mix one drop of lemongrass essential oil
with four to five drops of vegetable oil. Or, to regenerate nerve
tissue, Moon suggests substituting geranium oil for the lemongrass.

On the foot on the same side as your painful knee, put a
drop of the oil mixture on the knee reflex point and rub it in by
gently rolling your fingertips over the oil, advises Moon. If you
have trouble finding the reflex point, you can apply the diluted
oil all over your foot.

Use the oil once or twice a day until the pain is gone. After a
few days, the pain should be gone for good.

## ACUPRESSURE: *Keep Your Knee Pain-Free*

An acupressure point in the middle of the crease in the back
of the knee, called the commanding middle point, or BL54, releases a lot of inflammation from knee injuries, speeds healing,
and helps prevent subsequent injuries in people who have already injured a knee, says Alexander Majewski, a licensed mas-

sage therapist and director of the Acupressure Institute of
Alaska in Juneau.

"The results I've been getting with this point are tremendous,"
he says. "I treat a lot of snowboarders, who twist and turn more
than most folks and usually run into knee problems. When they
use this point, their injuries heal more quickly, and they're less
likely to reinjure themselves."

To find the point, bend your knee and place your thumb in the
crease located exactly between the two sides of the knee. (See
An Illustrated Guide to Acupressure Points on page 700.) Apply firm, steady pressure—not so hard that it's painful but not
so gently that you don't feel it—for 30 to 60 seconds. You can
also use your fingertips to rub gently in small circles around the
area of the point. You should treat the points on both knees.
Majewski recommends doing this throughout the day as needed
to relieve discomfort.

# *Easy Solutions for*
# Lactose Intolerance
# and Dairy Sensitivity

Ah, milk. It's right up there with Mom and apple pie as a national icon, a nutritional necessity (or so we're told) for strong
bones and sparkling teeth. Well, many alternative practitioners
say that all of those good things that you hear about milk are
white lies.

"Milk is not a perfect food, as is frequently advertised," says
Jacqueline Krohn, M.D., a physician in New Mexico. Milk, she
says, can cause allergic symptoms of all kinds, such as diarrhea, asthma, ear infections, rashes, and hives.

"Milk is a misunderstood and vastly overrated food," agrees
James Braly, M.D., an allergy specialist in Boca Raton, Florida.
"Ironically, while milk products are the most commonly con-
sumed foods, milk is one of the two or three most common
food allergens in the American diet," he says.

Most of the allergic symptoms caused by milk products don't

show up right away, which is why most people don't suspect milk as an allergen, he adds.

Along with the symptoms mentioned above, milk allergy can cause blood loss from gastrointestinal bleeding. At the same time, it can inhibit the absorption of iron, and iron deficiency is the most common nutritional problem in the United States. Plus, whole milk contains heart-hurting saturated fat.

Milk should not be part of the average person's diet, says Dr. Braly. "I believe that the greater majority of people worldwide are allergic to milk or are lactose intolerant, meaning that they lack the lactase enzyme necessary to digest milk sugar, called lactose," he explains.

So, if you have the digestive symptoms of lactose intolerance (bloating, cramping, diarrhea, and flatulence), or other symptoms that keep coming back, you may want to experiment with a dairy-free, lactose-free diet.

**DAIRY-FREE DIET:** *Try It for 10 Days*

To find out if you're sensitive to milk, cut out all dairy products for 10 days and see how you feel, says Elizabeth Lipski, a certified clinical nutritionist in Kauai, Hawaii. If your symptoms vanish during the 10 days and then return when you reintroduce dairy into your diet, you probably do have a sensitivity, she says.

You'll want to avoid obvious sources of lactose, such as milk, yogurt, ice cream, creamed soups, frozen yogurt, powdered milk, and whipped cream. But, says Lipski, you'll also need to be wary of dairy products used in bakery items, cookies, hot dogs, lunch meats, milk chocolate, most nondairy creamers, pancakes, protein powder drinks, and ranch dressing. Look at the ingredient lists on food packages and avoid anything that contains the dairy components casein, caseinate, lactose, sodium caseinate, or whey.

If you're not sure whether a food contains dairy, avoid it during the 10-day period. During the test, "it's probably best to eat all your meals at home or prepare all food yourself," Lipski says.

**MILK SUBSTITUTES:** *Satisfaction for the Sensitive*

If you find that you're lactose-intolerant or sensitive to milk but don't want to give it up entirely, try a milk substitute, says

## GUIDE TO PROFESSIONAL CARE

Lactose intolerance or dairy sensitivity is not usually a serious medical problem. As long as you avoid dairy in all its different forms, the symptoms will disappear. But many people don't know that they're lactose intolerant or sensitive to milk; all they know is that they feel lousy a lot of the time.

"In my experience, milk drinkers are often full of mucus," says Skye Weintraub, N.D., a naturopathic physician in Eugene, Oregon. "They tend to have more sinus infections, coughs, headaches, ear infections, postnasal drip, and colds than non-milk drinkers."

In some people, dairy foods may cause other, more serious problems, such as gallbladder attacks, irritable bowel syndrome, and even ulcers.

Since many of the symptoms of lactose intolerance and dairy sensitivity can mimic symptoms of serious illnesses, you should see your doctor to find out what's going on. Lactose intolerance can often be diagnosed in the office with a simple test called a hydrogen breath test. In addition, your doctor may give you a blood test for delayed milk allergy to see if you're reacting to something else in milk besides the lactose.

Lipski. Look for Lactaid milk, which includes the lactose-digesting enzyme, lactase. Or try soy milk, rice milk, almond milk, or any one of the many other milk substitutes on the market.

**LACTASE:** *Take It with Meals*
One way to enjoy dairy foods if you're lactose intolerant is to take a lactase supplement such as Lactaid in drops, tablets, or capsules. Take the supplement with any meal that includes dairy foods, following the directions on the label, says William B. Salt II, M.D., clinical associate professor of medicine at Ohio State University College of Medicine and Public Health in Columbus. The enzyme in the supplements will help you digest the lactose in dairy foods, he explains.

## LOWER-LACTOSE DAIRY: *You May Be Able to Eat It*

Some people with conditions such as lactose intolerance or milk sensitivity can tolerate small amounts of plain yogurt, processed cheese, goat's milk, or fat-free milk, all of which have smaller amounts of both lactose and some of the allergy-causing components of whole milk, says Skye Weintraub, N.D., a naturopathic physician in Eugene, Oregon.

## CALCIUM: *You Have to Get It*

"There are many sources of calcium other than cow's milk," says Dr. Braly. Good fish and seafood sources include canned salmon, sardines, shrimp, clams, crab, oysters, cod, and haddock. Good vegetable sources include kelp, collard greens, turnip greens, broccoli, cabbage, carrots, parsley, watercress, romaine lettuce, summer squash, and onions.

Among grains and nuts, you can get good amounts of calcium from pistachios, sesame seeds, sesame butter, oat flakes, buckwheat, and brown rice. White beans, pinto beans, chickpeas, dried figs, and soy products like tofu also offer adequate amounts.

Since milk is among the most concentrated sources of calcium, you may need to take a calcium supplement to replace what you're giving up, says Dr. Krohn. For maximum absorption, look for a chelated supplement that contains calcium and magnesium in a 2-to-1 ratio, she recommends. (Don't use calcium lactate if you are sensitive to milk, because it is milk-based.) People under the age of 50 need 1,000 milligrams of calcium a day, and those over 50 need 1,500 milligrams daily.

# *Nutrition Can Make a Difference for* **Macular Degeneration**

The cells in the center of your retina, an area called the macula, are responsible for your most acute vision—your central vision. If those cells slowly degenerate, your eyesight becomes more and more blurry. Eventually, there may be a black hole in the center of everything you see, and finally, almost all of your sight can fall into that black hole.

Most conventional doctors will probably tell you that there is nothing you can do about this disease. Nothing to slow the degeneration of the cells. Nothing to prevent the possibility of blindness. And certainly nothing to reverse the problem.

They're wrong, say alternative practitioners.

"Macular degeneration may be stabilized or reversed with nutritional intervention," says Marc Grossman, O.D., an optometrist, licensed acupuncturist, and codirector of the Integral Health Center in Rye and New Paltz, New York. And the single most important nutrient to prevent or treat it is lutein.

### LUTEIN: *The Best Nutritional Treatment*

"Everyone over the age of 50 should be taking lutein supplements," Dr. Grossman says. That's because many scientific studies have shown that regular intake of the nutrient, which is a pigment found in leafy green vegetables such as kale, collard greens, and spinach, can prevent macular degeneration, he says.

Besides preventing the condition, lutein may be able to stop or even reverse existing macular degeneration by increasing the density of the macula pigment. "By far, it's the number one nutritional treatment for the disease," Dr. Grossman says.

You can get all the lutein you need by eating five servings of leafy green vegetables a week. If you don't eat that amount (few people do), taking a supplement is the way to go. Dr.

---

# GUIDE TO
# PROFESSIONAL CARE

*Caution: You should use the alternative remedies discussed in this chapter only as part of a treatment program that is guided and monitored by a qualified medical doctor in partnership with a qualified alternative practitioner, both of whom are experienced in caring for your condition. Check with your conventional doctor before changing or stopping any conventional medical treatments or medications, and keep all of your doctors and/or alternative practitioners informed of all treatments that you are receiving.*

Anyone who has been diagnosed with macular degeneration needs to be under the regular care of either an ophthalmologist or optometrist, says Edward L. Paul Jr., O.D., Ph.D., an optometrist, holistic nutritionist, and director of Atlantic Eye Associates in Hampstead, North Carolina. He emphasizes, however, that professional care for the disease must include the type of nutritional interventions described in this chapter.

---

Grossman recommends a lutein supplement that supplies 6 milligrams a day.

## BILBERRY: *An Eye-Strengthening Herb*

Bilberry, a relative of the blueberry, is thought to improve circulation to the retina, helping to stop or reverse macular degeneration, Dr. Grossman says. He recommends taking the herb in a lutein-bilberry combination, which comes in a sublingual (under-the-tongue) spray that helps the ingredients be assimilated easily. This is a bonus for older people who may have digestive problems.

If you prefer to take a pill, Dr. Grossman recommends one that provides 6 milligrams of lutein and 180 milligrams of bilberry.

## TAURINE: *Regenerate the Retina*

This amino acid may help regenerate tissues in the retina, says Dr. Grossman. He recommends a liquid or sublingual form for best assimilation, or you can take 500 milligrams a day in pill form.

## ANTIOXIDANTS: *Stopping Retinal Rust*

Antioxidants such as vitamin C, vitamin E, selenium, and zinc can help stop the formation of free radicals. These unstable molecules cause oxidative damage (a kind of internal rust) to cells, including those in the macula.

A nutritional supplement that supplies high levels of antioxidants can help reverse macular degeneration, says John D. Huff, M.D., an ophthalmologist and codirector of the Prather-Huff Wellness Center in Sugarland, Texas.

Dr. Huff recommends a multivitamin/mineral product made specifically for eye health, which contains a high level of antioxidants. One that he uses with his patients is OcuDyne, manufactured by NutriCology. Take it according to the directions on the label.

## LIFESTYLE: *Make Some Changes*

A number of lifestyle factors are crucial in stopping or reversing macular degeneration, say alternative practitioners.

• Eat a low-fat, whole-foods diet. High cholesterol levels have been linked to macular degeneration, Dr. Grossman says. Also, since the health of your eyes depends on the health of your whole body, a diet that minimizes processed foods is the way to go.
• Stop smoking. Nutritional supplements won't work very well if you smoke, says Dr. Grossman.
• Ditto on the caffeine. Caffeine in any form—from coffee, cola, or chocolate—can worsen the disease.
• If you have macular degeneration, don't drink. Alcohol can damage the macula.
• Wear sunglasses. When you're outside, they protect the retina from further damage from ultraviolet radiation.

## *Natural Remedies*
## *Can Reverse*
# Male Menopause

What do you expect? You're 50.

That's how most conventional doctors respond to descriptions of vague but troubling symptoms that are commonly experienced by guys whose personal odometers are a few years or more past 40. Symptoms such as flagging energy. More pounds around the middle. A duller mind. Less drive and ambition. Sore muscles. A libido at half-mast.

"The most important health change that many men go through in their entire lives—male menopause, or the gradual decline in levels of the hormone testosterone—is not recognized or treated by most of the medical profession," says Eugene Shippen, M.D., a physician in Shillington, Pennsylvania. He believes that this change can be as dramatic in men as it is in women going through menopause.

As men age into what Dr. Shippen calls the gray zone, factors such as disease, stress, diet, obesity, and general health tend to change the signals that the pituitary gland sends to the testes, causing the production of testosterone to lessen.

This gradual decline in testosterone doesn't sabotage just your sex drive. "Every system in a man's body is impacted by a decline in testosterone, particularly the circulatory system, the muscles (including the heart), the bones, and the nervous system and brain," Dr. Shippen says.

Men can opt for testosterone replacement therapy, but there are also home remedies that can help stop or reverse testosterone decline. Using just one or two won't work, though, says Dr. Shippen.

"One self-care factor by itself is not powerful enough to maintain testosterone levels," he says, "but combining multiple factors can keep male menopause at bay." Here is the array of remedies that he recommends.

## GUIDE TO
## PROFESSIONAL CARE

Ideally, men should have their testosterone levels measured before they turn 40 to provide baseline readings. Then, from 40 on, they should have their levels checked at least once every 2 years, says Eugene Shippen, M.D., a doctor in Shillington, Pennsylvania. That way, they'll know when their testosterone begins to decline and by how much.

The prescription testosterone patch that's frequently used to replace the hormone is "very expensive and uncomfortable," says Jonathan V. Wright, M.D., a nutritionally oriented physician and director of the Tahoma Clinic in Kent, Washington. Instead, he recommends asking for a prescription for testosterone in cream, gel, or sublingual (under-the-tongue) form. Customized medications of this type are available from compounding pharmacies.

### EXERCISE: *A Must for Maintaining Testosterone*

"All overweight men have lower-than-normal levels of testosterone," Dr. Shippen says. That's because, as your body accumulates fat, it manufactures less testosterone and converts some of the testosterone you do have into estrogen. Yes, men have estrogen, but the balance between the two hormones is different from that in women.

Then the next domino falls: As your testosterone levels drop and your estrogen levels rise, your muscles become weaker and can't burn as much fat. In other words, being overweight leads to being even more overweight—and to even lower levels of testosterone.

Exercise is the one sure way to reduce body fat and stop the rise in estrogen and the decline in testosterone. And it doesn't take a whole lot of activity. Just a brisk 20-minute walk three times a week can help a middle-aged or older man maintain lean body mass, says Dr. Shippen.

"As the pounds fall off, so will your estrogen, allowing your testosterone levels to rise," he says. "Many of the symptoms of male menopause will vanish as well."

Of course, you can't overeat and expect to lose weight, even if you exercise. But Dr. Shippen says that no matter how healthy your diet, you won't lose weight unless you exercise regularly.

## ZINC: *Deactivate a Dastardly Enzyme*

The mineral zinc helps the body deactivate aromatase, an enzyme that converts testosterone to estrogen. "Many men will restore a proper balance of testosterone to estrogen just through supplementing their diets with zinc," Dr. Shippen says.

He recommends 50 milligrams twice a day until you see an improvement in your symptoms, which might take a month or two, at which point you should reduce your intake to 30 to 50 milligrams daily.

## VITAMIN C: *Low Levels Are a Midlife Risk*

When the body's level of vitamin C is low, levels of aromatase are high, possibly leading to lowered testosterone, Dr. Shippen says. He recommends 1,000 to 3,000 milligrams of vitamin C a day for a month or two. If you don't see any results by then, reduce your daily dosage to 1,000 milligrams or less.

## MULTIVITAMIN/MINERAL SUPPLEMENT: *Thrive into Old Age*

Along with zinc and vitamin C, Dr. Shippen recommends a high-potency multivitamin/mineral supplement (one that provides amounts that meet or exceed the Daily Value of the vitamins it contains) containing antioxidants such as beta-carotene and vitamin E to deactivate free radicals, the cell-destroying molecules that contribute to many age-related diseases.

The antioxidants will also help protect your pituitary gland (the body's "control panel" for hormone production) from free radical damage. That's important, says Dr. Shippen, because a problem with the pituitary gland often triggers a decrease in testosterone production in men over 75.

## CRUCIFEROUS VEGETABLES: *On Your Plate or in a Pill*

Memorize these words for more manliness: *broccoli, brussels sprouts, cabbage, cauliflower*. These are the cruciferous vegetables, and they're good for you in ways that your mother never imagined.

"All the cruciferous vegetables contain compounds called indoles, which help break down estrogen more efficiently so it doesn't build up in the system and depress or destroy testosterone," Dr. Shippen says. He recommends eating three or four servings of cruciferous vegetables a week.

He emphasizes that supplements are no substitute for the vegetables themselves, but if the thought of regular servings of those things curdles your taste buds, take heart. There is an alternative: You can take an indole-containing supplement. Follow the dosage recommendations on the label.

## SOY: *High in Estrogen-Replacing Isoflavones*

Found primarily in soy products, food chemicals called isoflavones rev up your liver's ability to process and excrete excess estrogen, so you end up with more testosterone. Dr. Shippen recommends that you drink one cup of soy milk a day, or use it on your morning cereal.

If you don't like soy milk, take a supplement that contains 30 to 50 milligrams of isoflavones, following the dosage recommendations on the label.

## ALCOHOL: *Ditch the Drinks*

If you drink too much alcohol, you have two strikes against middle-age male health: Alcohol decreases zinc levels (zinc, remember, is necessary for adequate testosterone) and cuts down the clearance of estrogen from the bloodstream.

If you drink, make sure you have no more than two drinks a day, says Dr. Shippen. If your estrogen level is high, any alcohol may be too much.

## GRAPEFRUIT: *Maybe Not for the Middle-Aged*

Grapefruit is a healthy food, but it can block the liver's breakdown of estrogen, says Dr. Shippen. If you're experiencing male menopause, you may want to take grapefruit off your shopping list.

# *Heal Brain Cells*
# *Naturally to Stop*
# **Memory Problems**

You're over 40, and you seem to have developed a Bermuda Triangle in your brain, a place where names, facts, and even recent events seem to mysteriously disappear.

That "triangle" is called age-related memory loss. If you ask most conventional doctors what you can do about it, they'll probably tell you that it's normal, it's inevitable, and you should learn to live with it.

Forget about it!

Memory loss is not a sad fact of getting older, says Steven J. Bock, M.D., a family practitioner, acupuncturist, and co-director of the Center for Progressive Medicine in Rhinebeck, New York. It's caused by damage to the cells of the brain, called neurons.

This damage, either oxidative (a kind of cellular rust) or inflammatory (a kind of cellular burn), can produce a range of memory problems, from a slight erosion of optimal memory all the way to Alzheimer's disease.

But you can slow, stop, or even reverse neuron damage, Dr. Bock says.

A good first step, he says, is to take the right brain-boosting nutrients and herbs. He cautions, however, that improving the cellular environment of your brain with such supplements is best done under the supervision of an alternative physician who understands natural medicine.

## MULTIVITAMIN/MINERAL SUPPLEMENT: *Nutrients for Neurons*

A high-potency multivitamin/mineral supplement will supply many of the antioxidant, anti-inflammatory nutrients that you need to help control memory loss, Dr. Bock says. Look for

# GUIDE TO PROFESSIONAL CARE

Most conventional physicians have no treatments for non-Alzheimer's, age-related memory loss, says Alan Brauer, M.D., founder and director of the TotalCare Medical Center in Palo Alto, California. But alternative doctors can use anti-aging medicine or cognitive enhancement therapies to improve memory capacity at any age, he says.

See your doctor if you forget important appointments, repeat the same stories in one conversation, forget the names of familiar objects, get lost while driving familiar routes, are confused about the time of day or where you are, are unable to manage simple finances such as balancing your checkbook (especially if you've done it with ease in the past), experience a personality change, or notice a sudden change in your artistic or musical abilities.

Ideal professional care for memory improvement should include the following, according to Dr. Brauer.

• Evaluation for illness and chronic pain. "In treating memory, the doctor should first look for physical disorders and attempt to correct them," he says.

• Hormone tests. Testosterone, estrogen, progesterone, cortisol, DHEA, and many other hormones affect memory, and unless those levels are healthy, you're not going to make any significant improvements in memory.

• Evaluation for clinical depression, which is the most common medical cause of memory loss.

• Evaluation of memory. Look for a doctor who has an in-office test that can evaluate your memory so you can repeat it during your treatment to track your progress.

• Prescription medications. Some are memory-enhancing in the proper (usually small) dosages, including ergoloid mesylates (Hydergine), selegiline hydrochloride (Eldepryl), vasopressin (Pitressin or Pressyn), and piracetam (Nootropyl).

• Evaluation of nutritional supplements. Dr. Bauer reviews his patients' supplement intake and revises it if necessary.

---

• Lifestyle factors. A good memory evaluation should include
questions about your exercise routine, diet, and levels of
stress as well as advice to help you establish a memory-enhancing lifestyle.

---

a supplement that delivers a daily intake of at least the following nutrient amounts.

• Vitamin A: 10,000 international units (IU)
• Beta-carotene and other carotenoids: 9 milligrams or more
• B vitamins: 50 to 100 milligrams of most of the Bs
• Vitamin C: 1,000 milligrams
• Vitamin E: 200 to 400 IU
• Zinc: 20 milligrams
• Copper: 2 milligrams
• Manganese: 2 to 3 milligrams
• Selenium: 200 micrograms
• Chromium: 200 micrograms

## PHOSPHOLIPIDS: *Crucial Compounds That Decline with Age*

Phospholipids help form the neurons' outer covering, or
membrane, and aid communication between brain cells. But
they decline with age, possibly hurting memory.

Since phospholipids aren't prevalent in the diet, the best way
to replace them is with a daily supplement, says James Hughes,
M.D., medical director of the Hilton Head Longevity Center in
Bluffton, South Carolina. Look for one that contains phosphatidylserine, choline, and inositol for a total of 200 to 300
milligrams of phospholipids.

## ESSENTIAL FATTY ACIDS: *Fats You Shouldn't Forget*

The essential fatty acids, or EFA, are also major components
of neuron membranes and can help protect memory, Dr. Bock
says. He recommends 2 tablespoons a day of flaxseed oil,
which is rich in EFA.

### ACETYL-CARNITINE: *Stop "Age Spots" in Your Brain*

The nutrient acetyl-carnitine can help improve memory, says Alan Brauer, M.D., founder and director of the TotalCare Medical Center in Palo Alto, California. Scientists theorize that it boosts energy production in the brain, improves function in the brain's glutamate receptors, which are responsible for learning, and may stop the formation of lipofucian, a kind of "age spot" of the neurons that can interfere with memory. He recommends 250 to 2,000 milligrams a day.

### DMAE: *A Boost for Your Neurotransmitters*

Neurotransmitters are the chemicals that relay messages between neurons, so when levels of neurotransmitters are low, memory suffers.

The supplement DMAE (short for dimethylaminoethanol) supplies a compound called methyl that your body needs to manufacture neurotransmitters, says Ross Hauser, M.D., director of physical medicine and rehabilitation at the Caring Medical Rehabilitation Service in Oak Park, Illinois. According to Dr. Hauser, DMAE may also help elevate mood and increase physical energy. Follow the dosage recommendations on the label.

### PERIWINKLE: *An Herb to Remember*

This herb can speed up brain activity. One of the extracts of periwinkle seeds works as a powerful enhancer of memory function by improving blood flow to the brain. In one study, secretaries who took periwinkle improved their ability to remember sequences of words by 40 percent. Take 20 to 40 milligrams a day, says Dr. Hauser.

### GINKGO: *Better Circulation for Your Brain*

The herb ginkgo can help protect memory in two ways, Dr. Brauer says. It improves circulation to the brain, and it is a potent antioxidant. He recommends 120 to 240 milligrams a day.

### ST. JOHN'S WORT: *Another Nudge for Neurotransmitters*

The herb St. John's wort increases a variety of neurotransmitters, Dr. Hughes says. Look for a product that is standardized for 0.3 percent hypericin, the most active ingredient in the herb, and take 900 milligrams a day in divided doses with meals. Do not take this herb if you are taking a prescription antidepressant.

## KAVA KAVA: *For Memory-Restoring Sleep*

This mildly sedative herb from the South Pacific helps you sleep better and allows your brain to produce more growth hormone, which is a substance that protects and improves memory, Dr. Hughes says.

Before bedtime, he recommends taking 500 milligrams of an extract of the herb standardized for 30 percent kavalactones, the active ingredient.

## FLOWER ESSENCES: *A Powerful Combination*

The right combination of three flower essences can help halt memory loss, says Patricia Kaminski, cofounder and codirector of the Flower Essence Society, based in Nevada City, California.

The essence rosemary is considered particularly good for age-related memory loss, she says. If you're easily distracted, a major cause of poor memory, use the essence called madia. Finally, the essence Shasta daisy is thought to help the brain find meaning in events. "The more something is meaningful to you, the more you will remember it," Kaminski says.

While you can use any one of these remedies to boost memory, it's ideal to use all three at once. "They are a wonderful combination for memory problems of all kinds," she says. Take four drops of each remedy four times a day.

### Seeing Is Remembering

The most reliable way to remember anything is to visualize it, says William Cone, Ph.D., a geriatric psychologist in Pacific Palisades, California.

Since most of our memory is stored in pictures, a decline in visual memory is a major contributor to age-associated memory impairment, he says. You can overcome this, he says, by learning to visualize better. "The basic technique is to turn anything you want to remember into a picture." Two examples will illustrate the idea.

If you were memorizing a sentence that included the word jealousy, you might visualize a bowl of Jell-O with two eyes in it: *Jell-O-see*.

If you wanted to remember the name of your new acquaintance Marlene, you might visualize a mark (*mar*) on a piece of steak (*lean*).

This method is particularly good for remembering names, which is one of the first abilities to disappear with age-related memory loss, but "you can teach yourself to remember anything with this technique," says Dr. Cone.

## Remember to Live Right

Any personal program to improve memory must include a good diet, regular exercise, and stress reduction, all of which strengthen the brain, Dr. Hughes says.

**FOOD:** *Make Your Meals Memory-Friendly*

What you eat either increases or decreases oxidation and inflammation in your brain, Dr. Bock says. Here are four food pitfalls to avoid.

• Refined sugar triggers the body to pump out the hormone insulin, which is a pro-inflammatory compound, says Dr. Bock. Limit your intake.
• Trans-fats are inflammation producers that are in processed foods whose labels list hydrogenated vegetable oil as an ingredient. Avoid them, says Dr. Bock.
• Food toxins can also inflame the brain. Consider using a water filter and maximizing your intake of organic foods.
• Food allergies may contribute to memory problems. The most common allergens are wheat, milk, and corn. If you're noticing some memory glitches, consider cutting down on these foods, which increase inflammation throughout the body, including the brain.

**EXERCISE:** *A Memory Tonic*

Go for a 1-mile walk shortly after you wake up, Dr. Hughes says. But rather than an aerobic, heart-pumping fitness walk, yours should be a solitary, peaceful walk in a natural setting, if possible. "Walk slowly and be aware of your surroundings, consciously taking in everything beautiful that you see and hear," he says.

Paying attention to natural beauty improves your mental attitude, which in turn improves mental functioning of all kinds, Dr. Hughes says. Taking your walk in the early morning resets your body clock for the day, a must for maximum alertness.

Also, by warming and loosening your muscles in the morning when they're typically stiff and tight, you develop better proprioception, which is your brain's awareness of the position of your body as it moves.

Dr. Hughes also recommends regular aerobic exercise for better health—and a better memory.

## MENTAL EXERCISE: *Push-ups for Your Memory*

Any activity that stimulates and challenges your mind, such as playing Scrabble, doing crossword puzzles, or learning a new language, is exceptionally good for retaining memory, Dr. Hughes says.

"People get lazy with their minds," he says. "Sitting in front of the TV for hours a day atrophies your muscle cells and your brain cells. Just as with your muscles, you have to use your brain in order not to lose your brain."

## STRESS REDUCTION: *Don't Let Cortisol Damage Your Brain*

During stress, the body pumps out high levels of the hormone cortisol, which damages the hippocampus, the part of the brain that turns short-term memory into long-term memory, says Dr. Hughes.

To combat stress, he recommends practicing a relaxation exercise daily, whether it's deep breathing, meditation, or contemplative exercises such as tai chi or yoga.

# *Natural Treatments Can Ease*
# **Menopausal Problems**

No wonder it's called The Change.

Every month since puberty, your body has ripened some of the half-million or so eggs stored in your ovaries. But now (usually around the age of 50), there are only a few eggs left. And the entire monthly cycle—the swelling and bursting of the egg sac, its release of the hormones estrogen and progesterone, the hormone-triggered thickening of the uterus with blood as it prepares to harbor and nourish a newly fertilized egg, and the menstrual shedding of uterine cells and blood if an egg isn't fertilized—is slowly coming to a halt.

Starting a few years before your final period (a time called peri-menopause), as your supply of eggs dwindles and reproductive hormones decline, you may begin to feel that *The Change* should be the title of a horror movie—with you as the unwilling star.

There can be hot flashes and night sweats. Fatigue and insomnia. Vaginal dryness and loss of sex drive. Depression, memory loss, or sudden mood swings. What's more, your intermittent periods may be the heaviest and most uncomfortable that you've ever experienced.

Of course, you can opt for hormone replacement therapy (HRT), and many women dealing with the symptoms of menopause can benefit from this type of medication. But it's likely that your doctor has told you that using HRT or enduring the symptoms are your only two choices.

"Few women learn about alternative therapies to reduce menopausal symptoms," says Susan Lark, M.D., a physician in Los Altos, California. As a result, she says, "many women do not get the treatment that's best suited to their needs." With the alternative home remedies offered here, however, which are recommended by doctors and healers who specialize in treating menopause, you don't have to be one of them.

# GUIDE TO
## PROFESSIONAL CARE

If you experience any vaginal bleeding after menopause, see a medical doctor as soon as possible.

The main medical question for any woman entering menopause, however, is whether to use hormone replacement therapy, or HRT. And, since every woman's experience is different, there's no right answer, says Susan Lark, M.D., a physician in Los Altos, California.

"Some women with severe menopausal symptoms certainly benefit from the use of HRT," she says, "and for other women, it can help prevent long-term health problems for which they're at genetic risk, such as osteoporosis or heart disease."

Many women, however, with the help of their physicians, choose not to use HRT, she says. The reason for their decision is that HRT can aggravate existing problems, such as uterine cancer, heavy bleeding from fibroid tumors, severe migraine headaches, or blood clots. It can also increase the risk of breast cancer as well as cause side effects, including depression, breast tenderness, and fluid retention.

Discuss the HRT option with your doctor to see if it makes sense for you, Dr. Lark says. If you do decide that you're going to use it, she offers the following guidelines.

• Pick a physician who will tailor HRT to your needs. Ask friends for referrals, then choose several doctors and interview them to determine if you are comfortable with their philosophy regarding HRT and their willingness to work with you.

• Choose the best form for you. You can use pills, a patch, or a cream. You will probably have to experiment with both the dosage and the formulation until you achieve the right results.

• Choose the regimen that suits you best. A daily regimen may be better than the on-off schedule used by many doctors.

> • If you stop HRT—because your symptoms have vanished or because of side effects—do it slowly and only under the supervision of your physician. Otherwise, symptoms can return.

## Cooling Hot Flashes and Night Sweats

In America, 75 percent of menopausal women experience hot flashes, and many seek medical care. It's not hard to understand why.

The "flash" usually begins in the chest, neck, or face and spreads to other parts of your body. You sweat—sometimes mildly, sometimes profusely. (If you have hot flashes at night, called night sweats, you may sweat so much that you have to change the sheets.) After you sweat, you shiver. Because you feel so uncomfortable—first hot, then cold—you may shed and then add clothes throughout the day.

Hot flashes typically last from 30 seconds to 5 minutes, and they can happen as infrequently as a few times a year or as often as 30 to 40 times a day. Here's how to get relief.

### VITAMIN E: *As Effective as Estrogen*

This nutrient can help control and even eliminate hot flashes, says Brenda Beeley, a licensed acupuncturist and director of Menopause and PMS Options for Women on Bainbridge Island, Washington. She recommends 400 to 1,200 international units (IU) daily. Start with 400 IU and gradually increase the dosage over 2 weeks until you obtain relief.

The best way to take the vitamin is in divided doses four or five times a day. (If you were taking 1,000 IU, for example, you would take 200 IU five times a day.) If you have night sweats, take one dose before bed and another during the night if you wake up.

"Once you're feeling well, you can gradually start reducing the dosage back to 400 IU," Beeley says.

Vitamin E may also help ease other symptoms of menopause, such as vaginal dryness, says Dr. Lark. "Various studies show that vitamin E can be an effective substitute for estrogen in the majority of women," she says.

**FOOD:** *Add E to Your Diet*

Foods that are good sources of vitamin E include avocado, flaxseed, and wheat germ, says Amanda McQuade Crawford, a medical herbalist and nutritionist in Ojai, California. She also urges women to regularly eat small quantities of E-rich seeds and nuts. "Sprinkle sunflower seeds over a salad, or chop a few Brazil nuts on a casserole or grain dish," she suggests.

**B-COMPLEX VITAMINS:** *To Reduce Stress*

The effects of stress on menopausal women can be reduced by being sure that the multivitamins they take contain adequate doses of B vitamins, says Joseph L. Mayo, M.D., cofounder of A Woman's Place Medical Center in Healdsburg, California. Take daily multivitamins that contain 25 to 100 milligrams of thiamin, riboflavin, niacin, pantothenic acid, and $B_6$ as well as 50 to 100 micrograms of $B_{12}$.

**BLACK COHOSH:** *For Hormonal Balance*

This herb attaches to estrogen receptor sites in the body, helping to correct hormone imbalances and reducing many of the symptoms of menopause, including hot flashes and night sweats, says Crawford.

She recommends using high-quality products such as standardized tinctures or tablets. If you want to make a tea, which is also helpful, buy some dried root at a health food store. Cut ½ to 1 tablespoon of root, place it in a pan with 2 cups of water, cover, and simmer for 10 minutes on low heat. Strain the tea, let it cool to room temperature, and drink ½ to 1 cup three times a day.

For tablets, she suggests taking 20 milligrams twice a day. If you use a tincture or liquid form of the herb, take ½ teaspoon as is or diluted in a small amount of water twice a day.

"Depending on the severity of your symptoms, you'll need to take the herb daily for anywhere from 5 days to 5 or 6 weeks before you feel better," Crawford says.

**MOTHERWORT:** *The "Cool" Herb*

If you don't see results from black cohosh, look for another "plant ally," says Crawford. Try motherwort, which cannot only help stop hot flashes but also alleviate irritability, a common problem during menopause.

To make motherwort tea, pour 1 pint of boiling water into a

pot containing 1 ounce of the leaves, steep for 10 minutes, strain, and drink at room temperature. Drink ½ to 1 cup of tea three times a day as needed.

As a tincture, take two droppers every 10 minutes until your symptoms go away, which usually happens after two or three doses. If you can't take it that often, take two droppers once an hour, either straight or with a small amount of water. "A tincture of this herb at these doses is quite safe," says Crawford.

## SAGE: *For Profuse Sweating*

"This herb works well for a woman who is having hot flashes throughout the day—taking her sweater off, putting it on, waking with night sweats, and driving everybody crazy, including herself," Crawford says. Make a sage tea, following the directions for motherwort tea, above.

## PROGESTERONE: *To Halt Hot Flashes*

In one study, 80 percent of women who used the hormone progesterone for 1 year reported improvement of their hot flashes, compared to only 20 percent who took a placebo (inactive substance). Crawford recommends Pro-Gest, a natural progesterone cream. Apply ¼ to ½ teaspoon of the cream twice daily, right after getting up in the morning and right before going to bed. You can rub it into any area of your skin.

## HYDROTHERAPY: *Sweat More to Sweat Less*

The body expels toxins during menstruation. When menstrual cycles decrease or stop, the body needs another outlet for the toxins, so it sweats or has hot flashes. By sweating intentionally in a sauna or steam bath, you provide an outlet for the toxins and can eliminate hot flashes.

That's the theory of Sydney Ross Singer and Soma Grismaijer, medical anthropologists and codirectors of the Institute for the Study of Culturogenic Disease in Hilo, Hawaii.

To test their theory, they asked 10 women who had hot flashes and had gotten no relief with HRT or any other therapy to take a 20-minute sauna or steam bath at a local YWCA 6 out of 7 days for a month.

The five women who completed the regimen experienced "significant or complete relief" from their hot flashes, while the five who didn't take daily sweats had no change in their symptoms, say Singer and Grismaijer. "If a sauna or steam room is not convenient, take a hot bath for 20 minutes a day," they say.

## Steps to More Energy and Better Sleep

Fatigue and insomnia are major problems for menopausal women, says Beeley. Here are some effective ways to solve them.

### SIBERIAN GINSENG: *An Herbal Energy Booster*

This herb helps restore energy and cool hot flashes, says Beeley. She recommends taking 200 to 1,000 milligrams in three divided doses throughout the day. Determine the size of the dose according to the severity of your hot flashes.

For some menopausal women, Siberian ginseng can cause increased menstrual bleeding, so if you experience this effect, discontinue the herb.

### SUPPLEMENTS: *Three for the Adrenals*

Worn-out adrenal glands are a common cause of fatigue in menopausal women, says Carolyn Dean, M.D., a physician in New York City.

To regenerate your adrenals, she recommends three adrenal-building supplements: 2,000 milligrams a day of vitamin C, 500 milligrams a day of pantothenic acid (a B vitamin), and 80 milligrams two to four times a day of desiccated adrenal extract. Take the extract for 2 to 3 months, then take a break for 1 to 2 months before restarting.

### LAVENDER ESSENTIAL OIL: *Give It the Nod*

Dabbing a few drops of lavender essential oil on your pillow can help you sleep, says Dr. Mayo.

### VALERIAN: *For a Good Night's Sleep*

Taking 300 to 500 milligrams of valerian extract 1 hour before bedtime is a safe, nonaddictive herbal option for better sleep, Dr. Mayo says.

### ACUPRESSURE: *Resting Points*

Stimulating two acupressure points on your feet once a day can help relieve insomnia and anxiety in menopausal women, says Dr. Lark. To do the exercise, sit comfortably and press firmly but gently on each point for 1 to 3 minutes with your middle and index fingers. (For the exact location of the points, see An Illustrated Guide to Acupressure Points on page 700.)

• KI6: Using your left hand, press the indentation on the inside of your right ankle, directly below the anklebone. Repeat, using your right hand on your left ankle.
• BL62: Using your right hand, press the indentation on the outside of your right ankle, directly below the anklebone. Repeat with your left hand on your left ankle.

## Dealing with Vaginal Changes and Lowered Libido

As perimenopause changes to menopause, early symptoms such as hot flashes and mood swings tend to go away.

Changes in the vagina increase, however. The tissues become thinner, drier, and less elastic, causing painful intercourse and reduced sexual desire. Sexuality itself is also estrogen-dependent, so after menopause, orgasms are less frequent and intense and clitoral sensitivity is lessened.

Don't think that you have to take a vow of celibacy, though. You can stay sexually active and enjoy it after menopause. Here are a couple of suggestions from alternative healers that will help.

### KEGELS: *Squeeze More Pleasure into Your Life*

This repetitive squeezing of the pelvic muscles improves vaginal elasticity and increases sexual pleasure. Kegel exercises can be done anywhere, while standing, sitting, or lying down. Ideally, you should practice them five times a day for the rest of your life. Here are instructions from Dr. Lark for performing these simple exercises.

Slowly draw up the vaginal muscles and hold for 3 seconds, then relax. Repeat 10 times. Next, squeeze the vaginal muscles firmly, then alternately contract and relax them as rapidly as you can. Repeat 10 times.

**CHASTEBERRY:** *Chases Away Symptoms*

This herb is believed to have a profound effect hormonally, not only helping to reverse vaginal changes and lowered libido but also relieving many of the symptoms of menopause, says Jason Elias, a practitioner of Traditional Chinese Medicine in New Paltz, New York. It takes about 3 months of daily use to see results.

He recommends using the herb in tincture form, following the dosage recommendations on the label. Chasteberry is often available in health food stores under the name vitex.

### Slowing Heavy Bleeding

As hormones shift, periods can become less frequent and lighter. For some, however, periods become longer and heavier before ceasing, says Dr. Lark. Fortunately, there are a number of nutrients that can help solve the problem.

**VITAMIN A:** *Helps Stem the Flow*

Dr. Lark says a study shows that women with excessive bleeding have lower-than-normal levels of vitamin A and that supplementing with the nutrient stops bleeding in almost 90 percent of women with the problem. She recommends eating plenty of sweet potatoes or drinking carrot juice, both of which supply beta-carotene, the most beneficial form of vitamin A.

**B-COMPLEX VITAMINS:** *Maintain Estrogen Levels*

Take 50 to 100 milligrams a day of B-complex vitamins, which can help stabilize estrogen levels, says Dr. Lark.

**VITAMIN C WITH BIOFLAVONOIDS:** *Reduce Bleeding*

Dozens of scientific studies show that these nutrients can reduce heavy bleeding, says Dr. Lark. She recommends 1,000 to 4,000 milligrams a day of vitamin C in combination with 500 to 2,000 milligrams of bioflavonoids.

## Natural Relief from Memory Problems, Mood Swings, and Depression

For many women, the emotional and mental effects of menopause—forgetfulness, wide mood swings, and depression—are worse than the physical ills, says Dr. Mayo. There are many simple solutions, however.

### GINKGO: *For Better Memory*

This herb is an antioxidant and improves blood flow to the brain, Dr. Mayo says. Look for a standardized product containing 24 percent ginkgo flavoglycosides with 6 percent terpene lactones as the active ingredients. Taking a 40- to 80-milligram capsule three times a day can provide significant improvement, especially for those over 50.

### ST. JOHN'S WORT: *For Anxiety and Irritability*

According to Dr. Mayo, St. John's wort has been shown in studies to be more effective than traditional antidepressants for mild to moderate depression. Take 100 to 300 milligrams of a supplement standardized for 0.3 percent hypericin three times a day.

### YOGA: *Pose As a Child*

The yoga exercise known as the child's pose is "excellent for calming anxiety and stress due to emotional causes and will also relieve menopause-related anxiety and irritability," says Dr. Lark.

Begin on your hands and knees with your knees hip-width apart and your elbows straight but not locked. Exhale and sit back on your heels, rest your torso on your thighs, and bring your forehead to the floor, stretching your spine. Rest your arms on the floor beside your torso with your palms up. Close your

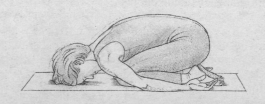

eyes, breathe easily, and hold the pose for as long as you're comfortable. You can do it for as long as you like without harm, says Dr. Lark.

## AFFIRMATIONS: *Be Positive*

Affirmations are positive statements that help change negative, unhappy emotional and mental states, says Dr. Lark. Here are some of her recommended affirmations for menopause. To do the affirmations, sit in a comfortable position and repeat each statement three times, slowly and clearly.

- My mood is calm and relaxed.
- I handle stress easily and effortlessly.
- I feel wonderful as I go through menopause.
- Menopause is a beautiful time of growth and change for me.
- I am enjoying my life more and more.
- My life brings me pleasure.

# *Natural Remedies Can Relieve*
# Menstrual Cramps

Conventional doctors know the biochemical cause of menstrual cramps. Hormonelike chemicals called series-2 prostaglandins trigger contractions in the muscular wall of the uterus, or womb.

They also know how to ease the problem with over-the-counter or prescription nonsteroidal anti-inflammatory drugs (NSAIDs), which cut down on the formation of those prostaglandins.

According to alternative physicians, however, certain nutritional factors stimulate the production of series-2 prostaglandins. By eliminating those factors, says Susan Lark, M.D., a physician in Los Altos, California, you can reduce the severity of cramps by 30 to 50 percent—and make painkillers a lot more effective (if you still need to take them).

Here are some nondrug remedies recommended by natural healers for both symptomatic and long-term relief.

## FOOD: *Cut the Fat*

"The kinds of fats you eat determine, in large part, your susceptibility to cramps," Dr. Lark says. "If you take drugs to reduce the severity of cramps, but you feed the biochemical pathways that cause the cramps, you're working at cross-purposes."

The nutritional factor in fats that does the dirty work is arachidonic acid, which is found in red meat, dairy products, and palm kernel oil (a common ingredient in processed foods). Cutting out those fats and emphasizing foods such as whole grains, legumes, vegetables, fruits, seeds, nuts, certain oils, and fish are key strategies in easing menstrual cramps, she says.

## HERBS: *A Relaxing and Balancing Formula*

An herbal formula using tinctures of black haw, ginger, valerian, and motherwort is very effective for relieving menstrual cramps, says Jason Elias, a practitioner of Traditional Chinese Medicine (TCM) in New Paltz, New York.

"Valerian is a general relaxant, black haw specifically relaxes the uterus, and ginger moves the life-energy, or what in TCM is called chi. Motherwort helps restore health in almost any situation of gynecological imbalance," Elias says. He recommends combining equal parts of the four tinctures and taking a teaspoon of the formula twice a day, every day that you have cramps.

---

### GUIDE TO PROFESSIONAL CARE

If you have chronic menstrual cramps that have not improved after 3 to 4 months of using a self-care program, see a medical or naturopathic doctor for a diagnosis. The cause of your cramps may be uterine fibroids or endometriosis, says Susan Lark, M.D., a physician in Los Altos, California.

If you have been menstruating for years without cramps and suddenly begin having them, see a medical doctor immediately. You may have pelvic inflammatory disease, which requires rapid diagnosis and treatment to prevent scarring of the reproductive organs, Dr. Lark says.

## MOTHERWORT: *Effective against Cramps*

Motherwort tincture alone can also stop menstrual cramps, says Susun Weed, an herbalist and founder of the Wise Woman Center in Woodstock, New York.

"I like to start with a small dose, say, five drops," she says. "If that doesn't relieve the cramps in 10 minutes, I take another five drops. I keep taking the tincture until my cramps stop, and I keep track of the total number of drops it took to stop them."

If you follow this routine, take your total dose once or twice more the same day and at least once or twice on each subsequent day that you have cramps. During subsequent periods, start with the total dose as soon as cramps start and continue taking motherwort several times a day during your period. "By the third month, many women are cramp-free," says Weed.

## OMEGA-3 FATTY ACIDS: *Control Cramp-Causing Chemicals*

While the arachidonic acid in red meat and dairy products stimulates series-2 prostaglandins and causes cramps, a component of another type of fat—the omega-3 fatty acids found in certain fatty fish and oils—keeps those prostaglandins trapped in cells so they can't get into muscle tissue and trigger spasms.

Flaxseed oil is rich in omega-3's, and Dr. Lark says that it is her favorite source. She recommends 2 tablespoons a day with meals.

## VITAMIN B₆: *For Less Pain*

This vitamin helps the body convert fatty acids to a form that helps produce pain-relieving chemicals, says Dr. Lark. She recommends taking a daily dose of 50 to 100 milligrams as part of a B-complex supplement, which can also help reduce cramping. Start taking the supplement 7 to 10 days prior to menstruation and continue throughout your period, she says.

## NIACIN: *Relief from Cramps*

This B vitamin is extremely effective at relieving cramps, Dr. Lark says. It works by dilating the blood vessels, bringing more circulation and oxygen to the uterine wall. She recommends that women take 25 to 200 milligrams a day, beginning 7 to 10 days before menstruation begins.

**VITAMIN C:** *Reduces Fatigue*

Vitamin C helps move nutrients to the uterine muscle and waste products away from it, Dr. Lark says. It can also reduce the fatigue and lethargy that often accompany cramps. She recommends 500 to 3,000 milligrams daily, especially when you're having symptoms.

**VITAMIN E:** *Crucial for Hormone Balance*

Women with cramps should take a daily dose of 400 to 800 international units of this vitamin, which helps balance the hormonal system, says Dr. Lark.

**CALCIUM:** *Tones the Muscles*

Calcium helps muscles stay relaxed and toned, preventing all kinds of cramps, including uterine cramps. While Dr. Lark suggests that you increase your intake of calcium-rich foods such as leafy green vegetables, some beans and peas, seeds, nuts, blackstrap molasses, and seafood, she also recommends taking 800 milligrams of supplemental calcium a day.

**MAGNESIUM:** *Lend Calcium a Helping Hand*

Magnesium helps the body absorb calcium and also has its own calming effect on muscles. Dr. Lark recommends supplementing your diet with 400 milligrams of magnesium a day.

# *Travel Free from the Nausea of* **Motion Sickness**

Airsick. Carsick. Seasick. Whatever you call motion sickness, one thing's for sure—you're definitely *sick*. You can turn pale, break out in a cold sweat, and just feel miserable. But the worst symptom by far is the intense nausea, which means that wherever you're traveling, the contents of your stomach may have their own Estimated Time of Arrival: Immediately.

You feel so awful because your brain has been double-crossed. Your body knows that it's moving, but your senses are saying it's stationary, and your brain reacts to this mixed message with a temporary short-circuit in the balance centers in your inner ear that causes the symptoms.

There are many different drugs that can help prevent or treat motion sickness. If you prefer a drug-free approach, however, here are some options.

## AROMATHERAPY: *Spray Your Car with Anti-Sickness Mist*

To help relieve the nausea of motion sickness during a car ride, you can prepare a mist spray of essential oils, say David Schiller and Carol Schiller, certified aromatherapy instructors in Phoenix. Here's how to make it.

First, you'll need a glass bottle with a fine-mist sprayer to hold the sickness-fighting formula. (Plastic or other material can change the scent of the essential oils in the spray, and it's the smell of the oils that can help relieve the nausea.) Next, fill the bottle with 4 ounces of distilled water. (Tap water can add its own odor, but water that's been filtered through a reverse osmosis process is okay, say the Schillers.) Then add the following essential oils to the water.

- 70 drops of lavender
- 40 drops of lemon
- 20 drops of dill
- 10 drops of cedarwood
- 10 drops of spearmint

The dill, lemon, and spearmint can help settle your stomach, the lavender can help calm your nervous system (anyone who's had motion sickness knows that the nervous system can get very nervous: shaky, sweaty, and weak), and the cedarwood helps keep the fragrances in the air to do their healing work.

To use the mixture, shake the bottle well (be sure the cap is tight). Then, say the Schillers, close your eyes and spray about 10 times above your head so that the mist will fall in front of but not onto your face. Breathe deeply. You can use the spray anytime you start to feel sick during your trip, and you can also spray the car before you leave, which may help prevent motion sickness.

A few extra tips and cautions from the Schillers: The mixture

---

# GUIDE TO PROFESSIONAL CARE

You should see a medical doctor if your symptoms, including headache, double vision, dizziness, and vomiting, last longer than 24 hours. If you have weakness or paralysis in any part of your body or hearing problems associated with the motion sickness, see your doctor immediately.

Even if your symptoms are mild, you should see a doctor if they last longer than 24 hours. You should also seek professional care for any case of motion sickness with symptoms that are so severe that you are unable to stand.

---

has a shelf life of 3 years, but to keep its ingredients active, be sure to store it in a dark, cool, dry place and, as with all therapeutic substances, out of the sight and reach of children.

## GINGER: *Tried-and-True Relief*

Ginger is the classic stomach-settling herbal remedy for the nausea of motion sickness, says Beverly Yates, N.D., a naturopathic physician and director of the Natural Health Care Group in Seattle. And ginger tea is one of the best ways to make sure that you get the right dose of the herb.

To make the tea, buy some fresh ginger at your supermarket. Cut a slice of the root approximately the same thickness and length as your pinky finger. Slice off the sides just a bit to expose more of the ginger, then place the root in 3 cups of water and boil for 10 minutes. Pour it over ice and add a little lemon juice. "You can drink this tea before and during travel to prevent or remedy nausea," says Dr. Yates.

Another easy way to get plenty of ginger is to eat ginger candy, says Pam Fischer, founder and director of the Ohlone Center for Herbal Studies in Concord, California. "Just suck on it before and during your trip."

## HOMEOPATHY: *Help from Cocculus Indicus*

Cocculus is effective for beating motion sickness, and it makes a great one-two punch when used with ginger, says Dr.

Yates. Put two pellets of the 6C or 12C potency under your tongue and let them dissolve.

"Have the pellets on hand and take them as soon as you feel any symptoms of motion sickness, up to four times a day," she says. One day's treatment is usually enough to provide relief, Dr. Yates adds.

### ACUPRESSURE: *Press Your Upper Lip*

The acupressure point above your upper lip, known as GV26, helps relieve nausea, says David Filipello, a licensed acupuncturist and director of the Acupuncture for Health Clinic in San Francisco. (For the locations of this point and the following ones, see An Illustrated Guide to Acupressure Points on page 700.) Using your index finger, press the indentation firmly (consistently but not painfully) for 30 seconds. You can do this technique every couple of minutes while you're traveling to prevent or help relieve nausea.

### ACUPRESSURE: *Relief Near Your Wrist*

Another acupressure point that can help relieve nausea is PE6, located on your forearm, Filipello says. It's on the inside of your arm, three finger-widths above the wrist crease closest to your palm, toward your elbow. If you start to feel nauseated, press the point firmly for 30 seconds every couple of minutes.

### ACUPRESSURE: *Tug Your Ears*

Simply grabbing your earlobes and gently but firmly tugging down on your ears increases circulation to the inner ears and helps prevent and relieve motion sickness, says Filipello. Do this as often as necessary before and during travel.

# *Hands-On Relief for*
# **Muscle Cramps and Spasms**

You exercised too hard. You exercised too fast, without warming up. You overused a particular muscle while typing, painting, raking, or doing some other repetitive activity. Your diet doesn't contain enough electrolytes, the minerals that help muscles relax. You don't drink enough water. You injured a muscle, either today or 10 years ago, and to protect itself from further injury, the muscle has constricted into a tight, painful mass.

All of these are possible causes of a cramp, which is a sudden constriction of a muscle, or a spasm, which is constriction that doesn't let up. Massage therapists say that your cramped or spasming muscle is just trying to let you know that it needs help—immediately—and they offer plenty of ways to find relief.

### PRESSURE: *Relief in Under 12 Seconds*

With your hands, find the center of the cramp—the area of maximum pain and tension. With your loosely clenched fist, the heel of your hand, or your thumb, press into the center of the cramp, exerting enough pressure to cause pain but not so much that it's excruciating. "The pain should be 5 to 7 on a 10-point scale," says Ralph R. Stephens, a licensed massage therapist and instructor of neuromuscular therapy and sports massage at Ralph Stephens Seminars in Cedar Rapids, Iowa.

Hold the pressure for 8 to 12 seconds. "The cramp will often vanish by doing nothing more than this exercise," he says.

### STRETCHING: *Instant Relief for Calf Cramps*

When you gently flex a muscle and then let it relax, it's easier to stretch the muscle and stretch out a cramp, providing instant relief.

Massage therapists call this type of stretch PNF, or proprio-

## GUIDE TO
## PROFESSIONAL CARE

Cramps and spasms are usually only annoying, not a severe medical problem. But if a cramp or spasm persists for more than a few days so that it becomes debilitating; if there's swelling, bruising, or bleeding around the area; or if a persistent cramp or spasm is accompanied by a fever, see your doctor.

Calf cramps while walking are symptoms of intermittent claudication, a type of circulatory disease. If you're having this type of cramp, see your doctor for diagnosis and treatment.

One of the best kinds of professional care for chronic cramps or spasms is regular massage therapy, says Ralph R. Stephens, a licensed massage therapist and instructor of neuromuscular therapy and sports massage at Ralph Stephens Seminars in Cedar Rapids, Iowa.

"Massage therapy can often resolve persistent cramps or chronic spasms by working on and releasing the chronic muscle tension that causes them," he says.

ceptive neuromuscular facilitation, says James Clay, a certified clinical massage therapist in Winston-Salem, North Carolina. Here's how to relieve a calf cramp (the most common kind) with a PNF stretch.

Sit up in bed (most calf cramps happen at night). Bend your leg and reach down to grasp the sole of your foot, between the ball of the foot and where your toes begin. Place your thumb in the corresponding spot on the top of your foot.

Using your fingers to provide resistance, gently press your foot down, using about a quarter of your strength. Count to five and stop, then relax for a five count. Straighten your leg and bend your ankle toward you, stretching out your calf for a count of five.

Return to the starting position. Then, using your thumb as resistance, pull upward. Count to five and stop. Straighten your leg and bend your ankle toward you, stretching out your calf for a count of five. Wait 5 seconds and repeat the exercise, and keep repeating it until the cramp vanishes.

### STRETCHING: *Halt a Hamstring Cramp*

If you get a cramp in your hamstring, the muscle on the back of your thigh, Stephens recommends this stretch.

While sitting, keep the foot of the cramped leg on the floor. Place your other foot on top of that foot, then pull up with the lower foot with about 10 percent of your strength. Then slowly straighten out the leg, get up, and walk around a bit. The cramp should go away.

### TENNIS BALL: *To Ease Back or Buttock Pain*

A tennis ball has just the right balance of "give" and firmness to help ease a cramp or spasm in your back or buttocks, says Clay.

Put the tennis ball on the floor and cover it with a towel. Lie on your back on top of the ball and move around until you can isolate it under the painful spot. Let the ball sink into the muscle, then lie there and wait for the cramp or spasm to ease—which it will. "You can give yourself a lot of relief this way," says Clay.

### ICE: *If the Cramp Won't Quit*

When you're cramping, the nerves in your muscles are firing away. Ice makes them a little more nonviolent and calms the cramp.

If you have a cramp that won't quit, says Stephens, put a cold pack or an ice pack over the area. Wrap it in a dry washcloth or kitchen towel, apply it directly to the cramped area, and keep it on for 20 minutes.

### MAGNESIUM: *Supplement to Stop Nighttime Leg Cramps*

The mineral magnesium is a natural muscle relaxant. Often, chronic, recurring cramps, such as nighttime leg cramps, are caused by reduced magnesium in the system, says Barry L. Beaty, D.O., an orthopedic physician and director of the DFW Pain Treatment Center and Wellness Clinic in Fort Worth, Texas.

"Magnesium supplements can help reduce or even eliminate cramps," he says. He recommends taking 100 milligrams of slow-release tablets twice a day. Continue the treatment for 2 to 3 weeks.

**POTASSIUM:** *Eat for Relief*

Low levels of another mineral—potassium—can also cause cramps, says Dr. Beaty. If you experience lots of cramps, eat more potassium-rich foods like bananas, potatoes, spinach, and cantaloupe. If you choose to take potassium supplements, do so only under the supervision of your doctor.

# *Simple Exercises Can Relieve*
# **Neck and Shoulder Pain**

You're sitting there quietly, reading a book, when someone sneaks up behind you and says "BOO!!!"

You're startled, of course. In fact, scientists would say that you had a "startle response": your neck muscles tightened, your shoulders lifted, and you breathed (gasped, really) from high in your chest.

With modern life being what it is—from the time the alarm goes off in the morning to the reports of murder and mayhem on the late-night news—many people get stuck in the startle response, says Hope Gillerman, a certified instructor of the Alexander Technique (a type of posture and movement re-education) in New York City.

"The tightening of the neck and shoulders in the startle response is the most basic way that we misuse ourselves every day," Gillerman says. "And because the startle response causes us to chronically breathe high in the chest, the neck and shoulder muscles tighten further to assist in the upward movement of the rib cage rather than being relaxed and allowing the breath to move into the abdomen."

And the problem doesn't stop there. Because your breathing is shallow, those tight, painful neck and shoulder muscles are deprived of oxygen, which causes even more tension and pain. No wonder neck and shoulder pain is a complaint that's almost as common as, well, necks and shoulders.

There's no reason, however, for you to stay stuck in startle mode, Gillerman says. Here are some simple steps to relieve the tension and pain.

## BREATHING: *Learning to Exhale*

"The best way to use breathing to reduce pain in your neck and shoulders—in fact, anywhere in your body—is to focus on completing the exhalation rather than assisting the inhalation," Gillerman says.

By exhaling completely, you reduce residual carbon dioxide in your lungs, leaving room for more pain-relieving, stress-reducing oxygen. Also, you don't create more tension in your neck and shoulders as you forcefully try to inhale more deeply.

"Extending the exhale is natural," says Gillerman. "It's exactly what we do when we speak." In fact, a simple way to complete the exhale is by speaking very quietly and counting to 10

# GUIDE TO PROFESSIONAL CARE

If you have sudden, acute neck pain, particularly after an accident or a fall, see a medical doctor as soon as possible for a diagnosis.

Movement therapies are some of the most effective ways to change muscular patterns that can cause chronic neck and shoulder pain, says Hope Gillerman, a certified instructor of the Alexander Technique (a type of movement and posture re-education) in New York City. Other widely available posture and movement education methods include Hellerwork and Feldenkrais.

Chiropractic treatments, in which the vertebrae are adjusted so that the spine is in its normal configuration, can also effectively relieve chronic neck and shoulder pain, says Michael D. Pedigo, D.C., a chiropractor in San Leandro, California, and past president of the American Chiropractic Association.

Other alternative therapies that may help relieve chronic neck and shoulder pain include acupuncture, massage therapy, and craniosacral therapy, an osteopathic technique that focuses on the muscles and bones in the head and neck area.

over and over until you have no more air left, then letting air come back in through either your mouth or your nose.

Be careful not to stressfully push the air out as your exhale is nearing completion, says Gillerman. Just count until the exhale is naturally finished, without squeezing or forcing air out of your lungs. Repeat five times in a row, she recommends. You can do this exercise as frequently as you like, "especially anytime your neck and shoulders feel tight," she says.

## RELEASE AND AFFIRMATION: *Learning to Let Go*

Breathing with a full exhalation helps release the painful tension in your neck and shoulder muscles, but it's only the first step, says Gillerman. The second is to discover the exact location of the tension. "You can't let go of tense muscles unless you feel the tension," she says.

Place one palm on the back of your neck. Tighten your neck muscles by jutting your chin forward. Hold for 2 seconds, then return your head and chin to their normal position while focusing on the muscles you've just tightened, and lift the back of your head off your shoulders.

"Put your attention on the tight area (neck muscles) and then say to yourself, 'I allow my neck to be soft and free.' The muscles there will immediately become less tense," says Gillerman.

Repeat this process each morning and at night before you go to bed.

## RELAXATION: *Melting Away Tension and Pain*

You'd think that lying flat on your back would be a great way to relax your tense neck and shoulders. Not so, says Gillerman.

"When you lie flat on your back, your neck arches, your chin lifts, and your forehead drops back, which is a constricting position for the neck and shoulder muscles," she says.

Instead, lie on a well-carpeted floor, a rug, or an exercise mat, and put between 1 and 3 inches of support under your head (your skull, not your neck). That's about the thickness of one or two paperback books.

"This places the chin and the forehead in line—in other words, the chin is not higher than the forehead, which relaxes the neck and shoulders," Gillerman says.

Bend your knees by resting your calves on the seat of a chair or a couch, or just put a couple of pillows under each knee. Then

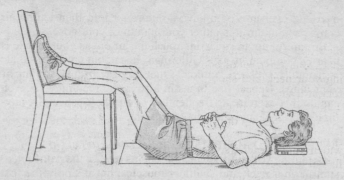

bend your elbows and place your hands on your ribs. (Lying with your hands by your sides rolls your shoulders forward, making it harder to let go of shoulder tension, says Gillerman.) As a variation, if you have a lot of tension between your shoulder blades, lie with your arms crossed over your chest.

"This is a great position for letting go of tension and relieving pain," says Gillerman. She recommends lying this way for 10 to 15 minutes a day (after work is a great time), focusing your attention on your tight neck and shoulder muscles and using affirmations such as "I allow my neck to be soft and free. I allow my shoulders and chest to be soft and wide." Gillerman suggests that you imagine large shoulder pads that are wider than your shoulders to help you visualize a wide chest and shoulders.

## SHOULDER SHRUGS: *Shaking Off Tension*

Shoulder shrugs are great for people with neck and shoulder pain, Gillerman says. Lift your shoulders easily and let them flop down a couple of times. "Don't push them down," she says. "There's very little muscular effort involved." She recommends doing these whenever you've been sitting for a long time.

### Tension-Relieving Strategies for Daily Life

There are many things that you can do—and not do—every day that can help prevent and relieve neck and shoulder pain, Gillerman says.

## LOOKING DOWN: *The Right Way*

"When most people look down, they bend from the middle of their upper backs, making their shoulders round," says Gillerman. This puts a lot of body weight in front of your spine, making your neck and shoulders "grip" to keep you from falling forward, she says.

Instead, keep your neck upright and look down by letting your nose and chin drop and the back of your neck muscles relax. Use the previous affirmations to soften your neck and widen your shoulders, says Gillerman. "This is really crucial for eliminating neck and shoulder pain. When people realize that that's all they have to do to look down, they say, 'Oh, that's so much easier on my neck and shoulders.'"

## TALKING ON THE PHONE: *Bring the Receiver to You*

"Talking on the phone is an activity where people develop a lot of neck tension," says Gillerman. The reason: You tilt your head to the receiver instead of keeping your head balanced and upright and bringing the receiver to your ear.

## BRUSHING YOUR HAIR: *Don't Bend Your Neck*

When you brush your hair, Gillerman says, keep your head balanced and move your arms and the brush up to your head.

## WORKING AT YOUR DESK: *Take a Break*

Here's a great way to rest your neck (and head) while working, says Gillerman: Fold your arms on top of each other genie-style and put them on the desk. Rest your forehead on top of your wrist; just let it sink into your arms, then feel your neck muscles relax as you repeat your affirmations.

## SLOUCHING: *Shrug It Off*

Maybe you've been told that your shoulder pain is caused by slouching. Well, that can worsen the pain, says Gillerman, but don't correct your posture by pulling your shoulders back. That tightens the trapezius muscles in your back, causing even more muscle pain and straining your neck, shoulders, and upper back.

Where should you hold your shoulders for maximum comfort? First, shrug your shoulders up and let them fall forward, then shrug them up and let them fall back. Finally, shrug them up and let them fall in between.

"That's where you want to leave them," Gillerman says, "just sitting there on top of your body. Think of them as large shoulder pads."

# *Change Your Life by Understanding Your* Nightmares

A chain saw–wielding vampire (who looks suspiciously like your new, aggressive boss) has you cornered and is about to cut you up and feast on your blood. You're terrified, and you wake up feeling anxious and upset.

You've just had a nightmare, of course—a dream so disturbing and frightening that it jars you out of sleep. But don't worry. Dream experts say that there's an alternative to being concerned about bad dreams, and also an easy way to stop them. The first step is understanding that they're often a good thing.

"Nightmares can be compared to a vaccine," says Alan B. Siegel, Ph.D., a psychotherapist in Berkeley and San Francisco. "You take a vaccine to build up antibodies so that you can fight off an infection. In the same way, a nightmare stimulates your psychological defenses, preparing you to cope with problems. It delivers an important, healthy message, telling you that you need to rebalance certain aspects of your life."

Nightmares are most common during major transitions or turning points, such as a new job, moving, the death of someone close to you, or a new relationship. "You'll deal with that transition more effectively if you remember and work with the nightmare than if you blot it out," Dr. Siegel says. Here is his step-by-step plan for doing just that.

## SELF-AFFIRMATION: *Frightening Dreams Are Normal*
First, says Dr. Siegel, you need to break the spell of the nightmare. (After all, it was scary.) You are not a uniquely hor-

# GUIDE TO
# PROFESSIONAL CARE

"When nightmares persist, when their content is consistently violent and disturbing, and when the upsetting conflicts in the dreams never change or achieve even partial resolution, it may be time to seek help from a mental health specialist who has training in dream analysis, nightmares, or sleep or dream disorders, such as a psychologist, psychiatrist, or psychotherapist," says Alan B. Siegel, Ph.D., a psychotherapist in Berkeley and San Francisco.

Also, some nightmares can be caused by a drug reaction or physical illness. See a medical doctor if recurrent nightmares don't seem to have a psychological cause, says Dr. Siegel.

---

rible person with uniquely horrible dreams. Tell yourself that upsetting dreams are normal. There is nothing wrong with you.

In fact, you are about to take your nightmare and make it into something healing by letting it show you exactly what is out of balance in your life that needs to be addressed.

## VISUALIZATION: *Write Your Own Ending*

Now that you are reassured about your dream, Dr. Siegel says to visualize it, to see it again in your mind's eye. Perhaps it was a dream of being chased—a very common plot for a nightmare.

In your imagination, rescript the dream with a different plot or outcome. Turn and confront the person (or monster) who is chasing you and tell the aggressor to go away. Or conjure magical tools, such as a wand to make the aggressor disappear or a net to capture the threatening character. Or fly away. Or say a magic spell that turns the aggressor into something harmless, like a rabbit. Or imagine bringing in reinforcements, such as police to jail the aggressor.

"This is assertiveness training of the imagination—a way to conquer nightmares," Dr. Siegel says. And you don't have to limit yourself to visualization when you rescript the dream.

"Use whatever form of expressive art you like," he says. Write a dialogue in a journal between you and the threatening character, writing assertive speech that subdues the aggressor. Or talk to a friend about the dream, describing different outcomes. Or create a dance in which you are powerful and victorious over your enemy.

Most nightmares will be resolved with this technique, Dr. Siegel says. In fact, doing this exercise will often stop recurring nightmares. His one caution is not to use violence to subdue the aggressor, which he says can create more internal conflicts and may not resolve the nightmare.

### REHEARSAL: *Do Your Visualization More Than Once*

Just as you need to practice assertiveness in real life to change your behavior, you need to rescript your nightmare more than once for it to be effective, says Dr. Siegel. As you practice, you may find yourself developing new and better ways to rescript your dream. And you may want to try a variety of rescripting approaches.

"You might try visualization the first time, writing in a journal the second time, and drawing a picture of a new ending the third time," says Dr. Siegel. "There are numerous ways to make assertiveness stick."

### RESOLUTION: *Connect the Dream to Your Life*

The final step is making a connection between the images in your nightmare and the changes in your life that are causing it, says Dr. Siegel. Ask yourself what is new in your life that is bothering you.

For instance, maybe you've figured out that your new boss, who has a habit of criticizing you in harsh tones, is the vampire in your dreams. Perhaps the nightmare is letting you know that you need to be more assertive, and you decide that rather than being quiet and submissive when the boss criticizes you, at least once a day, you will say more about what you feel to someone who will listen.

"The nightmare presents an opportunity to change the way you're dealing with an important aspect of your life," says Dr. Siegel. In fact, all dreams, not just scary ones that wake you up, convey clarifying, healing messages about your inner and outer lives. Keep a dream journal or talk to your family and friends about your dreams, urges Dr. Siegel.

"Dream images accurately reveal the essence of our fears, triumphs, and everyday concerns," he says. "If you remember and playfully explore your dreams, you will access heightened forms of creativity, intuition, insight, and emotional intelligence."

# *Natural Treatments to Rinse Away* **Oily Hair**

You've been told by health experts to eat a low-fat diet for lots of reasons, but probably never to solve the problem of oily hair.

"Oily hair is caused by an overly oily scalp," says Mary Beth Janssen, a beauty and wellness consultant and aromatherapist in Chicago. "One common cause of an oily scalp is a high-fat diet."

Just as the bulb of a tulip feeds the flower, so hair is fed through hair bulbs in the scalp. These bulbs are intertwined with sebaceous glands, which produce sebum, or oil. A diet loaded with fried foods and saturated fats from red meat and dairy products can trigger overproduction of sebum, Janssen explains, leading to an oily scalp and oily hair.

"To decrease the oil production from your scalp and reduce the oiliness of your hair, I think you should lower the amount of fried food and saturated fat in your diet," says Janssen. Then, once you're treating your oily hair internally, she believes that the best external way to reduce oil is with a natural rinse.

**LEMON RINSE:** *For Shiny, More Manageable Hair*
Rinsing after a shampoo closes down the cuticle, or outer layer of the hair shaft, creating shiny, smooth hair that feels thicker and is more manageable and less oily, says Janssen. One of her favorite

rinses for reducing the oiliness of hair is what she calls the Lemon Juice Highlighting Rinse. Here are her instructions.

Squeeze the juice from two lemons into 2 cups of distilled water and put the liquid in a plastic bottle with a spout (the kind used to dispense mustard or ketchup). Then, after showering, blot your hair dry with a towel and apply the liquid evenly to your hair and scalp, massaging it through the hair. Leave it on for 5 minutes, then rinse with cool to tepid water.

### Don't Overdo It

Many people with oily hair overcorrect by using shampoo that's too strong and has a harsh detergent that actually dries the scalp, perhaps causing flaking, says Mary Beth Janssen, a beauty and wellness consultant and aromatherapist in Chicago.

To avoid that result, be sure your shampoo doesn't include either sodium lauryl sulfate or NDELA (nitrosodiethanolamine). Earth Science and Aubrey Organics shampoos are two brands that are free of these detergents.

### HORSETAIL: *An Herbal Treatment*

Using the herb horsetail in a rinse is another effective remedy for oily hair, says Janssen. "Horsetail strengthens the internal bonds in the hair shaft and is excellent for cutting the oil."

First, boil 1 cup of distilled water. Then, put 2 tablespoons of dried herb in a stainless steel or glass pan, pour the water over it, and steep for 10 to 15 minutes. Drain off the liquid, let it cool, put it in a bottle with a spout, and use as a rinse according to the instructions for the lemon rinse, above.

### AROMATHERAPY: *Rinse with Essential Oils*

Essential oils can help cut the oil in hair, says Barbara Close, an aromatherapist and herbalist in East Hampton, New York. She recommends adding to your rinse three to four drops of rosemary, lavender, eucalyptus, cypress, or lemon oil in a base of 1 ounce of borage-seed or evening primrose oil. All of these oils are astringent, which means that they cleanse and tone the sebaceous glands.

# *Changing Your Diet*
# *Can Help Normalize*
# **Oily Skin**

If you have oily skin, with medium to large pores, a shiny appearance, and a tendency to have blackheads and blemishes, you may actually need more oil in your diet—the kind that contains fatty acids.

"There are two ways to deal with oily skin, externally and internally," says Joni Loughran, an esthetician, cosmetologist, and aromatherapist in Petaluma, California. Here are some treatments that alternative healers recommend.

## FLAXSEED OIL: *A Must for Healthy Skin*

"Every one of my clients is on a supplement of at lcast 1 to 3 teaspoons a day of flaxseed oil, an oil rich in fatty acids," Loughran says. These fatty acids, which are found in vegetable oils and seed oils, are a must for healthy skin cells no matter what type of skin you have.

## FOOD: *Cut Down on Saturated Fats*

"People who eat a lot of red meat and dairy products, which are loaded with saturated fat, can end up with oilier skin, clogged pores, and more blemishes," Loughran says. So, for healthier skin, maximize fresh fruits, vegetables, whole grains, beans, nuts, seeds, and fish, and minimize foods with saturated fat.

## LECITHIN: *Break Up the Fats in Your Body*

The food supplement lecithin can help emulsify, or break apart, the saturated fat in your body so that it doesn't make your skin more oily, says Loughran. Follow the dosage recommendations on the label.

## AROMATHERAPY: *A Natural Cleanser*

Adding a drop of the essential oil of neroli to a lavender floral water and spraying the mixture on your skin several times a day is an excellent treatment for oily, overactive skin, says Barbara Close, an aromatherapist and herbalist in East Hampton, New York.

"Lavender tones and cleanses skin," she explains, "and neroli is considered a skin tonic. It penetrates the skin and helps regulate the production of sebum, or oil. If there's too much sebum, neroli may help normalize production."

## HERBS: *Tea Is a Perfect Toner*

"I recommend using a gentle, astringent (pore-tightening) herbal tea, such as yarrow, sage, or peppermint, to remove left-over cleanser and dirt from oily skin," says Stephanie Tourles, a licensed esthetician, reflexologist, and herbalist in West Hyannisport, Massachusetts. Here are her instructions.

Boil 1 cup of water and remove the pan from the heat. Add 1 tablespoon of dried herb or 2 tablespoons of fresh herb, cover, and steep for 30 minutes. Strain the tea and let it cool, then use immediately. Store leftover tea in a squeeze bottle, which you can keep on your bathroom counter for 3 days or in your refrigerator for up to 5 days.

---

# GUIDE TO
# PROFESSIONAL CARE

The best practitioner to treat oily skin is an esthetician, a person trained in professional skin care, says Stephanie Tourles, a licensed esthetician, reflexologist, and herbalist in West Hyannisport, Massachusetts. If you also have moderate to severe acne, you should see a dermatologist, who should work with an esthetician to keep your pores deep-cleansed, says Tourles.

You may also want to consider a professional aromatherapist who specializes in skin care, says Joni Loughran, an esthetician, cosmetologist, and aromatherapist in Petaluma, California. "Aromatherapy treatments can be very beneficial for oily skin to help balance glandular activity, improve circulation, and detoxify," she says.

"Apply the toner with a cotton ball or square whenever your skin feels excessively oily or looks shiny," Tourles says. "This herbal remedy won't overdry your skin; you can use it up to 10 times a day." There's one caution, though: Keep it away from your eyes.

## AROMATHERAPY: *Try This Twice-a-Week Toner*

Astringent essential oils are excellent for oily skin, says Close. She recommends using this toner once or twice a week.

Dilute five drops of rosemary, geranium, or juniper essential oil with 1 tablespoon of an astringent base oil, such as apricot kernel or hazelnut. Put three to four drops of the oil onto a clean cotton pad and use it to gently dab any excess oil off your face.

These base oils are very lightweight and will not clog your pores, make your skin more oily, or add a shine to your skin.

## HYDROTHERAPY: *Sedate Your Oil Glands with Cool Water*

"Warm water activates the oil glands, while cooler water slows them down," says Loughran. After you clean your face (once in the morning and once in the evening—gently and never with soap), splash your face well with cool water.

## HYDROTHERAPY: *Steam Your Pores Clean*

"Steaming helps to deep-clean oily skin," Loughran says, and suggests doing it once or twice a week for 8 to 10 minutes. She prefers using a small facial steaming machine to the "face-over-the-pot" method.

"Putting your face over a pot does not provide continuous, gentle steam with a consistent temperature," she says. "The small facial steamers are much safer and more effective."

Start with a clean face, then apply eye cream and lip balm to protect those delicate areas. Follow the instructions for using the machine that you've purchased. After steaming, rinse with warm water, then splash with cool water and pat dry.

# The Natural Way to Prevent and Possibly Reverse
# Osteoporosis

Your skeleton is living tissue, just like your muscles or skin, and it's constantly wearing out and being rebuilt. Cells called osteoclasts dissolve old bone, leaving tiny spaces. Then cells called osteoblasts move into those empty areas, building new bone.

In osteoporosis, a disease that develops over decades, more bone is dissolved than is built. In other words, you lose bone. The cumulative result, particularly for American women, is a tragedy.

Each year, there are 1.5 million fractures caused by the skeletal erosion of osteoporosis. In fact, 50 percent of all white women in the United States will break an osteoporosis-weakened bone sometime during their lifetimes, says John Lee, M.D., a retired physician in Sebastopol, California

The real tragedy, though, is that osteoporosis is an "easily preventable or reversible disease," Dr. Lee feels. "I believe that age is not the cause of osteoporosis. Poor nutrition, lack of exercise, and progesterone deficiency are the major factors."

Here are the ways that alternative practitioners recommend to counter those major factors and keep your skeleton from ever scaring you.

## Eating to Beat Osteoporosis

The best place to begin your fight against osteoporosis is at the dinner table—not to mention the breakfast and lunch tables. Here's how.

### MEAT: *Six Ounces a Day Will Do*
Your body requires 1½ to 2 ounces of protein a day, which is the amount in a 6-ounce serving of red meat, poultry, or fish. Eat much more than that amount, Dr. Lee believes, and your

body produces "acidic protein waste products" that your kidneys can't eliminate until they're "buffered" with the mineral calcium.

Where do your kidneys get the calcium to do the job? From your body's biggest calcium reservoir—your bones. The result could be what doctors call a negative calcium balance.

"In osteoporosis," says Dr. Lee, "calcium is being lost from the bones faster than it is being added." He believes that's much less likely to happen if you eat no more than 6 ounces of meat daily.

## CALCIUM-RICH FOODS: *Not Necessarily Dairy*

You should be certain to include plenty of calcium-rich foods in your diet so that your calcium balance stays in the black. Three or four servings a day of low-fat dairy products, such as cheese or yogurt, or calcium-containing vegetables, such as bok choy, collards, or spinach, will do the trick. But is milk a must for meat eaters who want to beat osteoporosis? No, says Dr. Lee.

"It's important to remember that most of the people on Earth live where cow's milk is not used," he says. "And those people have better bones than we in the more northern industrialized areas have."

Brenda Beeley, a licensed acupuncturist and director of the Menopause and PMS Options for Women health center on Bainbridge Island, Washington, often tells her patients with osteoporosis not to rely on dairy products for calcium because many adult women are unable to digest lactose.

Instead, she recommends that people with osteoporosis emphasize foods that deliver all the nutrients that bones need, which include not only calcium but also magnesium, copper, zinc, manganese, silica, and boron. Those foods include soy products such as tofu and tempeh; dark green, leafy vegetables; broccoli; seaweed; salmon; sardines; beans; and almonds.

## BETAINE HYDROCHLORIDE: *Take with Meals*

As some people age, their stomachs produce less hydrochloric acid, which breaks down foods so that their nutrients can be absorbed. That means that their bodies absorb less calcium and other nutrients, such as vitamin $B_{12}$.

Alternative practitioners often test people with osteoporosis for low stomach acid. Those who are found to have it are advised

# GUIDE TO
# PROFESSIONAL CARE

Every woman age 35 or older and every man over the age of 60 should see a medical doctor to have a bone mineral density (BMD) measurement, which will show you and your physician the current state of your bones, says John Lee, M.D., a retired physician in Sebastopol, California.

If the BMD test shows bone loss, necessitating treatment for osteoporosis, you should repeat the test a year later to find out if the treatment is working.

Dr. Lee also advises women to take a yearly height measurement, starting at age 30. "A decrease in height caused by deterioration of the spinal bones is a likely indicator of osteoporosis," he says.

The most commonly recommended medical treatments for osteoporosis are estrogen preparations and calcium. However, Alan Gaby, M.D., a nutritionally oriented physician in Seattle, thinks that those treatments by themselves do not produce the best results and that treatment with natural remedies like those discussed in this chapter is far more likely to stop or possibly reverse bone loss.

"In my practice, I almost always begin treating osteoporosis with dietary modifications and nutritional supplements," he says.

He adds, however, that if a BMD test shows that the patient already has severe osteoporosis or is at high risk for developing the disease, estrogen and biphosphonate, a bone-protecting medication, may be necessary. Risk factors include having a close relative who has osteoporosis; being Caucasian; being thin and petite; not exercising; smoking; and regular use of antacids, diuretics, sleeping pills, or cortisone drugs.

to take one to three 10-grain capsules (tablets may be too hard to digest) of betaine hydrochloride with the first few bites of every meal, says Alan Gaby, M.D., a nutritionally oriented physician in Seattle.

Do not use these supplements unless a doctor has confirmed that you have low stomach acid, and then take them only with your doctor's supervision. If you experience heartburn, reduce the dosage. Also, if you take aspirin, ibuprofen, or other non-steroidal anti-inflammatory drugs, do not take betaine hydrochloride, because the combination could increase the risk of developing an ulcer.

## APPLE-CIDER VINEGAR: *To Pass the Acid Test*

Another way to keep your stomach acid levels high enough to aid absorption of nutrients is to drink apple-cider vinegar, Beeley says. Add 1 tablespoon to 8 ounces of water and drink it at the start of each meal.

### A Risk-Free Medicine
### That Can Reverse Osteoporosis

If you're a postmenopausal woman who's been diagnosed with osteoporosis, your doctor may have told you that it was the hormone estrogen produced by your ovaries that protected your bones when you were still ovulating and that you should consider a prescription for synthetic estrogen to slow the progress of the disease.

"Is your doctor telling you a fact, or are you hearing a scientifically dubious belief promulgated by the drug companies that sell estrogen?" asks John Lee, M.D., a retired physician in Sebastopol, California.

"Osteoporosis in women typically starts in their midthirties, often 15 years before menopause, with a bone loss rate of about 1 to 1.5 percent a year," Dr. Lee says.

At menopause, Dr. Lee says, that rate increases to 3 to 5 percent for about 5 years, then levels off and continues at about 1.5 percent per year. If estrogen prevents osteoporosis, he asks, "why does bone loss occur 10 to 15 years before menopause, when estrogen levels are still normal?"

The answer, he says, is that levels of the hormone progesterone (the other hormone manufactured by the ovaries of menstruating women) begin to fall during a woman's midthirties.

"I believe that the more important factor in osteoporosis is the lack of progesterone, which causes a decrease in new bone formation," says Dr. Lee. "Adding progesterone can actively increase bone mass and density and can possibly reverse osteoporosis."

Over a 10-year period, Dr. Lee used natural progesterone cream, along with a natural diet, vitamin and mineral supplements, and exercise, to treat hundreds of postmenopausal women with osteoporosis.

In a statistical analysis of 100 of his patients, he found that women with the worst cases of osteoporosis had an average 23.4 percent gain in bone mineral density after 3 years of treatment—a remarkable increase. Overall, the 100 patients had an average gain in bone of almost 13 percent, Dr. Lee says.

"With experiences such as these in patient after patient over a 10-year period, I cannot doubt that natural progesterone, along with a program of diet, a few vitamin and mineral supplements, and modest exercise, can effectively, inexpensively, and safely reverse osteoporosis in women," he says.

The key, he believes, is *natural* progesterone. Ask most doctors about progesterone, and they're likely to tell you about synthetic progesterone, called progestins, progestogens, and gestagens.

"These agents do not provide the full spectrum of natural progesterone's biological activity, and they may not be as safe," Dr. Lee says. Using natural progesterone products is easy.

To prevent or possibly reverse osteoporosis, Dr. Lee recommends that a woman use a 3 percent cream of natural progesterone, applied daily at bedtime, 24 days a month if she is postmenopausal or 2 weeks before her menstrual period if she is not menopausal. It's best to apply it to areas where people blush, such as the face, neck, chest, breasts, underarms, and palms of the hands, because there are more capillaries closer to the skin surface in those areas to increase absorption.

At that rate, you should be using ⅓ to ½ ounce a month. And you don't have to worry about side effects. Dr. Lee says there have never been any reported toxic effects from using natural progesterone at the recommended levels.

Two final tips: Dr. Lee recommends that you have a bone mineral density test before you start using natural progesterone and another a year later.

"If your bone mass hasn't stabilized or increased after a year of progesterone, good diet, and exercise, you and your doctor must address other factors in your life that can cause bone loss, such as cigarette smoking or the use of medications such as cortisone," he says.

Also, postmenopausal women who have very little body fat may need natural progesterone and estrogen supplements to preserve their bone. Those women may not produce enough estrone, a bone-protecting hormone generated by body fat both before and after menopause, Dr. Lee says.

## CALCIUM: *But Not Too Much*

Because calcium is so important for strong bones, Dr. Gaby recommends taking supplements of 600 to 1,500 milligrams a day.

If you take more than that, however, you may get so much calcium that it will interfere with the absorption of magnesium and certain trace minerals, possibly causing your bones to get weaker instead of stronger.

"Taking calcium supplements alone, particularly in large amounts, may not do as much good as it could unless several other nutrients are taken as well," Dr. Gaby warns.

## MAGNESIUM: *Calcium's Best Friend*

About half of the magnesium in your body is found in your bones, where it works with calcium to create a stronger bone structure and thus help prevent fractures.

Dr. Gaby cites a study in which postmenopausal women who took 500 milligrams of calcium and 600 milligrams of magnesium (along with other nutrients and hormone replacement therapy, or HRT), had an 11 percent increase in bone mineral density within 1 year, while postmenopausal women who took HRT but didn't take nutritional supplements had a 0.7 percent increase.

"If someone chooses to take supplemental calcium for osteoporosis, I strongly urge increasing magnesium intake as well," Dr. Gaby says.

How much magnesium? The typical guideline is to take twice as much calcium as magnesium, and most calcium-magnesium supplements contain this ratio. Dr. Gaby says, however, that there's no scientific research indicating the best ratio.

### Tap for Better Bones

"Percussion builds bone mass," says Rich Rieger, a licensed massage therapist in Morgantown, West Virginia.

He's talking not about playing the drums but about a massage technique called tapotement, a light tapping on the body that massage therapists believe mimics the bone-building stimulation from exercise. (Do this technique in addition to exercise, not as a substitute.) Here's how it works.

Bring the fingers of your right hand together so there's no space between them. Your hand should look as it would if you were about to swim freestyle. Next, bend your fingers and arch your palm so that your hand forms a cup shape. Do the same with your left hand.

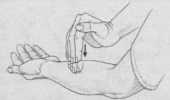

Using the tips of your fingers and the bases of your palms, tap very lightly over your hips, ribs, and (with one hand at a time) your forearms; these three areas are commonly weakened by osteoporosis. Or you can have your partner tap over your entire body, including the spine. Do tapotement once or twice a day for 5 minutes each time, Rieger recommends.

## VITAMIN D: *Stay on the Sunny Side*

Vitamin D is a must for the absorption of calcium, but most people don't get enough in their diets. Beeley recommends taking 400 international units of vitamin D daily.

You may have heard that you can get plenty of vitamin D by exposing your face to the sun for a few minutes each day, since Ol' Sol kindly turns a chemical in your skin into the vitamin. But Dr. Lee says that you'd need an hour a day of near-total body exposure to produce all the vitamin D you need. Since it's not advisable to do that much sunbathing, the simplest way to get plenty of calcium-helping vitamin D is by taking a supplement.

## VITAMIN K: *An Essential Building Block*

"A strong case can be made that vitamin K deficiency is one of the factors contributing to the development of osteoporosis and that vitamin K supplementation may be of value in preventing or possibly reversing bone loss," says Dr. Gaby. That's because vitamin K is necessary for the production of osteocalcin, a protein that functions as a foundation for calcium to construct bone.

The best food source of this nutrient is dark green, leafy vegetables. As added insurance, says Dr. Gaby, you may want to supplement your diet by taking 150 to 500 micrograms of vitamin K a day. Some nutritional supplements that are aimed at preventing or treating osteoporosis may contain this much vitamin K. If not, you may have to take a separate supplement.

## MANGANESE: *For a Strong Foundation*

Manganese is another foundation nutrient that helps build bone, and a deficiency of the mineral "may be one of the important factors related to the current epidemic of osteoporosis," says Dr. Gaby.

Nutritional deficiency may be rampant among Americans because our farming and food-processing techniques strip food of the mineral and because many food additives may block its absorption, Dr. Gaby says.

Manganese-rich foods include whole grains, nuts, seeds, and leafy vegetables. In his practice, Dr. Gaby also uses supplements that provide 5 to 20 milligrams of the mineral.

### Exercise Builds Bones

To understand why exercise is so crucial to strong bones, look to the skies. When astronauts live for a few weeks in a gravity-free environment, with little or no push-and-pull on their bones, they lose bone mass, says John Lee, M.D., a retired physician in Sebastopol, California. But if you look at the bone mass of a left-handed pitcher's left arm, you'll see big, thick bones.

Dr. Lee describes a study in which postmenopausal women who exercised regularly for 22 months increased the bone density of parts of their spines by 6.1 percent, while women who didn't exercise lost bone.

Almost any type of vigorous exercise will maintain or build bone. Dr. Lee recommends walking, biking, tennis, or weight lifting.

For maximum bone building, Beeley recommends weight-bearing exercise such as walking or jogging three or four times a week. And she believes that every woman should exercise her arms and upper body with light weights at least once or twice a week.

## OTHER SUPPLEMENTS: *What You Need*

Besides calcium, magnesium, vitamin K, and manganese, Dr. Gaby uses the following dosages for people who want to prevent or help reverse osteoporosis with nutritional supplements.

- Zinc: 10 to 30 milligrams
- Copper: 1 to 2 milligrams
- Boron: 1 to 3 milligrams
- Silicon: 1 to 2 milligrams
- Strontium: 0.5 to 3 milligrams
- Vitamin $B_6$: 5 to 50 milligrams
- Folic acid: 400 to 5,000 micrograms
- Vitamin C: 100 to 1,000 milligrams

**HERBS:** *A Bone-Building Brew*

For those who are willing to make and drink three cups of tea a day, Beeley recommends brewing a tea with one part horsetail, one part sage, one part alfalfa, one part oats, and one part peppermint (for taste) in 8 ounces of water. These herbs are rich in bone-building minerals, she says.

# *A Holistic Approach Is Key to Overcoming* **Overweight**

If you have a health problem, and you treat only the symptom and not the underlying cause, you may experience temporary relief. But the symptom will likely return . . . again . . . and again.

Sound anything like your extra pounds? The pounds you've lost and regained . . . again . . . and again?

"Overweight is the symptom of fundamental imbalances in your body, emotions, and mind," says Shoshanna Katzman, a certified acupuncturist, director of the Red Bank Acupuncture and Wellness Center in New Jersey, and cofounder of the Feeling Light weight-management program. These imbalances include:

- Emotional imbalance, in which food is used as a substitute for love or a way to "stuff" your uncomfortable feelings back inside you

• Nutritional imbalance, with the body crying out for the nutrients it needs for optimal functioning—nutrients that your food choices aren't supplying
• Physical imbalance, such as stored toxins in the digestive tract that drain your energy and cause you to eat "stimulating" foods like sugar that make you even more toxic in the long run
• Mental imbalance, in which your thoughts anxiously or angrily or sadly dwell on the past or future and you're never mindful of what you're doing now—including what you're eating

"When you're in balance, you naturally and easily make food choices that support your overall state of health," Katzman

---

## GUIDE TO
## PROFESSIONAL CARE

The best alternative health professional to help you lose weight is a person who understands and can help solve the various nutritional, metabolic, hormonal, immune, and lifestyle problems that actually cause overweight, says Julia Ross, executive director of Recovery Systems in Mill Valley, California. The practitioner should be able to medically investigate and correct each of the following eight factors that are possible underlying factors in weight problems, according to Ross.

• Depleted brain chemistry
• A low-calorie diet, which is a common cause of overeating
• Blood sugar problems, including medical problems such as hypoglycemia, diabetes, and exhaustion of the adrenal glands
• Low thyroid function
• Food allergies and addictions
• Hormone imbalances
• Yeast overgrowth with candida, which can cause carbohydrate cravings
• A deficiency of essential fatty acids

says. Here are some of her best client-tested methods for correcting the imbalances that she believes are the underlying cause of overweight.

## FOOD: *A Smoothie That Stops Cravings*

Having this Feeling Light smoothie or blender drink for breakfast is the most important balance-restoring step for many of her weight-loss clients, she says.

"The drink is a total infusion of essential vitamins, minerals, fatty acids, protein, and fiber," she says. "And it's a great way to cut down on food cravings, because, with the super-nutrition in the smoothie, you're actually giving your body the nutrients it needs."

Just put the following ingredients in a blender, mix, and drink:

1 cup rice milk; 1 cup soy milk; 1 cup apple juice, orange juice, or other fruit juice; 1 banana; 4 fresh strawberries; 1 teaspoon blackstrap molasses; 1 tablespoon aloe juice; 1 tablespoon black cherry juice concentrate; 1 tablespoon powdered "green" formulation; 1 to 2 tablespoons powdered brewer's or nutritional yeast; 1 teaspoon raw, organic bee pollen (loose, not in tablets or capsules); and 1 tablespoon flaxseed oil.

Be creative, says Katzman. Experiment with proportions to taste, or freeze the bananas or strawberries for a thicker, colder drink.

## AFFIRMATIONS: *Make the Right Food Choices*

Affirmations—positive statements of belief—can help you make the right food choices, Katzman says. "When you're confronted with food—while looking in the pantry, standing in front of the refrigerator, shopping at the supermarket, or eating at a restaurant—the whole key to making the right, healthy, balanced choice is what your mind is thinking at that moment," she says.

What's more, she says, if you regularly spend 5 to 10 minutes once or twice a day mentally affirming your intention to be balanced and healed, it's much more likely that you will make the right food choices. She recommends choosing one or two affirmations from the following list, memorizing them, and saying them to yourself on a regular basis.

- I am revealing a clearer, healthier, happier me.
- I am in control.
- I take responsibility for my physical self, my wellness, and my health.
- I eat to nourish my mind, body, and spirit.

## REBOUNDING: *The Best Weight-Loss Exercise*

Jumping on a rebounder or small trampoline is a particularly good exercise for those trying to lose weight, says Katzman. Alternative practitioners believe that it helps strengthen the lymphatic system, the body system that drains toxins and supports stronger immunity. She recommends a session of 20 to 30 minutes of rebounding three to five times a week.

### A Supplement Strategy
### That Cures Cravings

Julia Ross, executive director of Recovery Systems in Mill Valley, California, says that there often is a link between overeating and the levels of key chemicals in the brain.

"You are using food as self-medication because you are low in certain brain chemicals," she says, and your brain has to have these chemicals to function, she explains. Your food cravings, as well as depression, irritability, anxiety, and many other emotional and mental problems, are signs that your brain doesn't have enough of them.

When the brain is deprived of these chemicals, it sends out signals that overwhelm your willpower, triggering you to eat a druglike food (usually carbohydrate) that substitutes for the missing chemicals and makes you feel better—for a little while, says Ross.

These brain chemicals, which include dopamine, a natural energizer; GABA, a natural sedative; endorphin, a natural painkiller; and serotonin, a sleep promoter and mood and attention stabilizer, are deficient for a number of reasons, Ross says. They range from genetics and stress to overeating refined sugar and flours and eating too little protein.

You can easily correct those deficiencies with nutritional supplements that boost those brain chemicals, however. That in turn will stop your cravings, soothe your emotional and mental problems, and start you on the road to permanent weight loss.

Specifically, the supplements are amino acids, the building blocks of protein.

"Scientific studies have confirmed the effectiveness of using just a few targeted amino acid 'precursors' to the brain chemicals, thereby eliminating your cravings for food as well as your depression, anxiety, irritability, obsessiveness, and mental dullness," Ross says.

There are, of course, many factors that can cause overweight, says Ross. She believes that they include low-calorie dieting, blood sugar disorders, low thyroid function, food allergies, hormone imbalances, infection with the yeast candida, and a deficiency of fatty acids.

Correcting your brain chemistry with amino acids is the first and most important step in eliminating food cravings, Ross believes, so you can then address all the health problems that contribute to overweight. You can safely take all of the following supplements until you reach your goal weight or for a year, whichever comes first, Ross says.

### GLUTAMINE: *Balance Blood Sugar, Stop the Cravings*

Food cravings, particularly for sweets and starches, are often caused by low blood sugar, or hypoglycemia. But you can stabilize the delivery of blood sugar to your brain—and stop the cravings—by taking two 500-milligram capsules of glutamine three times a day between meals, says Ross.

If you want fast, emergency relief of carbohydrate cravings, Ross recommends opening a 500-milligram capsule of glutamine, pouring the contents under your tongue, and letting it dissolve.

### TYROSINE: *For Low Energy and Poor Concentration*

You feel fatigued and brain-fogged nearly all the time, and you use coffee and sweets (and maybe cigarettes) to give you a lift. If that description fits you, Ross recommends that you take 500 to 2,000 milligrams of tyrosine three times a day—before breakfast, at midmorning, and at midafternoon.

Start with 500 milligrams. If that doesn't seem to do the trick, increase your next dose by 500 milligrams, to 1,000. Continue to increase by 500 milligrams until you feel energized and alert, but don't exceed 2,000 milligrams per dose.

You may find that tyrosine is too stimulating, making you jittery or keeping you awake at night, or that it doesn't clear away your fatigue. If that's the case, eliminate it and use a similar amino acid, d-phenylalanine, at doses of 250 to 500 milligrams on the same three-times-a-day schedule.

## D-PHENYLALANINE: *If You Eat to Overcome Emotional Pain*

"If you overeat to help yourself deal with emotional pain—if you're sensitive, cry easily, crave comfort, and love certain foods—you may need the amino acid d-phenylalanine," says Ross.

That's because this supplement builds up your brain's reservoir of endorphins, the natural opiates that help to create feelings of pleasure and reduce physical pain. She recommends taking 500 milligrams of DLPA (a supplement that combines the d- and l- forms of phenylalanine), along with 500 milligrams of glutamine, three times a day—upon arising, at midmorning, and at midafternoon.

If you take DLPA regularly, you don't need to take phenylalanine to give you extra energy, as suggested above. Ross also recommends that you consume plenty of high-protein foods, which supply amino acids, since the body requires all of the amino acids in order to manufacture endorphins.

## GABA: *For Stress and Tension*

Your muscles are chronically tense. You feel stressed and burned out. Your doctor says that you should relax, but he might as well be telling you to levitate, because you just don't know how to calm down.

What's more, you chronically overeat sweets and starches (and perhaps smoke, drink, or use tranquilizers to help you cope). If this sounds like you, you may need gamma aminobutyric acid (GABA), says Ross. She recommends taking 100 to 500 milligrams whenever you feel the need to relax. (Experiment to find the dose that works for you, starting at 100 milligrams and increasing by increments of 100 milligrams, but don't exceed 1,000 milligrams a day.)

Don't take the supplement first thing in the morning, since it may make you too relaxed to drive. And you might want to look for a product that combines GABA with two other relaxation-inducing amino acids, taurine and glycine, Ross says.

"This combination can be even more calming for some people than GABA alone," she says.

## 5-HTP: *For Depression, Anxiety, or Low Self-Esteem*

If you have low levels of the brain chemical serotonin, you can have a host of emotional and mental problems that compel you to overeat sweets, starches, and chocolate. These problems include depression, anxiety, low self-esteem, obsessive thoughts, winter blues, irritability, and insomnia.

If you're experiencing any of those, Ross recommends that you take 50 to 100 milligrams of the serotonin-boosting supplement 5-hydroxytryptophan (5-HTP) three times a day.

### Imagine a Thinner You

Don't think of a purple elephant.

You immediately thought of a purple elephant, didn't you?

That's because your subconscious mind—the mind of desires, dreams, impulses, and urges—responds to words by forming images.

If you substitute the words *chocolate cake* or *pizza* for *purple elephant*, you'll have a very clear idea of what happens when you tell yourself again and again not to eat something. Your subconscious mind is overwhelmed with the desire to eat it, and eventually, you do.

That's why using positive imagery, or visualization, can succeed where willpower fails, says Debbie Johnson, author of *Think Yourself Thin: The Visualization Technique That Will Make You Lose Weight without Diet or Exercise*.

If you consistently imagine yourself thin, your subconscious will begin supporting everyday actions that help you become thin. Johnson calls it Focused Imagination, which goes beyond visualization to use all of your senses. Johnson herself lost 40 pounds and has kept it off for years using Focused Imagination. Here's her advice for making it work for you.

• Develop a "key image." Focus on an image of yourself as a thin person. "It anchors your mind to the ultimate fulfillment of your weight-loss goal," says Johnson. Use all of your senses—hearing, feeling, seeing, and smelling—to develop every aspect of the image. What does your body look like—exactly? What are you wearing? Where are you? At the beach, on the tennis court, dancing the night away? Imagine the happiness you feel with your new, thinner body.

"Picture the scene as if it were a movie or video about your new, thinner life—the life that you will be living very soon," Johnson says.

• Experience the Golden Minute. This is a time—twice a day, for 30 seconds when you wake up in the morning and 30 seconds before you fall asleep at night—when you intensively use your key image and other reinforcing mental exercises.

First, tell your body that you love and appreciate it just the way it is; that way, you won't feed your subconscious with negative images about yourself. Next, says Johnson, "tell your body that you are going to make some helpful changes."

Next, imagine that you are in a corner of the ceiling of your room, looking down at your new body. See your key image. Feel the wonderful, exhilarating sensation of being your thin self. If it's morning, get out of bed with the feeling of your new body and carry it with you throughout the day. If it's evening, fall asleep with this image so your subconscious, which never sleeps, can reinforce your key image overnight.

• Use a key phrase. Whenever you think of your key image, you should also say a key phrase to yourself, Johnson says. Her own favorite phrase is "I feel a little thinner today." Using a key phrase, she explains, helps bring your key image "into the moment" and also helps reinforce the image.

• Don't give up, says Johnson. If you persist, Focused Imagination will work. And don't worry about negative thoughts. "They're just part of being human," she says. "Every time a negative thought about you arises, use it as a springboard for visualizing and feeling your key image."

## Fats That Can Help You Lose

Fat supplements? For a person who's trying to lose weight, the idea of taking fat in a pill sounds like a cruel joke. But here's what you may not know: A deficiency of certain types of good fats, called essential fatty acids (EFA), that your body requires can lead you to crave and overeat the bad kinds of fats and put on extra pounds.

That's the opinion of Ann Louise Gittleman, a certified nutrition specialist in Bozeman, Montana. "Fat phobia is the cause of so much overweight in this country," she says. "Yes, saturated fats in animal products and trans-fats in processed foods are bad for your health. But not getting enough of the good fats—the essential fatty acids found in foods like fatty fish, certain oils, leafy greens, avocados, and nuts and seeds—is also bad for your health."

The different types of EFA, she believes, actually stimulate fat metabolism so that your body burns more fat, trigger the production of hormones that make you feel full, and balance your body's levels of insulin (the hormone that burns sugars) so you don't crave high-calorie sugars and other fattening carbohydrates.

Most Americans are deficient in various essential fatty acids, such as gamma-linolenic acid (GLA), alpha-linolenic acid (LNA), eicosapentaenoic acid (EPA), and docosahex-aenoic acid (DHA), Gittleman believes. The best way to make sure that you get enough of all of those types of EFA, each of which is crucial in helping you lose weight, is with EFA supplements, Gittleman says. Here's what she recommends.

## FLAXSEED OIL: *Reset Your Thermostat*

The LNA and other omega-3 fatty acids found in flaxseed oil help reset your body's thermostat to a normal level so you burn excess calories, Gittleman says. They also help normalize insulin metabolism, thus reducing sugar cravings. She recommends 1 tablespoon a day with a meal. Flaxseed is a great supplement, Gittleman says, and can be safely taken on a regular basis.

## GLA: *Activate Brown Fat*

GLA helps you lose weight by activating dormant brown fat, the type of fat that helps burn excess calories.

"Brown fat makes it possible to expend ingested fat as energy rather than storing it as excess white fat," Gittleman says. "Many of my clients who had 10 pounds or more to lose have reported dramatically successful results by taking four to eight 500-milligram capsules of GLA-rich evening primrose oil a day."

**CLA:** *Inhibit the Enzyme That Stores Fat*

The essential fatty acid conjugated linoleic acid (CLA) may help in your weight-loss efforts, says Gittleman. In a scientific study, people who took 3,000 milligrams of CLA daily lost 20 percent of their body fat in 3 months without dieting, she says.

The theory is that CLA interferes with the production of lipase, an enzyme that affects the way the body metabolizes fat. She recommends taking 1,000 milligrams three times a day before meals. As a bonus, CLA may have breast cancer–fighting properties and general immune-enhancing properties, Gittleman adds.

**FISH OIL:** *Balance Your Overall Fat Intake*

Although the fatty acids found in fish oil do not directly help with weight loss, they are crucial for balancing your overall intake of fats and maintaining good health, Gittleman says. She recommends taking 1,000 milligrams of the product Super-MaxEPA two or three times daily.

# Nutritional Supplements
## Can Help Slow
# Parkinson's Disease

With Parkinson's disease, connections between the brain and muscles deteriorate, resulting in tremors, a stooped and rigid posture, slow and difficult speech, a masklike facial expression, and eventually, dementia, as the process progresses in the brain. Conventional medicine can only respond with drugs that decrease the symptoms and perhaps slow (but never stop) the progress of the disease.

Truth be told, alternative medicine doesn't have a better answer. It does, however, offer powerful treatments that can lend prescription medicines a very big helping hand.

"There are various nutritional supplements that can help control or delay some of the movement-related and mental symptoms of Parkinson's disease," says Alan Brauer, M.D., founder and director of the TotalCare Medical Center in Palo Alto, California.

"Nutritional remedies have their greatest effect when Parkinson's first appears or has just begun to develop," says Philip Lee Miller, M.D., founder and director of the Los Gatos Longevity Institute in California. "Someone who's newly diagnosed with Parkinson's should ask himself, What can I do to slow the progress of this disease and reduce symptoms? In my opinion, the answer should include nutritional supplements."

## ANTIOXIDANTS: *E, C, and Glutathione to the Rescue*

One theory about the cause of Parkinson's disease says that free radicals (molecular monsters produced by a wide variety of biochemical and lifestyle factors) are oxidizing or destroying the receptor cells in the substantia nigra, a relay station in the brain between the body's muscles and the cerebellum, the area in the brain that controls movement.

Antioxidants can block that free radical damage and perhaps slow the progress of Parkinson's. But, says Dr. Miller, to be effective, several antioxidants must work together.

"The antioxidant process is like a team running a relay race," he says. "Vitamin C runs the first lap, becomes exhausted, and is replaced by vitamin E, which is then replaced by glutathione. Then so-called co-factors of glutathione take over." Here's how to outfit your team.

• Vitamin C: 1,000 to 4,000 milligrams daily in three divided doses with meals
• Vitamin E: 600 to 1,200 international units daily in three divided doses with meals
• Glutathione: The product Thiodox, from Allergy Research, which Dr. Miller recommends, provides a daily intake of 200 milligrams of glutathione and the nutritional co-factors necessary to make it work

## THIAMIN: *Boost Your Dopamine*

Dopamine is a chemical that enables messages to be sent from brain cell to brain cell. With Parkinson's, the availability of dopamine to the cerebellum plummets.

High levels of the B vitamin thiamin may help the brain produce dopamine, says Dr. Brauer. He recommends 3,000 to

---

# GUIDE TO
# PROFESSIONAL CARE

*Caution: You should use the alternative remedies discussed in this chapter only as part of a treatment program that is guided and monitored by a qualified medical doctor in partnership with a qualified alternative practitioner, both of whom are experienced in caring for your condition. Check with your conventional doctor before changing or stopping any conventional medical treatments or medications, and keep all of your doctors and/or alternative practitioners informed of all treatments that you are receiving.*

Tell your doctor if you notice an increase in one or more of the following symptoms of Parkinson's disease: muscle rigidity; tremor in the limbs, head, neck, face, or jaw; slow movement response; poor balance; or walking problems.

Philip Lee Miller, M.D., founder and director of the Los Gatos Longevity Institute in California, advises looking for a medical doctor who understands that drugs are not the only answer to disease and who will be open to using nutritional supplements to help slow Parkinson's and reduce its severity.

---

8,000 milligrams daily. You'll need to check with your doctor to find out which dosage is right for you.

## TYROSINE: *Another Dopamine Booster*

The amino acid tyrosine is an essential precursor of dopamine formation. Dr. Miller recommends taking 500 to 1,000 milligrams of the supplement once in the morning on an empty stomach.

## COENZYME Q$_{10}$: *A Potent Anti-Aging Nutrient*

This vitamin-like nutrient, found in every cell of the body, is crucial for sparking cellular energy. Dr. Miller recommends it for most patients to slow aging, and he says that Parkinson's patients should take at least 200 milligrams a day.

## PROTEIN SUPPLEMENTS: *Stop Muscle Wasting*

Muscle wasting—the decrease of muscle mass—is a common symptom of Parkinson's. Protein supplements can help maintain muscle mass, Dr. Miller says. Of the supplements available over the counter, he favors the product manufactured by Solgar called Whey to Go because it has the fewest harmful additives, such as artificial sweeteners, and has a pleasant taste. Follow the dosage recommendations on the label.

## DHEA: *A Helpful Hormone*

Parkinson's patients have low levels of this hormone, which is secreted by the adrenal glands, so supplementation may help reduce symptoms, says Dr. Brauer. He recommends 10 milligrams a day for women and 25 milligrams a day for men. Take this supplement only under the supervision of a knowledgeable medical doctor.

## Brain Food

The following nutritional supplements strengthen the brain and may help delay the onset of dementia in Parkinson's patients.

## NADH: *It's Usually Needed*

This coenzyme—a molecular key that opens biochemical doors and provides energy to the brain—is often deficient in people with Parkinson's, Dr. Brauer says. He recommends 10 to 20 milligrams of NADH (a form of the chemical nicotinamide adenine dinucleotide that includes hydrogen) a day, taken in the form of an oral spray, which improves absorption.

## PHOSPHATIDYLSERINE: *To Improve Memory*

This substance helps boosts the energy levels of the brain, improving memory and general mental functioning, Dr. Brauer says. He recommends 300 milligrams daily in three divided doses with meals.

## ZINC: *It's Good for the Brain*

Many people with Parkinson's are deficient in this mineral, and those low levels may contribute to dementia, Dr. Brauer says. He recommends taking a multivitamin/mineral supplement that supplies at least 30 to 50 milligrams of zinc.

**GINKGO:** *For Increased Blood Flow*

The herb ginkgo increases blood flow to the brain, helping to delay dementia, says Dr. Brauer. He recommends 200 to 300 milligrams a day in three divided doses with meals.

**VITAMIN B$_{12}$:** *Prevent a Shortfall*

A deficiency of this vitamin can compromise mental functioning in Parkinson's patients, says Dr. Brauer. He recommends 100 micrograms a day, either in a B-complex supplement or as part of a high-potency multivitamin/mineral supplement.

# Cleansing Herbs Head the List of Natural Remedies for
# Phlebitis

Phlebitis comes in two varieties: superficial and deep. Deep-vein phlebitis (thrombophlebitis) is inflammation and clotting in (you guessed it) a large vein deep in your leg. The vein becomes so taut and inflamed that you probably can't bend your foot without severe pain. And it may be infected, causing a fever.

With deep-vein phlebitis, you need to go the emergency room immediately. It can generate a blood clot that can break off, lodge in your heart or lungs, and even kill you. Your doctor will immediately put you on clot-dissolving medications.

In superficial phlebitis, a vein near the surface of the skin is inflamed. This generally happens when blood flow in varicose veins slows, stagnates, or starts to clot. Even though it's not an emergency, you should still see a doctor for an accurate diagnosis. Your doctor will probably recommend that you elevate your leg, put moist heat on the vein to relieve the pain and inflammation, and take a painkiller.

What conventional medical doctors probably won't recommend, though, is a way to prevent another bout of superficial phlebitis—a way to strengthen your weak, phlebitis-prone veins. But Virender Sodhi, M.D. (Ayurved), N.D., an Ayurvedic and naturopathic physician and director of the American School of Ayurvedic Sciences in Bellevue, Washington, says that there is a way to help stop new episodes of superficial phlebitis. It starts with your liver.

**AYURVEDIC HERBS:** *Cleanse Your Liver*

"The weakness in the veins that causes phlebitis is a sign that the liver has not been working properly for a long time," says

---

# GUIDE TO
# PROFESSIONAL CARE

Phlebitis, an inflammation in a vein that can leave it red, tender, and painful, always requires medical attention. Only your doctor can determine the seriousness of your individual case, because a clot deep within a leg vein may be difficult to see or diagnose. Your doctor will use ultrasound to see if you have deep-vein phlebitis or superficial phlebitis. If it's the latter, which is not life-threatening, he may prescribe a variety of nonpharmaceutical and medical treatments, including applying moist heat for the pain, elevating the leg, and taking anti-inflammatory drugs such as aspirin and antibiotics.

If these treatments do not eliminate your symptoms within 7 to 10 days, or if the phlebitis flares up again, call your doctor immediately. Even superficial phlebitis can turn into undetected, life-threatening, deep-vein phlebitis. The only symptoms that you may experience with deep-vein phlebitis are a feeling of heaviness in the leg, high fever, noticeable lumps, and pain and swelling in your ankle or leg. If any of these symptoms occur, have someone take you to the nearest hospital emergency room immediately.

None of the treatments for phlebitis addresses the cause of the problem, however, which is weak veins. "Only a naturopathic physician or naturally oriented doctor can help heal the problem by returning your veins to normal strength so you're less likely to get phlebitis again," says Mark Stengler, N.D., a naturopathic physician in San Diego.

Dr. Sodhi. How does a weak liver translate into weak veins? The job of your veins is to return blood to the heart and then the lungs, where carbon dioxide is dumped and oxygen is picked up, says Dr. Sodhi. On the way, the blood stops at the liver, where it's cleansed of toxins.

If the liver is already congested with toxins—from a fatty diet, pollutants, and many other possible sources—the blood can't flow easily into the organ. The result, Dr. Sodhi believes, can be a small but damaging backup of blood, which dilates the veins in the legs and weakens them over time. Eventually, the veins are damaged to the point that they become inflamed, and even infected—and you have phlebitis.

Thus, says Dr. Sodhi, the first step in preventing a flare-up of phlebitis is freeing the liver of congestion. The best way to do that is with one of four liver herbs recommended by Dr. Sodhi: *Eclipta alba*, *Terminalia arjuna*, *Picrorhiza kurrooa*, and *Solanum nigrum*.

"All of these herbs have shown really good results in cleaning the liver and helping to prevent episodes of phlebitis," he says. Choose any of the herbs and follow the dosage recommendations on the label.

**CARROTS AND RADISHES:** *Liver-Cleansing Vegetables*
Both of these foods are good liver cleansers because they increase bile flow, says Dr. Sodhi. He recommends eating a couple of radishes and a carrot or two every day.

**POSTURE:** *Pull Up a Chair*
Another way to clear a congested liver is by pulling up a chair—but not to sit in. Instead, lie on your back on the floor and put your feet and lower legs on the seat of the chair. This helps move blood out of the veins in your legs and into your liver, Dr. Sodhi says. Do this once a day, staying in the position for 5 to 10 minutes.

**GOTU KOLA:** *An Herb to Restore Elasticity*
"To heal phlebitis, you first need to free the liver of congestion and then work on the veins themselves," Dr. Sodhi says. The herb gotu kola can help restore normal elasticity to veins so they're not easy targets for inflammation. Look for gotu kola in

capsule or tincture form and follow the dosage recommendations on the label.

## BUTCHER'S BROOM AND BILBERRY: *Two Tonics for Your Veins*

Both of these herbs are venotonics, meaning that they help
strengthen veins and reduce inflammation, says Mark Stengler,
N.D., a naturopathic physician in San Diego. He recommends
taking 100 milligrams of butcher's broom three times a day to
prevent a recurrence of phlebitis. Use a product standardized
for 10 percent ruscogenin, the active ingredient in the herb.

He also says to take two 80-milligram capsules of bilberry
three times a day to help prevent future flare-ups. Look for a
product standardized for 25 percent anthocyanoside, the active
ingredient.

## VITAMIN E: *For Clot Prevention*

Vitamin E strengthens the veins in the legs and thins the
blood, helping to prevent blood clots, says Dr. Sodhi. He recommends two doses of 400 international units of vitamin E
daily for anyone with phlebitis.

## MASSAGE: *Improve Your Circulation*

If your doctor has diagnosed your phlebitis as the superficial
variety that doesn't involve a blood clot, you should massage
your legs once or twice a day, Dr. Sodhi says. Gently but firmly
knead each leg from your ankle to your midthigh. "You'll push
the pooled blood out of the legs and back into circulation, helping to relieve some of the pressure in the veins and prevent
worsening of the phlebitis," he says.

# *Warding Off*
# **Plantar Warts**

Your sole is possessed by a devilish problem—and exorcism won't be easy.

Yes, a plantar wart (a wart on the bottom of your foot) is a kind of possession. The virus that forms warts is a spooky invader, taking over genes (DNA) and forcing them to produce more viruses and virus-carrying cells. It even forces your body to supply the area with blood vessels and nerves.

The result is a wart that's covered with calluses and can be as small as a pinhead or as large as a quarter. It has tiny brown, black, or red spots, which are the blood vessels. It lives as a loner or in a herd, and it usually takes up residence on the ball or heel of your foot, which can make walking painful.

A podiatrist can remove the wart, but there's no guarantee that it won't return. In fact, many plantar warts do, because the viruses live inside you, just waiting for a chance to reinfect your foot.

Because of that, one effective way to get rid of plantar warts for good is to strengthen your immune system, say alternative foot specialists.

## GARLIC: *Dissolve Your Wart in 10 Days*

Putting garlic directly on a plantar wart can get rid of it, says Andrea Murray, a certified reflexologist and herbalist in Portland, Maine.

Mash a clove of garlic into pulp. Before you go to bed, put the pulp directly on the wart and cover it with a small adhesive bandage, then with a sock. In the morning, remove the bandage and clean the area. "Within a few days, you should notice the wart shrinking, and after 10 days to 2 weeks, it should be gone," says Murray. If the wart doesn't go away within 3 to 4 weeks discontinue the treatment.

# GUIDE TO
# PROFESSIONAL CARE

If natural methods have failed to remove your plantar wart, you've had it for 2 years or longer, or it is painful or bleeds, you should have it removed by a podiatrist. The most effective removal methods are liquid nitrogen (which freezes and kills the wart so that it falls off) or a surgical laser.

Do not use over-the-counter drops of salicylic acid to remove the wart yourself. They can damage the skin of your foot, says Steven Subotnick, D.P.M., a podiatrist in Berkeley and San Leandro, California.

An effective alternative treatment is to have a homeopathic doctor or a health professional trained in homeopathy prescribe a constitutional homeopathic remedy based on your body's needs. Although it's not a widespread practice, some doctors will make a customized homeopathic preparation from your wart by removing a small portion of it to extract a tissue sample. "I have had very good success with this treatment," says Gregory W. Spencer, D.P.M., a podiatrist in Renton, Washington.

**TEA TREE ESSENTIAL OIL:** *To Stand Tall Again*
This essential oil is antiviral and can help get rid of plantar warts, says Stephanie Tourles, a licensed esthetician, reflexologist, and herbalist in West Hyannisport, Massachusetts.

Apply a few drops daily. Stop using the treatment after 3 to 4 months if the wart doesn't disappear.

**VITAMIN C:** *For Immunity*
To strengthen your immune system, take 1,000 milligrams of vitamin C, an antiviral nutrient, daily, recommends Steven Subotnick, D.P.M., a podiatrist in Berkeley and San Leandro, California.

**ASTRAGALUS:** *A Helpful Herb*
Astragalus is one of the best herbs for strengthening the immune system and defeating plantar warts, says Dr. Subotnick.

Follow the dosage recommendations on the label of the bottle of capsules that you buy.


### HOMEOPATHY: *The Right Choices*

The homeopathic remedies Thuja occidentalis and Antimonium crudum can help banish plantar warts, says Dr. Subotnick. If the wart bleeds when washed, try Nitricum acidum (nitric acid).

Take a 6C potency of the specific remedy, following the dosage recommendations on the label. Stop using the remedy when the wart goes away.


*Medical Care Plus Alternative*
*Home Remedies Can Beat*
# Pneumonia


Pneumonia isn't just a cold with a bad attitude. It's an infection of your lungs, a blast of bacteria (or of viruses, fungi, or other organisms) that scatters a shrapnel burst of symptoms. You can have a hacking cough that produces rust-colored or greenish mucus, chest pain, aching muscles, shortness of breath, fever, sweating, chills, headache, and weakness so severe that just turning over in bed wears you out.

Even though medical care for pneumonia is a must, alternative home remedies can play an important role in your recovery.

"Supplements that strengthen the immune system can help shorten a bout of pneumonia, decrease its severity, and reduce symptoms that can hang on for weeks after the infection is over, such as a bad cough," says JoAnne Lombardi, M.D., a pulmonary specialist in Belmont, California.

The following list of remedies is similar to a menu: You don't have to take them all, but choose a few that suit your preferences.

## VITAMIN A: *Repair Your Respiratory Tract*

Vitamin A helps to strengthen the epithelium, the tissue that lines your lungs, so that your body is better able to fight off the pneumonia, Dr. Lombardi says. Use the liquid "mycelized" form of vitamin A, which is maximally absorbable. She recommends taking 25,000 to 50,000 international units (IU) a day during the first 3 to 5 days of the illness, then tapering to 10,000 to 25,000 IU until your symptoms are gone, but only under the supervision of a health care practitioner.

## VITAMINS C AND E: *A Winning Combination*

When your body fights infection, it produces free radicals, unstable molecules that can damage cells and make them more prone to bacterial invasion. Vitamin C helps stop free radicals,

---

### GUIDE TO
### PROFESSIONAL CARE

*Caution:* You should use the alternative remedies discussed in this chapter only as part of a treatment program that is guided and monitored by a qualified medical doctor in partnership with a qualified alternative practitioner, both of whom are experienced in caring for your condition. Check with your conventional doctor before changing or stopping any conventional medical treatments or medications, and keep all of your doctors and/or alternative practitioners informed of all treatments that you are receiving.

If a cold, flu, or bronchitis hangs on for more than 2 weeks or turns particularly nasty, with a cough, chest pain, aching muscles, shortness of breath, fever, sweating, headache, or weakness, you may have pneumonia.

In its cruelest forms, pneumonia can send you to the hospital and be potentially life-threatening, particularly for people who are at high risk. This group includes people whose immunity is weak, who have diabetes, heart or lung disease, a chronic condition of any kind, and those over age 65. See your doctor immediately for diagnosis and care, which may include antibiotics, oxygen, respiratory therapy, and intravenous fluids.

says Peter Holyk, M.D., director of the Contemporary Health Clinic in Sebastian, Florida.

As mentioned earlier, pneumonia requires a doctor's care. If you see an alternative doctor, he may recommend large doses of certain vitamins. Dr. Holyk recommends that his patients with pneumonia take 5,000 to 15,000 milligrams of vitamin C a day, taken in divided doses every 2 to 3 hours throughout the day. He also suggests 400 to 800 IU of vitamin E, which bolsters vitamin C with its antioxidant action.

In addition, Dr. Lombardi recommends taking 500 milligrams of bioflavonoids daily; these nutrients help make vitamin C more effective.

### BROMELAIN: *A Power Boost for Antibiotics*

The digestive enzyme bromelain helps thin mucus and boosts the bacteria-killing power of antibiotics, Dr. Lombardi says. She recommends taking 250 to 500 milligrams three times a day until you're feeling better.

### THYMUS EXTRACT: *To Make More Killer T Cells*

An extract from the thymus gland can help your own thymus release a chemical that activates the immune system's virus-and bacteria-slaying killer T cells, Dr. Lombardi says. She favors the product Bioprothymic A, and says to take one to three of the product's 4-microgram packets daily for the duration of your illness.

### GOLDENSEAL: *For Bacterial Pneumonia*

The herb goldenseal helps the immune system kill many of the germs that commonly cause bacterial pneumonia, Dr. Lombardi says. There are different forms of goldenseal, so Dr. Lombardi recommends taking the following dosages three times a day, depending on the form you choose: tincture in a 1:5 dilution, 6 to 12 milliliters; fluid extract in a 1:1 dilution, 2 to 4 milliliters; and capsules or tablets, 500 to 2,000 milligrams. Check the label of a tincture or extract for the dilution ratio.

### ECHINACEA: *The Classic Immune-Building Herb*

The herb echinacea boosts the production of macrophages and phagocytes, components of the immune system that fight bacteria and viruses, Dr. Lombardi says. Although there are many good brands of echinacea, she favors the product Esberitox, which includes two species of echinacea and other immune-boosting herbs. Take one tablet three times a day.

## SHIITAKE AND MAITAKE: *To Help with Recovery*

Shiitake, a type of mushroom from Japan, contains powerful immune-system enhancers that can help your body bounce back after a bout of pneumonia, says Dr. Lombardi. She recommends buying a liquid extract of the mushroom and adding a dropper to a bowl of soup once a day.

Maitake, another mushroom that's organically grown, then dried, can be eaten as a food. It also comes in capsule, extract, and tea forms. Take it according to the directions on the label until your vitality returns, usually within 2 to 4 weeks, says Dr. Lombardi.

## PROBIOTICS: *Stop the Damage from Antibiotics*

Antibiotics for bacterial pneumonia kill not only the bacteria that are making you sick but also the good bacteria in your digestive tract. To guard against possible long-term digestive problems, you can replace those good bacteria with probiotic supplements that include *Lactobacillus acidophilus* and *Bifidobacterium bifidum* bacteria, says Dr. Lombardi.

Take 1 to 3 teaspoons daily of a powdered probiotic supplement, mixed with lukewarm water or juice, on an empty stomach, or take one to three tablets containing 500 million live *L. acidophilus* and 250 million live *B. bifidum* bacteria.

*Herbs Offer Quick Relief for*
# Poison Ivy
# and Poison Oak

That itchy, weeping, blistering rash from poison ivy or poison oak is really an allergic reaction to urushiol, an oily resin in the leaves, stems, and roots of those nasty plants. But when you get a case of it, you're in no mood for chemical analysis. You just want relief—now. And instead of running to the drugstore for calamine lotion or cortisone cream, you can use alternative home remedies to get rid of that maddening itch.

### HYDROTHERAPY: *A Cold Shower—Right Away*
From her years of treating poison ivy, Norma Pasekoff Weinberg, an herbal educator in Cape Cod, Massachusetts, has discovered anti-rash remedies that work, such as showering in cool water immediately after you're exposed to the plant. "The sooner you shower, and the longer you shower, the better your chances of minimizing a rash." (This also works for poison oak, she says.)

### NATURAL TOOTHPASTE: *Clay and Peppermint Are Healers*
To soothe your rash, look for natural toothpaste with clay and peppermint as the primary ingredients, says Pamela Fischer, founder and director of the Ohlone Center for Herbal Studies in Concord, California. The mint in the toothpaste soothes hot, irritated skin. The clay draws out the toxins, speeding healing.

This product may be difficult to find, so you may want to make your own, Fischer says. Mix 5 to 10 drops of peppermint essential oil with ½ cup of green clay, then add enough water to make a thick paste. Spread the paste over the inflamed area in a thick, even layer, avoiding the eye area. Apply one to three times a day for 2 to 3 days.

---

# GUIDE TO
# PROFESSIONAL CARE

Although rashes from poison ivy and poison oak are extremely uncomfortable, they can usually be treated with home remedies. However, don't wait until you're miserable. If your rash is so bad that you can't sleep at night or can't work, or if it is very itchy, you should see a medical doctor for treatment with prescription cortisone and antihistamines, says Esta Kronberg, M.D., a dermatologist in Houston.

If the rash is near your eyes, has spread to most of your body, is weeping a cloudy fluid, or you develop a fever, see a doctor as soon as possible.

---

## EVENING PRIMROSE: *Fast Skin Repair*

The fatty acids in evening primrose oil stop the inflammatory process and help skin cells repair faster, Fischer says. She recommends taking 1,500 milligrams four times a day until your skin is completely clear.

"Evening primrose makes a bout of poison ivy or oak bearable," she says. "I'm often out in the wild in California, picking herbs, and I'm very susceptible to poison oak. I get it every 2 to 3 weeks. Within 2 hours of contact, it explodes onto my skin. But if I take evening primrose oil immediately and continue to take high doses, my skin doesn't even look like it's been touched by poison oak, and the entire episode clears up in 3 to 4 days."

## JEWELWEED: *Relief on the Rocks*

"My neighbors call me the Poison Ivy Lady," says Weinberg. That's because she regularly treats the rashes of children and adults in her neighborhood with an herb that she calls her plant ally against poison ivy: jewelweed.

And, she says, one of the best ways to use it is to make jewelweed ice cubes.

"You wash the affected area with a cube three or four times a day until the rash is gone," she says. "It not only feels good, it also works—in fact, I've seen cases of poison ivy dry up right in front of my eyes!" Here are her instructions for preparing the remedy.

• Look for jewelweed growing in moist ground near poison ivy plants. (After all, it's nature's antidote.) Jewelweed grows in shady wetlands from Canada to Georgia and west to Oklahoma and Missouri. It has tall, translucent stems and hanging, trumpet-shaped, yellow or orange flowers. Gather the stems and leaves after the dew is off the plants, usually around 10:00 to 11:00 A.M. You can also buy jewelweed seeds and grow your own to keep on hand in case you can't go where it's naturally found.
• Once you're home, cut the plants into 1- to 2-inch pieces, put them into a plastic bag, and flatten them with a rolling pin.
• Place the crushed pieces in a pot, adding enough water to cover the plant material. Bring to a boil and simmer until the water is reduced by half and is amber in color.
• Let the water cool and strain the plant material from the liquid.
• Pour the liquid into labeled ice cube trays.
• When the cubes are frozen, put them in a heavy-duty freezer bag and label the bag.

You can also keep the wilted, strained jewelweed in a covered container in the refrigerator for a week and use it to apply right on your poison ivy rash.

"You can't always have the wilted herb around," says Weinberg, "but you can keep the ice cubes for about 3 months."

## VITAMIN C: *Make a Paste*

If you don't have jewelweed handy, Weinberg has found that a paste made from vitamin C powder and water can minimize blistering. Make the paste by adding cooled, boiled water, a teaspoon at a time, to ¼ cup of vitamin C powder until the mixture is the consistency of paste. Apply it directly to the affected area and leave it on for 1 hour, then rinse it off with cool water and pat your skin dry. Do this three times a day until the rash improves.

**VITAMINS:** *Reduce the Stress of the Rash*

While you're spreading vitamin C on your skin, take the nutrient orally, too.

"Taking 500 milligrams of vitamin C four times a day can help the body cope with the severe stress of the rash," says Earl Mindell, Ph.D., a pharmacist and nutritionist in Beverly Hills. Take it for 1 to 2 weeks, depending on how quickly the rash disappears.

Also, taking 500 milligrams of pantothenic acid (sometimes labeled as vitamin $B_5$) once or twice daily for the duration of the rash will further support your body's stress-coping ability, he says.

# Healing the Pain of
# Post-Traumatic
# Stress Disorder

A driver slams into a tree. A woman is raped. A bystander witnesses a murder during a robbery. A child is abused.

If you've experienced this type of trauma—an abnormal situation in which you or others are threatened or harmed—you need to seek professional care. A doctor or therapist can help you deal with the after-effects. You usually don't get over it right away, says Reneau Z. Peurifoy, a marriage and family therapist and anxiety specialist in the Sacramento area. "If you have had a major trauma, it will mark you for a while," he says.

The marks of post-traumatic stress disorder (PTSD) may include:

• Hypervigilance, a state in which you're anxiously alert all the time, particularly around anything that reminds you of the original event.
• Depression, which makes you feel numb and uninterested in life.

• Flashbacks—usually not the full-scale, 3-D flashbacks you see in the movies, but frequent thoughts, feelings, or memories of the traumatic event.
• Physical problems such as digestive complaints, which can be stress-related.

Those symptoms all can interfere with everyday life, harming the ability to work or have normal relationships. With the help of a professional, someone with PTSD needs to understand what the disorder is and not beat himself up because he "can't handle" the trauma. He needs to recognize that he's a normal person who has been in an abnormal situation. Then he can learn how to heal, Peurifoy says. And one of the most effective ways to start that healing, he says, is to talk to yourself a little differently.

### AFFIRMATIONS: *Tell Yourself What's Real*
You can help yourself stay in the present rather than constantly reliving the past by talking to yourself in a different way, says Peurifoy. "This type of self-talk and realistic affirmation is very important in the healing process," he says. Whenever you start to have a flashback, ask yourself "What's happening? What's real?" You can then tell yourself "The trauma is not happening now. What's real is that the trauma was in the past. I am safe now. I am just sitting in my home."

### HERBS: *Calming Help for Recent Trauma*
A number of anti-anxiety herbs can help a person cope with trauma, particularly in the first few weeks after it has occurred, says Anu de Monterice, M.D., a practitioner of holistic medicine and psychiatry in Cotati, California. A calming herb may lose its effectiveness after several weeks, however, as the nerve receptors adapt themselves to its presence. If you choose an herb and later notice that it isn't working anymore, switch to another herb on the list. Dr. de Monterice always recommends herbal extracts, not ground herbs, except when making teas.

• Kava kava: Take a 500-milligram capsule of kava extract, standardized for 30 percent kavalactones, three times a day.

# GUIDE TO PROFESSIONAL CARE

If you have experienced a trauma, you need to be alert for signs that you may have post-traumatic stress. If you have any of the following symptoms that were *not* present before the trauma, you need to seek professional help, says Leah J. Dickstein, M.D., director of the division of attitudinal and behavioral medicine at the University of Louisville School of Medicine in Kentucky: difficulty falling asleep or staying asleep, irritability or outbursts of anger, difficulty concentrating, hypervigilance (always being "on alert"), or being extremely jumpy and easily startled.

Care for post-traumatic stress disorder (PTSD) includes a number of important elements that call for professional counseling, says Reneau Z. Peurifoy, a marriage and family therapist and anxiety specialist in the Sacramento area.

First, you need to understand what the condition is and that it's normal to have it if you've experienced a trauma. A counselor experienced in PTSD can help.

If you're severely traumatized, you may need to sit down with someone you trust, such as a friend, a family member, or a counselor, and have that person help you organize your life for a little while. That may even include scheduling meals so that you eat regularly.

"You also need medical evaluation that includes appropriate laboratory tests, because PTSD is a psychiatric diagnosis, and appropriate medication may be indicated," says Dr. Dickstein.

After you've had a medical evaluation, a counselor trained in cognitive-behavioral therapy can help you develop essential self-talk skills such as those in the discussion of affirmations in this chapter.

A technique called eye movement desensitization and reprocessing, or EMDR, is an excellent tool for healing from trauma, says Peurifoy. It utilizes specific eye movements to help you release emotions associated with the event. He says to look for a "level two" EMDR trainer who has treated people for the type of trauma that you've experienced.

Finally, you should consider group therapy. Talking in a group about your experience, particularly in a group of people who have had similar traumas, is very helpful, says Peurifoy.

• The Lotus Embryo: This Chinese herbal extract may be hard to find except in the Chinese districts of many cities. It's known as Lian Zi Xin, says Dr. de Monterice. Powdered versions are available from KPC products or from your health care practitioner. Dosages vary according to the individual, says Dr. de Monterice, so follow your practitioner's advice.
• Chamomile: Take two 350-milligram capsules of powdered chamomile extract three times a day or brew a strong tea by steeping a heaping tablespoon of chamomile flowers in a cup of water for 10 minutes. Drink a cup three times a day.
• Valerian: Take a 150-milligram capsule of powdered valerian root extract once or twice a day. At bedtime, increase the dose to 400 milligrams.

"There's a thin line between a dose that relaxes you and a dose that causes sleepiness," says Dr. de Monterice. "For some people, there's no such line." If valerian makes you nod off during the day, use it only at bedtime or try another herb.

## FLOWER ESSENCES: *Natural Medicine for the Emotions*
Flower essence remedies are liquid dilutions specially prepared from various flowers that affect the emotions by working on the "energy field" of the individual, says Nancy Buono, a registered Bach flower practitioner in Tempe, Arizona.
"In much the same way that you experience different types of feelings when you listen to different types of music—sometimes you're soothed, sometimes you're agitated—so the remedies affect your feelings, creating emotional balance and harmony," she says.
There are two ways to take the essences. You can buy a standard, commercially available "stock bottle" of one or more essences and take two drops of each essence four times a day. Or, if you're taking essences over a long period of time, you

can mix a "treatment bottle" by filling a 1-ounce amber bottle three-quarters full of spring water, then adding two drops each of one or more essences. Take four drops four times a day from the treatment bottle as long as symptoms remain.

You can take these remedies indefinitely, Buono says. As with all remedies for PTSD, see your health care practitioner for a complete evaluation before you begin.

### STAR OF BETHLEHEM: *Release the Trauma*

This flower essence helps release the trauma from your mind, feelings, and body, soothing and consoling you, says Buono.

### HONEYSUCKLE: *For Flashbacks*

"Honeysuckle helps put the experience into perspective and moves the person into present time," says Buono, so it's helpful for controlling flashbacks.

### CLEMATIS: *For "Spacing Out"*

If PTSD causes you to mentally go somewhere else because present reality is just too much to bear, try the flower essence clematis, says Buono.

### WHITE CHESTNUT: *For Torturous, Unwanted Thoughts*

If you're haunted by recurring thoughts of the traumatic event, this essence can help calm your mind, says Buono.

### AGRIMONY: *To Gain Emotional Balance*

People with PTSD sometimes bottle up or hide their emotions and try to act as if everything is okay, says Buono. Agrimony may help people integrate their true feelings with the outside world, thus becoming more emotionally balanced.

### CHERRY PLUM: *When You're Afraid of Losing Control*

Some people with PTSD feel that they're about to lose control, says Buono. "They feel they just can't take it, or their mind is going to snap, or they'll do something they don't want to do," she says. The flower essence cherry plum is for them.

## *Safe, Gentle, Alternative*
## *Remedies for*
## Pregnancy Complaints

There are pregnancy problems, and then there are pregnancy complaints.

Pregnancy problems are serious, mother- or baby-threatening conditions such as possible miscarriage, the swelling and high blood pressure of toxemia, or the skyrocketing blood sugar of gestational diabetes. They all require professional medical care, but their symptoms often go unnoticed. You should notify your doctor of any discomfort that you experience during your pregnancy in order to head off such problems before they harm you or your baby.

Pregnancy complaints, on the other hand, are those seemingly inevitable discomforts that go with having a brand-new human being growing inside of you. The heartburn as the swelling uterus pushes your stomach up. The backaches as the baby's weight strains your muscles. The varicose veins.

---

### GUIDE TO
### PROFESSIONAL CARE

The pregnancy complaints discussed in this chapter can usually be self-treated, says Aviva Jill Romm, a midwife and herbalist in Bloomfield Hills, Michigan. There are, however, many complaints and problems that arise during pregnancy that do require professional care. Romm counsels all pregnant women to be under the care of a midwife, nurse-midwife, obstetrician, or osteopathic obstetrician and to always seek immediate professional care if they have questions or concerns about any pregnancy complaint or problem.

The insomnia. The nausea. The . . . well, if you're pregnant, you can easily complete the all-too-long list on your own.

These complaints don't necessarily need continued professional care once your doctor is aware of them. In fact, self-care is often the best choice, says Aviva Jill Romm, a midwife and herbalist in Bloomfield Hills, Michigan. "There are many safe, gentle, natural remedies that a woman can use on her own to relieve the common complaints of pregnancy," she says—starting with the most common complaint of all: the nausea of early pregnancy.

## Homeopathic Remedies for Morning Sickness

No one knows why some future moms feel so nauseated and sensitive to smells and noise in the early months of pregnancy. But Seattle-based homeopath Miranda Castro recommends homeopathy as a safe and effective alternative solution that has benefits beyond simply stopping the nausea. "The correct homeopathic remedy will boost the general vitality of the pregnant woman so she is more resilient and less vulnerable to stresses, strains, and illnesses," she says.

Select your remedy by matching as many of your symptoms as possible with those listed for one of the following remedies, which are the four most commonly needed homeopathic remedies for this complaint, suggests Castro. The remedy you select can be taken in a 30C potency twice daily for up to 3 days.

"You should discontinue use once your symptoms diminish, although the remedy can be repeated if it was helpful and the same symptoms return," Castro says. If you have difficulty matching your symptoms to the following remedies, you'll need to consult a homeopathic practitioner for a remedy that fits your particular symptoms.

### Ipecacuanha
Use it if:

• You have constant, violent, and persistent morning sickness accompanied by empty belching, copious saliva, retching, and difficulty in actually vomiting.
• Eating and even the smell of food trigger your nausea, and you have no thirst and no appetite.

- Tobacco smoke and movement also trigger nausea.
- Headache often accompanies the nausea.
- Your tongue is unusually clean.
- You look pale and drawn, with dark rings under your eyes.
- You're very sweaty and sensitive to both heat and cold.
- You're extremely anxious when you're nauseated.

## Nux Vomica
Use it if:

- Your morning sickness is constant, accompanied by a lot of saliva, spasms of retching, and difficulty in actually vomiting.
- Your nausea is worse in the morning (especially when you're still in bed) and after eating and is triggered by tobacco smoke.
- You hate the cold and feel worse when you're cold and better when you're warm.
- You're very irritable, impatient, and snappish.

## Pulsatilla
Use it if:

- Your nausea is worse in the evening and is accompanied by vomiting.
- You can't tolerate hot, rich, or fatty foods, especially ice cream.
- The nausea is worse when you're in a hot, stuffy room and better when you're in the fresh air or you have a cold drink.
- You're not thirsty.
- You feel miserable and very emotional and are easily moved to tears or laughter.
- You want a lot of sympathy, which makes you feel better.

## Sepia
Use it if:

- You have intermittent nausea that is worse in the morning or when you eat dairy foods.
- You vomit easily (even vomiting bile) and feel better afterward.
- You have an empty, sinking feeling in your stomach that is only temporarily relieved by eating.
- You feel more nauseated when you think about food.
- Headache often accompanies the nausea.

• You generally feel chilly and worn out, but feel much better after aerobic or strenuous exercise.
• You feel apathetic and depressed and just want to be alone; nothing gives you joy, including your loved ones.

## Relieving Morning Sickness

Medical science hasn't figured out the exact cause of the nausea and (sometimes) vomiting that starts about 6 weeks into pregnancy and continues until the 12th week or so. And while no one seems to have hit on a cure, there are remedies to help ease the discomfort.

### GINGER: *Tea for Nausea Relief*
Ginger tea can help stop nausea by warming the digestive tract and improving sluggish digestion, Romm says. To make it, steep 1 teaspoon of freshly grated ginger in 1 cup of boiling water for 10 minutes, let it cool to room temperature, and sip it throughout the day. Do not prepare a stronger tea or drink more than 2 cups a day.

Alternatively, she says, you can take 1,000 milligrams of ginger in capsule form—two capsules every few hours, but not more than eight capsules a day—until the nausea subsides.

### DANDELION: *If You Can't Stand Ginger*
Some women with nausea find that they often have a bad taste in the backs of their throats, says Romm. For them, dandelion tea or tincture is an excellent option. "Dandelion sweetens the sour feeling, calms and strengthens the stomach, and improves the appetite," she says.

Put 4 to 6 tablespoons of dried dandelion root in 1 quart of boiling water and steep for 4 hours. Strain, let cool, and drink slowly throughout the day, up to two cups. Or take 30 drops of undiluted tincture three or four times a day until the nausea is gone.

### COMPLEX CARBOHYDRATES: *A Simple Solution*
Regular snacks and meals rich in complex carbohydrates, with foods such as whole-grain breads, pasta, and cereal, and the whole grains themselves, usually keep women with morning sickness feeling a whole lot better, Romm says. Among the

best choices are whole wheat, brown rice, oats, barley, and buckwheat.

## Soothing Indigestion and Heartburn

During pregnancy, says Romm, increased levels of the hormones estrogen and progesterone can slow digestion and relax the valve that keeps acid in the stomach. At the same time, the growing baby exerts great pressure upward on the stomach. Here are safe, natural ways to soothe heartburn, burping, gas, stomach upset, and acid indigestion.

### ALMONDS: *Shut Down the Acid Pipeline*
A natural chemical in raw almonds helps tone the sphincter between the esophagus and the stomach so that acid stays in the stomach and you don't experience heartburn, Romm says. She recommends eating a handful of almonds (about 12 to 15) after every snack and meal.

### MEADOWSWEET: *Excellent for Digestion*
Meadowsweet is one of the best digestive herbs for pregnant women, Romm says. She recommends using 15 to 45 drops of tincture diluted in a bit of water one to four times a day. You should experiment to see which dosage level provides relief.

You can also prepare a tea with meadowsweet. Put a heaping tablespoon of the herb in a cup, pour 1 cup of boiling water over it, steep for 20 minutes, strain, and drink. Drink three to four cups a day by sipping each cup slowly.

## Overcoming Insomnia

You can't get comfortable in bed. Even if you fall asleep quickly, the baby's movements wake you during the night, or you have to get up repeatedly to urinate.

"Insomnia is a common problem during pregnancy," says Romm. For many women, though, the solution is very simple.

**PROTEIN:** *Keep a Snack Handy*

Many pregnant women wake up in the middle of the night and can't fall back to sleep because they're hungry, Romm says.

"Most pregnant women are tired at night and don't think about eating right before bed," she says. "But the baby is growing, and your metabolism is burning up a lot more energy to support that growth, so you can easily find yourself starved in the middle of the night and wake up because of the hunger."

Her advice: Eat a protein-carbohydrate snack right before bed and keep one on your bedside table for when you wake up. "A snack with a little bit of carbohydrate and a little bit of protein helps women who wake up in the middle of the night fall right back to sleep," she says. Two good choices are a banana and a handful of almonds, or fruit yogurt.

**CALCIUM AND MAGNESIUM:** *A Supplement at Bedtime*

Taking a nutritional supplement with 500 milligrams of calcium and 250 milligrams of magnesium at bedtime can calm the nerves and muscles and help a pregnant woman sleep, Romm says. She recommends calcium citrate or calcium lactate for maximum absorption.

### Vanquishing Varicose Veins

A growing fetus puts more pressure on the circulatory system, so blood sometimes pools in the legs rather than returning to the heart, causing varicose veins. Natural remedies can help prevent or reduce these unsightly veins, Romm says.

**HORSE CHESTNUT:** *An Herb for Relief*

One of the best natural medicines for helping reduce varicose veins after the first trimester is the herb horse chestnut, says Romm. She recommends taking 5 to 15 drops of tincture diluted in ¼ cup of water two or three times a day.

**EXERCISE:** *Improve the Upward Flow*

Vigorous "pelvic tilting" during your second and third trimesters can improve the blood flow from your legs to your upper body, Romm says. Here are her directions.

Stand with your feet shoulder-width apart and your hands on

your hips. Slowly tip your pelvis forward, then backward, gradually increasing speed until you are swinging your hips forward and back vigorously. You can also roll and rock your hips and make figure-eights in belly-dancer fashion. Do this exercise for 5 to 10 minutes a day.

## Banishing Back Pain

"Backaches rank in the top five complaints of pregnancy, particularly in the last 3 months," says Elaine Stillerman, a licensed massage therapist in New York City.

The back muscles are stressed by weight gain, by the change in the center of gravity in the body, and by "displacements" in the body's structures as the growing baby takes up more room. Here are two remedies that Stillerman's clients have found helpful.

**EXERCISE:** *Pelvic Tilt*

To elongate the lower back, says Stillerman, get down on your hands and knees and round your back while holding in your abdominal muscles. Continue to breathe while holding this position for a count of 10. Release your muscles by flattening your back, but be careful not to make your back concave. Repeat 12 times. Since backaches can last long after childbirth, you can continue to do this exercise even after delivery if you find it helpful.

**REFLEXOLOGY:** *For Sciatica*

The growing baby can put pressure on the large sciatic nerve that passes from the lower back into the legs. The pressure inflames the nerve, causing severe lower-back pain that radiates into the legs. Reflexology, an alternative modality that says that every area of the body has corresponding "reflex points" on the feet, can help this condition, says Stillerman.

The reflex points for the sciatic nerve are on the heel. If you are in your second or third trimester, press gently and release with your thumbs to stimulate first one whole heel, then the other. Work each heel for a minute or two twice a day until your pain disappears.

## *Easy Exercises Help Avoid*
# Premature Ejaculation

Alan Brauer, M.D., is a psychiatrist, sex therapist, and coauthor of the 1980s bestseller *ESO (Extended Sexual Orgasm)*, which taught men and women how to have orgasms that last for a half-hour or more. And he has a very alternative perspective for men who reach orgasm quickly, a condition commonly known as premature ejaculation: They don't have a problem.

"In virtually every context that you can think of, faster reflexes are an advantage, and that includes ejaculation," says Dr. Brauer, founder and director of the TotalCare Medical Center in Palo Alto, California.

In evolutionary terms, for example, men who ejaculated faster during sex—a time of heightened exposure and

---

### GUIDE TO PROFESSIONAL CARE

Premature ejaculation is natural. It's not a medical problem, says Alan Brauer, M.D., founder and director of the TotalCare Medical Center in Palo Alto, California. Still, you can choose a medical solution, although many alternative-minded medical doctors would advise against it.

A medical approach may include the class of antidepressants known as selective serotonin reuptake inhibitors, or SSRIs. SSRI drugs such as fluoxetine (Prozac), paroxetine (Paxil), fluvoxamine maleate (Luvox), or sertraline (Zoloft) can slow or delay ejaculation. See your medical doctor if you're interested in discussing the use of these drugs for this purpose, says Dr. Brauer.

vulnerability—were more likely to survive, thus making so-called premature ejaculation a biological plus.

In fact, says Dr. Brauer, there wasn't even a condition called premature ejaculation until about 50 years ago, when sexual research first showed that women typically need more time than men do to achieve orgasm.

If you are prone to premature ejaculation, however (usually defined as ejaculating in 4 minutes or less, or earlier than your partner wants or needs for orgasm), you can learn to delay your natural ejaculatory reflex if you want to, says Dr. Brauer. By doing so, you'll be much more likely to help your partner reach orgasm, a goal that most men enjoy achieving.

"Think of changing your ejaculatory reflex as a challenge, similar to an athlete training to improve his reflexes," he says. The first step toward meeting that challenge is to learn a few variations on a tried-and-true exercise for strengthening your "sexual" muscles: Kegel exercises.

### KEGELS: *A Special Variety to Stop Ejaculation*

When you do Kegel exercises (named after the doctor who invented them), you squeeze the muscles in the anal area as if you were trying to stop the flow of urine. This helps you to be aware of and to strengthen the pubococcygeus (PC) muscle, which is a kind of muscular hammock or sling for the sex organs, the urethra (urinary tube), and the rectum.

"The more awareness and control you have over the PC and other sexual muscles, the more control you'll have over ejaculation," Dr. Brauer says.

There is a specific type of Kegel exercise to control ejaculation. Instead of tightening the muscles in the area of your anus, says Dr. Brauer, "push down moderately as if you're forcing out urine or a bowel movement."

You'll know that you're doing this exercise correctly if you feel your anus opening as you push down, relaxing afterward. "This pushing down movement can help stop ejaculation during sex," he says.

Here's how to practice both the "squeeze" and the "push-down" Kegels so you can do them easily during sex.

As you take a slow, deep breath, count from one to five and firmly clench and tighten your PC muscle. Then, as you exhale, count from five to one and push down, opening your anus.

Do both parts of this exercise as many times as possible in the course of a day, such as while you're driving, while you're waiting in line, while you're doing almost anything. Some people learn to do 50 repetitions within a 10- to 15-minute period, says Dr. Brauer.

At first, you may find that your PC muscle is too weak to clench repeatedly. It will strengthen over time as you do the exercise.

During sex, do the squeeze Kegel and hold it if you want to build arousal; do the push-down Kegel and hold it whenever you're so aroused that you think you're about to ejaculate, Dr. Brauer says.

### SELF-STIMULATION: *A Practice Session for Sex*

Top athletes practice their moves over and over until they can perform them effortlessly. You should do the same.

"The more practice a man has in getting near the point of no return but not actually cresting it, the more familiar that sensation will be and the less urgency it will have," Dr. Brauer says.

If you want to learn to slow your ejaculatory reflex, he recommends masturbating three or four times a week for 30 minutes each time, bringing yourself close to orgasm, but not ejaculating, at least six times during each session. Don't worry, though, if you go over the edge before you've reached your goal of six. Just enjoy yourself; there'll always be a next time, Dr. Brauer says.

### SCROTAL PULL: *Another Way to Stop*

During self-stimulation, try practicing what Dr. Brauer calls the scrotal pull technique, gently pulling down on your scrotal sac (which hugs your body when you're sexually aroused) before you reach the point of no return. During sex, you can do it yourself or ask your partner to do it.

"There's a not uncommonly held viewpoint among women that premature ejaculation is the man's problem, and therefore many women don't recognize the value in helping a man train to last longer," Dr. Brauer says. "Well, a man is not born knowing how to last longer, but he can learn. And he can learn faster with his partner's help."

**EXTERNAL PROSTATE SPOT:** *Press for More Pleasure, Less Urgency*

Pressing an area on your perineum, the space between the anus and the back of the scrotum, stimulates the prostate, the gland that supplies the fluid for semen during ejaculation. Pressing on this spot when you're highly aroused helps block the ejaculatory reflex, says Dr. Brauer. It can also be quite pleasurable.

The spot is an area in the middle of your perineum that indents more easily than the areas around it. To help delay ejaculation, press on it firmly and rhythmically at any point during sex after you've achieved a maximally firm erection.

It often takes some practice to find the amount of pressure that reduces the urge to ejaculate and is also pleasurable. Some men may find this a little uncomfortable at first, but with practice, they may experience heightened sensation.

**BREATHING:** *Go Slowly*

Taking a few slow, deep breaths when you're aroused helps "induce a sense of total body relaxation," says Dr. Brauer and decreases your sense of ejaculatory urgency.

# *Dietary Changes and Supplements to Ease* **Premenstrual Syndrome**

Most doctors call it premenstrual syndrome, or PMS.

Jesse Lynn Hanley, M.D., calls it a gift.

"The time before a woman's period is a time of heightened sensitivity, intuition, and creativity, a time when a woman feels intensely—bodily, emotionally, and psychically—what it means to be a woman," says Dr. Hanley, a specialist in women's health in Malibu, California.

Still, a number of nutritional, hormonal, and psychological factors can create an imbalance during this time, so that a woman feels the extremes of the premenstrual period.

Irritability, anxiety, mood swings, depression, headaches, bloating, weight gain, constipation, sugar cravings, cramps, acne, breast tenderness, and backache are just some of the 150 possible symptoms that are commonly experienced by the millions of women with PMS.

The first step in healing those symptoms, says Dr. Hanley, is to stop thinking that you're "crazy" or a "bad person" for being a woman.

The second step, she says, is to understand that the symptoms are wise messengers from your body and mind, guiding you to greater health and self-respect.

The third step is to begin to alleviate those symptoms by using a variety of remedies—starting, she says, with a change in diet.

### Breaking the Sugar Habit

During the premenstrual period, the body demands more sugar as fuel, says Susan Lark, M.D., a physician in Los Altos, California. The result, as many women know, is intense sugar cravings.

Satisfying those cravings with lots of fruit juice, chocolate, candy, cake, or cookies causes blood sugar levels to skyrocket and then plunge. That is what triggers much of the physical fatigue, mental fog, and emotional imbalance that are so characteristic of PMS.

"In my experience, getting women off sugar is the secret of curing many cases of PMS," Dr. Hanley says. Here are some ways to get off that sweet roller coaster. Use them during the premenstrual period and when sugar cravings strike.

### MISO SOUP: *To Halt a Sugar Binge*
Mildly salty foods can stop a sugar binge in its tracks, Dr. Lark says. Try a bowl of miso soup, made by stirring this delicious pastelike soy product into a bowl of hot water that's previously been boiled with celery, carrots, onions, and sometimes ginger.

## SEA SALT: *Dash Sugar Cravings*

Put ¼ teaspoon of sea salt in a cup of warm water and drink it down. "This should stop your sugar craving immediately," says Dr. Lark. Don't consume extra salt if you are salt-sensitive or on a salt-restricted diet, however.

## PICKLED FOODS: *Counter Chocolate Cravings*

Certain pickled or bitter foods can also stop sugar and chocolate cravings, says Dr. Lark. To head off a chocoholic rampage, eat umeboshi plums, which are Japanese plums that have been pickled with sea salt and dried. For a bitter taste, try a cup of either burdock or dandelion root tea.

## GINGER: *For a Sugarless Lift*

Stimulating ginger tea is a great substitute for the emotional lift of chocolate, says Dr. Lark. It also helps cure the fatigue of PMS. It's a much better choice than caffeinated drinks such as coffee, cola, or tea, all of which can worsen the anxiety, irritability, and insomnia that are common with PMS.

# GUIDE TO
# PROFESSIONAL CARE

If you see a doctor for PMS, "make sure that he works with you to personalize a treatment, rather than rushing you through the appointment," says Jesse Lynn Hanley, M.D., a physician in Malibu, California.

If your symptoms worsen, interfere with your work or keep you from getting to work, disrupt your life at home (you can't handle your children or you fight with your spouse), or you skip a period or have excessive bleeding, visit a doctor.

If you can't find a doctor who will recommend natural, self-help options and investigate possible underlying causes of PMS such as an infection, see a naturopath, acupuncturist, chiropractor, or herbalist, Dr. Hanley says.

**FOOD:** *Stabilize Your Blood Sugar*

Eating smaller, more frequent meals helps keep blood sugar stable and reduces sugar cravings, says Linaya Hahn, a licensed nutritional counselor and director of Hahn Holistic Health Centers in Buffalo Grove, Illinois.

You should eat three small meals and three snacks, making sure that each contains both a carbohydrate food (vegetables, fruit, or beans) and a protein food (meat, fish, tofu, nuts, or grains). A perfect complex carbohydrate–protein snack is whole-grain bread spread with sesame butter.

**ASPARTAME:** *A Must to Avoid*

Aspartame, the artificial sweetener found in NutraSweet, Equal, and other products, contains phenylalanine and is not the answer to sugar problems, says Hahn.

"Some people who consume products that contain aspartame or aspartic acid report symptoms such as depression, irritability, sugar cravings, poor sleep patterns, or headaches, which are all common PMS symptoms," says Hahn. "I recommend that all women with classic PMS stay off these products."

**LIGHT:** *Boost Hormones Naturally*

Preliminary research has indicated that PMS may be a sleep disorder related to a decrease in the hormones melatonin and serotonin that naturally occurs at ovulation, says Hahn.

"When melatonin is low, we don't sleep well," she says. "When serotonin is low, we feel tense, depressed, and crabby." These feelings may be chemically interpreted as a craving for sugar, bread and pasta, or alcohol.

Exposure to sunlight naturally boosts your body's levels of those hormones. "Classic PMS symptoms can be reduced by increasing exposure to full-spectrum light by going outdoors, opening shades, and buying full-spectrum light boxes or bulbs," says Hahn.

## Vitamins and Minerals for PMS

Every woman with PMS should take a daily multivitamin/ mineral supplement, says Dr. Hanley. "All the vitamins and minerals work together to help resolve PMS symptoms," she says.

Choose a high-potency multiple supplement with a minimum of 600 milligrams of calcium, 600 milligrams of magnesium, and 50 milligrams of most of the B vitamins. You may also want to consider taking additional amounts of the following nutrients during your premenstrual phase.

## VITAMIN B₆: *To Control Excess Estrogen*

This vitamin helps the liver eliminate excess estrogen, a primary cause of PMS symptoms, says Dr. Hanley. It also works as a natural diuretic, helping to relieve the bloating of PMS.

"Daily doses of between 50 and 300 milligrams can help to regulate many premenstrual symptoms, including mood swings, irritability, fluid retention, breast tenderness, bloating, sugar cravings, and fatigue," Dr. Lark says.

## CALCIUM: *For Better Moods*

In a study that compared women who took 1,200 milligrams of calcium to women who did not take the nutrient, "twice as many women on calcium said they felt less moody and depressed than women not on calcium," says Susan Thys-Jacobs, M.D., an endocrinologist at St. Luke's–Roosevelt Hospital in New York City.

Dr. Thys-Jacobs, who was lead author of the study, theorizes that the calcium helps to reduce the fluctuation of calcium-reducing hormones that are being stimulated by estrogen and progesterone during the latter half of the menstrual cycle.

## VITAMIN E: *To Reduce Food Cravings*

Vitamin E can reduce PMS symptoms such as food cravings, anxiety, irritability, depression, and breast tenderness, Dr. Lark says. She recommends 400 to 600 international units daily.

### Natural Relief for PMS Symptoms

A number of food supplements, herbs, and the natural hormone progesterone may help with PMS symptoms, say alternative practitioners.

## PYCNOGENOL: *For Bloating*

This food supplement, derived from pine bark or grape seeds, can reduce bloating, fluid retention, and breast tenderness, says Dr. Lark. She recommends 50 milligrams once or twice daily.

## BIOFLAVONOIDS: *For Headaches*

Genistein and daidzein, two bioflavonoids found in soy products, can help control excess estrogen, thus decreasing PMS symptoms such as headaches, mood swings, and fluid retention. Dr. Lark recommends taking a bioflavonoid supplement of 1,000 to 2,000 milligrams daily.

## EVENING PRIMROSE OIL: *For Breast Tenderness*

This oil is a rich source of omega-3 fatty acids, which can reduce breast tenderness as well as fluid retention and mood swings, says Dr. Hanley. Take 2,000 to 3,000 milligrams a day for as long as needed.

### Zap Excess Estrogen

Some alternative practitioners believe that using plastic in the microwave can allow chemicals that act like estrogens in your body to leach into your food—and too much estrogen is one cause of PMS symptoms.

"To avoid this problem, use wax paper in the microwave whenever you would normally use plastic wrap," says Jason Elias, a practitioner of Traditional Chinese Medicine in New Paltz, New York.

## HERBS: *Four Symptom Relievers*

Jason Elias, a practitioner of Traditional Chinese Medicine in New Paltz, New York, recommends the following herbs to relieve PMS symptoms: sage for headaches, St. John's wort for depression or irritability, cleavers for breast tenderness, and dandelion leaf for bloating. Follow the dosage recommendations on the labels.

## PROGESTERONE: *For Desperate Times*

If a woman is truly desperate—overwhelmed by her PMS symptoms—she should consider adding the hormone progesterone to her remedy list, Dr. Hanley says. One of the best products to use, she says, is the progesterone cream Pro-Gest, which contains standardized amounts of the hormone in a natural rather than a synthetic form.

"I usually recommend using ¼ to ½ teaspoon of the cream once or twice a day from midcycle to menses," she says. Rub the cream anywhere—on your face, stomach, breasts, arms, or legs. The progesterone is absorbed as soon as the cream touches your skin.

As the additional progesterone brings your estrogen-progesterone levels into balance, your breasts may feel more tender and you may have some spotting for the first few cycles, but these symptoms will go away. The natural hormone, Dr. Hanley says, is "incredibly safe," and there are few, if any, side effects. In fact, the main side effect is feeling calm to the point of tiredness.

## *Alternative Remedies May Be Powerful Weapons against* Prostate Cancer

Each year, about 185,000 men are diagnosed with cancer of the prostate, the walnut-size gland below the bladder that supplies the fluid to carry sperm during ejaculation.

"I believe every one of those men should use alternative cancer treatments," says Michael Schachter, M.D., director of the Schachter Center for Complementary Medicine in Suffern, New York.

Alternative cancer therapies include treatments outside the realm of current conventional treatments (surgery, radiation, chemotherapy, and anti-hormone therapies). While the focus of conventional therapy is to get rid of the cancer at all costs, alternative treatments emphasize strengthening the body's defenses to control its spread.

The assumption of alternative treatments is that under the proper circumstances, the body has the ability to heal itself, says Dr. Schachter.

Alternative cancer therapy may reduce your risk of dying from other conditions such as heart disease or diabetes while possibly extending your survival time, although there aren't any definitive studies that show this.

Dr. Schachter also recommends alternative therapies for those who are already receiving conventional prostate cancer treatment such as surgery, radiation, or hormone therapy. Adding alternative treatments may reduce some of the side effects associated with conventional treatments.

Dr. Schachter has found that alternative therapies help conventional treatments work better and speed recovery from these treatments. In general, most supplements are much safer than conventional drugs, even when taken for long periods of time, he says. For best results, however, an individualized dietary and supplement program should be developed by an experienced practitioner.

## COENZYME $Q_{10}$: *A Potential Cancer Fighter*

Coenzyme $Q_{10}$ (co$Q_{10}$), is a chemical spark plug that helps every cell in your body generate energy. In one study, researchers gave 15 patients with advanced prostate cancer 600 milligrams a day of oil-based co$Q_{10}$ and followed the progress of their disease. After one year, co$Q_{10}$ had halted prostate cancer in 4 cases and reversed it in 10 others.

Although attempts to replicate this study are being made by other researchers, Dr. Schachter thinks that since co$Q_{10}$ is relatively safe and potentially beneficial, all patients with prostate cancer should be aware of its benefits. His prostate cancer patients generally take 200 milligrams three times a day.

## SELENIUM: *A Powerful Antioxidant*

"Selenium is a crucial mineral in the battle against prostate cancer," says Dr. Schachter. In one study of hundreds of men, a daily intake of 200 micrograms of selenium cut the incidence of prostate cancer by 60 percent.

Selenium is a potent antioxidant, a nutrient that helps control free radicals, the renegade molecules that damage cells and DNA, triggering cancer and other diseases.

Although more studies need to be done to corroborate these results, Dr. Schachter says that selenium is very safe and that it's also inexpensive. His patients with prostate cancer take 400 to 600 micrograms of selenium daily—a large, therapeutic dose that should be taken only with the approval and supervision of a doctor.

## VITAMINS C AND E: *More Antioxidant Help*

Dr. Schachter also says that prostate cancer patients generally benefit from a variety of antioxidants, including 1,000

# GUIDE TO PROFESSIONAL CARE

*Caution: Cancer is a complex and life-threatening disease that requires professional medical care. Some alternative remedies may actually worsen cancer if they are not used appropriately. Therefore, use the alternative remedies discussed in this chapter only as part of a cancer treatment program that is guided and monitored by a qualified physician who is experienced in cancer care and alternative medicine. If you are being treated by a conventional doctor, check with him before changing or stopping any conventional medical treatments or medications, and keep all of your doctors and/or alternative practitioners informed of all treatments that you are receiving.*

Conventional treatment for prostate cancer varies according to the severity of the disease and the age and general condition of the patient, says Michael Schachter, M.D., director of the Schachter Center for Complementary Medicine in Suffern, New York.

A typical recommendation for a man age 65 or younger whose cancer is confined to the prostate gland is radical prostatectomy (removal of the entire gland), which carries a moderate risk of urinary incontinence and a high risk of permanent impotence. Another possible treatment, especially for older men with cancer confined to the prostate area, is external beam radiation, which also has severe side effects, including impotence.

If the cancer has spread beyond the gland, patients often undergo anti-hormone therapy, which reduces the amount of available testosterone, the major male sex hormone, and can help stop or reverse the growth of the tumor for a year or more. Unfortunately, the tumor generally returns, Dr. Schachter says.

Because the treatments are so harsh, and improved diagnostic methods now detect so many prostate cancers at very early stages, some physicians prefer "watchful waiting," giving treatment only if there are symptoms or if the cancer begins to spread. This approach is generally reserved for elderly or debilitated men with relatively low-grade prostate cancers.

Dr. Schachter, however, recommends a different type of professional treatment for those diagnosed early with prostate cancer. It involves immediately beginning a program of alternative cancer therapy with a physician experienced in the alternative treatment of cancer patients. These patients must be monitored closely so that if a treatment is not working, other alternative or conventional therapies may be offered.

His alternative treatment includes lifestyle changes; avoiding toxic environmental substances in water, food, and air; individualized dietary recommendations according to a person's metabolic type; oral nutritional supplements such as vitamins, minerals, enzymes, amino acids, fatty acids, herbs, phytonutrients, and concentrated foods; a detoxification program; an exercise program; stress management; body energy techniques such as acupuncture; body manipulative therapies such as massage; natural hormone balancing, and homeopathy.

milligrams of vitamin C taken three times a day and 400 to 800 international units of vitamin E daily.

## ZINC PICOLINATE: *To Replenish the Gland*

"With their physicians' approval and supervision, prostate cancer patients should consider taking a daily supplement of 30 to 50 milligrams of zinc picolinate, the most absorbable form of the mineral," says Patrick Quillin, R.D., Ph.D., director of nutrition for the Cancer Treatment Centers of America in Tulsa, Oklahoma. The prostate gland has the highest concentration of zinc in the body, he says, and additional amounts help the organ battle cancer cells and heal.

## SAW PALMETTO: *An Herb to Shrink Prostate Tissue*

"I have had many patients with prostate cancer who have started alternative treatment at the time of diagnosis and whose tumors have stopped growing," says James Forsythe, M.D., medical director of the Cancer Care Center in Reno. One of the ways that Dr. Forsythe helps stop prostate cancer is with saw palmetto.

"This herb is known to help shrink prostate tissue," he says. "It also blocks the effect of male hormones such as testosterone, which can 'feed' prostate cancer."

Dr. Forsythe recommends that his prostate cancer patients take 80 milligrams of saw palmetto twice a day, along with 25 milligrams a day of pygeum, another herb that may reduce prostate swelling.

## FISH OIL: *Tap Its Anti-Cancer Power*

Fish oil contains high levels of fatty acids, a component of fat that helps fight cancer, says Dr. Quillin. It's also rich in vitamins A and D, nutrients that help control the development of cells—and cancer is a disease in which cell development is out of control.

Dr. Quillin recommends that prostate cancer patients (and anyone who is interested in optimal health) use old-fashioned cod-liver oil. "It's unfiltered and unrefined, so it contains the optimal levels of fatty acids and vitamins A and D," he says. For better taste, he uses an emulsified, flavored version. Take 2 teaspoons a day, but use it only under the supervision of your doctor.

For those who prefer not to take cod-liver oil, he suggests a daily dose of 2 tablespoons or four 1,000-milligram capsules of flaxseed oil, which is rich in fatty acids. He also advises prostate cancer patients to take 1,000 to 2,000 milligrams daily of pumpkin seed oil, which helps supply the prostate gland with the nutrients, such as zinc and magnesium, that it needs to heal.

### Five Ways to Prevent Prostate Cancer

What's the ultimate "remedy" for prostate cancer? Don't get it in the first place. Here are five simple steps that may prevent the disease, says Dan Labriola, N.D., a naturopathic physician in Seattle.

1. Cut back on saturated fats, which weaken the immune system and increase your risk of prostate cancer. This means eating less red meat and dairy products, which deliver a big dose of saturated fats.
2. Ditto for coffee, tea, and alcohol, which irritate the prostate and may put you at risk.
3. Take an antioxidant supplement. Men with higher intakes of antioxidants such as vitamin C, vitamin E, and the trace mineral selenium have lower levels of prostate cancer.

**4.** Use your prostate regularly. The gland supplies the fluid (called semen) for ejaculation. Some research suggests that frequent ejaculation reduces the risk of prostate cancer.

**5.** Think twice about a vasectomy, as studies show that this operation may increase your risk. That doesn't mean that you shouldn't have a vasectomy, says Dr. Labriola, but if you do, be extra careful to minimize your other risk factors.

## LYCOPENE: *A Protective Pigment*

One study showed that men who ate more pizza had less prostate cancer, Dr. Quillin says. The protective factor in pizza may be a pigment in tomatoes called lycopene, which blocks free radicals, strengthens the immune system, and may help regulate cancer genes.

Lycopene is a type of phytochemical, an anti-disease compound in food. It is also found in red grapefruit.

Robert Rountree, M.D., cofounder of the Helios Health Center in Boulder, Colorado, "prescribes" a teaspoon a day of tomato paste for his patients with prostate cancer. "Lycopene has more potent antioxidant properties than beta-carotene, and it has anti-cancer properties," he says.

## ISOFLAVONES: *Keep Cancer Cells from Multiplying*

Isoflavones, anti-cancer phytochemicals found in soy products, "inhibit a biochemical process that can cause cancer cells to proliferate," says Elizabeth Ann Lowenthal, D.O., an osteopathic physician and cancer specialist in Alabaster, Alabama. She advises her prostate cancer patients to take two 70-milligram tablets with each meal.

# *The Natural Plan to Relieve*
# **Prostate Problems**

Sometime after age 40, many men notice that urinating isn't as simple as it once was. They have difficulty starting the flow. When it does start, it's weak. There's the embarrassment of dribbling, and they find themselves getting up several times a night to go to the bathroom.

These symptoms are caused by benign prostatic hyperplasia (BPH), a disorder of the prostate gland. In Germany, most men who see a doctor for BPH are prescribed an extract of the herb saw palmetto, a safe and powerful treatment that relieves the symptoms. In the United States, however, men with BPH who see a doctor are likely to get a prescription for the drug finasteride (Proscar). This drug doesn't work any better than saw palmetto, it can cause side effects such as loss of sex drive, and it may even contribute to prostate cancer in high-risk men, says Jonathan Wright, M.D., a nutritionally oriented physician and director of the Tahoma Clinic in Kent, Washington.

Why the transatlantic disparity? It's not hard to figure out, Dr. Wright says. "Drug companies drive health care practices in America, and drug companies can't make big money on an unpatentable herb such as saw palmetto."

Fortunately, saw palmetto and other natural treatments that help relieve BPH are readily available without a prescription. But, says Dr. Wright, you should use them only under the supervision of a health professional who is knowledgeable in natural and nutritional medicine.

## SAW PALMETTO: *The Best Natural Treatment*
Medical science doesn't know exactly why saw palmetto works to banish the symptoms of BPH, says Dr. Wright. Like finasteride, it is thought to help stop a cascade of prostate-damaging enzymes that may spark the problem.

## GUIDE TO
## PROFESSIONAL CARE

The symptoms of benign prostatic hyperplasia (BPH), including a weak urine stream, a bladder that doesn't empty completely, hesitancy or the inability to start urinating even when you have the urge, dribbling, and frequent nighttime urination, can also be the first symptoms of prostate cancer.

If you're experiencing BPH symptoms, you must see your medical doctor for a rectal prostate exam and a test for elevated levels of prostate specific antigen, which may signal cancer. (Although the early symptoms of BPH and prostate cancer are the same, having BPH does not increase your risk for prostate cancer.)

It also occupies "binding" sites on the prostate that are typically occupied by an enzyme that may trigger BPH. It may reduce prostate swelling and inflammation, and it may block estradiol, a type of estrogen that can cause prostate cells to multiply.

Whatever the reason for its effectiveness, taking 160 milligrams of saw palmetto extract twice daily can do the trick, but you need to talk to your doctor before starting this treatment, and you will have to continue taking this dosage in order to control BPH. Look for a product whose label states that it contains 85 to 95 percent fatty acids and sterol, says Dr. Wright. "Anything less may not have the potency to do any good."

### NETTLE: *Boosting the Effectiveness of Saw Palmetto*
While you're locating the right saw palmetto product, you may want to consider a supplement that contains saw palmetto and other herbs that can help defeat BPH, says Michael Janson, M.D., consultant physician at Path to Health in Burlington, Massachusetts.

One of those herbs is nettle. "An extract of stinging nettle may enhance the action of saw palmetto when the two are combined," he says. Look for a product that provides 300 milligrams of nettle extract.

**PYGEUM:** *For Extra Help*

This herb, derived from the bark of an African tree, can also reduce the symptoms of BPH, and it may work particularly well in combination with saw palmetto and nettle, says Eva Urbaniak, N.D., a naturopathic physician in Seattle. She recommends 25 to 100 milligrams a day until symptoms subside.

## Stimulate Your Prostate by Using Your Feet

No, this isn't as kinky as it sounds. We're talking about using foot reflexology, the alternative therapy that says that the feet are covered with "reflex points" corresponding to various parts of the body and that stimulating specific reflex points sends healing energy to specific body parts.

"There are reflex points on your feet that can send a surge of energy to the prostate, clearing out congestion and helping restore it to health," says Eva Urbaniak, N.D., a naturopathic physician in Seattle. Here are her instructions for massaging those points.

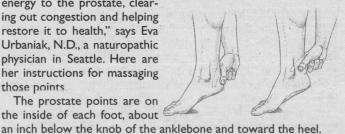

The prostate points are on the inside of each foot, about an inch below the knob of the anklebone and toward the heel.

Sit in a chair, bend over or lift both feet to the edge of the chair, and "pinch" the base of each heel with the thumb and forefinger of the corresponding hand, applying firm, steady pressure (above left). Then, using a milking-type motion, slowly move from the base of your heel toward your anklebone (above right).

"Be sure to cover the entire area of the heel below the ankle, paying more attention to tender spots," Dr. Urbaniak says. Do this massage for a few minutes two or three times a day.

## The Hidden Cause of BPH?

While the three herbs just discussed can be wonderfully effective for eliminating the symptoms of BPH, a "deficiency" of the herbs is definitely not the cause of the disease. Dr. Wright theorizes that in some men, BPH may actually be a nutritional disease: the result of a dietary deficiency of the trace mineral zinc and of the fatty acids found in good-for-you oils such as flaxseed.

## ZINC: *Your Prostate Loves It*

The prostate gland contains more of the trace mineral zinc than any other organ in the body, so it's not surprising that a supplement of the mineral can help reduce the symptoms of BPH.

Dr. Wright recommends taking 90 milligrams of zinc daily (in the highly absorbable form of either zinc picolinate or zinc citrate) in three 30-milligram doses. Taper slowly to 60 milligrams daily and then to a maintenance dose of 30 milligrams as symptoms recede. And, since too much zinc can cause a copper deficiency, take 2 milligrams of copper with every 30 milligrams of zinc, he advises.

## FATTY ACIDS: *Oil Your Gland*

"In my clinical experience, fatty acids and zinc are the most important parts of a supplement program designed to reverse BPH and its symptoms," Dr. Wright says. He recommends that men eat a handful or two a day of unroasted sunflower seeds and pumpkin seeds, which are excellent sources of both nutrients.

He also recommends a tablespoon of organically grown, carefully processed (the label will say "processed under nitrogen"), high-lignan flaxseed oil twice a day, along with 400 international units of vitamin E, which is thought to help flaxseed oil work in the body.

# *A Dietary Approach That Can Clear Up* Psoriasis

John O.A. Pagano, D.C., a chiropractor in Englewood Cliffs, New Jersey, maintains that he has spent more than 30 years doing what conventional medicine says is impossible: healing patients of the scaling, itching, bleeding, disfigurement, and other symptoms of the skin disease psoriasis.

"Conventional doctors say that this disease is incurable because they have no concept of the cause of psoriasis," Dr. Pagano says. "They use either topical, external treatments to keep the lesions under control or powerful systemic drugs that can often clear the skin but wreak havoc on the rest of the body. The fact is that although psoriasis is viewed as a disease of the skin, in which skin cells proliferate and shed at an abnormally fast rate, its cause does not originate in the skin. It originates within the intestinal tract."

Although psoriasis is a chronic inflammatory disease of the skin, Dr. Pagano explains, it is the result of a condition, widely acknowledged by alternative healers, known as intestinal permeability, or leaky gut syndrome. In this syndrome, alternative practitioners believe that the walls of the small intestine become thin and permeable, allowing toxic elements (such as fats, yeast, acids, and bacteria) that would normally be eliminated by the digestive tract to enter the bloodstream in large quantities. The toxin overload can become so great that the poisons build up in the body faster than they can be eliminated. The body then tries to eliminate them through the skin via the sweat glands, which results in the lesions of psoriasis, Dr. Pagano says.

"When you understand the true cause of psoriasis, you understand that the disease can be healed in a perfectly natural way using dietary therapy," he says.

Harold Mermelstein, M.D., a dermatologist in Westchester County and Riverdale, New York, says that the dietary regimen developed by Dr. Pagano works.

"There is no question in my mind that Dr. Pagano's diet can work to clear up psoriasis, particularly in patients with severe cases," he says. "I have seen patients with psoriasis get better on this diet. In severe cases, I think a patient would be wise to try the diet first as an alternative before using powerful medicines that can cause side effects. If I had psoriasis, I would definitely try Dr. Pagano's diet to control the problem."

Dr. Mermelstein says that Dr. Pagano's dietary recommendations are virtually risk-free. but he counsels any patient with psoriasis to develop a total approach to the disease under the supervision of a medical doctor or other qualified health care professional.

Dr. Pagano recommends following this approach for at least 3 to 6 months, under the supervision of your health care practitioner, until your skin is completely clear. Then continue for another 3 to 6 months before introducing foods that you have been avoiding to see if there's a reaction.

If a reaction does occur, Dr. Pagano suggests going back on the diet. If the diet still doesn't appear to be effective at that point, talk to your doctor about using conventional measures that are available to help control the disease.

## WATER: *For Internal Cleansing*

The first step in Dr. Pagano's program is cleansing your body of toxins so they don't keep pouring out through your skin. Water is the best internal cleanser. He recommends drinking six to eight 8-ounce glasses every day.

## STEWED FRUITS: *Good for the Bowels*

Eat a serving or two a day of stewed figs, apples, raisins, apricots, pears, peaches, or prunes, says Dr. Pagano. Their laxative effect will help clean your bowels.

## EXERCISE: *A Vital Part of the Cleansing Regimen*

"Exercise is a vital part of the regimen for clearing psoriasis," Dr. Pagano says. "It stimulates the internal structures of the body, increases circulation, activates the glands, oxygenates the blood, opens the pores, and filters the blood through the liver and kidneys." He recommends a daily period of 30 to 40 minutes of any aerobic activity such as walking, swimming, bicycling, or tennis.

# GUIDE TO
# PROFESSIONAL CARE

Psoriasis is a serious, often severe, condition that requires professional care. In the United States alone, there are more than 7 million people with psoriasis. Unfortunately, a dermatologist, who may not understand the cause of the disease—or the cure—will likely recommend treatments that provide only symptomatic relief and may saddle you with a host of side effects.

"The psoriasis patient needs to find a medical doctor, naturopath, osteopath, or chiropractor who understands nutrition and who will help to implement a natural approach to the disease, which is the only truly curative approach," says John O. A. Pagano, D.C., a chiropractor in Englewood Cliffs, New Jersey.

Even if you decide to go the conventional route, you can choose a treatment regimen that minimizes the risk of side effects, says Harold Mermelstein, M.D., a dermatologist in Westchester County and Riverdale, New York.

He recommends that patients start with cortisone-based topical medication or light therapy before relying on nutrient-based, topical medications such as a vitamin D– or vitamin A–based ointment, both of which can have long-term side effects.

For very severe cases of psoriasis, Dr. Mermelstein advises patients to try the dietary regimen discussed in this chapter before beginning oral medications that treat the disease by suppressing the immune system and can damage the liver.

## OILS: *Moisturize Your Skin Naturally*

Rubbing castor oil on thick skin lesions or a 50-50 mixture of olive oil and peanut oil on thinner lesions can help moisturize your skin without further irritating it, says Dr. Pagano.

## ANTIPERSPIRANTS: *A Must to Avoid*

Choose a regular deodorant over an antiperspirant, Dr. Pagano advises. Antiperspirants block normal elimination through the sweat glands; deodorants don't.

## HYDROTHERAPY: *A Bath for the "Healing Crisis"*

As the body is cleansed, it will begin to throw off years of accumulated toxins, and your psoriasis may get worse for a few days before it gets better. Dr. Pagano calls this period the healing crisis.

To cope with the increased burning and itching, he recommends taking a bath in lukewarm water to which you've added 1 cup of apple-cider vinegar (if your skin isn't cracked from scratching) and 1 cup of rolled oats and cornstarch (⅔ cup oats to ⅓ cup cornstarch, blended to a powder). A pound of baking soda added to the water often helps as well. "Taking a bath in this alkaline mixture for 15 to 20 minutes a day will soothe the nerve endings," he says.

## FOOD: *Emphasize These*

"Without following the right diet, efforts to cure are fruitless," Dr. Pagano says. The diet should be 70 to 80 percent fruits and vegetables, whose high fiber content helps cleanse the colon, or large intestine, of toxins, he says. It's essential to include many leafy green salads.

The other 20 to 30 percent should be grains, poultry, fish, lamb, and low-fat, low-sodium dairy products. This ratio maintains an alkaline (rather than acid) chemistry in the system, which is a must for healing psoriasis.

## FOOD: *Avoid Saturated Fats*

Saturated and hydrogenated fats cause inflammation and must be avoided, Dr. Pagano says. That means no red meat in any form and no products with hydrogenated fats, which are common ingredients in processed foods. Instead of cooking with butter or margarine, use olive oil, he suggests.

## FOOD: *Turn Off the Nightshades*

Plants in the nightshade family are also toxic for people with psoriasis. "Every psoriasis patient must stay away from these foods if he wants to heal," Dr. Pagano says. Nightshades include eggplant, white potatoes, peppers, and paprika, but the worst for those with psoriasis is tomato, says Dr. Pagano. That means ketchup, tomato juice, pizza, and other tomato-based foods are off-limits. You also need to avoid smoking, since tobacco is a nightshade.

**FOOD:** *These Are Forbidden*

Other foods that block the healing of psoriasis, says Dr. Pagano, are shellfish, junk foods such as soda or potato chips, fried foods, alcohol, pickled and smoked foods, and processed foods with coconut oil or palm oil. He also recommends avoiding excess sweets such as sodas, candy, pastries, and pies.

**SLIPPERY ELM:** *30 Minutes before Breakfast*

The herb slippery elm coats the inner lining of the intestinal wall, promoting healing, says Dr. Pagano. To prepare a tea, put ½ teaspoon of slippery elm powder in a cup of warm water, let stand for 15 minutes, then stir and drink. Don't eat for the next 30 minutes. Use the tea every day for the first 10 days of the program, then every other day until your psoriasis clears.

**YELLOW SAFFRON:** *Flushes Out Toxins*

American yellow saffron tea helps heal the lining of the intestinal walls as it flushes the liver and kidneys of toxins, says Dr. Pagano. To make the tea, put ¼ teaspoon of saffron in a cup, add boiling water, and let stand for 15 minutes. Drink it 5 days a week until your psoriasis clears. If you experience excessive urination or bladder irritation, stop using the tea.

**FISH OIL:** *More Healing for the Intestines*

The omega-3 fatty acids found in fish oil or flaxseed oil can help heal the "compromised" intestinal walls, Dr. Pagano says. Follow the dosage recommendations on the label.

**LECITHIN:** *Gives Many Benefits*

The nutritional supplement lecithin (also called phosphatidyl choline or choline) helps alkalinize the body and is a natural laxative, says Dr. Pagano. He recommends taking 1 tablespoon of granular lecithin three times a day 5 days a week.

# *Alternative Therapies*
# *Ease the Pain of*
# **Repetitive Strain Injury**

Repetitive strain injury, or RSI, is an epidemic, says Robert E. Markison, M.D., a hand surgeon in San Francisco. Millions of Americans are experiencing inflammation and injury in some part of their upper extremities—fingers, hands, wrists, forearms, elbows, or shoulders—caused by repetitive action at work, school, or play.

This "cumulative microtrauma" can come from activities such as entering data at a keyboard, using a mouse to click your way around the Internet, sweeping bar codes over a laser at a checkout counter, or cutting hair with scissors in a beauty salon.

What's worse, many people with RSI are misdiagnosed and often don't receive either the correct professional treatment or natural self-help therapies, says Scott M. Fried, D.O., director and chief surgeon at the Montgomery County Hand Center and Upper Extremity Institute in East Norriton, Pennsylvania.

But even when an RSI diagnosis is correct, medical treatment may not be the answer. "There are many effective alternatives to drugs and surgery for RSI," says Dr. Fried. "Usually, the body will naturally heal if it is allowed to do so." Here are the best ways to help it along.

**MODIFY OR ELIMINATE:** *Make Tasks Painless*
"First and foremost, if at all possible, stop or modify the activity that is causing the problems," says Dr. Fried. "For example, change your workstation or use a headset for the phone."

**POSTURE:** *Pain-Free Positions*
Your posture throughout the day and night can help relieve the pain of RSI. Here are Dr. Fried's and Dr. Markison's recommended pain-free positions.

# GUIDE TO
# PROFESSIONAL CARE

If you feel any numbness or tingling in your arms or hands or have constant pain that interferes with your activities for more than a week, you should see a health professional who specializes in repetitive strain injury (RSI). He will conduct a full evaluation—from your neck to your fingertips—to provide an accurate diagnosis, says Scott M. Fried, D.O., director and chief surgeon at the Montgomery County Hand Center and Upper Extremity Institute in East Norriton, Pennsylvania.

You also need to develop a relationship with the professional you choose so that he can help you change or eliminate the factors in your life that might be contributing to your problem and help you develop a healing plan.

That plan should be tailored to whether you have swelling, inflammation, or both. It also should change or modify the activity that is causing the problem and use a combination of conventional and natural treatments—both professional and self-help—to reduce the pain. Such pain-relieving professional care can include acupuncture, reflexology, massage, tai chi, yoga, ultrasound, a custom-made splint, or pain-relieving medications.

Finally, you need to realize that you're not going to get better overnight. RSI problems can take weeks, months, or even years to heal, Dr. Fried says, so don't be quick to give up and opt for surgery. "Surgery is not a cure," he says. "It is often just a temporary fix."

• While sleeping, don't lie on your stomach with your head turned to the side, sleep with your arms overhead, or lie on the affected side. Instead, lie on the unaffected side with one pillow under your head and another pillow in front of you to support the affected arm. Or lie on your back with one pillow under your head and a pillow under each arm up to the shoulders. The three pillows should form an inverted U.
• While driving, steer with your hands low on the wheel in a secure but relaxed grip. For long trips, put a pillow in your lap to support your forearms. You may also need a lower-back pillow for support.

• At the computer, sit with the keyboard and mouse as close to you as possible. The more you lean forward or extend or lift your arms, the more you are likely to cause or worsen RSI.

Also, the monitor should be directly in front of you and at eye level so you don't have to look down. Use a large typeface on the screen so you don't have to lean forward to see it. You should have a copy stand, an adjustable keyboard tray, and a wrist rest. Type with a gentle touch.

• While using a mouse, tilt it outward at an angle of 30 degrees or so to avoid a relentless, nerve-binding, muscle-straining, palms-down position. Put the mouse pad on a clipboard with an object (such as a foam wedge) underneath to tilt it. The top of the clipboard provides a "rail" so the mouse won't slide off.

## STRETCHING: *Flex Your Wrists*

At minimum, you should take a break for a minute or two every half hour, particularly if you're working at a keyboard. Stretch your wrists and neck during the break, Dr. Fried says. Here's how.

First, loosely close both hands into fists, then bend both wrists forward and backward a couple of times. Then bend one wrist forward and gently stretch it with the other hand. Switch hands and repeat. Next, bend one wrist backward and stretch with the other hand. Switch hands and repeat.

Next, stretch your neck. While seated and facing forward, slowly lean your right ear toward your right shoulder, then pause and return to the original position. Repeat on the left side. Then slowly bend your head forward to move your chin to your chest, then return to the upright position. Finally, gently look upward, then return.

## STRETCHING: *A Super-Slow Shoulder Roll*

Doing the following shoulder roll two or three times a day can significantly reduce the stress in your shoulders, arms, wrists, and hands, reducing or preventing the pain of RSI, says Sharon Butler, a certified practitioner of Hellerwork (a structural bodywork and movement therapy) in Paoli, Pennsylvania.

Raise your shoulders toward your ears and let your arms hang loosely by your sides. Very slowly, rotate your shoulders toward the front of your body. Continue rotating them to the lowest point, reverse direction and rotate them toward the back, then return to the starting position.

Take at least 30 seconds to do this exercise, making the widest circle possible, then do another complete revolution in the opposite direction.

### GLOVES: *A Practical Fashion Statement*

At work, warmer hands are freer of pain, Dr. Markison says. He recommends finding a local seamstress to make cotton knit gloves that run from just above or below your elbows to the midjoints of your fingers, leaving your fingertips free for use.

"The time to use this type of glove is whenever you touch your cheek with your hand and your hand feels cool," he says. That means that your hands are too cool to work, and your RSI problem will go from bad to worse. People who use this type of glove regularly to keep their hands warm at work are usually delighted because their hands feel so much better, he says.

### GINKGO: *Improve Your Peripheral Circulation*

The herb ginkgo can improve the circulation to your arms and hands, thus reducing the symptoms of RSI, Dr. Markison says. He recommends 60 milligrams in the morning, taken with 16 ounces of water.

### GLUCOSAMINE AND CHONDROITIN: *For Older Workers*

The supplements glucosamine and chondroitin can help decrease the aches and pains of RSI, particularly in older data-entry workers, Dr. Markison says. He recommends a supplement with 500 milligrams of glucosamine and 400 milligrams of chondroitin; take three a day if you weigh more than 110 pounds and two a day if you weigh less.

### WATER: *64 Ounces a Day Is Essential*

Staying well-hydrated boosts the circulation of the body, pushing pain-relieving oxygen and nutrients into the areas hit by RSI, Dr. Markison says. He recommends a minimum of 64 ounces a day, but more is better.

### CAFFEINE: *You're Better Off Without It*

"If you have RSI, you should eliminate caffeine from your diet," Dr. Markison says. Caffeine is a diuretic that drains water out of your body, and less water means poorer circulation to your arms and hands. If you must have a morning cup of coffee, he says, drink twice as much water at the same time.

## NICOTINE AND ALCOHOL: *A Must to Avoid*

"Nicotine is forbidden for RSI patients," Dr. Markison says. "There is no hope for smokers with RSI." A single puff of a cigarette can shut down blood flow to the hands by as much as 60 percent, he says.

Alcohol is discouraged because it increases inflammation. "Tendons and other areas typically inflamed by RSI only get worse if you drink alcohol," he says.

## VEGETABLE JUICE: *A Great Anti-Inflammatory*

The huge dose of inflammation-beating antioxidant nutrients in an 8-ounce glass of homemade carrot-celery-beet-parsley juice is as good as any anti-inflammatory pill for RSI, Dr. Markison says. Have a glass every morning, adjusting the proportions of the four juices to taste.

## WEIGHT CONTROL: *Being Overweight Quadruples the Risk*

Twenty to 30 pounds of extra weight can quadruple your chances of the nerve problems that cause RSI, Dr. Markison says. For example, the bony passageway that houses the median nerve as it passes through the wrist can be crowded by fat, causing the wrist-stabbing, hand-numbing form of RSI called carpal tunnel syndrome.

"I've seen many cases of carpal tunnel that have been controlled by weight loss alone," he says. To lose weight, he recommends a primarily vegetarian diet (which also helps to reduce the inflammation of RSI); avoiding fatty foods, starches, and junk foods; and walking 2 miles or more three or four times a week. To get the protein that your body needs, Dr. Markison suggests eating tofu and fish.

## VISUALIZATION: *Counter the Stress That Chokes Your Hands*

Stress reduces blood flow to the upper extremities, worsening RSI. Here's a visualization technique that counters stress and improves blood flow to your hands. Use it anytime you're feeling tense, Dr. Markison says.

Sit up straight with your hands in your lap. Take a few deep breaths. Close your eyes and let your eye muscles relax. Feel concentric waves of relaxation, like the ripples in a calm lake when a leaf falls on the surface, move down your face and neck, spread above and below your collarbone, and move down your chest.

Next, feel that you are at a safe, warm place such as a beach and, with every breath, feel oxygen-rich, nutrient-rich blood flowing into and warming your hands. Continue feeling your hands warm with every breath for 2 to 3 minutes.

## *Massage, Essential Oils, and Herbs Can Help Reduce* **Scarring**

Scar tissue is as necessary as a patch on a flat tire or new shingles on a damaged roof. It is the skin's new connective tissue. If you've had an injury— a cut, wound, or surgical incision—scar tissue allows the injury to close. But scar tissue can have a downside.

Scars can form into keloids, which are large, hard growths above the skin surface. Although they are harmless, keloids can be unsightly, tender, and sometimes itchy. Many young children as well as African-Americans and other dark-skinned people are particularly at risk for keloids.

Also, scar tissue from a surgical incision or other trauma or infection can form an adhesion, an area where tissue binds to tissue. This problem can be painful and limit normal movement. Worse, it's not typically addressed by conventional medicine.

"The degree of adhesion that forms as a result of scar tissue can cause many physical imbalances, including pain," says Edward Rosen, a physical therapist in Cotati, California. He says, however, that home massage therapy offers a way to help minimize painful adhesions and relieve them when they do occur.

Other alternative remedies, such as essential oils, herbs, and acupressure, can help keep scarring to a minimum and relieve the discomfort of keloids.

## LAVENDER ESSENTIAL OIL: *Apply It Right Away*

Putting a few drops of undiluted essential oil of lavender on the skin immediately after an injury can help prevent excessive scarring, says Norma Pasekoff Weinberg, an herbal educator in Cape Cod, Massachusetts. You can also mix a few drops of lavender oil with aloe gel, apply it to the injured tissue, and cover it with a sterile pad, she adds.

## MASSAGE: *Rub Out Pain After Surgery*

After an operation, when the stitches have been removed and the incision is completely closed, you can use a self-massage technique to help prevent adhesions, says Rosen.

Place the flat of your fingers (not your fingertips, but the pads where your fingerprints are) on either side of the incision. Then, without lifting your fingers or actually touching the incision, gently move the tissue around. Normal tissue should glide with ease in all directions. When there are adhesions, you'll

---

## GUIDE TO PROFESSIONAL CARE

Scars are usually not a threat to physical health, but if you have a scar that you feel is unattractive, you may want to see a dermatologist or plastic surgeon to discuss cosmetic surgery, including laser resurfacing procedures.

Keloids are hard, firm masses of scar tissue that grow above the skin surface and may be painful or itchy or, in some cases, even restrict movement. If you develop a keloid, see a dermatologist about treatments for removal, which include silicone gel products such as ScarEase (also available over the counter), steroid injections, surgery, and laser therapy. The recurrence rate of treated keloids is high, but the sooner they are treated after they appear, the less chance there is of recurrence, explains Esta Kronberg, M.D., a dermatologist in Houston.

reach a point where you'll feel a rapid increase in resistance, and the gliding motion of the tissue will stop.

"Respect that, and don't pull hard against it," Rosen says. "Go to that limit and maintain a gentle tension, and you'll begin to feel a softening and release in the tissue under your fingers. Go to that limit, maintain the tension, and allow the tissues to release in all directions around the incision. Until the surgical site is well-healed, usually after 2 to 3 weeks, be careful never to pull on or across the incision itself." Do this for a few minutes every day or every other day, he says.

### CHICKWEED: *To Promote Healing and Reduce Scarring*

As a wound or incision starts to crust over or scab, a compress made with the herb chickweed, which has a softening quality, can help keep scarring to a minimum, Weinberg says. Here's how to make the chickweed oil and have it ready to use as a compress.

You'll need enough fresh chickweed to fill an 8-ounce jar (about 1 cup). Wrap the herb in cheesecloth and crush it with a rolling pin. Fill the jar with the crushed herb, packing it firmly so there's as much in the jar as possible. Add enough sunflower seed oil to cover the chickweed, with at least ½ inch of oil at the top of the jar (the herb will swell slightly as it absorbs the oil). Put a lid on the jar, label it with the date, and put it in a cool, dark place.

After 2 weeks, use a paper coffee filter to strain the oil. Pour it into a tinted glass bottle, cap the bottle, label it, and store in the refrigerator. It should keep for at least 6 months, Weinberg says.

Before using a compress, be sure that the wound is no longer raw or open, she says. To prepare it, saturate a clean cotton cloth with the chickweed oil and put the cloth over the injured area for 15 to 20 minutes once a day. You can use it for as long as you like. This remedy is also good for boils, rashes, and eczema, she adds.

### ST. JOHN'S WORT: *Relieve Keloid Pain*

To reduce the discomfort of a keloid, use St. John's wort oil, says Weinberg. This herb is both antiseptic and analgesic, she explains. "Smooth a small amount of the oil over the painful area once or twice a day," she says. You can safely use the oil for as long as you like.

**MASSAGE:** *For Incision Scars*

In Traditional Chinese Medicine, life-energy, or chi, flows through the body in currents called meridians. An incision made during surgery interrupts one or more of those currents, and the energy flows around or underneath the incision.

The less chi that is present in the area of the incision, the larger, harder, and more inflexible the scar will be, says David Filipello, a licensed acupuncturist and director of Acupuncture for Health in San Francisco. Here's his advice to increase the flow of chi.

Within a week after the surgery—after the bandage is off and the wound is no longer open—use a warming herbal compound such as Tiger Balm around (never on) the incision. Gently work the liniment into the skin in a 1-inch area all around the incision with the tip of your finger, using a repeating circular motion that moves close to the incision and then away from it. Do this for 5 minutes or so once a day until the incision is completely healed.

# *Shedding Light on*
# **Seasonal Affective Disorder**

It's winter. The days are darker—and so is your mood.

You feel heavy and dull when you wake up. You drag your body around all day like a ball and chain. You find it hard to focus on your work or even on simple chores at home. You crave sweet, starchy food. Your constant snacking is piling on the pounds.

Worst of all, you feel depressed: Sad, with a capital S.

Well, add a capital A and a capital D to spell S-A-D, and you'll know a little bit more about why you feel so down. You're probably one of 10 million Americans with seasonal affective disorder (commonly known as SAD), says Norman E. Rosenthal, M.D., clinical professor of psychiatry at Georgetown University

Medical School in Washington, D.C. He is a SAD sufferer who has overcome the problem.

Genetics, stress, and other factors can play a role, but the main cause of SAD is a lack of light, says Dr. Rosenthal. Although no one knows the exact mechanism, it's theorized that less light disrupts the functioning of serotonin, a brain chemical that influences mood, energy, sleep, appetite, and concentration. That in turn causes one or more SAD symptoms: fatigue, overeating, sleep disturbances, decreased sex drive, foggy thinking, physical problems such as headaches and backaches, and, of course, sadness.

These symptoms vary in severity. The intense, winter-long depression of SAD requires professional care, Dr. Rosenthal says. But the milder variety that he calls the winter blues is self-treatable. And the first treatment to banish those blues is not necessarily antidepressant medication. It's the most natural treatment of all: Light.

## LIGHT: *Let the Sun Shine In*

Light therapy simply replaces the light that's missing during the short, dark days of winter. "It helps people with winter blues attain a more energetic and cheerful state of mind, similar to the way they feel during the summer," Dr. Rosenthal says.

Simple ways to get more light include spending more time outdoors on bright days and using more lamps in your home and office, Dr. Rosenthal says. But the most effective way, he says, is to use a special light fixture called a light box, which simulates a summer dawn on a winter morning. Here's what you need to know to use light therapy.

Light boxes are usually about 2 feet long and 1½ feet high, with white fluorescent bulbs behind a plastic screen. (Fluorescent lights spread light over a wider area. Incandescent bulbs are not acceptable or suitable for this use, says Dr. Rosenthal.) Look for a unit that delivers 2,500 to 10,000 lux (a measurement of intensity). The most effective units cost $300 to $500, which is an amount that many people with the winter blues have found to be well worth the investment, he says.

It's necessary to customize the amount of light you use to your symptoms and the time of year. "If you are starting light

# GUIDE TO
# PROFESSIONAL CARE

If you have moderately severe symptoms of depression during the winter, you shouldn't try self-help methods. You need the help of a professional, says Norman E. Rosenthal, M.D., clinical professor of psychiatry at Georgetown University Medical School in Washington, D.C.

Dr. Rosenthal suggests light therapy, supervised by a qualified professional who has had experience with the treatment, for the following problems.

• Impaired functioning, such as frequent difficulty getting to work on time or an inability to perform tasks that you normally do with ease.
• Feelings of depression, such as feeling guilty and pessimistic and thinking that life isn't worthwhile, having negative thoughts about yourself that you don't have at other times of the year, and feeling sad or having crying spells.
• Markedly disturbed physical functions, such as the need for more sleep, a desire to lie around during the day, and a lack of control over eating.

therapy at the beginning of the winter season, just when you're having your first symptoms, 10 minutes a day may be sufficient," Dr. Rosenthal advises. In the depths of winter, however, you may need 45 minutes twice a day. If you're somewhere between these two extremes, use your judgment and choose a time between 10 and 90 minutes daily. If that amount reverses your symptoms, stick with it. If symptoms continue for longer than 2 weeks, however, increase to 90 minutes, which is the maximum treatment time. If that doesn't work, seek professional care.

When you're using a light box, there's no need to stare at it directly; just position yourself 1 to 3 feet away and face it with your eyes open. You can do paperwork, make phone calls, read, or exercise. "I have a light box set up in front of a treadmill and find the combination of light therapy and exercise to be particularly energizing," Dr. Rosenthal says.

While it's uncommon, it's possible to have mild side effects from the therapy, says Dr. Rosenthal. If you experience headaches or eyestrain, decrease your exposure to 15 minutes and build up to the therapeutic amount in increments of 5 minutes or so a day over a week or two. If you become irritable, decrease your exposure. If you have insomnia, which usually occurs in people who use the lights late at night, shift the treatment to the morning.

If you have dry eyes or nasal passages, use a humidifier and drink warm beverages during the exposure. If you have sensitive, easily sunburned skin, put on sunblock before you start. Finally, if you have a history of eye disease, such as macular degeneration or retinitis pigmentosa, see an eye doctor before beginning light therapy.

### Adding Extra Voltage to Your Therapy

"Although most people with the winter blues will benefit from light therapy, many still don't feel as well in the winter as they do in the summer," Dr. Rosenthal says. Here are other ways that he recommends to help fight the symptoms of light deprivation.

### WARMTH: *Turn Up the Heat*
"Many patients have told me that warmth, in conjunction with light, seems to help combat the winter blues," Dr. Rosenthal says. Turn up the thermostat, use an electric blanket, and drink warm beverages.

### ST. JOHN'S WORT: *Beat the Blues*
The antidepressant herb St. John's wort may help the winter blues, says Dr. Rosenthal. He recommends 300 milligrams three times a day. The best brand is Kira, he says, because it's the brand that was used in European studies that proved the effectiveness of the herb. He also advises that you use St. John's wort only under the supervision of a qualified professional.

### MELATONIN: *Small Amounts Work Best*
The hormone melatonin can help reset your biological clock, thus decreasing the symptoms of winter blues. The trick is to take a very small amount in the afternoon, says Dr. Rosenthal. Use

100 micrograms ($\frac{1}{10}$ milligram). If you can't find melatonin in this dose, Dr. Rosenthal suggests that you break a 200-microgram tablet in half. Do not take this supplement unless under the supervision of a knowledgeable medical doctor.

# Quick Relief from the Pain of
# Shingles

When you were a kid, you probably had a bout of chicken pox, a rashy infection caused by the Varicella zoster virus, also called herpes zoster. (It's a variety of the virus that causes oral and genital herpes.) Unfortunately, the virus didn't disappear even when you were better. Instead, it hibernated in nerve tracks along your spine. At some point, like an unexpected visit from a distant and very annoying relative whom you haven't seen in 40 years, it may re-emerge.

There are many reasons that the virus can reactivate years—even decades—later and cause shingles. Among them are aging or physical trauma such as injury or surgery, which can weaken the immune system and cause shingles, explains Kenneth A. Bock, M.D., codirector of the Rhinebeck Health Center in Rhinebeck, New York, and the Center for Progressive Medicine in Albany, New York.

Shingles show up as an itchy and sometimes painful rash, immediately followed by blisters that can break out anywhere above the waist. They typically form a rectangular band that extends from the spine to the chest. The blisters appear over a period of 3 to 5 days, during which you're likely to be feverish, headachy, and weak, and they take anywhere from 2 weeks to a month to heal.

Alternative practitioners recommend many drug-free and effective home remedies to relieve the severe pain of an attack. There are also things that you can do to shorten outbreaks and help prevent them from coming back.

# GUIDE TO
# PROFESSIONAL CARE

Shingles is a painful but relatively harmless infection that can usually be treated with either medications or home remedies. Most people suffer only one attack, but in the worst-case scenario, episodes recur, sometimes one after another. Also, in some people (particularly those over 70), the pain of shingles never leaves, a condition called postherpetic neuralgia.

If you have shingles blisters anywhere on or near your head, or you are immuno-compromised (meaning that you have AIDS, cancer, or any other immune-weakening disease), see a medical doctor immediately.

Contact your doctor if you have difficulty eating or drinking during an attack, or if you're having trouble with hearing and balance, says Kenneth A. Bock, M.D., codirector of the Rhinebeck Health Center in Rhinebeck, New York, and the Center for Progressive Medicine in Albany, New York. These symptoms may mean that you have internal blisters, which can be very serious. You should also see a doctor if you have a second attack, recurrent attacks, or pain that doesn't go away after the first attack.

Alternative physicians suggest a number of nondrug methods for treating serious cases of shingles, particularly for recurrent episodes. Injections of vitamin $B_{12}$ "get incredible results in my practice," says Mark Stengler, N.D., a naturopathic physician in San Diego. He also recommends acupuncture for pain relief during an outbreak. He suggests that you can benefit from seeing a homeopathic or naturopathic physician, who may recommend a homeopathic remedy called Varicella, a diluted version of the virus that causes the disease.

Another alternative treatment may include injections of a neutralization vaccine, which is created from a diluted mixture of the virus, says John M. Sullivan, M.D., a physician in Mechanicsburg, Pennsylvania. Some alternative doctors treat shingles by giving diluted, intravenous hydrogen peroxide, which may help kill the virus.

## FRENCH CLAY AND TEA TREE OIL: *Dry the Blisters*

Available in health food stores, French Green Clay is a topical treatment that is thought to help dry up moist, weeping shingles blisters. Adding tea tree oil to the clay can give it antiviral properties, says Guillermo Asis, M.D., director of Path to Health in Burlington, Massachusetts.

To prepare a poultice, mix a teaspoon or so of water with enough French Green Clay to make a paste. Add one to two drops of tea tree oil. Wearing plastic or latex medical gloves, gently apply a thin covering of the paste directly to the blisters. Cover the paste with a double thickness of gauze and secure the gauze to the skin.

Leave the poultice on for 2 to 3 hours, Dr. Asis advises, then remove the gauze and gently clean the area with a warm cloth. You can apply the paste again if you want; Dr. Asis says that you can use it once or twice a day.

Be aware, though, that if you've never had chicken pox, you can get it from the viral material in shingles blisters. If you're applying a poultice to someone, avoid touching the blisters directly with your hands or any other part of your skin, says Dr. Bock. Immediately discard or wash any treatment materials that touched the blisters.

## ACTIVATED CHARCOAL: *Removes the Virus*

Activated charcoal is a tremendously helpful home remedy that draws the herpesvirus out of the skin, quickly drying and healing blisters, says David A. Darbro, M.D., a physician in Indianapolis. Used properly, it can also help lessen the pain, he says.

Add enough water to a small amount of activated charcoal, plus the same amount of cornstarch or ground flaxseed, to make a paste. Let stand for 20 minutes, then apply the paste to the blisters with a piece of muslin.

Follow the same directions and precautions as for French Green Clay, but leave the paste on for 12 hours. Wash it off, then keep reapplying it until the blisters are completely dry and healing, Dr. Darbro says.

## HYDROGEN PEROXIDE: *Speeds Shingles Healing*

A gel of hydrogen peroxide contains high levels of oxygen, which is believed to kill viruses and can help shorten an episode of shingles, says Vijay Vijh, M.D., Ph.D., director of the

Cherry Hill Wellness Center in New Jersey. He recommends applying the gel to the blisters every 2 to 3 hours until they've dried and healed.

## HOMEOPATHY: *Fast Pain Relief*

The homeopathic remedy Rhus tox is thought to quickly reduce pain and speed healing, says Mark Stengler, N.D., a naturopathic physician in San Diego. He recommends using a 6X potency during the blister stage, taking two pills every 3 to 4 hours until the blisters heal.

## CAPSAICIN: *More Pain Relief*

Capsaicin, which is found in chile peppers, is a compound that blocks the buildup of substance P, a chemical in the body that sends pain signals from the nerves to the brain.

Capsaicin cream is an outstanding treatment for postherpetic neuralgia, a condition that occurs mainly in people over age 70 in which the pain of shingles lingers long after the attack, says Dr. Stengler.

When treating the neuralgia after an outbreak, follow the label directions for applying the cream to painful areas, says Dr. Stengler. (Remember to wear medical gloves or to wash your hands immediately after the application.) Don't expect it to work right away, however. It may take a few weeks to block all of the substance P and fully relieve your pain.

## MULTIVITAMIN/MINERAL SUPPLEMENT: *Health from the Inside*

"The immune system has to be weak for a breakout of shingles to occur," says Dr. Asis. And since almost every vitamin and mineral contributes to the strength of the immune system, he recommends taking a high-potency multivitamin/mineral supplement if you've ever had a bout of shingles and want to prevent another.

## VITAMIN C: *The Immune Booster*

Of all the nutrients you can take, vitamin C is perhaps the most important for healthy immune functioning. Adding a bit extra to your supplement regimen is a good way to prevent an encore of shingles, says Dr. Asis. He recommends taking 2,000 milligrams twice a day.

**ALPHA-LIPOIC ACID:** *Jail the Free Radicals*

Your body contains out-of-control molecules called free radicals, which oxidize (or "rust") the cells of your body, including the cells of your shingles-fighting immune system. Alpha-lipoic acid has powerful antioxidant properties, meaning that it helps stop this process from occurring, says Dr. Asis. He suggests taking 50 milligrams twice a day to help prevent shingles outbreaks.

**LYSINE:** *Starve the Virus*

Taking 1,000 milligrams a day of the amino acid lysine can help decrease the recurrence of shingles. This is because lysine prevents the absorption of the amino acid arginine, which appears to be vital for the virus to stay active, says Rashid Ali Buttar, D.O., an osteopathic physician who practices emergency and preventive medicine in Charlotte, North Carolina. Take this supplement only under the supervision of a knowledgeable medical doctor.

## *Recover Quickly from*
# Shin Splints

You overdid it. Too many miles of jogging on hard roads while training for that 5-K. Too many aerobics classes while trying to trim a few inches off your tummy. All that pounding tore tiny sections of tendon or muscle off your shin, the area of skeleton between your knee and ankle.

A shin splint hurts either in the front of or on the side of the leg, usually a few inches above the anklebone. If you want it to heal, you have to reduce or stop the activity that caused it for at least 2 to 4 months, says Steven Subotnick, D.P.M., a podiatrist and naturopathic doctor in Berkeley and San Leandro, California. But if you want to heal as quickly as possible, say alternative practitioners, these remedies can help.

## HOMEOPATHY: *Your First Line of Defense*

The first sign of a shin splint is pain and swelling. Your first response should be the homeopathic remedy Arnica montana, says Dr. Subotnick. Take it as soon as you notice the pain and continue until the pain goes away. He advises taking the 30X potency four times each hour.

## MSM: *For Pain Relief*

The nutritional supplement MSM (methylsulfonylmethane) is a form of sulfur that can help reduce muscle soreness and inflammation, says Stanley W. Jacob, M.D., professor of surgery at Oregon Health Sciences University in Portland.

He cites the case of a college track-and-field athlete who developed shin splints in both legs that caused throbbing pain after her workouts. She began taking 1 gram of MSM a day, and her pain vanished after 2 weeks. When she ran out of the supplement and stopped taking it for a while, the pain returned, but it subsided when she started taking MSM again. One gram a day is a good therapeutic dose for pain relief, says Dr. Jacob.

## HOMEOPATHY: *Ruta Grav for Healing*

Ruta graveolens is the most effective homeopathic remedy for relieving the pain of shin splints and speeding healing, says Dr. Subotnick. He recommends using the 30X potency four times a day until the pain subsides.

---

## GUIDE TO PROFESSIONAL CARE

If you have shin splints, see a sports medicine specialist for x-rays and lab tests to rule out a medical cause of the problem, says Steven Subotnick, D.P.M., a podiatrist in Berkeley and San Leandro, California. Pain in the front of the shin that develops gradually can be caused by a stress fracture, circulatory disease, back problems, or, in rare cases, a bone tumor. You should also see a podiatrist about orthotics, shoe inserts that correct problems with your gait that may be causing the shin splints, he says.

## MASSAGE: *Stimulate the Chi*

In Traditional Chinese Medicine, the pain of shin splints is believed to be partly caused by the body's life-energy, known as chi, flowing up rather than down the leg, says David Filipello, a licensed acupuncturist and director of the Acupuncture for Health Clinic in San Francisco.

To correct that flow, gently but firmly push your thumbs down both sides of your calf or along the shinbone, starting at the knee and ending at the ankle. Use your left thumb on the left side and your right thumb on the right side. Repeat four or five times, then do the same technique on the other leg. Do this massage two or three times a day.

## VISUALIZATION: *Prepare Yourself to Return to Activity*

When you have shin splints, you have to rest. But even while you're resting, you can move healing chi into your legs and speed your recovery with a visualization technique, says Alexander Majewski, a licensed massage therapist and director of the Acupressure Institute of Alaska in Juneau. Visualize yourself performing the activity that you'll be resuming, whether it's running, basketball, or ballet. Next, visualize energy from your hara, the energy source of the body that is located just below the navel, flowing to your legs while you're performing the activity.

"I have had great success recommending this technique to dancers who over-rehearse and develop shin splints," he says. "While injured, they rehearse in their minds, imagining chi flowing to their legs, and their healing and pain relief is almost always much quicker than in similar cases where this technique isn't used."

# *Learning to Relax Is a Must in Overcoming* Shyness

Is there a cure for shyness? Some conventional doctors would have you believe that by popping an antidepressant pill, you can metamorphose from a wallflower into a social butterfly.

According to Jonathan Berent, a psychiatric social worker and director of the Berent Associates Center for Social Therapy in Great Neck, New York, however, medication is useful in only about 25 percent of people he treats for shyness, or what health professionals now call social anxiety.

"Medication should never be the first or only treatment, and it is not a cure," he says. To truly cure social anxiety, you need to resolve low self-esteem, face the specific situations that you fear, and overcome that breathless, sweaty-palmed hypersensitivity.

The first two components require professional guidance, Dr. Berent says. The third you can tackle on your own by practicing the following relaxation techniques for 15 to 20 minutes every day, gradually making them a way of life.

## BREATHING: *Make Friends with Your Diaphragm*

"Diaphragmatic breathing, which is breathing into your stomach area rather than into your chest, is the basis of all relaxation and internal self-regulation," says Dr. Berent. When you're anxious, consciously take slow, deep, rhythmic diaphragmatic breaths by inhaling through your nose, drawing the oxygen down into your abdomen, and holding it for a few seconds. Exhale through your mouth, mentally counting 5 . . . 4 . . . 3 . . . 2 . . . 1.

"Don't push or force the air in and out of your body," Dr. Berent says. "Breathe slowly and deliberately until the pace feels natural."

**VISUALIZATION:** *Increase the Temperature of Your Hands*

Increasing the skin temperature of your hands by 3 to 4 degrees can abort anxiety, Dr. Berent says.

First, do your breathing exercise. Then, focus your attention on your right arm and say to yourself, "My right arm is warm; I feel the warmth flowing through my right arm." Repeat this phrase for about 30 seconds. Notice the heaviness and limpness in your right arm and hand.

Next, picture yourself lying on your back in the warm sun at the beach. Hear the waves. Smell the salty air. Feel the sun's rays warming the palms and fingers of your right hand. Do this for a minute or so, then repeat the entire process with your left hand.

**AFFIRMATION:** *Use It to Take Control*

In facing situations where you typically feel anxious, use the following affirmation: "My social anxiety symptoms are temporary, and eventually they will diminish significantly and may well disappear altogether."

"This sentence must become a regular part of your daily routine," Dr. Berent says. Repeating it many times a day, every day, particularly in anxiety-producing situations, will help you remember that you are in control of your anxiety rather than it having control of you.

---

### GUIDE TO PROFESSIONAL CARE

Most people with shyness or social anxiety do not get professional help, even though they would benefit from it, says Jonathan Berent, a psychiatric social worker and director of the Berent Associates Center for Social Therapy in Great Neck, New York. Those who do seek help go to traditional therapists, who, says Dr. Berent, "really do not know how to treat the problem." Instead, he recommends seeing a psychologist, psychotherapist, or psychiatrist who specializes in anxiety.

*Complete Relief, with
No Side Effects, from*
# Sinusitis

Join the club. The very large club. Each year, nearly 35 million Americans visit doctors, hoping for relief from one or more of the symptoms of sinusitis: facial pain, tooth pain, headache, cough, and a nose more clogged than an LA freeway at rush hour.

That stuffed-up scenario is caused by a bacterial infection in the sinuses around the nose. Sinusitis can be acute, usually a result of a secondary bacterial infection that sneaks in behind the nasal congestion of a cold and sticks around for a miserable week or two. Or it can be chronic, lasting for a few weeks or even occurring again and again.

The strongest weapons in the anti-sinusitis arsenal of conventional doctors are antibiotics. Though they usually slay the bug that's biting you, they can backfire.

"I'm unhappy with the side effects that frequently accompany the use of antibiotics," says Kenneth A. Bock, M.D., codirector of the Rhinebeck Health Center in Rhinebeck, New York, and the Center for Progressive Medicine in Albany, New York.

Antibiotics destroy friendly bacteria in the gut that keep digestion normal, which leads to diarrhea, inflammation, and increased gut permeability. This in turn can trigger all kinds of other health problems, possibly including serious autoimmune diseases such as rheumatoid arthritis, Dr. Bock says.

Also, the more antibiotics you take, the tougher the bacteria become as they evolve quickly to resist the drug—which means that your next bout of sinusitis may be a doozy.

"Recurrent doses of antibiotics for sinusitis usually make things worse," says Guillermo Asis, M.D., director of Path to Health in Burlington, Massachusetts. Alternative doctors have their own anti-sinusitis remedies that kill bacteria (and relieve your symptoms) without the side effects of antibiotics.

# GUIDE TO PROFESSIONAL CARE

Alternative practitioners believe that most cases of chronic sinusitis are caused by an allergy or sensitivity to either food or an environmental allergen, such as pollen, dander, or dust mites, says Mark Stengler, N.D., a naturopathic physician in San Diego. That's why he and many other alternative practitioners suggest that a person with chronic, recurring sinusitis be tested and treated for food and inhalant allergies.

An intestinal yeast infection called candidiasis can also cause chronic sinusitis, says Guillermo Asis, M.D., director of Path to Health in Burlington, Massachusetts. This infection sparks increased production of mucus—and chronic sinusitis. If you have this problem, he recommends finding a naturally oriented practitioner with experience in detecting and treating candidiasis.

In some cases, sinusitis is caused by nasal obstructions such as nasal polyps or a deviated septum (the tiny wall of cartilage inside your nose that divides the nostrils). If your physician has ruled out all other causes of chronic sinusitis, these should be investigated, Dr. Asis says.

## GARLIC: *Peel Away Symptoms*

The most potent remedy for acute sinusitis is raw garlic, Dr. Asis says. Peel a clove and take one a day until your sinusitis clears, he recommends. Chop large garlic cloves into smaller pieces that are easy to swallow. To aid the digestion of small cloves, slice off both ends after peeling to perforate the thin film that surrounds the garlic.

"The garlic will disintegrate in the small intestine and release its bacteria-killing medication," Dr. Asis says. Take the garlic after a meal and drink 8 ounces of water with each clove to avoid stomach upset.

## VITAMIN C: *Every 2 Hours*

Take 500 milligrams of vitamin C every 2 hours during the day until the infection is cured, says Dr. Asis. This will help increase your immune system's bacteria-fighting power.

If you develop gas or diarrhea (harmless side effects of high intakes of C), cut the dosage by 1,000 milligrams a day until the intestinal upset goes away, he advises.

### NAC: *To Help Clear Sinuses*

N-acetylcysteine, or NAC, is a form of the amino acid cysteine that helps liquefy mucus so that it can drain. That's really good news, since sinus mucus can solidify like concrete.

Take 500 milligrams twice a day for the duration of the infection, says Mark Stengler, N.D., a naturopathic physician in San Diego.

### GOLDENSEAL: *Mother Nature's Infection Fighter*

The herb goldenseal is tailor-made by Mother Nature to fight sinus infections, says Dr. Stengler. It kills bacteria; helps dry up thick, wet mucus; and stimulates sinus drainage. It is available as capsules or tincture; follow the dosage recommendations on the label.

### COLLOIDAL SILVER: *A Healing Spray*

This liquefied form of silver is a powerful natural antibiotic that can help knock out an acute sinus infection, says John M. Sullivan, M.D., a physician in Mechanicsburg, Pennsylvania. Buy a bottle of colloidal silver, put some full-strength into a spray bottle, and use one or two squirts into your nose twice a day until the infection has been noticeably gone for 3 days.

## For Chronic Sinusitis, an Ocean of Relief

Salt water kills bacteria, says Carla Wilson, executive director of the Quan Yin Healing Arts Center in San Francisco. That's why she recommends spraying salt water into your nose.

This technique can help heal sinusitis in all but the most acute, severe cases, she says. Even if you choose to take antibiotics, spraying your nose every day while you take the drugs will help keep the infection from recurring, she says.

First, buy a nasal douche (also known as a neti pot), which is a small glass pipe with a hole in the side. Make a solution of ½ teaspoon of sea salt per cup of distilled water, then taste it to see if it's salty enough (it should be "half as salty as the sea," says Wilson).

Fill the douche with the salt water, hold one finger over the hole in the douche, then snort and move your finger. The salt water will shoot into your sinus. Do this twice a day. The environment inside your sinuses will quickly start to change for the better, says Wilson. Instead of being a "mushy mess" that's like a compost pile for bacteria, your sinuses will be clean and clear.

If you have chronic sinusitis, there will be a foul discharge from your nose as old mucus clears out. After a few days, you'll experience noticeable, or even complete, relief, she says.

## GRAVITY: *Hang Your Head for Relief*

"There are a variety of ways to drain your sinuses without antibiotics," Dr. Asis says. One of the simplest is to use gravity by positioning your head so that your sinuses drain naturally.

Lie flat on your back across your bed and let your head hang slightly over the side. Stay in that position for 5 to 10 minutes as your sinuses drain into your pharynx and eventually into your digestive system.

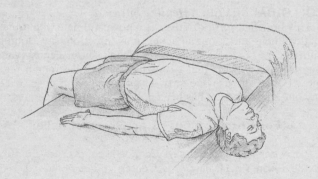

## HYDROTHERAPY: *To Relieve Facial Pain*

Place a warm, wet washcloth over the painful area for 60 seconds, then switch to a cold, wet washcloth for 30 seconds, says Dr. Stengler. Repeat the applications three times.

"Alternating warm and cold washcloths over the sinus area pumps in circulation and moves out congestion," says Dr. Stengler. You can use this remedy as often as you like during the day to relieve the pain.

**EUCALYPTUS ESSENTIAL OIL:** *Breathe Deeply*

Inhaling steam with eucalyptus oil really helps open the sinuses, says Dr. Stengler. First, boil some water in a large pot and add a few drops of eucalyptus essential oil. Place the pot on a table or counter, drape a towel over your head, lean over the water (about 12 inches away to avoid burns), and breathe deeply. Repeat a few times during the day.

# *Fast, Long-Lasting Relief from* **Sprains and Strains**

You tripped when you stepped off the curb and sprained your ankle, overstretching the bands of tissue (ligaments) that hold your ankle joint in place. Now your ankle is swollen, bruised, hot, red, and painful.

Or maybe you raked leaves all day Sunday and strained your back, which basically means that you asked your muscles to do more work than they could handle.

A sprain involves an injury to ligaments, which connect bone to bone. A strain involves an injury to tendons, which connect muscle to bone. In both cases, the classic treatment that conventional doctors recommend is known as RICE: rest, ice, compression, and elevation.

Alternative doctors recommend many additional remedies, which they say can provide immediate relief and enhance the RICE treatment. Just as important, these remedies can also help prevent long-term joint and muscle problems, such as a joint that's a bit unstable, a muscle that's chronically stiff, or an old injury that keeps being reinjured.

The following recommendations are for immediate first aid. If they give relief, you're probably on your way to recovery. If not, you should seek medical attention.

**YOUR COMFORT POINT:** *Takes the Strain Off Sprains*

A sprain is a sudden injury, usually accompanied by a stab of pain. Your first reaction will probably be panic. Instead, try to take a deep breath and stay calm, says James Clay, a clinical massage therapist in Winston-Salem, North Carolina.

What you need to do for immediate relief is find a position of maximum comfort, says Clay. Gently move the injured area until you find the position that hurts the least. Leave it there for 2 minutes, keeping your breathing deep and regular, then very slowly return it to its normal position.

"In many cases of minor sprain, this will immediately solve the problem," says Clay. The technique works, he believes, because right after the painful injury, the tissue is shouting "Sprain!" to the central nervous system. If you can put it in a painless position where it stops shouting, you "re-establish non-sprain as the baseline for the nervous system, the tissue relaxes, and the pain vanishes," he says.

He believes that this technique works better and faster than RICE for relieving painful sprains and has used it to send many dancers, basketball players, and other sprain-prone people right back into action.

## The RICE Plan

When you sprain a ligament or strain a muscle, you tear the microfibers of the tissue, and where there's tearing, there's bleeding. The blood and injured and dead cells can bind together to create a soupy mixture called a hematoma around the injury. This blocks healing oxygen from getting to the area and also stops toxic waste products from leaving. Once the swelling goes down, true healing can begin.

Getting rid of the hematoma as quickly as possible is the best way to relieve pain and heal a sprain or strain, says Ralph R. Stephens, a licensed massage therapist and instructor of neuromuscular therapy and sports massage at Ralph Stephens Seminars in Cedar Rapids, Iowa. A good way to do that is with RICE—rest, ice, compression, and elevation.

- Rest: "Using the injured area will cause further damage," says Stephens, so stop using it.
- Ice: "Ice helps control the internal bleeding," says Stephens. As

soon as possible after the injury occurs, apply a cold pack wrapped in a towel. Keep it on for 20 minutes, then take it off for 40 minutes, and continue with these cycles during your waking hours. Do this treatment for 2 to 3 days, or as long as there's swelling. Do not use heat, which will only flood the area with more fluid.

Even if you've had a bad sprain or strain and are headed to the emergency room, pick up a bag of ice on the way. "You may sit in an ER for 2 to 3 hours without treatment, and this is the crucial time to be icing your injury," Stephens says.

• Compression: Putting an elastic compression bandage, such as an Ace bandage, around the area also helps stop internal bleeding. Make the bandage snug, but not too tight. It should be loose enough to allow normal circulation.

• Elevation: Elevating the injured area drains fluid so there's less swelling. If you can't keep the injury elevated during the day, try to do so for most of the evening and at night for 2 to 3 days after the injury, says Dennis Courtney, M.D., director of the Courtney Clinic for Pain Relief and of the Center for Complementary Health, both in McMurray, Pennsylvania.

## PRESSURE: *Breaks the Tension*

After you've found your position of maximum comfort, probe gently with a thumb or finger for tender points around the area of the injury. These are spots that hurt a little (or a lot) more than the surrounding area. When you find a tender point, press it—not so hard that you're in agony, but hard enough to put you on the edge of bearable pain.

"Hold the tender point and wait for the pain to ease," says Clay. (It should take about a minute. If the pain doesn't ease within that time, the injury may be too severe for this type of treatment, and you need to see a doctor.)

This technique works, Clay believes, because whenever a ligament or muscle is injured, it tightens to defend itself from further injury. The tender point is the spot of maximum contraction, and pressing that point can persuade the ligament or muscle to relax, he says.

## DMSO: *Deep Relief*

You can speed healing by applying DMSO, a gel that is thought to penetrate the skin and reduce inflammation, says Barry Beaty,

D.O., an osteopathic physician and medical director of the DFW Pain Treatment Center and Wellness Clinic in Fort Worth, Texas.

"It can reduce the time a sprain or strain takes to heal," he says. He recommends spreading the DMSO gel on the sprained area three or four times a day for 2 to 3 days after the injury.

Two precautions: Be sure that your hands and the injured area are clean before you use the gel. Otherwise, dirt on your skin may be absorbed into your body along with the DMSO. Also, you can expect to smell slightly garlicky during the treatment, since once it's absorbed, DMSO has a very strong odor.

## HOMEOPATHY: *To Reduce Swelling*

Right after an injury, apply homeopathic Arnica salve, suggests Ted L. Edwards Jr., M.D., a physician in Austin, Texas, and former team physician for the U.S. Cycling Team. Apply the salve three or four times a day. It can help decrease swelling and inflammation from sprains and strains.

Along with the ointment, you should use homeopathic Arnica tablets. Take two tablets of the 6X potency every 15 minutes for the first hour after the injury, Dr. Edwards suggests. After that, take two tablets every 4 hours. Continue using both the tablets and the salve for 2 to 3 days, he suggests.

## AROMATHERAPY: *Help Speed Healing*

Within 24 to 72 hours after your sprain or strain, begin applying essential oils, advises Dr. Edwards. "The oils can speed the healing process of any muscle injury," he says. He recommends choosing either lemongrass, birch, or marjoram oil. Put a few

---

## GUIDE TO PROFESSIONAL CARE

If you sprain your knee, ankle, or other joint so badly that you experience extreme pain and cannot take even three steps on it, or if the injured joint looks disfigured, go to a hospital emergency room or an urgent care center. You may have a fracture.

drops of oil on the area of the injury and rub it in three or four times a day for as long as you have pain.

## ICE: *Good for Lower-Back Pain*

Maybe you were raking or shoveling or pushing the vacuum cleaner and you sprained your sacroiliac joint, an area in your lower back that's dense with ligaments. Now it seems that your low backache never goes away.

One way to treat this chronic inflammation is with aggressive icing, says Adela T. Basayne, past president of the American Massage Therapy Association and a licensed massage therapist in Portland, Oregon.

Put ice on the area five or six times a day in the following cycles: Hold the ice in place for 20 minutes, remove it for 40 minutes, then apply it again, she advises. During icing, touch the injured area. If it's numb, take the ice off.

Obviously, it would be inconvenient to stop what you're doing six times a day to lie down with an ice pack. Basayne recommends wrapping a bag of frozen peas in a kitchen towel and tucking it in the waistband of your pants or skirt, right on top of the painful area.

"Ice for 4 days in a row, even if your back stops hurting," she says. "It's very hard to heal this kind of sprain without regular icing."

## MASSAGE: *Relief for Knee Sprains*

It's best to wait 24 hours before you massage directly over an injury, says Basayne.

After that, however, a massage technique called effleurage can reduce the pain and speed the healing of a knee sprain, says Ralph R. Stephens, a licensed massage therapist and instructor of sports massage and neuromuscular therapy at Ralph Stephens Seminars in Cedar Rapids, Iowa. Effleurage means a "light, gliding touch." Here's how to do it.

First, put massage oil or lotion on the top, sides, and back of your knee. Use enough oil so that your hands will slide easily over the skin without pulling any hair, but not so much that it drips.

Then, using effleurage, work all around the patella, the bony knob on the top of the knee. Stroke above it, below it, and around the sides, always gliding in the direction of the heart. Light to moderate pressure is appropriate. Effleurage is one of the best strokes to use over areas where there is significant swelling.

In areas with little or no swelling, a massage stroke with deep circular friction works well, says Stephens. This stroke uses pressure to move the skin over the deeper layers of tissue. Using the tips of your fingers, your thumbs, or your palm, press on the skin and move it in a circle. Make 5 to 10 circles, release, and move an inch or so. Repeat until you have worked all around the patella and the front and sides of the joint. Use firm, not painful, pressure, and never apply pressure behind the knee between the two cordlike tendons, where there are large nerves and blood vessels close to the surface that can be easily injured.

Repeat deep circular friction a second time over the most sensitive areas, then finish with three or four long, gliding effleurage strokes. Do this knee massage once a day, Stephens says.

## FOOT WRITING: *For Ankle Injuries*

Think of your elementary school days, when you learned to write the alphabet in cursive script. Well, it's time to trade in handwriting for foot writing.

You can do this exercise either seated or standing. If you stand, hold on to a table for support. Then, while moving your foot from the ankle (not the knee), pretend to trace every curvy, capital letter of the cursive alphabet as if your big toe were the tip of a pen.

"This exercise works all the ligaments of the ankle," says Dr. Edwards, "possibly preventing the formation of adhesions"— stiff areas formed from scar tissue that are easily reinjured. Do this A-to-Z exercise once a day, he suggests.

## TOE PICKUPS: *For Extra Flexibility*

Here's another exercise to help keep your ankle flexible, strong, and free of adhesions after a sprain.

Take off your shoes and socks, stand near a table, and lay a kitchen towel lengthwise on the floor in front of you within reach of your foot. Next, put one hand on the table for balance, extend your foot, and use your toes to grab one section of the towel. Release it, then grab the next section with your toes and release. Continue to grab and release as you slowly pull the entire towel along the floor. Do this exercise twice a day, once in the morning and once in the evening, says Basayne.

## CIRCLE AND TOUCH: *Eases Thumb Sprains*

If you've sprained your thumb, this exercise will help restore flexibility. About a week after the injury, make broad circles in both directions with the thumb. Move it clockwise three times, then counterclockwise three times, and continue alternating for a minute or two.

Next, moving your other fingers as little as possible, reach with your thumb so that it touches the tip of each finger—little, ring, middle, and index. Repeat the exercise a few times several times a day, says Dr. Edwards.

## THE NEWSPAPER CRUMBLE: *Builds Thumb Strength*

To help restore strength to your thumb after a sprain, get a sheet of newspaper and, with the injured hand, try to ball up the sheet until it fits into your hand, Basayne suggests.

## ARM CIRCLES: *Help for the Shoulder*

To help keep a sprained shoulder free of adhesions, bend over slightly at the waist so that there's no strain on your back and the injured arm can swing freely. Place your other hand on a table or the back of a chair for support. With your injured arm, make gentle circles, both clockwise and counterclockwise, Basayne says. Next, swing your arm gently like a pendulum, then do figure-8s.

After a week or two, do the same exercise while holding a can of soup. Do the exercise twice a day for 1 minute, she says, then slowly increase your time, but don't go any longer than 3 minutes.

# *Use Nutrients and Your Mind to Recover from a* **Stroke**

You know all about heart attacks. Well, think of a stroke as a brain attack.

In a stroke, an artery to the brain is obstructed or small blood vessels inside the brain burst. Both scenarios sound deadly, and they are. Only heart disease and cancer kill more Americans than strokes.

Moreover, those who survive a stroke may sometimes wish they hadn't. Of the more than 4 million stroke survivors in the United States, many suffer from speech problems, paralysis, and diminished mental capacity, all caused by the death of oxygen-deprived brain tissue during the stroke. What's more, second strokes are very common.

The best way to prevent a stroke is by lowering high blood pressure, the number one risk factor. But if it's too late for prevention—that is, if you're recovering from a stroke—alternative practitioners offer many ways to help speed your recovery and decrease the odds of a second stroke.

Contact your physician before taking any of these supplements or vitamins, especially if a stroke has impaired your ability to swallow or caused excessive choking or coughing when you eat.

## BROMELAIN: *To Dissolve Blood Clots*

Bromelain is a digestive enzyme that can help dissolve a blood clot, preventing a second stroke, says Glen P. Wilcoxson, M.D., director of the New Beginnings Medical Group in Gulf Shores, Alabama. Take 1,500 milligrams of bromelain three times a day (a total of 4,500 milligrams) between meals, starting no sooner than 1 day after a stroke.

"If taken sooner, it could cause mild bleeding in the brain and worsen the situation," Dr. Wilcoxson says. Once you start

# GUIDE TO
# PROFESSIONAL CARE

*Caution: You should use the alternative remedies discussed in this chapter only as part of a treatment program that is guided and monitored by a qualified medical doctor in partnership with a qualified alternative practitioner, both of whom are experienced in caring for your condition. Check with your conventional doctor before changing or stopping any conventional medical treatments or medications, and keep all of your doctors and/or alternative practitioners informed of all treatments that you are receiving.*

Immediate hospitalization and allopathic medications that help dissolve clots—some of which can even abort a stroke while it's happening—are the best ways to deal with a stroke, says Glen P. Wilcoxson, M.D., director of the New Beginnings Medical Group in Gulf Shores, Alabama.

Call 911 or have someone take you to the nearest hospital emergency room if you suddenly experience the following symptoms: numbness or weakness on one side of your body (face, arm, or leg), confusion or trouble speaking, vision problems, dizziness or loss of balance, or severe headaches that come on for no apparent reason.

Some alternative professional treatments can help in the recovery process. One alternative modality for stroke recovery is a specialized type of acupuncture: scalp acupuncture. "This is the number one treatment for stroke in China," says Mark Stengler, N.D., a naturopathic physician in San Diego. It works by increasing blood flow into the small blood vessels of the brain.

A hyperbaric oxygen chamber, in which the atmospheric pressure is artificially raised, and you breathe pure oxygen, can also help with stroke recovery, says Dr. Wilcoxson.

"After a stroke, there are areas of the brain that are not really dead but are thought to be in a kind of hibernation," he says. "Hyperbaric oxygen allows these areas to thrive again. It also increases the speed of repair of all damaged brain cells by causing an increase in the total oxygen supply that allows cellular recovery and new blood vessels to grow into the blood-starved areas."

If a stroke leaves a person inactive for a long period, the inactivity raises the threat of osteoporosis. "Most doctors who treat stroke patients don't remember that disuse and a lack of weight-bearing activity results in a loss of calcium, which leads to osteoporosis," says David Steenblock, D.O., an osteopathic physician in Mission Viejo, California. Calcium loss affects not only the bone but also the muscles, causing pain, spasms, and discomfort.

To prevent osteoporosis, Dr. Steenblock says to ask your doctor for a prescription for calcitonin (Miacalcin), a calcium-containing nasal spray. "Calcitonin can help prevent osteoporosis and helps with brain repair processes as well," he says.

taking bromelain, you can continue using it on an ongoing basis as a preventive measure.

**PHOSPHATIDYLSERINE:** *A Brain-Cell Stimulator*
"Certain nutritional supplements can protect and stimulate brain cells, making the most of what hasn't been killed or damaged by the stroke," says Phillip Minton, M.D., a homeopathic physician in Reno. The nutrient phosphatidylserine, which is a component of cellular membranes, is among them. Take 100 milligrams three times a day for at least a year following a stroke.

**DMAE:** *Helps with Brain Chemistry*
The nutrient DMAE, or dimethylaminoethanol, is a precursor of chemicals that are essential to brain function, Dr. Minton says. Take a supplement for an extended period of time, following the dosage recommendations on the label.

**ACETYL-CARNITINE:** *Energize Your Brain Cells*
This is another nutrient that helps energize brain cells, Dr. Minton says. Take a 500-milligram supplement three times a day for at least a year following a stroke.

**GINKGO:** *Improves Blood Flow to the Brain*
This herb can help you recover from a stroke and prevent a second one by improving blood flow to the brain, says Mark

Stengler, N.D., a naturopathic physician in San Diego. He recommends 180 to 240 milligrams daily of a standardized 24 percent extract of the herb.

## SUPPLEMENTS: *A Regimen to Prevent a Second Stroke*

"I've found in my practice that these nutrients can reduce the likelihood of a second stroke by helping to open and repair arteries and strengthen the heart," says Emily Kane, N.D., a naturopathic physician and acupuncturist in Juneau, Alaska.

- Vitamin E: 400 to 600 international units daily
- Omega-3 fatty acids: 1 tablespoon of flaxseed oil daily
- Coenzyme $Q_{10}$: 30 to 100 milligrams daily
- Vitamin C: 3,000 milligrams daily

## Mind/Body Healing through Medical Hypnosis

Self-hypnosis is a rehabilitation technique that stroke victims can use without assistance from a therapist. Not only can it help restore a positive mental attitude, it may also boost healing by helping to return feeling and strength to the injured parts of the body. Here's how to do it.

### BREATHING: *Enter the Therapeutic Trance*

Start with what's called a therapeutic trance. "This is a special, fully conscious state of mind characterized by feelings of peacefulness and freedom and a sense of being in communication with your body and your life-force," says Gerard Sunnen, M.D., associate clinical professor of psychiatry at New York University–Bellevue Medical Center in New York City and an expert in medical hypnosis.

To enter the trance, sit comfortably in a chair, letting your body relax as much as possible. It takes about a minute to tone the body down after normal activity. Close your eyes sometime during this body slowdown.

Next, begin to count very slowly from one to seven. With each number, feel yourself going deeper and deeper into a special state of awareness, where there is no future and no past but only an awareness of the present.

At the count of seven, take three deep, slow, consecutive

breaths. This will propel you even deeper into the trance. After these three breaths, let your breathing assume its own rhythm, but continue to meditate upon it for approximately 3 to 5 minutes. As you breathe, send your awareness into the bottoms of your lungs; you should actually feel the air filling the bottoms of your lungs and experience the sensation of your lungs coming in contact with your abdominal organs.

When you are in the trance, you will feel as if you are in a state of profoundly relaxed and peaceful communication with your body. You should experience very few thoughts even though your mind remains active. At the same time, you will have a sense of coming in contact with your life-energy forces and may sense an internal glow, diffused light, or a melodious sound.

## AFFIRMATIONS: *A Positive Outlook*

Stay in the trance for 5 to 10 minutes. During the time you are in the trance, gently meditate on positive affirmations, visualizations, or energizing feelings to activate healing. If possible, do these exercises once or twice a day to ensure steady progress, says Dr. Sunnen.

"You are asking your mind and nervous system to follow a pathway in the direction of health and well-being," he says. "And these affirmations will work automatically, because your mind and body need that guidance." Here are some examples of positive affirmations.

* I am speaking more clearly each and every day.
* My muscles are feeling stronger each and every day.
* I am more and more motivated to do my exercises.

Create your own affirmations, says Dr. Sunnen. That way, there will be real feeling behind the words, which is key to activating your nervous system. Always phrase the affirmations positively, stating what you want to achieve, not what you want to avoid.

## VISUALIZATION: *See Your Future*

You can use visualization in addition to or instead of affirmations while within the trance state. For example, rather than saying, "I will walk better each and every day," you should actually *see* yourself walking better.

"In your mind's eye, picture yourself as an actor or actress in a movie performing these types of actions more efficiently every day," says Dr. Sunnen.

**FEELINGS:** *Get in Touch With Your Emotions*
Experiencing corrective feelings during the trance is of tremendous therapeutic value, says Dr. Sunnen. Imagine how it would feel to speak normally again or to walk without a limp. Expand upon and maintain these feelings for as long as you can during the trance.

Whatever method you determine is right for you, continue to develop your trance power. Devote 10 minutes or even longer once or twice a day. "Once you start expanding your self-hypnotic abilities, your subconscious mind will work to propel your healing intentions into reality," he says.

# *Alternative Remedies Are*
# *Your Best Bet to Soothe*
# **Sunburn**

You've heard it before: Sunburn is very bad for you. It ages your skin and may increase your risk of skin cancer.

"The best advice for sunburn is: Avoid overexposure to the sun," says Beverly Yates, N.D., a naturopathic physician and director of the Natural Health Care Group in Seattle.

Once you've been burned, though, your best options for relief are alternative remedies, says Norma Pasekoff Weinberg, an herbal educator in Cape Cod, Massachusetts.

"Many typical drugstore remedies for sunburn numb the pain but do little to support the body's own healing systems," Weinberg says. Alternative remedies that use natural substances such as herbs and flowers not only help reduce symptoms, she says, but may also bring the body back to a state of balance.

**ALOE:** *The Best Natural Remedy*

"There's no better remedy for minor burns than aloe gel," says Therese Francis, Ph.D., an herbalist in Santa Fe, New Mexico. "Use the gel as needed to relieve the pain, heat, and redness, and keep slathering it on until your skin stops absorbing it," she says. "A new burn soaks up aloe gel extremely fast; it's amazing how much you may have to put on before your skin can't absorb any more," Dr. Francis adds.

If you have an aloe plant handy, you can get the gel directly from the leaves. Break a leaf, squish out the gel, and spread it on the burn. Apply as much as your skin will absorb three to five times a day until the burn is healed.

If you're buying aloe gel, find a product whose label states that it contains a very high percentage of aloe—99 or even 100 percent, says Dr. Francis.

"A lot of gel products contain only 45 or 50 percent aloe. The rest is filler," she says. "They are not as effective." Also, she points out that real aloe gel is not neon green (that's artificial coloring added to the gel) but a pale, almost transparent green.

## GUIDE TO PROFESSIONAL CARE

Most sunburns are first-degree burns; you've roasted your epidermis, the outer layer of skin, and it's red, painful, and hot. You can treat this type of sunburn with the remedies in this chapter. Moreover, taking high daily doses of antioxidant vitamins for 1 week and of zinc for 2 to 3 weeks after the burn may speed recovery, according to Bradley Bongiovanni, N.D., a naturopathic physician in Cambridge, Massachusetts. This should be done only under medical supervision, he adds.

If you have a second-degree burn, which involves the dermis, or underlying skin layer, and causes swelling, blisters, intense pain, and perhaps nausea, chills, and fever as the body tries to cope with the shock, you need to seek immediate medical care.

## LAVENDER ESSENTIAL OIL: *Combine It with Aloe*

"Combining aloe gel with a few drops of the essential oil of lavender works so well to soothe the pain and speed the healing of a sunburn that these are usually the only two remedies I use," Dr. Francis says.

Lavender, she explains, encourages new skin growth and is thought to be a superb healer for first-degree burns. It's also one of the few essential oils that you can apply directly to the skin without diluting it in a carrier oil.

To use the oil, add a drop or two to the aloe gel, then spread the mixture over the burned skin and several inches of the surrounding area, Dr. Francis says.

## YOGURT: *Relief in the Refrigerator*

If you don't have aloe or lavender essential oil in the medicine cabinet, check the refrigerator for plain yogurt.

"Yogurt is very cooling and a natural moisturizer," says Weinberg. Apply it liberally to the burned area and leave it on for about 10 minutes. "Then rinse with water that has been boiled and cooled so it is sterile and pat dry with a clean cloth," she says. Repeat this three or four times during the first day and then as needed.

## GREEN TEA: *Better Than Benzocaine*

Compresses made from green tea can reduce the swelling of a minor burn and relieve the sting, Weinberg says. "This remedy works better than benzocaine, an ingredient in many over-the-counter products for sunburn relief," she says.

To prepare a compress, make a pot of tea by bringing 6 to 8 ounces of water almost to a boil, then pouring it over 1 teaspoon of loose green tea. Cover and steep for 5 minutes, then dilute with an equal amount of cool, distilled water. Soak a clean cotton cloth in the tea water once it has cooled, lay the cloth on the sunburned skin, and leave it on for 5 to 10 minutes. Reapply three or four times a day or as needed, advises Weinberg.

## HYDROTHERAPY: *A Soothing Tea-and-Cider Bath*

To use water to help soothe a sunburn, add soothing, anti-inflammatory ingredients to a bath and soak for 10 to 20 minutes, says Brigitte Mars, an herbalist and nutritional consultant in Boulder, Colorado.

Twice a day until the sunburn is gone, add 1 cup of black tea (for its anti-inflammatory tannins) and 1 cup of apple-cider vinegar (a time-tested, soothing sunburn remedy) to bathwater that's a comfortable, not-too-hot, not-too-cold temperature, and soak. You can also put seven drops of lavender essential oil in the water, adds Mars. To make the tea, bring 4 cups of water to a boil, then remove from the heat. Add 6 tea bags, cover, and steep for 10 minutes.

## HOMEOPATHY: *For Painful Skin*

You can use a homeopathic remedy for red and painful skin, says Bradley Bongiovanni, N.D., a naturopathic physician in Cambridge, Massachusetts. He recommends dissolving three pellets of the 6C or 12C potency of Belladonna under your tongue three times a day until symptoms are relieved.

For skin that's blistering and peeling, you must seek medical care. But after you've seen a doctor, you can also help heal the problem with the homeopathic remedy Cantharis. Use the same potency, dose, and frequency as for Belladonna until the pain is gone and healing is under way.

## ANTIOXIDANTS: *To Speed Healing*

Antioxidant vitamins will help the skin heal more rapidly from a sunburn, Dr. Bongiovanni says. "The sun causes oxidative damage to skin cells, and antioxidants speed recovery," he says. Dr. Bongiovanni recommends the following doses daily for 1 week.

• Vitamin A: 10,000 international units (IU)
• Vitamin C: 1,000 milligrams
• Vitamin E: 400 IU

# *Whole-Body Relief for Pain of*
# Temporomandibular Disorder

Jaws. Pain circles your skull, pulses in the muscles of your face, and sears your neck, shoulders, and back.

No, we're not describing a shark attack. We're talking about some of the different kinds of pain that can be caused by your jaws if you're one of the estimated 44 million Americans who experience symptoms of temporomandibular disorder, or TMD. In TMD, the joint that connects the lower and upper halves of the jaw is damaged or out of alignment. The resulting cascade of symptoms can range from headaches to numb, tingling hands, dizziness, or a jaw that stays painfully locked in one position.

TMD can have many causes: stress, trauma to the head from a car accident or blow, poor posture, or a malocclusion (a bite problem), to name just a few. Most dentists treat TMD by making the patient a customized plastic mouthpiece that relieves stress in the jaws.

TMD should be treated not just as a dental problem, however, but as a "whole-body problem," says David Lerner, D.D.S., a holistic dentist in Cold Spring, New York. And he speaks from personal experience.

After graduating from dental school, he developed severe head, face, neck, and back pain from TMD. He was treated by several dentists, some of whom made the problem worse, he says. Finally, he turned to the whole-body healing methods of chiropractic, physical therapy, osteopathy, and acupuncture. He was cured of his TMD problem—and his nearly constant pain.

Finding the best whole-body care for TMD may take a while—and you are in pain now. Once a dentist has diagnosed your pain as TMD, try these six techniques that Dr. Lerner found were ideal for relieving his pain and that he now teaches to his TMD patients.

# GUIDE TO
# PROFESSIONAL CARE

If you have pain or have trouble chewing or opening your mouth, you should see a dentist.

TMD is a complex problem that must be treated professionally, but not just by a dentist, says James Kennedy, D.D.S., a dentist in Littleton, Colorado, who specializes in craniomandibular disorders such as TMD. "TMD affects the entire body, so the entire body must be addressed during the healing process," he says.

He recommends that you first find a dentist who specializes in TMD and who will use custom-made mouthpieces, orthodontia, and other dental techniques to help realign your jaw and heal the damaged joint.

But, he says, that dentist should also work with an osteopath who knows cranial manipulation, a technique that can help correct many TMD symptoms; a chiropractor who can correct hip and spinal imbalances that may be affecting your jaw; and a nutritionist who can recommend a dietary and supplement program that will help relieve pain naturally and maximize your body's natural healing power. Massage therapy can also be helpful in reducing muscle spasms and tightness associated with TMD problems, he says.

In addition, you may want to see an acupuncturist for pain relief while your body is healing, says David Lerner, D.M.D., a holistic dentist in Cold Spring, New York.

**ICE AND STRETCH:** *For Head and Jaw Pain*

"This technique is a real godsend for TMD pain," says Dr. Lerner. He explains that tense neck muscles are often the source of head and jaw pain in TMD. The best remedy for any tense muscle is to stretch it.

You can make stretching easier and more effective if you first rub ice over the tight muscle. "The cold sends a signal to the nervous system that overrides the pain signal, making it easier to stretch the aching muscle," says Dr. Lerner.

To ice and stretch, hold an ice cube in a washcloth, leaving one side of the cube uncovered. Rub the uncovered part of the cube down the left side of your head and neck, starting near the top of your head and moving the cube from behind your ear, down the muscle on the side of your neck, and onto the shoulder area. Repeat three or four times.

Then, says Dr. Lerner, stretch the left side of your neck by bending your head toward your right shoulder. Hold the stretch for about 10 seconds. Put your left hand on your neck to keep the muscle warm. (The purpose of the ice is to interrupt pain signals, not to cool the muscle.)

After each session, warm the muscle with your hand. Then switch to the right side and repeat in the same way for 2 to 3 minutes.

"The signal of cold from the skin to the brain should block the signal of pain from the muscle as it is being stretched," he explains, "allowing it to be stretched more. This method, done once a day, should provide significant relief for jaw and head pain."

## REVERSE STRETCH: *For Neck Pain*

In TMD, the neck muscle that begins behind the ear and extends to the collarbone is often painful. An easy way to relax it is to pull both ends of the muscle toward the center, says Dr. Lerner.

To do that, place the index, middle, and ring fingers of your right hand behind the lobe of your right ear. Next, put the thumb of the same hand just above your collarbone, about an inch from the notch in the center of your neck (*a*). Pull the ends of the muscle together by moving your thumb and

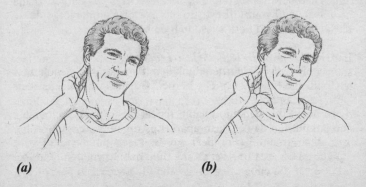

*(a)*                    *(b)*

fingers toward the middle of the muscle, sliding them along your skin (*b*).

Do this several times, then repeat on the left side. Perform this reverse stretch for as long as you'd like whenever your neck is painful, says Dr. Lerner.

### "RUBBER BAND" STRETCH: *For Facial Pain*

The facial muscles on the side of your jaw are frequent targets for TMD pain, says Dr. Lerner. To help relax those muscles, wash your hands and hook the index finger of each hand inside the corresponding corners of your mouth. Insert the fingers down to the middle knuckles.

Pulling gently, stretch out your cheeks as you would a rubber band, stopping the stretch when you feel a fair amount of pull in your cheeks but before you feel any pain. Release. Repeat this stretch three or four times a few times a day.

### THE PINKY POINT: *For Pain behind the Eye*

TMD sufferers often have pain and pressure deep behind their eyes, says Dr. Lerner. The source of this pain is a spasm in the muscle that opens the jaw and moves it from side to side. "The following maneuver can relieve the muscle spasm," he says.

If the pain is in your right eye, slide your right pinky finger along the upper gum on the right side of your mouth until the pad of the finger is behind your last molar and the tip of your pinky is pointing to the center of your skull, behind the eye. Gently press up and into the area behind the molar four or five times and hold for a couple of seconds, says Dr. Lerner. If the pain is behind your left eye, do this exercise on the left side. If the pain is behind both eyes, do it on both sides.

### TMD MANTRA: *To Relieve Jaw Tension*

"People with TMD often think that it's natural to clench their teeth all the time," says Dr. Lerner. But this only keeps their jaws tense and painful.

To break the clenching habit, repeat this phrase to yourself throughout the day: "Teeth apart, lips together, tongue on the roof of the mouth." (For ideal "jaw posture," put the tip of your tongue on the roof of your mouth right behind your front teeth.)

"These corrections help to center the jaw and eliminate TMD problems," says Dr. Lerner.

## ISOMETRIC EXERCISE: *To Balance Jaw Muscles*

Misaligned muscles in your jaw are the cause of a lot of TMD pain, says Dr. Lerner. To help balance those muscles, place your elbow on a solid surface, bend your arm, and hold your chin in the palm of your hand.

Gently try to open your jaw, but resist with your hand so it won't open. Do this isometric (resistance) exercise for 30 seconds four or five times a day, says Dr. Lerner. Then press on one side of your chin in an attempt to move your jaw sideways. Resist the movement with your jaw muscles, keeping your jaw in line. Repeat on the other side.

## Point Yourself to Pain Relief

You can relieve all kinds of TMD pain by pressing on specific acupressure points, say experts. These points are like way stations on paths of energy called meridians. By pressing one point on the meridian, you can help relieve pain in other parts of the body.

The first point that you might want to press is point M, says Albert Forgione, Ph.D., chief clinical consultant at the Gelb Orofacial Pain Center at Tufts University School of Dental Medicine in Boston.

## THE M POINT: *Pressing Away Cheek Pain*

The cheek, or masseter, muscle stretches from the cheekbone to the lower edge of the jaw. Typically, it's loaded with more chronic TMD tension and pain than any other muscle. The acupressure point that can relieve the pain—point M, in Dr. Forgione's TMD pain-relief system—is on your outer forearm, three finger-widths below the elbow crease. To locate it, place your forearm and hand palm down on a table, place three fingers on your forearm at the fold of the elbow, and search for a painful point in this area.

To stimulate the point (which may be intensely painful itself), put your index finger or knuckle on the area and press downward in a rotating manner with as much pressure as you can tolerate for 30 to 40 seconds. Repeat on the other arm. "The more you do it, the less pain there will be in the M point, and the less pain there will be in your face," says Dr. Forgione. If the pain is too severe, rub the area with ice first or use a vibrating massager on the point.

## *Natural Boosters for* **Thyroid Problems**

See if the following description—either all or some of it—sounds familiar.

You're overweight and have been for years, in spite of your best efforts to shed pounds. You feel sluggish a lot of the time, especially first thing in the morning. Your hands and feet often feel cold. Your skin and hair are dry. You're constipated. You have trouble concentrating. You're depressed.

All of those symptoms (and many more) can be caused by an underactive thyroid gland, or hypothyroidism. The hormones pumped out by the thyroid gland regulate your body's temperature, so when thyroid hormones are low, so is your temperature, usually by a degree or two.

When your temperature is low, many of the body's energy-producing enzymes can't do their job. When they don't work, your body doesn't work very well, either, and every system, from your brain to your bowels, is stuck in first gear.

Blood tests, which are used by conventional doctors to screen for underactive thyroid, are not reliable for ruling out the problem, say alternative practitioners.

"More and more, I'm seeing patients who have so-called normal blood tests but who do have an underactive thyroid," says Ralph Lee, M.D., a family physician specializing in preventive medicine and nutritional therapy in Marietta, Georgia.

Healing your thyroid requires professional care, but there are alternative home remedies that you can use to assist your physician in the healing process.

**ENERGY EXERCISE:** *Express Yourself*

The thyroid gland, one of the seven organs of the hormone-generating endocrine system, is located in the throat just below the larynx, or voice box. This is also the location of the throat chakra, one of the seven centers of subtle energy in the body

# GUIDE TO
# PROFESSIONAL CARE

If you experience fatigue, dry hair, bloating, muscle soreness and cramps, painful joints, abdominal pain, mood swings, depression, and decreased concentration, you may have an underactive thyroid, and you should see your doctor right away for a diagnosis.

"What conventional doctors are taught about thyroid problems is fundamentally wrong," says Kenneth Blanchard, M.D., Ph.D., an endocrinologist in Newton, Massachusetts. "There are many symptoms and conditions that have hypothyroidism as their cause, but the problem is usually missed by most doctors because people with underactive thyroids often have 'normal' blood tests."

The standard tests used to detect thyroid deficiency are not sensitive enough to uncover most cases of underactive thyroid, says Ralph Lee, M.D., a family physician specializing in preventive medicine and nutritional therapy in Marietta, Georgia. That means that many people who have the symptoms of hypothyroidism are told that they don't have the condition, Dr. Lee says. Moreover, even when thyroid problems are treated, it is usually with the synthetic thyroid hormone Synthroid, which supplies only one of the range of thyroid hormones, says Dr. Lee.

If you suspect that you have an underactive thyroid, you should try to find an alternatively oriented medical doctor or naturopathic physician who is willing to do the range of medical tests that can accurately detect the problem and who will consider treating the condition with Armour Thyroid, a nonsynthetic extract of animal thyroid that provides the full complement of thyroid hormones, Dr. Lee advises.

whose locations correspond to the endocrine glands, says Julie Claire Holmes, N.D., a naturopathic physician and clinical hypnotherapist in Kuli, Hawaii.

"To really bring the thyroid gland back into balance, a person must be willing to balance the energies associated with the throat chakra, which are the energies of expression," she says.

Here's a simple energy exercise from Dr. Holmes to do just that.

Lie flat on a comfortable surface such as a bed or a blanket folded on a carpeted floor. Relax and warm your diaphragm—the source of your breath and your voice—by gently massaging your upper abdominal area for a minute or so. Next, put one hand over your throat and, as you exhale, start to make a sound—any sound—allowing it to emerge from your throat.

"It might start as a groan or a grunt, like something constricted and caught that wants to be free," Dr. Holmes says. Continue to make a sound (it's very important to remember that any sound is okay) with every exhalation. At the same time, imagine that the sound is coming directly out of your thyroid and that the cells of the organ are vibrating with the sound like the strings of an instrument. Do this exercise for 5 to 10 minutes every day.

"People with hypothyroidism often suppress their speech and natural expressiveness, fearing what others may think about them," Dr. Holmes says. By doing this exercise, the suppressed energies of the voice are loosened and released, and the thyroid is nourished at a deep level, she says.

## SUNLIGHT: *Catch It Early*

In the early morning, go outside and look toward the sun. Light stimulates the pineal gland (the endocrine gland in the center of your brain), which in turn positively affects the thyroid as well as all the other endocrine glands, Dr. Holmes says.

She recommends that you go outside within the first hour after sunrise and look toward the sun (not directly at it) for 10 minutes.

This technique won't work if you look through a window or through your glasses; the light has to directly enter your eyes, Dr. Holmes says.

## Take the At-Home Test

Only a doctor with experience in treating hypothyroidism can tell you for sure whether you have an underactive thyroid. But if you have many of the common symptoms, such as overweight, constipation, dry skin and hair, fatigue, depression, and cold hands and feet, you can conduct a simple at-home test to see if a thyroid problem is the likely cause, says Ralph Lee, M.D., a family physician specializing in preventive medicine and nutritional therapy in Marietta, Georgia.

Just take your basal (or core) body temperature every day for a few days. Your thyroid regulates body temperature, so a basal temperature that's consistently a degree or two below normal is a sure sign that your thyroid may not be functioning properly.

First, you'll need a glass mercury thermometer. Before you go to bed, shake it down and put it on the nightstand. Then, when you wake up in the morning, don't move; simply reach over, get the thermometer, and tuck it in your armpit for 10 minutes. "This is the best measurement you can get of your core body temperature," says Dr. Lee.

Do this every morning for 6 days. If your temperature is consistently low—in the low 97° or 96° range—"it's a good indication that you have an underactive thyroid, even if previous blood tests have indicated that your thyroid is normal," says Dr. Lee. And, he says, it's time to see a knowledgeable doctor about treatment.

## FOOD: *Choose Organic or Free-Range*

Most meat, dairy products, and eggs contain synthetic hormones that can affect the balance and functioning of the thyroid, Dr. Holmes says. Choose free-range or organic meats, dairy products, and eggs, which don't contain synthetic hormones.

## PROGESTERONE: *Ease the Symptoms*

If you have premenstrual syndrome or have entered perimenopause (when periods are irregular but haven't stopped), using a cream that contains natural progesterone can help reduce the symptoms of hypothyroidism, says Dr. Holmes. (The hormones progesterone and estrogen control the menstrual cycle.) "A deficiency of progesterone, which is very common, can affect the thyroid gland, and vice versa," she says.

Follow the application instructions and dosage recommendations on the label, starting about 14 days before the start of your menstrual period.

**TYROSINE:** *A Balanced Approach*

The amino acid tyrosine combines with iodine to make thyroxine, a thyroid hormone, Dr. Holmes says. You should get 500 to 1,000 milligrams of tyrosine from a pure amino acid supplement balanced with good protein in your diet, she says, since tyrosine by itself can cause side effects in large doses. She recommends using tyrosine for 3 to 6 months and then being re-evaluated by your medical practitioner.

**FATTY ACIDS:** *Help for Hormones*

These components of fat are involved in the production of thyroid hormones, says Dr. Lee. Take either flaxseed oil or fish oil, both of which are rich in fatty acids. Follow the dosage recommendations on the label, shooting for between 3,000 and 6,000 milligrams a day, he says. "In colder weather, you should take the higher dosage. It's also okay to take both oils together to get each one's subtle benefits, but be sure not to exceed the total dosage."

# *Alternative Remedies Can Quiet* **Tinnitus**

After conventional medicine has ruled out the possibility of an underlying cause, such as a drug side effect or a brain tumor, it has almost nothing to offer the person with tinnitus.

That means nothing to quiet the internal sound—the ringing (or whistling, chirping, clicking, or hissing) in the ears that can be soft or loud, intermittent or constant, mildly annoying or so maddening that some people choose suicide as the only way to get relief.

"A conventional doctor usually says, 'I can do nothing about this problem,' and the patient is usually hugely frustrated and unhappy," says Michael D. Seidman, M.D., an otolaryngologist (ear, nose, and throat specialist) and medical director of the tinnitus center at the Henry Ford Health System in West Bloomfield, Michigan.

But Dr. Seidman is also the co-chair of the complementary and alternative medicine initiative at the Henry Ford Health System. Instead of showing his tinnitus patients the door, he offers them alternative remedies to help reduce the sound. It's safe to take the following supplements long-term, but if your tinnitus goes away, you may be able to stop using them.

## B VITAMINS: *Getting What You Need*

"A deficiency of these vitamins can cause tinnitus, and supplementation may improve symptoms," Dr. Seidman says. He recommends a high-potency B-complex supplement that supplies 50 milligrams of most of the B vitamins.

In addition to the multivitamin, Dr. Seidman recommends supplementing at higher levels for three key B vitamins: thiamin, niacin, and $B_{12}$.

"Some patients find that thiamin supplements relieve their tinnitus," Dr. Seidman says. The nutrient may work by "stabilizing the nervous system, especially the nerves of the inner ear," he says. He recommends 100 to 500 milligrams a day, taken with your doctor's approval and supervision.

Niacin may work by improving the circulation to the cochlea, or inner ear. "Many patients with tinnitus who have used niacin have had significant benefit," says Dr. Seidman. He recommends taking 50 milligrams twice a day. If there is no improvement after 2 weeks, increase the dosage by 50 milligrams every 2 weeks until you reach 500 milligrams twice a day.

A deficiency of vitamin $B_{12}$, which is present in an estimated 5 to 10 percent of people over 65, may be a common cause of tinnitus in that age group, Dr. Seidman says.

"Several of my patients over 65 who supplemented with $B_{12}$ had significant improvement in their tinnitus," he says. He recommends taking 1,000 micrograms daily for the first 6 months, then dropping to 100 micrograms a day.

## ZINC: *Nip Tinnitus in the Bud*

Some patients with tinnitus have a deficiency of the mineral zinc. For them, taking a combination of zinc and niacin can sometimes cure the tinnitus, particularly if the onset of symptoms is recent, Dr. Seidman says.

"Complete resolution is possible if the tinnitus is recent," he says. "If it's longstanding, the tinnitus can frequently be diminished." He recommends combining niacin treatment with 25 milligrams of zinc gluconate twice a day.

### Walkman Away from Tinnitus

Kevin Hogan, Ph.D., was contemplating suicide. He had not one or two but three sounds in his head: a 24-hour-a-day siren at 85 decibels (about as loud as a TV), a sound like a crackling fire, and behind that, a constant 60-decibel whistle.

"It was a living hell," says Dr. Hogan, a psychologist and doctor of clinical hypnotherapy in Burnsville, Minnesota. And every doctor he saw for the problem told him the same thing: "There is nothing I can do for you."

So he started to treat himself. One of the most effective techniques that he found to help rid himself of the condition was "auditory habituation," a process of slowly but surely teaching his brain not to listen to the internal sound or sounds of tinnitus.

---

### GUIDE TO PROFESSIONAL CARE

If you have tinnitus, you must be evaluated by a medical doctor for a possible brain tumor, which causes the problem in less than 1 percent of all cases.

You should also be evaluated by an audiologist, who can do hearing tests to determine whether the problem is caused by damage to your cochlea, or inner ear, which can sometimes result from over-the-counter or prescription medications, or to an auditory error in the brain itself.

The audiologist can also work with your doctor to prescribe a masking device, a hearing aid—like device that generates background noise to cover the tinnitus sound and provide relief.

Anyone can do this technique at home, says Dr. Hogan. Here's his advice.

"Buy a portable cassette player or CD player, something in which you can play pleasant background music, like classical or New Age or environmental sounds. Play the music at a slightly lower volume than your tinnitus for at least 90 minutes a day. During this time, the brain has to choose between the external and internal sounds instead of listening exclusively to the tinnitus, and the neural pathways that are keeping the tinnitus in place will slowly start to atrophy."

It may take 1 to 2 years before the technique significantly reduces (or even eliminates) the tinnitus, Dr. Hogan says. But for him and the 2,000 or so patients he has instructed in the technique, the time invested is well worth it.

"Auditory habituation can provide a lot of relief, particularly in the long term," he says. "And for someone who could be tortured for the rest of his life by tinnitus, long-term relief is crucial."

## MAGNESIUM: *For Symptom Relief*

Many patients with tinnitus reduce symptoms by supplementing their diets with the mineral magnesium, says Dr. Seidman. He recommends 400 milligrams daily.

## GINKGO: *Reduce the Noise*

The herb ginkgo, which is well known for enhancing memory by improving circulation to the brain, may also help reduce tinnitus symptoms by improving circulation to the inner ear, says Dr. Seidman.

Look for a ginkgo extract standardized to 24 percent ginkgo-flavoglycosides. He recommends 120 to 240 milligrams twice a day, once in the morning and once in the evening.

## FOOD: *Banish the Noisemakers*

Caffeine, salt, sugar, and alcohol can each cause or worsen tinnitus, Dr. Seidman says. "Some people give up caffeine or sugar or alcohol and find that the tinnitus goes away," he says.

# *Easing the Pain of*
# **Toothache**

The cavity is deep. The crack is wide. The gum is infected. For whatever reason, you have a toothache—and that's why dentists have emergency phone numbers on their answering machines. Until you can see the dentist for diagnosis and treatment, though, here are some alternative home remedies to muffle the throb.

## HYDROGEN PEROXIDE: *Kills Ache-Causing Bacteria*

This is the first and best alternative home remedy for killing the pain from an infection in the gum or the nerve of a tooth, says James Hardy, D.M.D., a holistic dentist in Winter Park, Florida. As a germ-killing way to reduce discomfort and pain, hydrogen peroxide (used safely) can be a big help.

Floss first, then swish a mouthful of a 3 percent solution of hydrogen peroxide in your mouth for a few seconds. Let it stay in your mouth for about a minute, then spit it all out and rinse thoroughly with water. Do this once a day for 2 or 3 days in a row.

There are a few precautions, however. First, don't swallow the peroxide, as it can burn your esophagus and cause stomach cramps, says Dr. Hardy. Second, don't use this treatment for more than 3 days; used too often, peroxide can burn tender gums.

## HOMEOPATHY: *Choose the Right Remedy for You*

If your toothache pain is worse at night, dissolve one tablet of homeopathic Arnica 30X under your tongue every 15 minutes, says Flora Parsa Stay, D.D.S., a dentist in Oxnard, California.

If your tooth throbs more when it's exposed to hot liquids like coffee, dissolve one tablet of Chamomilla 30X under your

## GUIDE TO
## PROFESSIONAL CARE

If you have isolated instances of tooth pain—from biting down on a peach pit, for example—it may not be a problem. But if there's a pattern to your pain—if it comes and goes or is constant—you need to see a dentist as soon as possible. He will diagnose the cause, whether it's a cavity, a cracked tooth, a gum infection, a sinus problem, or some other factor, and recommend treatment to solve the problem and eliminate the pain.

Also, if you have a toothache and facial swelling that spreads to your neck, see your dentist immediately or go to the emergency room. This type of swelling can be life-threatening, says James Hardy, D.M.D., a holistic dentist in Winter Park, Florida.

---

tongue as needed until the sensitivity decreases. If the pain doesn't subside or gets worse, see your dentist. You can use the remedy during your dental visit to enhance healing.

If your toothache is more sensitive to cold beverages like soda, use the 6X potency of Plantago major, dissolving one tablet under your tongue three times a day until the pain goes away. You should visit your dentist, and you can continue to take this remedy while you're being treated.

For a tooth that aches after a cavity has been filled, dissolve one tablet of Hypericum 30X under your tongue three times a day until the pain subsides.

### ECHINACEA AND ALOE: *Powerful Pain Relief*

Buy capsules of powdered echinacea and a bottle of pure aloe gel at a health food store (check the label to be sure you're getting gel that can be used internally). Aloe reduces pain and inflammation, and echinacea battles the infection that may be causing the ache, says Edward M. Arana, D.D.S., a retired dentist in Carmel Valley, California, and past president of the American Academy of Biological Dentistry.

Open two capsules of the echinacea and mix the contents with enough aloe gel to form a paste about the consistency of toothpaste. Put a wad of the paste on the gum next to the aching tooth and let it dissolve. Use this poultice as often as needed for relief.

### ECHINACEA: *Help in a Capsule*

If the preceding remedy seems like too much work, Dr. Arana recommends taking a closed gelatin capsule of echinacea and putting it between your cheek and the gum next to the aching tooth, then letting it dissolve. Use this remedy only before you go to bed, however, as it may temporarily turn your mouth green.

### CHAMOMILE OR CALENDULA: *The Toxin Avengers I, II*

Applying chamomile or calendula can help draw toxins out of an infected tooth and reduce the pain, says Dr. Hardy. Once a day, moisten a small amount of either herb or an herbal tea bag and place it on the painful area for 15 minutes; you can use this treatment for up to 3 days.

### ACTIVATED CHARCOAL: *The Toxin Avenger III*

Activated charcoal can also help draw out the toxins, says Dr. Hardy. Mix a teaspoon of activated charcoal powder with enough water to make a paste. Place some of the paste on a small piece of gauze, put the gauze on the sore area, and bite down so that the paste surrounds your tooth. Leave it on for up to 5 minutes, then remove the gauze and excess paste and rinse your mouth with water. You can use this remedy three or four times a day as needed.

### BLACK TEA: *The Toxin Avenger IV*

The pain is intense, and you don't have time to go to the health food store for chamomile, calendula, or activated charcoal. If you have any tea bags around the house (black tea, the kind you get when you buy Lipton, not green or herbal tea), relief may be near. The tannins in black tea can help draw toxins out of the tooth or gum, says Dr. Hardy.

### OIL OF CLOVES: *For Cavity Relief*

If there's a hole in your tooth—a cavity that you can see— take a small piece of a cotton ball or gauze pad and put one to two drops of clove bud oil on it. Then stick it right in the hole. The piece should be large enough to fit the hole snugly without falling out.

This will calm the nerve and reduce the toothache, says James Kennedy, D.D.S., a dentist in Littleton, Colorado. Use a new pellet each time you reapply the clove oil.

## The Anti-Toothache Diet

When you eat foods that contain white flour or white sugar, including soft drinks, particles left on your teeth are gobbled up by bacteria and converted into toxins, explains Flora Parsa Stay, D.D.S., a dentist in Oxnard, California. These toxins are highly acidic and can cause cavities if the food residue is not removed daily by brushing and flossing.

Furthermore, once a cavity forms, eating acid-forming foods can irritate the nerve in the tooth and cause a toothache. If you suspect that you have a cavity, or your dentist confirms that you do, not eating foods made with white sugar and white flour can help you avoid a toothache until the tooth is fixed, says Dr. Stay.

### ARNICA: *A Swell Remedy*
Use a tincture of the herb arnica to help reduce swelling. Tear off a small piece of a cotton ball and apply a dropper of the tincture to the cotton, says Dr. Arana, then place the cotton next to the swollen gum. You can use this remedy as needed for relief.

# *Getting to the Root of* **Tooth Decay**

Is there anything about cavities that you didn't learn in first grade? You eat sugary foods. The bacteria in your mouth eat the leftovers. The bacteria thrive and produce a sticky film called plaque on your teeth. The plaque coats your teeth with acid, stealing minerals from enamel, the tooth's surface. You can fill in (no, make that *fillings*) the rest.

So, to prevent cavities, all you have to do is limit your intake of sugary foods and brush and floss regularly to control plaque.

Plus, see your dental hygienist regularly for professional plaque control, advises Michael Olmsted, D.D.S., a biocompatible dentist in Del Mar, California.

Well, those habits are definitely a must for healthy teeth. But a discovery being touted by alternative dentists shows that reducing the sugar in your diet may be more important than ever, because sugar may rot your teeth from the inside out.

### SUGAR: *A Must to Avoid*

A tooth isn't a tiny mineral monolith but a complex unit of living tissue. For example, inside a tooth are thousands of microtubules, small tubes that lead from the nerve deep inside the tooth to the enamel on the outside. (If all the tubules in a single tooth were laid end to end, they'd stretch for 7 miles.)

Research shows that these tubules are the "circulation" of the tooth, says Burton Miller, D.D.S., director of Health-Centered Dentistry in Anchorage. The tubules contain a cleansing, nourishing, watery fluid that flows from deep inside the tooth to the outside in a process similar to sweating.

But, says Dr. Miller, alternative dentists believe that if you eat lots of sugar (which he calls a negative nutrient), your body chemistry becomes unbalanced, and the flow is reversed. With no normal inside-to-out flow, the bacteria-created acids on the outside of the tooth begin to eat away at the enamel. The abnormal reverse flow also moves bacteria deeper into the tooth, causing large cavities.

This is why Dr. Miller believes that good dental hygiene can't prevent tooth decay in people who eat diets loaded with sugar. To protect yourself from decay, he recommends eliminating sugar from your diet. That includes not only sucrose (table sugar) but also all forms of refined sugar, such as fructose, dextrose, maltose, and glucose.

### Are Mercury Fillings Poisoning Your Health?

You probably know that mercury is a poison. Maybe you've read newspaper stories in which people were advised not to eat fish caught in a lake that was contaminated with mercury.

Despite that, however, you figure that the silver-mercury fillings in your mouth are safe. ("Silver" fillings, called dental amalgam, contain about 50 percent mercury, along with copper, zinc, silver,

# GUIDE TO
# PROFESSIONAL CARE

"You should have your teeth professionally checked at least once a year for signs of decay," recommends David Kennedy, D.D.S., a dentist in San Diego.

That's because tooth decay is usually painless until it's well-advanced, he explains. A cavity starts as a tiny flaw that is slightly whitish and feels soft when the dentist probes it with his pick; it is almost always completely painless. It will later mushroom into the softer inner tooth and hollow out the inside of the tooth, eventually invading the nerve and killing the tooth. Often, it's only at this point that the tooth becomes painful and sensitive; then you need to see your dentist as soon as possible, advises Dr. Kennedy.

But what's causing the cavity? That's the question posed by Burton Miller, D.D.S., director of Health-Centered Dentistry in Anchorage.

"The mouth is a barometer for the body's total health," he says. He believes that tooth decay is a sign that the body is suffering from a chronic degenerative condition, which can only be reversed by natural methods such as a diet that creates optimal biochemistry.

Dr. Miller recommends that you see a naturopath, a chiropractor, a licensed nutritionist with experience in alternative diets and the use of supplements, or an alternative-minded M.D. to help guide you to the best health-restoring diet, one that will help you prevent not only cavities but other degenerative diseases as well.

"You can brush and floss until your arms fall off," he says. "But if you have tooth decay, there is a deeper, whole-body problem—an imbalance in your biochemistry—that is causing it. You must deal with that problem, not just receive fillings and other types of dental care."

and sometimes tin.) After all, your dentist wouldn't poison you, right? Well, here's what you probably don't know about your mercury fillings, courtesy of David Kennedy, D.D.S., a dentist in San Diego.

• Chewing gum puts friction on mercury fillings, which causes the level of mercury vapor in your mouth to rise.

• Experimental rats that inhaled the same level of mercury present in the mouths of some people with numerous amalgam fillings developed lesions similar to those found in patients with Alzheimer's disease. And some studies have concluded that "mercury must be considered as a potential source for the [cause] of Alzheimer's disease."

• The use of fillings containing mercury is now restricted in several countries, including Sweden, Germany, Austria, and England. Why? Because those governments declared that the fillings may be dangerous for some parts of the population, especially pregnant women.

• Symptoms of mercury poisoning include fatigue, headache, depression, irregular heartbeat, insomnia, high blood pressure, and allergies, among others.

If you have mercury fillings, what can you do to protect your health? Since the mineral selenium displaces mercury in your body and helps usher it out of your system, Dr. Kennedy suggests taking 200 micrograms a day.

A daily dose of 1,000 milligrams of vitamin C can also help protect your body from mercury poisoning from fillings, says James Hardy, D.M.D., a holistic dentist in Winter Park, Florida.

He also recommends eating a lot of cilantro. "I think it's the best herb for removing heavy metals such as mercury from your system," he says. Every day, put about ½ ounce of the herb in salads, burritos, or wherever you use greens. (Make sure the herb is fresh, says Dr. Hardy.) Toss some garlic in those recipes, too. The sulfur in garlic binds to heavy metals and ushers them out of your system, he believes. He recommends two cloves daily. Other significant food sources of sulfur include milk, eggs, and all protein foods.

To help minimize problems with mercury, ask your dentist for non-mercury-containing fillings in any cavities that need fillings, says Dr. Kennedy.

## SODA: *Not Even Sugar-Free Will Do*

Unfortunately, even sugar-free soft drinks have a tooth-destroying ingredient: phosphoric acid. This acid, also found in nondiet soft drinks, can eat away at the enamel of your teeth just like the acid produced by decay-causing bacteria, says Dr. Olmsted. If you must drink soda, down it quickly, he recommends. Prolonged sipping is the last straw for your teeth.

## LIQUID MINERALS: *Build Stronger Teeth*

Teeth are made of minerals, so, if your teeth are prone to decay, you may need more minerals in your system, says Beverly Yates, N.D., a naturopathic physician and director of the Natural Health Care Group in Seattle.

Dr. Yates believes that liquid minerals are better absorbed than tablets. "The liquid easily crosses the gut lining and becomes available to the cells of the body, including the teeth, very rapidly," she says.

Be sure that calcium, magnesium, boron, manganese, and silica are in the supplement. They all contribute to strong teeth. Dr. Yates recommends taking 20 drops daily. Avoid colloidal mineral products, however, because they contain aluminum, which is toxic.

## WATER: *If You Can't Brush, Rinse*

Sure, we're supposed to brush after every meal. But who does?

For an easy alternative, simply rinse your mouth with water 3 to 5 minutes after eating or drinking anything, then spit. "This will decrease the particles in the mouth that feed decay-causing bacteria," says Dr. Olmsted. "This habit, consistently practiced, will definitely reduce the incidence of tooth decay."

# *Dealing With Stress Roots Out* **Tooth Grinding**

Grinding, clenching, or gnashing your teeth—a health problem known as bruxism—often has an emotional cause, says William Payne, D.D.S., a dentist in McPherson, Kansas.

"In my 20 years of experience as a dentist, I've found that those individuals who are emotionally and spiritually self-aware have much better control of their bruxism than those who aren't," Dr. Payne says.

By being emotionally self-aware, he means understanding that you're grinding your teeth, or bruxing, instead of dealing with the stress in your life. When you've figured this out, you can decide to constructively handle the stress rather than destroy your teeth. But Dr. Payne believes that reducing stress isn't all that it takes to fully overcome the problem.

"The people in my practice who are most able to overcome bruxism not only reduce stress in their lives," he says, "they also develop spiritual self-awareness. They know that there is a spiritual presence within—an inner voice, an intuition, a constant guidance—that is deeper than their emotional ups and downs. And if they begin to listen to their inner voice, they will be able to truly overcome the anxiety, tension, frustration, and emotional pain that are the causes of bruxism because they will have profound and stable guidance from their souls."

Bruxism commonly occurs at night, as your subconscious mind "chews over" your problems. But whether you do it by moonlight or sunlight or both, the results can be a nightmare for your teeth. You can wear them to a nub or damage them where they enter the gum and jawbone so that they loosen and even break off. And even if you're not ruining your teeth, bruxing may cause head, face, and neck pain.

If stress is putting the bite on you, alternative healers recommend many different ways to end the daily grind.

## RELAXATION: *Putting Stress to Sleep*

To help prevent grinding while you sleep—the most common time for unconscious, tooth-eroding gnashing—don't do anything stressful for at least 30 minutes before bedtime, says Beverly Yates, N.D., a naturopathic physician and director of the Natural Health Care Group in Seattle. What should you do during that half hour? Listen to soft music (choose a tune without lyrics; the words might disturb you) or a relaxation tape. Or take a warm bath.

## HERBS: *To Calm Your Nerves*

Chamomile, hops, valerian, and skullcap are each believed to relieve anxiety and provide deeper sleep, says Michael Olmsted, D.D.S., a biocompatible dentist in Del Mar, California. Experi-

# GUIDE TO
## PROFESSIONAL CARE

Although tooth grinding has different causes, the symptoms are the same. According to Beverly Yates, N.D., a naturopathic physician and director of the Natural Health Care Group in Seattle, you should see a dentist for bruxism if you experience unexplained headaches or jaw pain, have difficulty chewing food thoroughly, or notice a change in the shape of the lower half of your face. Other warning signs include a clicking or popping sound when you open your mouth to yawn or laugh and sore jaw and facial muscles, especially around your temples and in front of your ears.

Bruxism isn't always caused by stress. Sometimes, a malocclusion, or misaligned bite, can cause you to clench and grind your teeth. It can also be a result of temporomandibular disorder, or TMD, a misalignment of the joint in the jaw.

"There is one simple medical treatment for nighttime tooth grinding caused by stress," says Michael Olmsted, D.D.S., a biocompatible dentist in Del Mar, California. It's a night guard, a mouthpiece similar to those worn by professional athletes.

The guard, made of clear, hard acrylic, prevents you from clenching and grinding your teeth while you sleep. If you have bruxism, ask your dentist about having a guard made for you. It has to be customized to your bite in order to be effective; an off-the-shelf product will only create more dental problems, Dr. Olmsted warns.

Tooth grinding may also be a symptom of other physical problems—problems that in some cases, conventional dentists don't even think exist.

Some cases, for example, may be caused by electrical currents created by a multiplicity of metals in the mouth, says William Payne, D.D.S., a dentist in McPherson, Kansas. Dr. Payne says that it may be caused by allergies, and grinding your teeth may be an unconscious attempt to massage your clogged and inflamed sinuses.

If self-care techniques don't work, Dr. Payne counsels any person who has a problem with tooth grinding to see a bio-

> compatible or biological dentist (one who thinks that many of
> the substances used in conventional dentistry are harmful to
> health and who uses only dental materials that he believes to
> be safe), who can evaluate the full array of possible causes,
> make a diagnosis, and recommend the proper treatment.

ment with teas containing each of them and see which one gives
you the best results. For even better results, take a tincture of any
one of these herbs before bedtime, stirring the dose recommended on the label into 1 to 2 ounces of hot water.

"Tinctures can have an even more beneficial effect than teas,"
he says. This is because they are more concentrated and are absorbed more quickly by the body.

## HOMEOPATHY: *To Relax Your Face*

The homeopathic remedy Magphos is believed to help relax
the muscles of the face. People who regularly grind their teeth
should take a 12X potency of the remedy three times a day for
a week and see if it helps, says James Kennedy, D.D.S., a dentist in Littleton, Colorado. If you notice that you are grinding
less, cut your dose to once a day right before bedtime. If the
remedy doesn't work or if your symptoms stop, discontinue
treatment. If symptoms continue for more than 6 weeks, see
your dentist.

If you grind only when you're under a lot of stress, try this
remedy when you feel tense, taking it three times a day. It might
help prevent a bout of stress-induced grinding, Dr. Kennedy
says.

## RELAXATION: *Enunciating for Relief*

Say each vowel—A, E, I, O, U—out loud, exaggerating the
sound of each. This stretches and relaxes your facial muscles,
relieving pain and helping to prevent bruxing, says Dr. Payne.
Do the exercise four times a day in front of a mirror to be sure
that you're really stretching your muscles as you say each letter. Do it every day until bruxing is under control, then continue practicing it as a reinforcement therapy.

### BIOFEEDBACK: *Listening to Your Native Tongue*

Just realizing that you grind your teeth is the first step toward breaking this unconscious habit, says Dr. Payne. "Seventy-five percent of my patients who become aware that they are bruxing are able to stop bruxing," he says.

For daytime bruxing, keep your tongue between your top and bottom teeth, for instance, so you'll know instantly when you start to clench (it will hurt a bit). When you feel the slight twinge of pain, tell yourself "I don't need to do this."

"This technique is very effective," says Dr. Payne.

### EATING: *Not Before Bedtime*

To prevent bruxism, you want your body to be as rested as possible during sleep, Dr. Olmsted says. Eating an hour or less before you go to bed increases digestion and metabolism, making it more likely that you'll grind your teeth during the night. "Don't eat late," he advises.

### CARBOHYDRATES AND CAFFEINE: *Never at Night*

Okay, maybe you will raid the refrigerator now and then during *The Late Show with David Letterman*. But if you do eat late at night, don't include any sugar, honey, maple syrup, or other carbohydrates in your snack, says Dr. Olmsted. Don't have any caffeine-containing tea or coffee, and alcohol is also a definite no-no, as it can disturb the sleep cycle. Dr. Olmsted believes that these foods keep the body very active during sleep and are bad news for people who want to prevent bruxism.

## *Gentle Ways to Reduce*
# Tooth Sensitivity

"Don't be so sensitive!"

Maybe you can get away with saying that to your spouse, but it won't have any effect on your sensitive, painful teeth. They can't stop being sensitive, because some of their protective

---

# GUIDE TO
# PROFESSIONAL CARE

If areas of your teeth are damaged and sensitive, you need professional dental care. Your dentist will recommend either fillings or crowns and will also work with you to determine the cause of the problem, from improper oral hygiene (too-vigorous brushing) to ill-fitting dentures, so that other areas of your teeth don't become sensitive.

---

enamel has been worn away (by too-vigorous brushing, an imbalance in your bite, habitual chewing on hard objects such as pencils, or many other possible causes), leaving an open "wound" that only professional dentistry can repair.

In the meantime, you could use commercial rinses designed to mute the pain, but most of them are loaded with preservatives and alcohol, two ingredients that don't do the rest of your body any good, says Harold Ravins, D.D.S., director of the Center for Holistic Dentistry in Los Angeles. Here's his alternative "solution."

### HERBS: *A Soothing, Healing Mouthwash*

Mix equal parts of liquid extracts of white oak bark, horsetail, and fennel. Then you can either put eight drops of the mixture directly on the sensitive tooth or dilute the eight drops in a cup of water and use the solution as a rinse. Swish it in your mouth for about a minute each morning and night, says Dr. Ravins.

"Fennel root has been used since ancient times for soothing the nervous system," he says. It contains potassium, sulfur, and sodium, three minerals that are crucial for quieting the nerves of the teeth.

This herbal rinse actually does double duty, since it also helps heal inflamed gums. The horsetail is rich in selenium, which helps decrease bleeding, says Dr. Ravins, and the white oak bark contains tannins, herbal astringents that tighten and clean gum tissue.

**THIAMIN:** *To Reduce Sensitivity*

This B vitamin can help reduce your sensitivity to pain, says Flora Parsa Stay, D.D.S., a dentist in Oxnard, California. She recommends 100 milligrams a day.

**CALCIUM HYDROXYAPATITE:** *For Added Protection*

This form of calcium helps to regenerate the enamel, thus making your teeth less sensitive, says Edward M. Arana, D.D.S., a retired dentist in Carmel Valley, California, and past president of the American Academy of Biological Dentistry. Follow the dosage recommendations on the label.

## The Clove Connection

Clove is a classic emergency remedy for toothaches, and it also helps calm down sensitive teeth until you can see the dentist, says Dr. Stay.

To make an herbal salve to soothe your sensitive teeth, mix ¼ teaspoon of clove powder with a few drops of water. After every meal, apply just enough to cover the sensitive area, but don't put it on a tooth that is cracked or has a hole in it.

**HOMEOPATHY:** *For Heat and Cold*

Maybe your sensitive teeth only hurt when you eat very hot or very cold foods. To reduce sensitivity to hot foods, Dr. Stay recommends dissolving two tablets of Chamomilla 30X under your tongue as needed until the sensitivity goes away. For sensitivity to cold foods, she says to use one tablet of Plantago major 6X three times a day until the sensitivity subsides.

In either case, if the pain doesn't lessen or gets worse, see your dentist. You can continue to use these remedies to enhance healing during treatment by your dentist.

# The Antibiotic-Plus Plan for Healing
# Ulcers

Most alternative practitioners agree: The best treatment for a peptic ulcer is . . . antibiotics.

Wait a second. Don't most practitioners avoid using antibiotics? Don't those drugs destroy the helpful bacteria in the colon, causing all sorts of digestive difficulties? Don't many other chapters in this book warn against using them?

The answers are yes, yes, and yes.

Nevertheless, both conventional and alternative doctors agree that using antibiotics is the best way to kill *Helicobacter pylori*. This common bacterium causes up to 70 percent of peptic ulcers, which are painful sores in the lining of the stomach or duodenum (the section of small intestine right next to the stomach).

Ulcers must be treated. Along with pain, they can cause weight loss, bloating, burping, and nausea. Some ulcers bleed. Others cause a perforation, or hole, that goes right through the stomach or intestine.

Once doctors determine that an ulcer is caused by *H. pylori* infection, a diagnosis that's made with a blood test that shows the *H. pylori* antigen and with a tissue sample taken from the stomach, they can quickly and effectively cure the problem by prescribing a week or two of antibiotic therapy. They'll usually accompany the antibiotics with bismuth subsalicylate or other acid-controlling drugs to protect the stomach lining. This therapy cures the ulcer and prevents recurrence in 90 percent of people. That's a very successful cure rate by any standard, conventional or alternative.

That doesn't mean, however, that alternative home remedies aren't important in the treatment of ulcers. You can use them following your course of antibiotics to help the stomach and duodenum heal and to help keep ulcers from coming

---

### GUIDE TO
### PROFESSIONAL CARE

If you suspect that you have an ulcer (the main symptom is a dull, gnawing ache in the stomach that occurs 2 to 3 hours after a meal or in the middle of the night, comes and goes for several days or weeks, and is relieved by food), you need to see your medical doctor.

If you've been diagnosed with an ulcer, and you start having sharp, persistent stomach pain, black and bloody stools, or vomit that is bloody or looks like coffee grounds, you probably have a bleeding ulcer or a perforation in the stomach or duodenum. This is an emergency; see a doctor immediately.

---

back. You can also use them to minimize the side effects during treatment.

Also, if your ulcer isn't caused by *H. pylori*, these remedies can be more effective at controlling symptoms and healing the problem than prescription or over-the-counter acid-blocking drugs, says Mark Stengler, N.D., a naturopathic physician in San Diego.

### FISH OIL AND CORN OIL: *Help Keep Ulcers from Coming Back*

One scientific study found that corn oil and fish oil can inhibit the growth of *H. pylori* bacteria, says Duane Smoot, M.D., lead scientist for the study and associate professor of medicine in the department of gastroenterology at Howard University College of Medicine in Washington, D.C. "Diets rich in these oils may help reduce ulcer recurrence," he says.

You can get enough of these oils just by cooking with corn oil and using it in salad dressings and by having two or three servings of fish a week, Dr. Smoot says.

If you don't like fish, you can take fish-oil supplements, following the directions on the label, says Elizabeth Lipski, a certified clinical nutritionist in Kauai, Hawaii.

### HIGH-FIBER FOODS: *Get as Many as You Can*

Increasing your intake of dietary fiber can help prevent ulcer recurrences, Dr. Stengler says. Foods such as apples, oat bran, broccoli, brussels sprouts, cabbage, carrots, whole-grain breads and cereals, and green leafy vegetables all supply plenty of fiber. Or you can take a fiber supplement that contains psyllium seeds, he advises. Once a day, take two or three capsules with an 8-ounce glass of water.

## GAMMA ORYZANOL: *Good for Healing*

A compound called gamma oryzanol can help most ulcers heal, Lipski says. Whether or not you're using antibiotics, taking 300 milligrams of gamma oryzanol a day will speed healing and also help prevent ulcers from coming back, she says.

## DGL: *More Powerful Than Medication*

Deglycyrrhizinated licorice, or DGL, is a form of licorice from which the compound glycyrrhizic acid, which can cause high blood pressure, has been removed. Scientific studies have shown that it is more effective than some over-the-counter antiulcer medications at controlling the symptoms of a peptic ulcer, says Dr. Stengler. He recommends taking 1,000 to 1,500 milligrams of DGL daily in capsule form, or 30 drops of DGL tincture three times daily on an empty stomach, for up to 2 months.

### Germs to the Rescue

Even though antibiotics are very effective at treating and curing most types of ulcers, the antibiotics themselves often cause side effects because they kill good bacteria along with the bad. This can be a problem because good bacteria in the intestine help regulate digestion and maintain a healthy environment.

When the friendly bacteria are killed, you may develop a condition called dysbiosis, a surge of bad bacteria and fungi. This can cause bloating, indigestion, constipation, diarrhea, flatulence, fatigue, and yeast infections.

You can help prevent dysbiosis during antibiotic therapy by taking a daily dose of one to three capsules, or ¼ to ½ teaspoon, of probiotics a day. Probiotic supplements contain healthful bacteria such as acidophilus, bifidum, and faecium, says Elizabeth Lipski, a certified clinical nutritionist in Kauai, Hawaii. These bacteria help replace those killed by the antibiotics, she explains.

When you're buying probiotics, check the label for the terms *freeze-dried*, which ensures that the various bacteria in the supplement won't compete for food and starve each other out while they're in the package, and *FOS*, which is a sugar that feeds the bacteria as they travel through the digestive tract. With it, the bacteria reproduce more effectively.

It's also a good idea to buy probiotics that are refrigerated in the store, because cold temperatures keep the bacteria alive and ensure potency. Also check the expiration dates on the bottles.

### GLUTAMINE: *The Healing Secret of Cabbage Juice*

Cabbage juice is considered a traditional folk remedy that can help peptic ulcers heal—but the taste of the juice is vile, says Lipski. Fortunately, the ulcer-healing compound in the juice is available in supplement form.

One of the active ingredients is glutamine, an amino acid that nourishes and repairs the lining of the digestive tract. Lipski recommends taking 8,000 milligrams of glutamine a day for 4 weeks.

## *Restoring Chemical Balance Can Clear Up* **Vaginitis**

Think of the vagina as an ecosystem. Living on the inside and the outside are many different types of flora—strains of good-for-you bacteria that protect you against bacteria and other organisms that are not so good. These "bad" bacteria can invade the area, causing one or more of the symptoms of infectious vaginitis: soreness, irritation, inflammation, discharge, burning, swelling, redness, urinary discomfort, and pain during sex.

Conventional doctors try to solve the problem by killing the bad organisms with drugs, which is a must if the infection is severe or chronic. Alternative doctors, however, prefer remedies that improve the vaginal ecosystem so that the bad organisms can't live there. These remedies help the good flora return to the vagina; restore the normal pH, or chemical balance, of the tissues; and decrease inflammation and irritation as well as kill off the infecting organisms.

Correct treatment depends on knowing which organism is causing your problem; it's usually either bacteria, the fungal yeast *Candida albicans*, or the protozoa *Trichomonas vaginalis*. Thus, the following remedies should be used only after having a diagnostic test to identify the infecting organism, says Tori Hudson, N.D., a naturopathic physician and medical director of A Woman's Time clinic in Portland, Oregon.

## SUGAR: *A Must to Avoid*

"When you want to feed bacteria in a scientific experiment, you coat the petri dish with glucose, or sugar," says Amy Rothenberg, N.D., a naturopathic physician in Enfield, Connecticut. That's why she tells her patients with bacterial vaginosis, or BV, to avoid sugar as well as refined carbohydrates and alcohol, both of which turn into glucose in the body. You should also avoid these foods if you have vaginitis caused by candida or a trichomonas infection.

## YOGURT: *The Most Important Food for Healing*

"Nothing is more key to the health of the ecosystem of the vagina than the bacteria lactobacillus," Dr. Hudson says—and no food is richer in lactobacillus than yogurt.

She recommends that for 2 weeks, women with BV, candidiasis, or trichomoniasis eat 8 ounces daily of unsweetened yogurt with *Lactobacillus acidophilus* bacteria and take three capsules of a supplement of the bacterium between meals. You can use the same regimen to help prevent a recurrence.

Dr. Hudson also advises women with BV to use the capsules of *L. acidophilus* as vaginal suppositories, inserting one capsule each morning for 2 weeks. Look for capsules that contain 1 to 5 billion live organisms each, she says.

## GARLIC: *A Strong Infection Fighter*

Garlic is antibacterial and antifungal, so it can fight both BV and candidiasis, Dr. Hudson says. Look for a garlic supplement that's high in allicin—one that contains about 5,000 micrograms of allium, the major infection-fighting chemical in the herb. She recommends taking one capsule once or twice daily for as long as needed.

# GUIDE TO PROFESSIONAL CARE

The first and most important step in treating acute or chronic infectious vaginitis is an accurate diagnosis, says Tori Hudson, N.D., a naturopathic physician and medical director of A Woman's Time clinic in Portland, Oregon.

"See a licensed health care practitioner who knows the different symptoms of the various forms of the problem, can perform a physical exam, knows what to test for to diagnose the problem, and can collect those samples during your exam," she says.

See your doctor if you notice any of the following symptoms: pain or itching in your vagina and vulva (the area outside the vagina); reddening of your vulva; pain that is especially noticeable when you urinate or during sex or that worsens upon urination or during sex; greenish yellow, frothy, foul-smelling discharge (which suggests trichomoniasis, a sexually transmitted organism); foul-smelling, thin, white or blood-streaked discharge (which may signal atrophic vaginitis); heavy, white, thick, odorless vaginal discharge (which could mean a yeast infection); or white or gray, fishy-smelling vaginal discharge (which suggests bacterial vaginosis).

Once you know what type of infection you have, you can choose self-treatment. If you have infections more than three times a year, however; if you have a chronic infection that never completely goes away; or if you're pregnant, you should seek professional care. Untreated vaginitis can lead to pelvic inflammatory disease, which can result in infertility.

## GOLDENSEAL: *Rich In Immunity-Building Berberine*

The chemical berberine in goldenseal fights off bacteria and candida in the mucous membranes of the vagina, Dr. Hudson says. It also strengthens the immune system. She recommends taking two 500-milligram capsules once or twice a day.

## BORIC ACID: *A Suppository for Yeast Infections*

"Nothing impresses me more than the success rate of boric acid suppositories for the treatment of candida infections," Dr.

Hudson says. She cites a study in which 100 women with yeast infections who hadn't been helped by antifungal medications were given the suppository twice a day for 2 to 4 weeks; 98 percent were cured. Regular use of the suppositories also helps prevent recurrences. "Clinical effectiveness doesn't really get any better than this," she says.

If you have been diagnosed with an acute yeast infection, insert a 600-milligram capsule of boric acid powder into your vagina twice a day, in the morning and evening, for 3 to 7 days, says Dr. Hudson. For a chronic yeast infection, use this regimen for 2 to 4 weeks. To prevent a recurrence, insert one capsule daily at bedtime for 4 days a month, during your menstrual period, for 4 months.

Over-the-counter boric acid suppositories, such as Yeast Arrest, are available in drugstores. Or you can ask a pharmacist to fill size "0" gelatin capsules with 600 milligrams of powdered boric acid each.

The suppository can cause burning in tissue that's already irritated by an infection, Dr. Hudson warns, but you can prevent this by coating the irritated tissues with vitamin E oil before inserting the suppository. If you want to try this treatment, be sure to inform your doctor first, and don't use it if you're pregnant, says Dr. Hudson.

## VITAMIN E: *Soothe Your Symptoms*

Using a gelatin capsule of vitamin E as a suppository is very soothing to vaginal tissue, decreasing irritation, redness, swelling, and congestion, Dr. Hudson says. Insert a capsule once or twice daily for 7 days.

## TRIPHALA: *Get the Toxins Out*

The Ayurvedic herb triphala helps remove toxins from the body and restores a normal flow of body fluids, both of which are important in treating a yeast infection, says Robert E. Svoboda, a faculty member at the Ayurvedic Institute in Albuquerque, New Mexico, and visiting faculty member at Bastyr University in Kenmore, Washingtron.

Soak ½ teaspoon of dried herb in 1 cup of hot water for 5 minutes, then drink the tea before bed. If you don't like the taste, you can take two 500-milligram tablets or capsules before bed.

A once-a-month douche with triphala will help prevent recurrent yeast infections, Svoboda says. Put 1 tablespoon of triphala in 1 pint of water and bring it to a boil. Remove from the heat, let cool to lukewarm, then strain. Use a regular douche bag to douche with the tea. "The longer you keep the triphala tea in contact with the vaginal mucosa, the better," Svoboda says.

If you want to try this remedy, check with your health care practitioner. Douching can dry the vagina and upset its natural balance.

# Alternative Remedies
# Can Vanquish
# Varicose Veins

Each vein in your legs has delicate valves, which open to let blood flow to the heart and then close so gravity can't pull blood back into the leg. If these valves break, blood pools in the vein and you've got what doctors call a varicosity—a varicose vein.

Varicose veins come in all shapes and sizes, from small spider veins to larger veins that may be swollen and achy, not to mention unsightly. They can make your legs feel heavy or tired. Medical doctors treat most varicose veins with a prescription of compression hose—bulky, hard-to-put-on, expensive hosiery that relieves pain by reducing the fluid in the veins.

Natural doctors say they can do a lot better—that they can greatly improve varicose veins.

"Alternative, natural remedies enhance the integrity of the wall of the vein, including the valve, helping to reverse the varicose vein process," says Amy Rothenberg, N.D., a naturopathic physician in Enfield, Connecticut. And even if all your varicose veins don't vanish, natural medicines will help relieve pain, reduce the size of existing veins, and stop new ones from forming.

## QUERCETIN: *A Vein-Strengthening Bioflavonoid*
Bioflavonoids act as plant pigments, providing the palette for many fruits and vegetables. But these handy nutrients don't just

> # GUIDE TO
> # PROFESSIONAL CARE
>
> If you have varicose veins, you should see a medical doctor whenever you notice new symptoms or if the aching and fatigue in your legs worsens. You are at higher risk than others for developing phlebitis (vein inflammation), and you especially want to watch for signs of possible clotting. Let your doctor know right away if you notice hard lumps on your veins that won't go away, burning sensations in your leg, or a painful, red swelling in a localized area.
>
> If you don't have severe varicose veins, however, see a naturopathic physician for treatment, says Amy Rothenberg, N.D., a naturopathic doctor in Enfield, Connecticut. "In all but the most severe cases, using natural medicines will decrease pain and help heal existing veins," she says.

paint, they do construction work, too, strengthening the walls of veins to prevent and heal varicosities.

The most skilled bioflavonoid of all may be quercetin, says Walter Crinnion, N.D., a naturopathic physician and director of Healing Naturally in Kirkland, Washington.

"Quercetin is fantastic for treating and preventing varicose veins," he says. "Legs that are totally blue and painful with swollen varicosities heal completely with just this nutrient." Depending on the severity of their problem, his patients take one or two 500- to 600-milligram capsules of quercetin three times a day with meals.

**GRAPE SEED OR PINE BARK:** *For Even Stronger Veins*

These extracts are rich in anthocyanidins and proanthocyanidins, bioflavonoids that are "excellent" at strengthening the vein wall, says Mark Stengler, N.D., a naturopathic physician in San Diego. He recommends a daily dose of 150 to 300 milligrams of either of these extracts taken indefinitely to prevent the varicosities from worsening and to actually help improve their appearance over time.

Cherries, blueberries, and blackberries are also loaded with these two bioflavonoids, so eat as much of these foods as possible.

**VITAMIN C:** *Another Source of Strength*
This nutrient strengthens vein walls, says Dr. Stengler. He recommends 2,000 to 3,000 milligrams daily for an indefinite period.

**HORSE CHESTNUT:** *Tone Your Veins*
A vein that's not toned is an easy target for a varicosity. A venotonic strengthens the elastic fibers in the vein wall and improves its tone—that is, its ability to tighten or contract. The herb horse chestnut is a great venotonic, Dr. Stengler says.
He recommends taking a 300-milligram capsule or 30 drops of tincture twice a day on an ongoing basis. Look for a product standardized for 60 milligrams of escin, the venotonic in the herb.

**BUTCHER'S BROOM:** *To Prevent Inflammation*
Many varicose veins can become inflamed, turning into a condition known as phlebitis, which is why they hurt. You can help prevent inflammation with the herb butcher's broom, Dr. Stengler says. He recommends 100 milligrams three times a day on an ongoing basis. Look for an extract of butcher's broom standardized for 10 percent ruscogenin, the herb's active ingredient.

**BILBERRY AND GOTU KOLA:** *Vein Protection*
These two herbs also have vein-protecting, vein-healing power. Dr. Stengler recommends taking 80 milligrams of bilberry three times daily when you first notice varicose veins. Look for a product standardized for 25 percent anthocyanoside, the active ingredient. If you notice marked improvement, you may be able to cut the dosage in half.
Seth Baum, M.D., an integrative cardiologist and founder of the Baum Center for Integrative Heart Care in Boca Raton, Florida, gives the herb gotu kola to patients with varicose veins. He recommends taking capsules that supply 60 to 120 milligrams daily of a standardized extract of gotu kola that provides 50 milligrams of triterpenic acids, the active ingredient in the herb. Try this for about a month to see if your condition improves.

**BROMELAIN:** *To Prevent Hard, Lumpy Veins*
Bromelain, a digestive enzyme from the pineapple plant, also "digests" fibrin, a protein in the body that crowds around varicose

veins, turning them hard and lumpy. Dr. Rothenberg recommends a 500-milligram supplement three times a day to prevent hardening of the veins. Take the supplements between meals so the enzyme will dissolve fibrin, not your dinner.

**EXERCISE:** *Take a Walk—in a Pool*

Any exercise that works your legs is helpful, but Dr. Rothenberg believes that the best exercise for people with varicose veins is walking in water. "The exercise and the pressure of the water on the outside of the legs is especially effective in pushing the blood out of the legs and into circulation," she says. She recommends walking or gently jogging in a swimming pool for 30 minutes a day 5 or 6 days a week.

**SLEEPING POSITION:** *For Nighttime Pain Relief*

Elevating the foot of your bed, Dr. Rothenberg suggests, will relieve pain by improving circulation in your legs during the night. An easy method is to insert a brick under the foot of the bed.

**HYDROTHERAPY:** *Take a Hot-and-Cold Foot Bath*

A hot-and-cold foot bath before bed improves circulation to the legs, preventing varicosities and helping them heal, says Dr. Rothenberg. Fill two large basins, one with ice-cold water and one with very warm water. Put your feet in the cold water for 30 seconds, then in the very warm water for 2 minutes. Repeat three times, ending with a final 30 seconds in the cold water.

# Find the Right Natural Remedy to Get Rid of
# Warts

Warts are unsightly and painful colonies of viruses that can take up residence anywhere on the surface of the body. Among their more unpleasant characteristics are itching, burning, and oozing.

# GUIDE TO
# PROFESSIONAL CARE

"Warts should be diagnosed accurately and treated appropriately," says Esta Kronberg, M.D., a dermatologist in Houston. That's particularly true of warts in the genital area, which can be sexually transmitted and may be a risk factor for cervical cancer in women.

Once the warts are diagnosed, they should be removed. "It's important to treat them early rather than waiting until they spread and enlarge and are more difficult and expensive to eliminate," Dr. Kronberg says.

Warts are easily removed by cryosurgery, or freezing, and electrocautery, a procedure that burns the wart off with an electrified surgical tool.

"My first choice of treatment is to freeze them with liquid nitrogen," says Dr. Kronberg. It is the most effective, quickest, easiest, and least expensive treatment, she says.

---

If you're looking to get rid of a wart, an experienced alternative healer—a person committed to natural, nonmedical treatments—has this advice: See an M.D.

"The easiest, best way to get rid of a wart is to have it frozen off by a medical doctor," says David E. Molony, Ph.D., a licensed acupuncturist and director of Lehigh Valley Acupuncture Center in Catasauqua, Pennsylvania.

If you'd prefer to treat your wart with natural methods, though, breathe easy. Many exist. "When it comes to warts, different remedies work for different people," says Norma Pasekoff Weinberg, an herbal educator in Cape Cod, Massachusetts. "I would try every wart remedy I could find until I found one that worked."

## HOMEOPATHY: *Alternate These Two Remedies*

For those who want to go the natural route, Dr. Molony recommends two homeopathic remedies to get rid of any kind of wart: Thuja occidentalis and Antimonium crudum, both in 30X potency.

For 3 days, alternate doses of the two remedies, taking one

dose of Thuja in the morning and late afternoon and one dose of Antimonium at noon and in the evening. Wait 2 weeks, then repeat the treatment. Use the dosage specified on the product.

Take the remedy on the same schedule—3 days every 2 weeks—until the wart disappears. You can use a 6C potency if 30X is not readily available, says Dr. Molony.

## HOMEOPATHY: *An Alternative Approach*

Bradley Bongiovanni, N.D., a naturopathic physician in Cambridge, Massachusetts, prefers a 6C potency of Thuja occidentalis "if the wart is soft, fleshy, and oozes or bleeds easily." Use the dose recommended on the label two or three times a day until the wart goes away.

For a smaller wart that itches or stings and may also ooze or bleed, use Calcarea carbonica. For hard warts that burn and throb, use Sulfur. In both cases, take three pellets of the 6C potency two or three times a day until the wart goes away.

## GENTIAN VIOLET: *Purple Virus Eater*

Gentian violet is an antiseptic over-the-counter preparation that contains the herb gentian. "I've seen it work really well to kill wart viruses," Dr. Molony says.

## GARLIC: *A Potent Antiviral*

Garlic oil is a traditional remedy for warts, Weinberg says. You can buy garlic oil or make your own by covering a chopped garlic bulb with olive oil, refrigerating it overnight, and straining out the garlic the next day. Swab the oil on the wart or on a bandage applied to the wart on a daily basis, she says.

## MULTIVITAMIN/MINERAL SUPPLEMENT: *Check the Dosages*

Dr. Bongiovanni counsels his patients with warts to take a daily multivitamin/mineral supplement that includes at least 200 micrograms of selenium, which is thought to be a strong antiviral nutrient, and at least 10,000 international units (IU) of vitamin A, 500 milligrams of vitamin C, 15 milligrams of zinc, and 400 IU of vitamin E, all of which can help to strengthen the immune system so that it can more easily defeat the virus.

## Watch Your Wart Melt Away

Mind-body techniques such as self-hypnosis can be very effective for healing warts, says Ted Grossbart, Ph.D., a clinical psychologist in Boston and faculty member at Harvard Medical School. "The treatment of warts is where mind-body techniques have made the greatest inroads into the mainstream of dermatology," he says.

For example, you might sit comfortably in a chair, relax your body with a few deep breaths, and form a mental picture of a patch of snow over your wart, which creates a pleasant, refreshing tingling in the area, then melts the wart as it melts away. As you visualize, say to yourself, "My wart is melting away." Do this visualization technique every day for 5 minutes or more.

**OLIVE LEAF:** *Fights Infections of All Kinds*

An herbal extract from the Mediterranean olive tree contains powerful anti-infectious compounds and may help get rid of a wart, Dr. Bongiovanni says. Look for a product with 17 to 23 percent oleuropein, the active ingredient, and follow the dosage recommendations on the label.

# *Safe Strategies for Relieving*
# Water Retention

Maybe your legs look thicker than they should, your belly has suddenly gotten larger, or your breasts feel swollen and tender. These are all symptoms of fluid retention, also called edema, which occurs when fluids that normally flow through your body pool in tiny spaces between the cells. It is more common in women than in men because women have larger spaces between cells, which is nature's way of allowing for expansion during pregnancy.

Almost every woman is familiar with the extra fluid that accumulates and then disappears over the course of the menstrual cycle. But some women have fluid retention all the time, and it may be caused by serious health problems. That's why it's important for anyone who has fluid retention that lasts for more than a week to see a doctor for diagnosis and treatment.

Conventional doctors usually try to control the condition with diuretics, drugs that flush water out of the body. The problem is, diuretics also flush out potassium and magnesium, minerals that keep your muscles contracting, your heart beating, and your nerves communicating with one another. And the drugs can have plenty of other nasty side effects, like raising blood sugar levels and lowering sex drive.

No wonder alternative doctors recommend other, all-natural methods to relieve fluid retention, starting with the most natural substance of all.

### WATER: *Flushes the Kidneys*

It's hard to believe that drinking more water would help fluid retention. Isn't the problem that you already have too much fluid

---

## GUIDE TO PROFESSIONAL CARE

Pre- and postmenopausal women may hold excess fluid because they're not eating enough protein, have a high-salt diet, or aren't getting enough vitamin $B_6$. Food or chemical sensitivities may also contribute. While short-term fluid retention isn't necessarily serious, a long-standing problem could be a sign of a hormone imbalance or even acute heart or kidney failure.

If it isn't a natural part of a monthly menstrual cycle or if it's accompanied by shortness of breath, palpitations, pain in the calf muscles, or a decrease in urination, you should see a doctor right away.

You may want to see a doctor who's attuned to natural medicine, says Betty Sy Go, M.D., a naturally oriented doctor in Bellevue, Washington. A naturally oriented doctor will focus on discovering and eliminating the cause of the problem, rather than just treating symptoms with drugs, she says. Even if a diuretic is necessary, there's a good chance you'll be able to use a natural product, which won't have the side effects of medications, she says.

in your body? Well, when you're dehydrated because you're drinking too little water to meet your body's needs, your kidneys may decide to conserve water. This is one cause of bloating and fluid retention, says Betty Sy Go, M.D., a naturally oriented doctor in Bellevue, Washington. To stop your kidneys from treating your body like a reservoir, she recommends drinking 2 quarts of water a day, or eight 8-ounce glasses.

## FOOD: *Try Natural Diuretics*

A number of foods act as natural diuretics by removing excess fluid from the body, says Mark Stengler, N.D., a naturopathic physician in San Diego. Parsley, celery, and watermelon are the best, he says.

Other good choices include asparagus, carrots, artichokes, and alfalfa sprouts, says Dr. Go. Try to have at least one serving of one of these foods every day, she advises.

## DANDELION: *Nature's Best Medicine*

The leaf of the dandelion is considered nature's best natural diuretic, says Dr. Stengler. And unlike pharmaceutical diuretics, it doesn't rob your body of potassium. He advises people with fluid retention to take 250 milligrams of dandelion leaf extract three times a day. You can also take 30 to 60 drops of tincture in ½ cup of juice or water three times a day, he says.

You can take dandelion indefinitely if you're using it to relieve water retention from high blood pressure, says Dr. Stengler. For water retention during pregnancy or for leg swelling due to water retention, take the recommended dosage until the symptoms are under control, then cut the dosage in half, he advises.

Other herbs that act as diuretics include astragalus, buchu, burdock, horehound, and meadowsweet, says Dr. Stengler. You can use any one of these as a tea, extract, or tincture. Drink two to three cups of tea or take 30 to 60 drops of tincture a day. For extracts, which are in capsule form, it's best to follow the directions on the label, he says. When water retention is under control, reduce the dosage by half. These herbs may be taken indefinitely, says Dr. Stengler.

## VITAMIN B$_6$: *Help for the Liver*

The liver manufactures proteins that combine with water and escort it out of the body, but if it isn't working effectively, you can develop fluid retention, says Dr. Stengler. Taking 100 milligrams of vitamin $B_6$ a day can help strengthen the liver and reduce edema, he says.

The best way to get vitamin $B_6$ is by taking a B-complex supplement, Dr. Stengler adds, which will give you a balanced intake of all the B vitamins.

### EXERCISE: *Jumping Jolts Fluid Movement*

Bouncing on a mini-trampoline is thought to stimulate the lymphatic system, the series of vessels that moves and drains fluids. The up-and-down motion may help rid your body of excess fluid, says Virender Sodhi, M.D. (Ayurved), N.D., an Ayurvedic and naturopathic physician and director of the American School of Ayurvedic Sciences in Bellevue, Washington. He recommends doing it for 10 to 15 minutes every day as long as the fluid retention is present. Remember to bend your knees while jumping, he cautions.

## *Rejuvenating Natural Remedies Can Reduce* **Wrinkles**

Conventional medicine has lots of ways to fix a wrinkled face. Collagen injections to fill small wrinkles. Laser surgery to "resurface" lined areas. A brow lift for your forehead.

Maybe cosmetic surgery doesn't appeal to you, though. If that's the case, alternative beauty care experts have a wealth of natural options for reducing wrinkles and "implanting" more youth in your skin.

### AROMATHERAPY: *A Rejuvenating Mask*

"A facial mask can have a wonderfully rejuvenating effect on aging skin," says Joni Loughran, an esthetician, cosmetologist, and aromatherapist in Petaluma, California. She recommends the following homemade mask, which contains essential oils

---

# GUIDE TO
# PROFESSIONAL CARE

While wrinkled skin alone is not a life-threatening problem, it can be considered a form of scarring from the ravages of our environment, such as radiation and other toxins, says Lawrence Green, M.D., assistant professor of dermatology at George Washington University in Washington, D.C. Wrinkled skin may also signify that conditions are right for the development of precancerous and cancerous growths.

For natural skin care, you may want to seek the services of a licensed esthetician. "While an esthetician can't turn back the hands of time, she can rehydrate and deep-cleanse your skin, leaving it smoother and more supple than when you arrived," says Stephanie Tourles, a licensed esthetician, reflexologist, and herbalist in West Hyannisport, Massachusetts.

---

that are thought to stimulate the production of new skin cells, thus helping to reduce fine lines and wrinkles.

In a bowl, mix 1 teaspoon facial-quality clay, 1 teaspoon instant oatmeal or oat flour, ½ tablespoon powdered milk, 2 teaspoons honey, 1 teaspoon avocado or olive oil, and enough water to make a paste. Add two drops of essential oil of frankincense and two drops of essential oil of neroli, lavender, or rose.

Apply the paste in an even layer to your clean face, avoiding the eye area, and leave it on for 10 minutes. If it begins to dry before 10 minutes, mist it to keep it moist. While the mask is on, lie down with your feet slightly elevated and cover your eyes with eye pads moistened with water.

After 10 minutes, rinse with warm water and follow with a cool-water splash. Use the mask two to four times a month.

## MISTING: *To Reduce Fine Lines*

Aside from exposure to the sun, the main reason that skin wrinkles is that it loses moisture, says Loughran. "The components in our skin that have the ability to hold moisture decrease with age," she says. But misting the skin—spraying it with a fine mist of water—can help moisturize your face and reduce fine lines.

"This technique works extremely well," she says. "Just as dried fruit plumps up and softens when it's soaked, so misting can help soften and plump the surface of dried, wrinkled skin, reducing fine lines."

To mist, you'll need an 8-ounce bottle with a pump sprayer that emits a very fine spray that won't disturb makeup. The moisturizing element that you choose to put in the bottle can be plain water, 10 drops of an essential oil (or blend) in water, or an aromatherapy hydrosol (the water left over after a plant has been distilled to remove the essential oils).

If you add essential oils such as neroli, lavender, or rose, shake the mixture vigorously before use, and be careful not to spray it into your eyes, since essential oils can irritate them.

For maximum benefit, you should mist while wearing a moisturizer that contains humectants. "Humectants attract and hold water," says Loughran, "so if you mist while they're on your face, your skin will continue to receive moisture throughout the day."

Mist a minimum of three times a day: in the morning, at noon, and in the evening. Since misting is so good for wrinkled, aging skin, however, feel free to mist as often as possible, she says.

## AROMATHERAPY: *A Toner for Sagging Skin*

For a toner that firms and enlivens sagging skin, combine one drop each of essential oils of neroli and everlasting in 1 ounce of evening primrose oil or borage oil, says Barbara Close, an aromatherapist and herbalist in East Hampton, New York. Put the mixture on a cotton pad and wipe your face with it after your cleansing routine.

These essential oils are believed to help skin regenerate, and evening primrose and borage oils are rich in gamma-linolenic acid (GLA), one of the fatty acids involved in collagen production.

## MASSAGE: *To Ease Forehead Lines*

You can help reduce the lines on your forehead with a gentle massage from Ayurveda, the ancient system of natural healing from India, says Pratima Raichur, an Ayurvedic practitioner in New York City. Use a massage oil containing four essential oils that nourish, soothe, and energize the skin, she says.

To a base of 1 ounce of sesame or almond oil, add two drops

each of sandalwood and geranium essential oils and one drop each of lemon and cardamom oils.

"With your fingers, gently massage your forehead, using horizontal strokes," she says. Do this once a day for 3 to 4 minutes.

## MASSAGE: *Reduce Crow's-Feet*

Here's a technique from Traditional Chinese Medicine that tones the entire eye area and helps to prevent and eliminate crow's-feet, Loughran says.

Apply a small amount of moisturizer or massage oil to the area around your eyes so that your fingertips will slide easily without pulling the skin. Next, using the middle finger of each hand, massage around both eyes simultaneously. Starting at the inner part of your eyebrows, use slight pressure as you glide over the eyebrows toward your temples and underneath the eyes along the bones. Circle the eyes 30 times. Use this massage once a day.

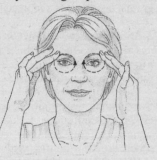

## LIFESTYLE: *It Makes All the Difference*

Lifestyle is the major determinant of how you wrinkle as you age, says Loughran.

"What you do for your overall health from day to day will prevent or reduce wrinkling much more than anything you do directly to your skin," she says. Here are five key factors.

• Avoid overexposure to sunlight. "The sun breaks down the collagen and elastin in your skin, causing wrinkles," says Loughran. When you're out and about, wear a hat and a chemical-free sunscreen (made with titanium dioxide or zinc oxide) that has an SPF of 15 or higher. Then wash it off when you're not in the sun.
• Don't smoke, since cigarette smoking deprives your skin of oxygen and nutrients. Even the act of smoking can cause lines around the corners of your mouth and vertical lines in your upper lip.

• Choose cleansing lotions instead of soap. Soap or any other product that foams up and makes your skin feel squeaky clean strips your skin of natural oils and ages it prematurely, says Loughran.

• Limit coffee and alcohol to one cup or drink a day. More than that can rob your body of water and nutrients, which in turn can age and wrinkle your skin. For some people, even those small amounts may be too much.

• Eat naturally. "I believe that the further away from natural foods your diet gets, the worse it is for your skin," Loughran says. Emphasize whole foods such as vegetables, fruits, grains, beans, nuts and seeds, fish, and low-fat dairy products.

## MASSAGE: *The "Big Washing Face Massage"*

This technique can help prevent wrinkles, Loughran says. First, wash and dry your hands. Then, rub your hands together rapidly 36 times to put chi, or energy, on your palms.

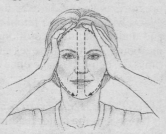

Move your hands over your face in an upward motion, covering your entire face, including your ears. Your hands should touch the skin gently, without pulling. Move each hand in a circle, beginning at the chin and moving up alongside the nose, over the eyes to the forehead, along the hairline, over the ears, and back to the chin again. Do this circular motion 36 times. Do the technique every day as part of your skin care routine.

### Part 2

# Alternative Healing At-a-Glance

# Acupressure

## WHAT IS IT?

Acupressure is a branch of Traditional Chinese Medicine, which also includes acupuncture, herbal therapy, and other modalities. The goal of acupressure is to balance chi, the flow of life-energy that travels throughout the body.

## HOW DOES IT WORK?

Chi normally flows along specific paths in the body called meridians, which are like roads. The chi travels along these roads to major organ systems such as the lungs, heart, and liver. When chi flows freely along the meridians, there is health. When it is blocked or stagnant, there is disease.

It's possible to alter the flow of chi by pressing points on the skin called acupoints, which are located along the body's meridians. Acupressure involves pressing and rubbing these points with the fingers. This helps to restore the free flow of chi, not only in those specific areas but also within organs that are "controlled" by those meridians. (In acupuncture, a practitioner stimulates the acupoints with needles.)

## WHAT CAN IT DO FOR YOU?

Acupressure is considered particularly effective for treating problems with the soft tissues, such as the muscles, tendons, and ligaments. It's also good for back pain, joint problems such as arthritis, and gynecological problems.

You can buy mechanical devices that are designed to stimulate the body's acupoints. Most professional acupuncturists believe the devices are unnecessary, however, and that you'll get better results with genuine hands-on attention. When looking for a practitioner, it's best to find someone who has been certified by a national organization.

## IS IT SAFE?

Since acupressure isn't an invasive technique, it's extremely safe for most conditions. There are times, however, when it shouldn't be used.

Pregnant women should not have acupressure unless it's performed by a licensed practitioner, as pressing certain acupoints can stimulate uterine contractions.

Although acupressure is thought to be highly beneficial to those with cancer, it should not be administered on or near a tumor because stimulating acupoints there can cause cancer cells to spread in the bloodstream.

It should not be used in areas where there's been a recent injury, sore, or skin ulcer or where there is a prolapsed or varicose vein.

It should not be used by or on anyone who has had a stroke within the past 30 days, since pressing certain acupoints can trigger brain activity that may be harmful to people who have recently had strokes.

Finally, acupressure should never be the sole treatment for any serious medical condition. Rather, it should always be used as a supportive therapy.

# Affirmations

## WHAT ARE THEY?

An affirmation is simply an upbeat, snappy statement or phrase that conveys a desire that you want to realize. Common affirmations include statements such as "I'm going to have a wonderful day today" or "I am prosperous" or "I am healthy."

## HOW DO THEY WORK?

The goal of creating and repeating affirmations is to "reprogram" your mind. Repeating affirmations several times a day will allow you to replace common but self-destructive ways of thinking with ideas that are positive and constructive.

The key to making affirmations successful is to practice them consistently for at least 2 to 3 weeks. That's about how long it takes to form new mental habits.

There are many ways to use affirmations. You can write them on cards or slips of paper, for example, and carry them with you all the time. Then you can periodically take out your positive notes and read them, either silently or out loud. Many people like to post their affirmations in places where they'll see them all the time, such as on the refrigerator, for example, or on the bathroom mirror. Some people even record their affirmations and listen to them whenever they need a little lift.

## WHAT CAN THEY DO FOR YOU?

Affirmations can be used for any health problem. People who are ill often spend a lot of time thinking about their illness and how uncomfortable they feel. After a while, they start *expecting* to be ill. With affirmations, you can replace these negative thoughts with positive ones. For example, you might repeat to yourself, "I am happy and healthy," "I am well," "I feel healthy," "I feel strong," "My body is vibrantly healthy," "All the cells in my body are healthy," or "I am healed." Replacing negative thoughts with positive ones can actually help the body combat illness.

Affirmations aren't used only for physical problems, of course. You can use them to achieve any goal. Maybe you want to be more prosperous, or perhaps you want to succeed at work or have better relationships. Affirmations can help you achieve these goals.

## ARE THEY SAFE?

Since affirmations are nothing more than positive thoughts, their effects can only be beneficial. The one exception might be for those who have some form of mental illness, such as schizophrenia or a manic-depressive condition. For them, affirmations may cause additional problems.

# Aromatherapy

## WHAT IS IT?

Aromatherapy is the use of aromas for physical, mental, and emotional healing. The primary sources of healing aromas are essential oils distilled from herbs and flowers.

## HOW DOES IT WORK?

Essential oils are volatile, which means that their molecules quickly evaporate into the environment. When you inhale an essential oil molecule, its unique tapestry of active components reacts with the olfactory membranes in your nose, which is directly linked to the limbic system and hypothalamus in the brain. These two areas play a crucial role in regulating your emotions, mind, and body.

You can also apply certain essential oils directly to the skin. This is doubly effective, since the oil is not only inhaled but also absorbed into your bloodstream.

Like gems or wines, essential oils vary tremendously in cost, depending on their availability and the methods necessary to produce them. An ounce of lavender oil might cost $5 and a half-ounce of rose oil, $250. An initial supply of the most useful therapeutic oils—the types of oils included in the remedies in this book—is approximately $80, and it can last for years.

A diffuser—the device used to disperse the oil into the air—can be very inexpensive. Basic atomizers work fine. An aromatherapy pottery ring that fits over a lightbulb costs about $5.

## WHAT CAN IT DO FOR YOU?

Aromatherapy is particularly useful for digestive complaints; skin problems (including burns); infections; stress and emotional upset; hormone imbalances, particularly in menopausal women; and respiratory complaints (with the exception of asthma).

You can also use essential oils around the house as natural air fresheners and as ingredients in cleansers.

## IS IT SAFE?

Essential oils are extremely potent—much more so than dried herbs—and most cannot be applied to the skin undiluted. Read the package directions. If the label says that you can use the oil on your skin, follow any instructions for diluting it, then test cautiously to see if you are sensitive to it. Put a drop of oil on a cotton ball, wipe it on the inside crease of your elbow, and close your arm for 5 minutes. If, after that time, you notice a stinging sensation or there is redness where you applied the oil, do not use it.

Women should not use essential oils during the first 3 months of pregnancy, since many oils contain thujone, a chemical that has been shown to have an abortive action.

# Ayurvedic Medicine

## WHAT IS IT?

Ayurveda is an ancient system of natural and medical healing that originated in India. *Ayur* means "life," and *veda* means "science." Ayurveda, then, is the science of life—a total approach to health, healing, and longevity. It includes a wide range of modalities, such as the use of diet, herbs, massage, purification regimens, exercise, music therapy, aromatherapy, color therapy, meditation, yoga, and astrology, among others.

## HOW DOES IT WORK?

According to Ayurveda, everything in nature—the body, foods, the seasons, the time of day, and even colors and music—is composed of five elements. They are space, air, fire, water, and earth.

Ayurvedic practitioners group these five elements into three categories, or doshas. The doshas are vata, or space and air; pitta, or fire and water; and kapha, or earth and water. Practitioners believe that disease is caused by an excess of one or more of these elements. Someone with a cold, for example, might be found to have an excess of kapha. Heartburn, on the other hand, is an excess of pitta.

The treatments in Ayurvedic medicine are aimed at restoring balance by decreasing excessive elements and increasing the others. Someone with a cold might be given a fiery herb such as garlic and instructed to stop consuming kapha-producing dairy products.

Ayurveda emphasizes the psychological, social, and spiritual causes of disease. Practitioners believe that almost all illnesses are based in unhappiness, usually in the form of stress and confusion about life's purpose. Many of the techniques of Ayurveda, such as meditation, are aimed at relieving stress and restoring clarity of purpose.

When choosing a practitioner, look for someone who has received extensive training at an Ayurvedic school in the United States or India and who is qualified to do "pulse diagnosis." The practitioner should provide extensive lifestyle recommendations along with herbal treatments.

## WHAT CAN IT DO FOR YOU?

Ayurveda can be used for any health problem, but it seems to be uniquely effective for treating problems that Western medicine has difficulty solving. Conditions that may be effectively treated with this healing system include diabetes, arthritis, anemia, allergies, and other problems involving the immune system.

## IS IT SAFE?

Since it's a natural approach to health, Ayurveda is generally safe. Some Ayurvedic techniques may be harmful, however, when used without proper supervision. It's best to use Ayurvedic herbs and techniques only under the care of a qualified practitioner.

# Breath Therapy

## WHAT IS IT?

Also called breath work, breath therapy incorporates a variety of techniques to help us breathe in a freer, more natural, and healthier way. Breath therapy not only supports our overall health and well-being, it can also be used to help specific physical and emotional problems. It's based on the principle that most adults tend to breathe in unnatural, constricted ways and that such breathing has a negative influence on almost every aspect of our lives. Learning proper, unrestricted breathing is a natural way to achieve better health.

## HOW DOES IT WORK?

Proper breathing supports our health in many ways. It efficiently oxygenates tissues and energizes the body, calms and balances the nervous system, massages and helps cleanse our internal organs, improves lymphatic circulation and helps remove wastes from the body's cells, and helps us release our negative emotions and experiences.

Breath therapy works by helping our breathing find its natural harmony and coordination in relation to the changing demands of our lives. Although there are many approaches to breath therapy, one of the most fundamental is breath awareness. Through breath awareness techniques, you learn to observe the restrictions and imbalances in your breathing. Without this awareness, many breathing therapy techniques fall far short of their potential and may even make problems worse.

Another important approach is focused breathing, in which you consciously "direct" each breath into a particular part of the body for healing. Still another is controlled breathing (called pranayama in yoga). Here, different breathing techniques, including fast breaths and breath holding, are used not only to assist physical, mental, and emotional health but also to aid in spiritual development.

In addition, there are a variety of breathing therapy approaches that are used in combination with other healing modalities. In movement-supported breathing, you move in ways that can stimulate new, healthier patterns of breathing, and in touch-supported breathing, you use touch or pressure to help focus your breaths and reduce any restrictions or tensions that inhibit your breaths. In posture-supported breathing, you use certain postures to expand your breaths and support fuller breathing. In sound-supported breathing, you utter sounds that can help lengthen your exhalations, strengthen your diaphragm, and release unnecessary tension.

The best way to learn is to find a competent breath therapist, teacher, or coach. There are also many good alternative practitioners who use breath therapy as part of their treatment programs.

## WHAT CAN IT DO FOR YOU?

Breath therapy is great for stress reduction, pain relief, and relaxation. It can help us maintain our health and live longer, healthier, more vital lives. It is useful for people with respiratory disorders such as asthma, chronic bronchitis, and emphysema. Breath therapy is also thought to help heal (and prevent) a variety of stress-related conditions, such as headaches, insomnia, digestive problems, back pain, high blood pressure, immune system disorders, heart disease, anxiety, depression, and fatigue.

## IS IT SAFE?

Although most simple types of breath therapy can safely be done at home without professional supervision, it is sensible to get the help of a qualified practitioner for more advanced breath work. Breath-control exercises involving breath holding and fast breathing, for example, can weaken and disharmonize your breathing unless they're done properly under a professional's supervision.

It's important to remember that if any breathing exercise makes you feel more tense or uncomfortable instead of more relaxed, you should stop doing it. It probably won't do you any good, and it may cause harm. Also, if you've had recent surgery, be sure to wait until you've healed before beginning breath work that might affect the area of your surgery.

# Energy Healing

## WHAT IS IT?

There is a fundamental energy that permeates and animates our bodies and minds. This energy has different names in different traditions: *chi* in China, *ki* in Japan, *prana* in India, *mana* in Hawaii, *wakan* among the Lakota Indians, and *bio-energy* among Western healers who (unlike most Western scientists) acknowledge this subtle but universal phenomenon. Energy healing involves directing and intensifying this life-force energy to make the body stronger.

## HOW DOES IT WORK?

Different cultures have a variety of explanations for how energy healing works. In Traditional Chinese Medicine, it is thought that energy healing removes blockages in meridians, the energy pathways that run through the body. Some healers believe that the technique works by balancing and stabilizing chakras, a series of energy centers in the body that roughly correspond to the endocrine glands. Other healers believe that energy healing is nothing less than the force of God.

Some scientists believe that energy healing works through *resonance* and *entrainment*. According to this theory, things (or people) in close proximity to each other actually resonate together. This would explain, for example, why disembodied animal hearts, when kept alive in a lab and placed near each other, entrain—that is, the individual hearts begin to beat in unison. On a more familiar level, people often feel sad or happy when a person nearby is feeling sad or happy.

In energy healing, a practitioner uses his hands to set up a high-vibration energy field. The person receiving the therapy then begins to resonate and entrain in response to that energy. It is not the practitioner who is doing the healing, however. Rather, when the body is provided with additional life-energy, it naturally heals itself according to its own miraculous and spontaneous wisdom.

## WHAT CAN IT DO FOR YOU?

Energy healing is uniquely effective for relieving pain, especially back and neck pain. It appears to work well for treating internal problems, such as those in the glands, organs, and various systems of the body. It's also particularly well suited for treating psychological and spiritual problems—by turning distressed emotions into gratitude and joy, for example.

## IS IT SAFE?

People who practice energy healing need to be careful that they don't absorb someone else's low energy state. Apart from this, energy healing is entirely safe, although some healers won't work on people who have had organ transplants or are taking medications to suppress immunity. This is because energy healing is thought to boost immunity, which could be counterproductive to the medical treatments.

When you first meet with an energy healer, it's worth asking how he feels at the end of the day. If he says he is happy and energized, he is probably effective. If, on the other hand, he says that he feels drained and that he suffers for the good of his clients, he probably isn't effective.

# Flower Essences

## WHAT ARE THEY?

Flower essences are liquid extracts prepared from wildflowers or garden blossoms. Flowers have been used for healing since ancient times, but a complete system of flower healing was developed by an English physician, Dr. Edward Bach, in the 1930s.

## HOW DO THEY WORK?

When flower essences are prepared, the specific energy pattern of each flower is transferred to the extract. This unique energy pattern has the ability to affect the energy of the person who takes the essence. Flower essences calm and balance the mind and emotions. They bring awareness of your "soul patterns," revealing new possibilities for creativity and emotional, mental, and physical growth.

This phenomenon is similar to hearing a particularly moving piece of music. Just as the sound waves awaken an experience within us that's similar to the emotions felt by the composer, the energy patterns of the flower awaken a healing and emotionally fulfilling type of energy.

## WHAT CAN THEY DO FOR YOU?

Flower essences are often used to calm, stabilize, and energize—when a person is under stress, for example, or is in a situation of intense suffering. The essences help bring awareness. They may be used to help resolve mental and emotional problems that are causing physical illness. They can also "unblock" problems that are interfering with the full expression of human potential.

Imagine, for example, a mother who is always yelling at her children. Flower essences can help her understand why she responds that way and also give her the ability to choose more constructive (and more effective) responses.

Flower essences are often used to help people uncover entirely new parts of their personalities. The proper flower essence might help someone discover previously unrealized artistic potential, for example.

The essences are frequently used as a type of preventive medicine because they help create positive emotional states. Someone who often feels cynical around the holidays, for example, might feel more loving after using a flower essence.

## ARE THEY SAFE?

It's impossible to take an overdose of flower essences, and they don't cause side effects. They do, however, intensify the mind and emotions at first. People need to be aware that their emotions may be heightened for several days after starting to use a new essence.

# Herbal Therapy

## WHAT IS IT?

Herbal therapy is the use of medicinal plants for health and healing. It is one of the oldest forms of what is now called alternative medicine.

## HOW DOES IT WORK?

Plants contain a variety of chemicals that are beneficial to health. In fact, a large number of modern drugs contain compounds that were originally found in plants. Consider saponins. Found in many plants, these compounds break down excess mucus and improve elimination from the bowels. Other common compounds, called tannins, can slow bleeding from wounds, and some are now known to have antimicrobial properties.

Medicinal herbs can be taken in many forms. One of the most common is herbal tea. Another preparation, a tincture, is a concentrated liquid extract of the herb. There are also herbal tablets and capsules, fresh herbs as food, and, for external use, poultices, compresses, creams, and salves. External preparations often utilize essential oils.

## WHAT CAN IT DO FOR YOU?

Medicinal herbs can be taken for any condition, but they're often used in mainstream culture as a supportive treatment, taken in combination with other types of conventional or alternative care. Herbs can reduce the side effects of certain medications, for example. But while some herbal and nutritional treatments interact beneficially with prescription drugs, others have negative interactions.

Herbal therapy is often recommended for treating chronic conditions such as cardiovascular disease, diabetes, memory

problems, and arthritis. It's also helpful for acute illnesses such
as colds and for healing skin, muscle, or other problems.

## IS IT SAFE?
Just because herbs are natural does not mean that they are always safe. While some people may assume that if a little bit of
an herb is good, more must be better, the fact is that large doses
of herbs may cause problems. Ginkgo, for example, has been
shown to improve memory by affecting circulation, but large
doses of the herb may cause problems for an elderly or sensitive person who is taking a blood-thinning medication at the
same time. For maximum safety, herbs should be used under
the guidance of a qualified herbal practitioner.

# Homeopathy

## WHAT IS IT?
Homeopathy is a system of alternative medicine that was developed in the 1800s by the German doctor Samuel Hahnemann.
This system of medicine is based on an ancient principle called
the Law of Similars. The essence of this "law" is that any substance that can produce symptoms of disease in a healthy person
can help someone who is ill and has the same symptoms.

Homeopathic medicines (or remedies) are FDA-approved
and derived from many natural sources, including plants, metals, and minerals. These substances are used in diluted forms—
so diluted, in fact, that in some cases, there is not a single
molecule of the original substance remaining. Paradoxically,
the strength of the medicines depends on the dilution: The more
dilute the remedy, the more powerful it is.

## HOW DOES IT WORK?
Homeopathy is used worldwide because it clearly works.
How it works, however, remains a mystery. One theory is that

the unique method of diluting the remedies imprints the "energy pattern" of the active ingredient onto the water being used to dilute it. It's thought that this energy pattern can stimulate the body's self-healing energy.

## WHAT CAN IT DO FOR YOU?

Homeopathy can be used for virtually any condition, including acute problems ranging from sudden back pain to infections such as colds and flu. Homeopathy is also effective for digestive problems and for treating minor injuries requiring first aid, such as insect bites or mild burns, sprains, or bruises.

When used under professional supervision, homeopathy is equally effective for treating chronic conditions such as heart disease, arthritis, diabetes, allergies, or long-standing emotional problems such as depression. To be effective for serious conditions, however, homeopathic remedies must be tailored to the individual by a trained practitioner. You really can't treat these problems on your own.

## IS IT SAFE?

Homeopathic medicines are completely nontoxic. They can be safely given to children and used by pregnant women and the elderly. If you are using homeopathy for home health care, however, there are some guidelines that you need to follow.

Always check with your primary health care provider to be sure that your condition does not require immediate medical attention. Take the remedies one at a time, as combining remedies reduces their effectiveness. Be sure to follow dosage instructions carefully, and stop taking the remedy as soon as you see improvement because, in rare cases, taking too much of a remedy may make symptoms worse. If symptoms persist after self-treatment, see a professional homeopath or your health care practitioner. Finally, never treat chronic, serious conditions without professional supervision.

# Hydrotherapy

## WHAT IS IT?

The prefix *hydro* means "water," and hydrotherapy is a technique in which water is applied to the body in order to stimulate and redirect the flow of blood and lymph. (Lymph is the filtered portion of blood that carries waste products away from the cells. There is three times more lymph in the body than blood.) By encouraging the flow of fresh blood and lymph to an area, hydrotherapy helps nourish cells and promote the regeneration of tissues, which allows the body to heal from illnesses or physical damage.

## HOW DOES IT WORK?

Water is the most efficient vehicle for transporting heat and cold. The application of warm or hot water causes arteries and veins to expand, bringing additional blood and lymph to an area. Cold, on the other hand, makes the arteries and veins constrict, which pushes blood and lymph away. This in-and-out movement of blood and lymph brings in fresh oxygen and nutrients and removes toxins and waste products.

There are many techniques for using hydrotherapy. It may involve the use of showers, baths, water-soaked towels, water-soaked sheets, and other methods.

Some people use hydrotherapy as a preventive. Taking a daily shower in which you alternate hot and cold water along the spine, for example, will help stimulate the nervous system. This in turn triggers improved circulation to the abdomen, lungs, and heart.

## WHAT CAN IT DO FOR YOU?

Almost all diseases can be helped by hydrotherapy because many diseases involve inflammation, infection, or both. The application of hot and cold water improves circulation, which is essential for relieving infection and inflammation. Naturopathic physicians, who are trained in hydrotherapy, think that most health care professionals greatly underestimate the importance of improving circulation as a way of healing disease.

## IS IT SAFE?

Since hydrotherapy involves nothing more than applications of water, it's safe for most people. Those who have reduced sensation in their limbs (a common symptom of diabetes), however, should not use this therapy. Since people with this problem may be unable to tell when applications of heat are too hot, there is increased possibility of burns.

When using hydrotherapy, it's important not to end the treatment when you're chilled; this can make the illness worse. You should always end a session when you're feeling warm.

# Magnet Therapy

## WHAT IS IT?

Each cell in your body has an electrical charge that produces a magnetic field. Applying a magnetic field to the body to achieve a healing effect, either by putting a so-called permanent magnet (similar to a refrigerator magnet) on your skin or by treatment with a medical device that emits an electromagnetic field, is magnet therapy.

## HOW DOES IT WORK?

No one knows for sure. It may be that the magnetic field affects the movement of ions, the positively and negatively charged particles that constantly move in and out of cells. It may be that placing a permanent magnet on certain areas increases the body's production of painkilling chemicals called endorphins. Scientists do know, however, that some oft-repeated popular explanations for the potency of magnet therapy are incorrect. Magnets do not work, for example, by affecting the iron in hemoglobin, the molecules that carry oxygen throughout the body, nor do they improve circulation in the areas over which they're placed.

## WHAT CAN IT DO FOR YOU?

Applying a permanent magnet can relieve pain, reduce inflammation, and speed the healing of bones and injured soft tissues (muscles, ligaments, and tendons). Permanent magnets are applied directly in bandagelike devices that cover large or small areas of the body, in mattresses, in shoe insoles, and many other forms. They are used for back, neck, and shoulder pain; carpal tunnel syndrome; arthritis; headaches; postsurgical pain; fibromyalgia; sprains, fractures, and other muscle and bone injuries; and diabetic neuropathy, among other types of pain problems. Medical devices that emit electromagnetic fields are used for the same conditions as well as for insomnia, drug addiction, depression, anxiety, high blood pressure, osteoporosis, glaucoma, and neurological disorders such as Parkinson's disease, Alzheimer's disease, and epilepsy.

## IS IT SAFE?

Doctors who are familiar with magnet therapy say that it is safe and that trying out a permanent magnet on your own is virtually risk-free. It's theoretically possible that magnets could harm a pregnant woman or someone who has a pacemaker or other implanted electrical device; those individuals should talk with a doctor before using this therapy.

# Massage Therapy

## WHAT IS IT?

Massage therapy is a technique in which muscles and other soft tissues are pressed, rubbed, and otherwise manipulated. There are several forms of massage. Swedish massage, for example, is a gentle form of muscular manipulation that's used primarily for relaxation and stress relief. Clinical massage therapy (which includes dozens of approaches) treats specific health problems.

## HOW DOES IT WORK?

Pain causes the nervous system to stimulate muscles to contract. The contractions cause more pain, which results in more contractions. Unless the pain-contraction cycle is interrupted, it's hard to find relief.

Massage is a way of breaking this cycle. It "persuades" muscles to relax and lengthen. It brings pain-relieving oxygen and blood to the muscles and may remove irritating waste materials. In addition, just being touched has a deeply relaxing and therapeutic effect on the body, although the mechanisms of this effect are not fully understood.

## WHAT CAN IT DO FOR YOU?

Massage therapy is effective for any type of pain in the body's soft tissues. This includes back, neck, and shoulder pain; headaches, which are often caused by tense muscles in the face and scalp or tightness and trigger points in the neck muscles; bursitis and tendinitis; repetitive strain injury; and sports injuries such as shin splints.

It's best if your therapist has experience in treating the kinds of health problems you're dealing with. Be cautious about therapists who guarantee results; it's unrealistic, and it may be a sign they aren't entirely trustworthy.

When looking at advertising for massage therapists, look for phrases such as *deep tissue massage, neuromuscular therapy, trigger point therapy*, and *myotherapy*. These are all types of clinical therapeutic massage that have been proven to be effective in relieving pain.

## IS IT SAFE?

Since massage therapy involves manipulating parts of the body, there's always the possibility that it will make things worse. If you have any type of pain, it's important to see a medical doctor before turning to massage. Also, massage should never be done on areas where there is extensive bruising or other kinds of tissue damage. If you are pregnant, have circulatory problems, or any unusual condition, get clearance from your physician before starting massage therapy. Always let your massage therapist know about your condition; most are trained to work conservatively in such situations.

# Movement Education

## WHAT IS IT?

Movement education is a general term that refers to a number of different techniques, such as Alexander Technique, Aston-Patterning, Feldenkrais Method, and Hellerwork.

What these techniques have in common is the use of physical movement (and sometimes deep massage and other methods) to help release stress from the body and expand your normal range of movement. Having a freer, more balanced body allows you to experience more of your natural potential for health, energy, and creativity.

## HOW DOES IT WORK?

A practitioner of movement education begins by observing your patterns of movement, including how you sit, stand, and walk. After that, you'll be taught specific exercises and skills that will help you to be more aware of your habitual physical patterns of tension and constriction. At the same time, these skills will give you more flexibility and balance. You'll find yourself moving in new, more comfortable ways.

A full movement education treatment usually requires a series of sessions over a period of weeks or months. After all, the habitual patterns of the body cannot be changed quickly.

## WHAT CAN IT DO FOR YOU?

Each type of movement education has a different philosophy. Practitioners of the Feldenkrais Method and the Alexander Technique say that their techniques are not therapies but learning processes that will help enhance your feelings of well-being. On the other hand, practitioners of Aston-Patterning offer their technique for specific physical problems, such as chronic pain or helping injuries heal.

Regardless of the technique, you want to find a movement therapist who is willing to tailor his approach to your specific needs, rather than someone who dogmatically insists on using a particular system of exercises on your body.

In general, movement education is used therapeutically for all kinds of muscle problems, such as back, neck, and shoulder pain; bursitis and tendinitis; and repetitive strain injury.

### IS IT SAFE?

Movement education is almost always safe because it's tailored to your individual needs, but you need to trust your intuition (and your common sense) when using it. If a movement feels wrong or causes pain, don't do it. If you've recently had a severe injury or illness, you may want to take time to heal completely before starting movement training sessions. Also, if you're pregnant or have a specific health problem such as high blood pressure, be sure to get your doctor's approval before beginning movement education.

# Music Therapy and Sound Healing

### WHAT ARE THEY?

Sound and music have been used in traditional cultures for thousands of years to promote healing on many levels of the body, mind, and spirit. Music therapy and sound healing are the two modern schools of thought that scientifically apply these ancient practices.

Music therapy, which is prescribed by board-certified music therapists, uses primarily western European classical music and live performance to effect positive psychological, physical, cognitive, or social changes. Sound healing, on the other hand, relies on rhythmic drumming, chanting, and recordings composed specifically to bring about a higher level of balance and self-healing.

## HOW DO THEY WORK?

The principle behind the therapeutic use of music and sound is quite simple. These techniques use certain sounds to induce a state of deep relaxation called the relaxation response. In this state, your breathing becomes deeper and slower, your heartbeat slows, your brain waves shift in frequency, your muscles relax, and your circulation works more efficiently. These responses are exactly the opposite of those caused by stress. Thus, music therapy and sound healing can be effective choices to help the body resist stress-related health conditions.

Certain sounds and types of music stimulate the relaxation response because of a scientific phenomenon known as rhythm entrainment. What happens is that your heart spontaneously changes its rhythm to correspond with the rhythm of the music or sounds you're listening to. This is why fast music is generally not therapeutic.

In some cases, the therapy utilizes sounds that don't have an expected melody or rhythmic pattern. (This is particularly true of various types of New Age music.) Because there is no anticipated pattern, your analytical mind essentially shuts down, creating a deep sense of relaxation because you're able to enjoy the sounds or music without trying to analyze them.

## WHAT CAN THEY DO FOR YOU?

Because they promote deep relaxation, these therapies may be useful for stress-related conditions, including muscle pain, tension headaches, high blood pressure, insomnia, depression, anxiety, and fatigue. While there is a great deal of evidence supporting the use of music and sound to encourage relaxation, however, it is too early to prescribe these therapies to heal specific illnesses, and legitimate practitioners in these fields never make such claims.

## ARE THEY SAFE?

According to the principle of entrainment, listening to rap, heavy metal, or other types of music with heavy, rapid beats could cause the heart to speed up, creating additional stress on the mind and body. It's fine to enjoy these types of music, but they are definitely not therapeutic. In fact, you may want to avoid them at times when stress is a serious factor in your life.

# Naturopathic Medicine

**WHAT IS IT?**

Also called naturopathy, naturopathic medicine is a very broad system of scientifically based healing. It emphasizes disease prevention and wellness and incorporates a wide range of alternative or traditional techniques.

Naturopathic physicians (N.D.'s) attend 4-year naturopathic medical schools before being licensed. The techniques they use in their practices include (but are not limited to) nutritional therapy, herbal medicine, homeopathy, Traditional Chinese Medicine, and many types of physical therapies.

**HOW DOES IT WORK?**

Naturopathic physicians believe that the body is a self-regulating mechanism that has the natural ability to maintain a state of homeostasis, or balance. When people are ill, naturopaths attempt to restore or enhance homeostasis. They do this by supplying the body with what it needs for optimal functioning, such as dietary supplements, herbal remedies, and other natural medicines. Once the body is back in balance, it has the ability to better resist disease and maintain a state of health and wellness.

This approach is very different from that used by conventional, or allopathic, physicians. The goal of conventional medicine is generally to suppress or eliminate disease by using drugs or surgery. Naturopathic physicians believe the conventional approach actually may interfere with the body's natural ability to heal. While allopathic techniques can suppress symptoms in the short run, they may actually weaken the body over time.

**WHAT CAN IT DO FOR YOU?**

Since naturopathy is a complete healing system, it's well-suited for treating virtually every type of illness. Many naturopathic physicians believe that it's best used in partnership with allopathic medicine. Conventional techniques are uniquely effective for treating acute and emergency situations, such as a heart attack. Naturopathy, on the other hand, is well-suited for providing long-term protection. Thus, the two approaches naturally complement each other.

Suppose, for example, that you're about to undergo surgery. The techniques used in naturopathy can help ease the pain and discomfort of the surgery, reduce the length of your hospital stay, shorten your postoperative recovery time, and generally improve the outcome of the surgery.

## IS IT SAFE?

Licensed naturopathic physicians undergo extensive postgraduate training at accredited naturopathic medical schools; they are trained diagnosticians and primary care providers. They know the strengths and limitations of their approach, and they don't hesitate to recommend conventional intervention when it's appropriate.

Keep in mind, however, that some practitioners who call themselves N.D.'s may have received their "degrees" from mail-order organizations. They are not scientifically trained, licensed physicians.

# Qigong

## WHAT IS IT?

Qigong is one aspect of Traditional Chinese Medicine. The name comes from the Chinese word for vitality, or life force, and also the word meaning to practice, cultivate, or refine. Qigong, then, is the practice of cultivating your life force or vital energy. It typically involves the use of gentle exercises that combine physical movements, deep breathing, and mental focus directed at certain parts of the body.

## HOW DOES IT WORK?

When practicing qigong, you breathe deeply and direct attention to various parts of the body. This process increases the strength and energy in vital organs and the blood. It oxygenates tissues and opens up the body's meridians, the pathways that carry energy throughout the body. It also balances yin and yang, which are the contracting and expanding energies within the body.

In the simplest qigong exercise, you sit in a relaxed but erect posture. You close your eyes, concentrate your mind on your abdomen, and consciously feel your breath flow in and out of your nostrils. This exercise stimulates the "Lower Tan Tian point," a potent center of healing energy in the body.

Some exercises involve moving the arms, while others are performed in a stationary position. The arm exercises stimulate and open the meridians—typically those affecting the lungs, large intestine, small intestine, and heart—that flow through these areas. This helps to increase and balance energy within these meridians, promoting vitality in these organs.

The best way to learn qigong is by using a video or working with a teacher, which allows you to actually see how the routines flow and progress. A teacher (whether in real life or in a video) should be someone who has learned qigong from a "master" and who is practicing within a "lineage," a traditional school of qigong. One of the best clues is appearance: The teacher should appear to be balanced, calm, and full of energy and clarity.

## WHAT CAN IT DO FOR YOU?

Many exercises in qigong are specifically therapeutic—that is, they're designed to affect certain parts of the body, such as the heart or the digestive, respiratory, or reproductive system. Others are not organ- or condition-specific; they're designed to have an overall effect on the body, rejuvenating energy and preventing illness.

## IS IT SAFE?

In general, qigong is very safe. If you are pregnant or have a chronic health problem of any kind, however, be sure to consult a medical, osteopathic, or naturopathic doctor before doing the routines on your own. Also, you should always do qigong at your own pace. Never do an exercise that you feel is too strenuous.

# Reflexology

## WHAT IS IT?

This field of therapy uses specific touch techniques to stimulate "reflex points and areas" on the feet, hands, and ears. Reflexologists believe that each of these points corresponds to a specific part of the body. (The toes, fingers, and earlobes, for example, correspond to the head.) By using touch techniques on these areas, you can apply reflexology to yourself or receive it during a session with a trained reflexologist. Either way, it can help maintain or improve the health of corresponding areas in the body.

## HOW DOES IT WORK?

There are many theories about how reflexology works, but none has been scientifically proven. The most likely explanation is that using reflexology on the feet, hands, or ears stimulates specific pathways of sensory nerves. The nerves then send messages to the brain, which in turn sends messages to the corresponding area of the body to produce relaxation. Reflexology improves blood flow and increases supplies of oxygen and nutrients to areas of the body, resulting in better health.

## WHAT CAN IT DO FOR YOU?

Reflexology is best suited for reducing the accumulation of stress in the body. This is an important benefit because stress has been found to cause or complicate a large percentage of all health problems.

Reflexology does more than reduce stress in common areas of accumulation, such as the neck, shoulders, and lower back. It also reduces stress inside the body, such as in the lungs, heart, kidneys, or entire intestinal tract.

Reflexology seems to be most effective in relieving muscular and skeletal pain in the jaw, shoulders, neck, back, and hips. It's also commonly used to help relieve conditions that are stress-related and involve the heart, lungs, digestive tract, and other organs.

## IS IT SAFE?

Reflexology is a gentle technique, so it's safe. There are situations, however, in which it shouldn't be used. You should never have reflexology on an area in which the skin is broken, there is infection, or a fracture is healing. If you've had reconstructive surgery of the feet, hands, or ears, you should not undergo reflexology in that area for at least 1 year after the surgery. Women who are in the first trimester of pregnancy should not have reflexology that stimulates the uterine points on the hands, feet, or ears. In general, it's best for pregnant women to receive reflexology that uses light, gentle pressure.

# Relaxation Therapy

## WHAT IS IT?

The goal of relaxation therapy is to induce the relaxation response—a calm, rested state of body and mind that relieves tension and stress. Since scientists have estimated that stress plays a role in a large percentage of health problems, relaxation therapy can be an integral part of treating and preventing disease.

Stress takes an emotional as well as a physical toll, and relaxation therapy is often used to help people cope more effectively with the inevitable difficulties and frustrations of life.

## HOW DOES IT WORK?

There are many methods of achieving the relaxation response. Deep breathing, for example, calms and balances the nervous system. Many therapists utilize mantras (meaningless phrases) or rhythmic, soothing words (such as *peace*). Repeating these words over and over again harmonizes the electrical activity of the brain, imparting a sense of calm and well-being.

Another form of relaxation therapy is progressive relaxation, which involves systematically tensing and relaxing muscle groups throughout the body. Then there is the technique called mindfulness, which involves giving peaceful attention and acceptance to whatever is happening at the moment. These techniques are typically done while sitting or lying in a comfortable, quiet place where you won't be disturbed.

In addition to the "quiet" forms of relaxation therapy, there are also more active forms. These include the stretching of yoga and the slow, gentle movements of the Chinese-based exercise called tai chi.

## WHAT CAN IT DO FOR YOU?

Relaxation therapy is best used for common stress-related complaints such as high blood pressure, insomnia, headaches, fatigue, arrhythmia (irregular heartbeat), digestive problems, allergies, skin disorders, anxiety, depression, and chronic anger or hostility.

## IS IT SAFE?

When you begin to practice relaxation therapy, you may find yourself even more anxious at first. This is because, with no external distractions such as television, you may become acutely aware of anxious thoughts and feelings.

If you're just starting out with relaxation therapy, you may want to choose a technique that is not meditative and is more body-based, like deep breathing or yoga.

People with a history of mental illness or mood disorders should not practice relaxation therapy without the approval and supervision of a practitioner who is trained in the various techniques.

# Traditional Chinese Medicine

## WHAT IS IT?

Unlike conventional Western medicine, which views disease as affecting certain parts of the body, Traditional Chinese Medicine (TCM) views it as a sign of imbalance in the whole person—the body, mind, and spirit. The goal of TCM is to restore balance and harmony, not only within the individual but also between the individual and the environment.

## HOW DOES IT WORK?

TCM is a complex system of healing that utilizes many different modalities to help restore balance. These techniques include dietary therapy, acupuncture (insertion of sterile needles into specific points on the body in order to control the flow of chi, or life-energy), moxibustion (burning an herb, called moxa, over acupuncture and other points), herbal medicine, and qigong (a combination of exercise and meditation).

Each technique that's used in TCM is meant to balance various systems in the body, mind, and spirit. These systems include chi, shen (spirit), the 12 organ systems, and the meridians, or channels of energy that connect the organ systems.

## WHAT CAN IT DO FOR YOU?

As a complete system of medicine, TCM can be used to treat any physical or emotional problem. It is thought to be particularly effective for chronic conditions that Western medicine is unable to reverse, such as heart disease and arthritis. It is considered effective for treating gynecological problems, such as menopausal and menstrual difficulties, and for relieving problems with the immune system, such as sinusitis and allergies. It's also used to treat chronic fatigue syndrome and fibromyalgia.

## IS IT SAFE?

Since TCM is generally practiced by licensed practitioners who have undergone years of training, it's an extremely safe system of healing. It's not a system that should be used without professional supervision, however.

Licensed TCM practitioners almost unanimously agree that people shouldn't use Chinese herbs on their own. Chinese herbal medicine utilizes thousands of herbs. Using the correct herbal prescriptions, which usually consist of customized formulas combining multiple herbs, requires getting an accurate diagnosis. And since these herbs, just like the drugs of Western medicine, have many limitations and possible side effects, TCM practitioners advise using them only with the supervision and approval of a trained practitioner.

# Visualization

## WHAT IS IT?

Imagine being on a beach, feeling the warm sun shining on your skin, hearing the slap of the waves, and smelling the salty tang of the breeze. You've just visualized—that is, you've pictured a mental reality, complete with sight, sound, touch, and smell.

Visualization is a technique for using the natural, image-making capacity of your mind in order to achieve desired life goals such as better health, stronger relationships, or more fulfilling personal growth.

## HOW DOES IT WORK?

When you create a strong mental image, neurons in your brain secrete chemicals. These chemicals literally change the nervous system, which in turn sends messages to all parts of your body, helping to improve mental and physical health.

Suppose you suffer from heartburn. You might create a mental image of a fire-breathing dragon. This image becomes a link between your mind and the problem that allows you to more easily release emotional tensions that may be causing or complicating the problem.

Visualizing the problem is just one approach. Some people create a healing image in response to the problem. In the case of heartburn, for example, you might visualize an even more powerful animal chasing away the "dragon." Or you might simply form a mental image of yourself in a wonderfully healthy state rather than focusing on how uncomfortable you feel.

For visualization to work, you have to do it many times, because you're training the nervous system to behave in a new way. Thus, you can't expect instant results; it may require weeks or months of practice.

## WHAT CAN IT DO FOR YOU?

You can use visualization to achieve virtually any goal. For physical problems, it seems to be most effective when it's used to combat muscle pain or problems with circulation or immunity. Allergies, for example, respond well to visualization.

## IS IT SAFE?

Since visualization requires deep relaxation, you don't want to practice this technique when you're driving or doing any other task that requires a lot of vigilance. In addition, since using visualization may decrease the need for medications for diabetes, high blood pressure, or depression, it's important to tell your doctor if you're using this technique. Finally, people with any serious mental illness should talk to a doctor before practicing visualization on their own.

# Vitamin and Mineral Therapy

## WHAT IS IT?

You may be getting your government-recommended three to five servings of fruits and vegetables a day and eating plenty of other good foods besides. But alternative practitioners agree: No matter how well you eat, you're likely to be deficient in certain key vitamins and minerals.

The problem is partly environmental, since the soil has been depleted of crucial nutrients by modern agricultural practices. As a result, fruits and vegetables don't have access to these nutrients as they did years ago, and they can't provide us with the same amount of vitamins and minerals. Stress also plays a role. All kinds of stress, whether physical, emotional, or mental, drains your body of nutrients.

By supplementing your diet with vitamins and minerals, it's possible to provide a kind of insurance that will help prevent disease. And when you're actually sick, taking additional nutrients can help relieve symptoms and speed healing.

## HOW DOES IT WORK?

Vitamins and minerals act as cofactors in thousands of cellular reactions inside your body. Each nutrient is like a key that opens biochemical doors. In small doses, nutritional supplements will help maintain these essential reactions. In larger doses, vitamins and minerals act as natural medications, optimizing your body's ability to heal itself.

## WHAT CAN IT DO FOR YOU?

There are very few health conditions that won't be helped by the appropriate vitamin and mineral therapy. Taking certain nutrients will help speed healing and prevent recurrences. Consider vitamin E, which has been shown to help relieve symptoms of angina, diabetes, intermittent claudication, menopausal discomfort, premenstrual syndrome, prostate problems, shingles, varicose veins, and many other health problems.

## IS IT SAFE?

Compared to medications, which almost always cause some side effects, vitamins and minerals are extremely safe. Nevertheless, there are many decisions that you'll need to make before using these nutrients therapeutically. Important considerations include the best form to take (capsules, tablets, liquid, or powder), the right dose for the best therapeutic effects, and the best daily nutritional supplements for maintaining health and preventing disease.

Vitamin and mineral therapy will provide the best (and safest) results when it's used under the supervision of a health professional. Experts in nutritional therapy include naturopathic physicians and nutritionally oriented, alternative-minded registered dietitians; M.D.'s and D.O.'s; and holistic healers who have had extensive experience using vitamins and minerals to treat disease.

# Yoga Therapy

## WHAT IS IT?

Yoga is an ancient and comprehensive form of spiritual self-discovery. In the broadest sense, yoga practitioners use physical and mental techniques to purify and vitalize the body and mind in order to open them to a type of universal reality. Yoga therapy is the art and science of healing according to yogic principles. It uses specific techniques designed as a form of therapeutic intervention specifically directed at an individual's interrelated systems for balance and harmony.

## HOW DOES IT WORK?

A yoga therapist begins by looking for physical, mental, and social-behavioral obstacles to your wellness. In order to restore balance, the therapist might recommend changes in your diet and behavior patterns, lifestyle, and social relationships. The therapist might also suggest physical postures (asanas) to develop balanced strength and flexibility, pranayama to optimize your flow of breath, and meditation or reflection to help focus your understanding of the source of tensions that contribute to your symptoms.

Regardless of which techniques are used, yoga therapy aims to calm the nervous system, which, optimally, helps to balance the body, mind, and emotions. This in turn helps to reduce or eliminate physical pain and mental and emotional suffering.

## WHAT CAN IT DO FOR YOU?

Yoga therapy can be very effective in treating all types of muscle and skeletal problems, such as neck and shoulder pain and various lower-back disorders. Yoga therapists also have been successful in helping to treat fibromyalgia, arthritis, high blood pressure, insomnia, diabetes, asthma, digestive problems, and many of the common complaints of aging.

Yoga therapy has the potential to relieve the discomfort caused by almost any health problem. The reason for this is that nearly all health problems are complicated by stress and tension, which are readily treated with yoga.

## IS IT SAFE?

Provided that any particular health concerns you may have are taken into consideration, yoga therapy should always be safe. For maximum safety, you should always work with a yoga therapist to learn the proper techniques for treating your specific problems.

The relationship between student and teacher is very important. You should seek the guidance of someone who has not only the experience but also, when appropriate, the specific knowledge base for your particular needs. The therapist should be trained in one of the established yogic traditions and should exemplify a lifestyle of balance and harmony in keeping with the moral and ethical aspects of yogic philosophy.

Yoga sessions should be offered with compassion and gentle guidance so you feel safe. In short, you want a therapist whom you can trust. It's the only way that you will be able to relax and feel confident with the therapy.

# Part 3

# Resources

# *An Illustrated Guide to* **Acupressure Points**

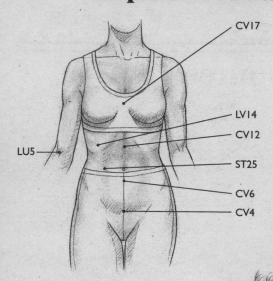

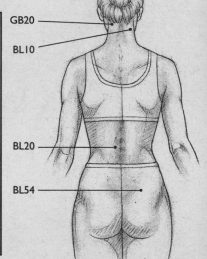

| Key | |
|---|---|
| BL | Bladder |
| CV | Conception vessel |
| GB | Gallbladder |
| GV | Governing vessel |
| HE | Heart |
| KI | Kidney |
| LI | Large intestine |
| LU | Lung |
| LV | Liver |
| PE | Pericardium |
| SI | Small intestine |
| SP | Spleen |
| ST | Stomach |
| TB | Triple burner |
| TW | Triple warmer |

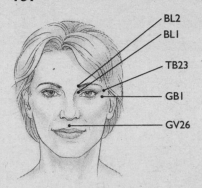

BL2
BL1
TB23
GB1
GV26

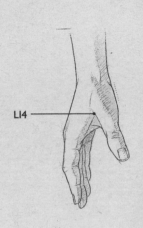

LI4

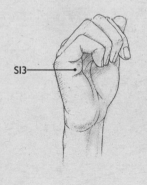

SI3

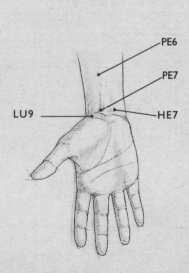

PE6
PE7
LU9
HE7

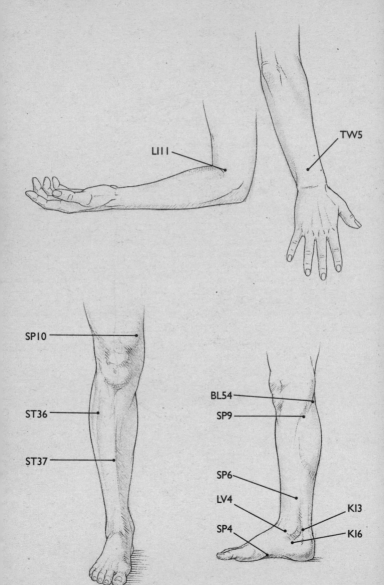

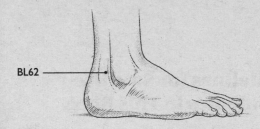

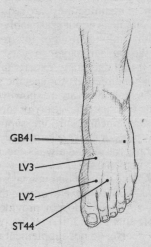

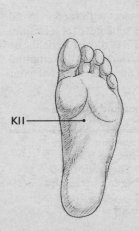

# Guidelines for Safe Use
# of Remedies in This Book

## EMERGING SUPPLEMENTS

Reports of adverse effects from emerging supplements are rare, especially when compared to prescription drugs, and supplement manufacturers are required by law to provide information on labels about reasonably safe recommended dosages for healthy individuals. For this reason, and because the potency and dosing strategy can vary significantly among products, you'll find that many experts in this book advise you to follow the label directions for specific supplements.

You should be aware, however, that little scientific research exists to assess the safety or long-term effects of many emerging supplements, and some supplements can complicate existing conditions or cause allergic reactions in some people. For these reasons, you should always check with your doctor before taking any supplements.

We recommend that you take supplements with food to avoid stomach irritation. Never take them as a substitute for a healthy diet, since they do not provide all the nutritional benefits of whole foods. And, if you are pregnant, nursing, or attempting to conceive, do not supplement without the supervision of your doctor.

| Supplement | Safe Use Guidelines and Possible Side Effects |
|---|---|
| Activated charcoal | If taken regularly over time, may interfere with absorption of nutrients or pose a risk of gastrointestinal obstruction. If taken within 2 hours of oral medications or other supplements, may interfere with their absorption. At high doses, may cause stomach upset, diarrhea, constipation, or vomiting. |

| Supplement | Safe Use Guidelines and Possible Side Effects |
|---|---|
| Adrenal extract | If you experience irritability, restlessness, and insomnia at the recommended dose, switch to a lower dose. |
| Alpha-lipoic acid | Experimental. Do not take more than 800 milligrams a day for a maximum of 4 months. Dosages of as much as 600 milligrams a day have been used for treatment of diabetic neuropathy with no serious side effects. |
| Arginine | Take only under the guidance of a knowledgeable medical doctor. High doses may cause nausea and diarrhea. Do not take if you have genital herpes; may increase herpes outbreaks. Do not take arginine and lysine at the same time, as they can over-balance each other. Long-term effects are unknown. |
| Beta glucans | Experimental. Possible risks are unknown, and more study is required. |
| Betaine hydrochloride | Use only if you have been diagnosed as having low stomach acid, and then only with medical supervision. If you experience heartburn, reduce the dosage. Do not take in combination with aspirin, ibuprofen, or other nonsteroidal anti-inflammatory drugs; the combination may increase the risk of developing an ulcer. |
| *Bifodobacterium bifidum* | *See Lactobacillus acidophilus* |
| Bromelain | May cause nausea, vomiting, diarrhea, skin rash, and heavy menstrual bleeding. May also increase the risk of bleeding in people taking aspirin or anticoagulants (blood thinners). Do not take if you are allergic to pineapple. |
| Carnitine | Take the "l" form only; the "d" form may displace the active form of carnitine in tissues and lead to muscle weakness. Doses above 2 grams may cause mild diarrhea. |

| Supplement | Safe Use Guidelines and Possible Side Effects |
| --- | --- |
| Choline | Daily doses exceeding 3.5 grams should be taken only under medical supervision. Excess choline can cause low blood pressure and a fishy body odor in some people. |
| Cod-liver oil | Use only under the supervision of a knowledgeable medical doctor. May be toxic in high amounts. |
| Coenzyme $Q_{10}$ | Supplementation for more than 20 days at a daily dose of 120 milligrams or more should be used only with medical supervision. Side effects are rare but may include heartburn, nausea, and stomachache, which can be prevented by taking the supplement with a meal. Rarely, a slight decrease in the effectiveness of the blood-thinning medication warfarin (Coumadin) has been reported. |
| Conjugated linoleic acid | Experimental. No side effects have been reported in animal studies. |
| Curcumin | May cause heartburn in some people. |
| Cysteine | If you have diabetes, check with your doctor before using supplements; may inactivate insulin. If supplementing for more than a few weeks, take with a multivitamin/mineral supplement that supplies the Daily Value of zinc and copper; may deplete these minerals. High doses may cause kidney stones in people who have cystinuria. |
| Dehydroepiandrosterone (DHEA) | Take only under the supervision of a physician such as an endocrinologist, who is familiar with the way hormones work in the body. May cause liver damage, acne, irritability, irregular heart rhythms, accelerated growth of existing tumors, altered hormone profiles, increased cancer risk (prostate in men and breast in women), hair loss in men and women, and growth of facial hair and deepening of the voice in women. Men and women under 35 should not take supplements, as they suppress the body's natural production of DHEA. |

| Supplement | Safe Use Guidelines and Possible Side Effects |
|---|---|
| Dimethylaminoethanol (DMAE) | Do not exceed the dosage recommended on the label. |
| d-phenylalanine | Experimental. Use only under the supervision of a qualified medical doctor; long-term effects are unknown. It is known that this supplement can raise blood pressure to dangerous levels, especially in people taking MAO inhibitors as antidepressants. Do not take if you have phenylketonuria. Large amounts decrease antioxidant levels, thereby encouraging disease. |
| Fatty acids | Do not take if you have a bleeding disorder, uncontrolled high blood pressure, or an allergy to any kind of fish, or if you are taking anticoagulants (blood thinners) or use aspirin regularly. Supplements increase bleeding time, possibly resulting in nosebleeds and easy bruising, and may cause upset stomach. |
| Fish oil | Do not take if you have a bleeding disorder, uncontrolled high blood pressure, or an allergy to any kind of fish, or if you are taking anticoagulants (blood thinners) or use aspirin regularly. If you have diabetes, check with your doctor before taking fish oil because of its high fat content. Increases bleeding time, possibly resulting in nosebleeds and easy bruising, and may cause upset stomach. (Do not take fish-liver oil; it is high in vitamins A and D, which can be toxic in high amounts.) |
| 5-hydroxytryptophan (5-HTP) | Experimental. May contain a contaminant called peak X, which may cause serious symptoms associated with eosinophilic myalgia syndrome (EMS). The following brands claim to perform tests confirming the absence of peak X: Natrol, Nature's Way, TriMedica, Country Life, and Solaray. Supplements are also reported to cause gastrointestinal distress, muscle pain, lethargy, and headaches. |

| Supplement | Safe Use Guidelines and Possible Side Effects |
|---|---|
| Glutamine | Do not take if you have end-stage liver failure or kidney failure. |
| Huperzine A | Use only under the supervision of a knowledgeable medical doctor. |
| Isoflavones | Safety of doses exceeding 100 milligrams a day is unknown. |
| Lactase | If allergic, do not take supplements derived from mold or fungus. Supplements made from bacteria are considered safe. |
| Lecithin | Doses exceeding 23 grams a day should be taken only with medical supervision. Doses close to 5 grams may cause upset stomach, nausea, and diarrhea. High doses may cause sweating, salivation, and loss of appetite. Some people report a fishy body odor after taking high daily doses. |
| *Lactobacillus acidophilus* | If you have any serious gastrointestinal problems that require medical attention, check with your doctor before supplementing. Amounts exceeding 10 billion viable organisms daily may cause mild gastrointestinal distress. If you are taking antibiotics, take them at least 2 hours before supplementing with lactobacillus. |
| Lutein | Do not exceed the dosage recommended on the label. Take with a meal to lessen the chance of stomach upset and to increase digestion and absorption. |
| Lysine | Experimental. Use only under the supervision of a knowledgeable medical doctor; long-term effects are unknown. Do not take arginine and lysine at the same time, as they can overbalance each other. |
| Melatonin | Use only under the supervision of a knowledgeable medical doctor; long-term effects are unknown. Causes drowsiness; take only at bedtime and never before driving. May cause headaches, |

| Supplement | Safe Use Guidelines and Possible Side Effects |
|---|---|
| Melatonin (cont'd) | nausea, morning dizziness, depression, giddiness, difficulty concentrating, and upset stomach. May interact with prescription medications, including hormone replacement therapy. May have adverse effects if you have cardiovascular disease, high blood pressure, an autoimmune disease such as rheumatoid arthritis or lupus, diabetes, epilepsy, migraine, or personal or family history of a hormone-dependent cancer such as breast, testicular, prostate, or endometrial cancer. May cause infertility, reduced sex drive in men, hypothermia, and retinal damage. |
| Methylsulfonylmethane (MSM) | Do not use if you are allergic or sensitive to sulfur-containing drugs. Do not take without medical supervision if you are taking anticoagulants (blood thinners). |
| NADH | Nervousness and loss of appetite have been reported in the first few days of supplementing; may cause upset stomach. |
| Progesterone cream | Intended only for external use and only for women 16 and older. Consult a medical doctor if you experience irritation, any changes in breast symptoms, or menstrual irregularities with continuous use. |
| Protein powder | Doses above 0.5 gram per pound of body weight could lead to imbalances in other aspects of the diet (for example, a 150-pound person should not exceed 75 grams a day). If you have liver or kidney disease, use only under the supervision of a knowledgeable medical doctor. |
| S-adenosylmethionine (SAM-e) | May increase blood levels of homocysteine, a significant risk factor for cardiovascular disease. |

| Supplement | Safe Use Guidelines and Possible Side Effects |
| --- | --- |
| Taurine | May affect people with a tendency to have increased stomach acid. If you have diabetes, use only under the supervision of a knowledgeable medical doctor. |
| Thymus extract | Use only under the supervision of a knowledgeable medical doctor. |
| Tyrosine | Do not take if you are taking MAO inhibitors. May cause sweating and elevated blood pressure. |
| Whey protein | See Protein powder |

## ESSENTIAL OILS

Essential oils are inhaled or applied topically to the skin, but with few exceptions, they are never taken internally.

Of the most common essential oils, lavender, tea tree, lemon, sandalwood, and rose can be used undiluted. The rest should be diluted in a carrier base, which can be an oil (such as almond), a cream, or a gel, before being applied to the skin.

Many essential oils may cause irritation or allergic reactions in people with sensitive skin. Before applying any new oil to your skin, always do a patch test. Put a few drops of the essential oil, mixed with the carrier, on the back of your wrist and wait for an hour or more. If irritation or redness occurs, wash the area with cold water. In the future, use half the amount of essential oil or avoid it altogether.

Do not use essential oils at home for serious medical problems. During pregnancy, do not use essential oils unless they're approved by your doctor. Essential oils are not appropriate for children of any age.

Store essential oils in dark bottles, away from light and heat and out of the reach of children and pets.

Flower essences are not essential oils, but they are not recommended for use in the eyes, on mucous membranes, or on broken or abraded skin. Most flower essences contain alcohol as a preservative, so if you are sensitive to alcohol, check with your doctor before using them.

| Essential Oil | Safe Use Guidelines and Possible Side Effects |
|---|---|
| Basil (*Ocimum basilicum*) | Do not use while nursing. Do not use for extended periods of time. Do not use more than three drops in bathwater. |
| Bergamot (*Citrus bergamia*) | Avoid direct sunlight while using; can cause skin sensitivity (except bergapten-free types). |
| Black pepper (*Piper negrum*) | Do not use more than three drops in bathwater. Do not use at the same time as homeopathic remedies. |
| Cedarwood (*Cedrus atlantica*) | Do not use for more than 2 weeks unless under the supervision of a qualified practitioner; may cause skin irritation, especially in high concentrations, and allergic reaction. If irritation occurs, use more carrier base to further dilute it. Do not use more than three drops in bathwater. |
| Clary sage (*Salvia sclarea*) | Do not use while consuming alcohol; can cause lethargy and exaggerate drunkenness. |
| Coriander (*Coriandrum sativum*) | Do not use for more than 2 weeks unless under the supervision of a qualified practitioner; can cause lethargy and unconsciousness in large amounts. |
| Cypress (*Cupressus sempervirens*) | Do not use if you have high blood pressure, cancer, or breast or uterine fibroids. |
| Eucalyptus (*Eucalyptus globulus*) | Do not use for more than 2 weeks unless under the supervision of a qualified practitioner. Do not use more than three drops in bathwater. Do not use at the same time as homeopathic remedies. |
| Garlic (*Allium sativum*) | Do not use more than three drops in bathwater. Do not use pure essential oil in the ears; use only infused oil. |
| Ginger (*Zingiber officinale*) | Do not use more than three drops in bathwater. Avoid direct sunlight while using; can cause skin sensitivity. |
| Juniper (*Juniper* spp.) | Do not use for more than 2 weeks unless under the supervision of a qualified practitioner; may be toxic. Do not use if you have kidney disease. |

| Essential Oil | Safe Use Guidelines and Possible Side Effects |
|---|---|
| Lavender (*Lavandula officinalis*) | If using undiluted oil, keep away from your eyes. |
| Lemon (*Citrus limon*) | Do not use more than three drops in bathwater. Avoid direct sunlight while using; can cause skin sensitivity. |
| Myrrh (*Commiphora myrrha*) | Do not use for more than 2 weeks unless under the supervision of a qualified practitioner because of toxicity levels. |
| Peppermint (*Mentha piperita*) | Do not use more than three drops in bathwater. Do not use at the same time as homeopathic remedies. Keep away from your eyes. Ingestion of peppermint oil may lead to stomach upset in sensitive individuals. If you have gallbladder or liver disease, do not use unless under the supervision of a knowledgeable medical doctor. |
| Rosemary (*Rosmarinus officinalis*) | Do not use if you have high blood pressure or epilepsy; has a powerful effect on the nervous system. |
| Sandalwood (*Santalum album*) | May be used undiluted as a perfume, but keep away from your eyes. |
| Spearmint (*Mentha spicata*) | Do not use more than three drops in bathwater. |
| Thyme (*Thymus vulgaris*) | May irritate the skin in high concentrations; if irritation occurs, use more carrier base to further dilute it. Do not use more than three drops in bathwater. Do not use if you have high blood pressure. Red thyme is toxic and should never be used. |
| Turmeric (*Curcuma domestica*) | Do not use for more than 2 weeks unless under the supervision of a qualified practitioner; may be toxic. May irritate the skin in high concentrations; if irritation occurs, use more carrier oil to further dilute it. Do not use more than three drops in bathwater. |

| Essential Oil | Safe Use Guidelines and Possible Side Effects |
| --- | --- |
| Ylang-ylang (*Cananga odorata*) | May be used undiluted as a perfume, but keep away from your eyes. Use in moderation; the strong smell can cause nausea or headaches. |

## HERBS

While herbal home remedies are generally safe and cause few, if any, side effects, herbalists are quick to caution that botanical medicines should be used cautiously and knowledgeably.

Most important, if you are under a doctor's care for any health condition or are taking any medication, do not take any herb or alter your medication regimen without informing your doctor. Do not administer herbs to children without consulting a physician. Also, if you are pregnant, nursing, or attempting to conceive, do not self-treat with any natural remedy without the consent of your obstetrician or midwife. Some herbs may cause adverse reactions if you are allergy-prone, have a major health condition, take prescription medication, take an herb for too long, take too much, or use the herb improperly. Homeopathic remedies are generally considered safe.

The guidelines in this chart are intended for adults only and usually refer to internal use. Be aware that some herbs may cause a skin reaction when used topically. If you are applying an herb for the first time, it is always wise to do a patch test. Apply a small amount to your skin and observe the exposed area for 24 hours to be sure that you aren't sensitive. If redness or a rash occurs, discontinue use.

Due to reports that some Chinese-made products contain potentially harmful contaminants, it is recommended that you obtain Chinese herbal remedies from a qualified practitioner of Traditional Chinese Medicine. While Ayurvedic herbs do not pose the same concern, it is best to consult an Ayurvedic practitioner to obtain the highest-quality herbs and receive personalized recommendations regarding their safe use.

| Herb | Safe Use Guidelines and Possible Side Effects |
|---|---|
| Aloe (*Aloe barbadensis*) | May delay wound healing; do not use gel externally on any surgical incision. Do not ingest dried leaf gel; it is a habit-forming laxative. |
| Arnica (*Arnica montana*) | Do not use on broken skin. |
| Ashwaganda (*Withania somnifera*) | Do not use with barbiturates; may intensify their effects. |
| Asian ginseng (*Panax ginseng*) | May cause irritability if used with caffeine or other stimulants. Do not use if you have high blood pressure. Siberian ginseng is considered safe. |
| Ayurvedic herbs | Consult an Ayurvedic practitioner to obtain quality herbs and receive personalized recommendations regarding their safe use. |
| Black cohosh (*Actea racemosa*) | Do not use for more than 6 months. |
| Black haw (*Viburnum prunifolium*) | Use only under the supervision of a knowledgeable medical doctor if you have a history of kidney stones; contains oxalates, which can cause kidney stones. |
| Black tea (*Camellia sinensis*) | Not recommended for excessive or long-term use; may stimulate the nervous system. |
| Bloodroot (*Sanguinaria canadensis*) | May cause nausea and vomiting in doses higher than 5 to 10 drops of regular-strength tincture more than twice a day. Safe when used in commercial dental products or under the supervision of a knowledgeable medical doctor or qualified herbalist. |
| Buchu (*Barosma crenulata*) | Do not use if you have kidney disease. |
| Cascara sagrada (*Rhamnus purshianus*) | Do not use if you have an inflammatory condition of the intestines, intestinal obstruction, or abdominal pain; may cause laxative dependency and diarrhea. Do not use for more than 14 days. |

| Herb | Safe Use Guidelines and Possible Side Effects * |
|---|---|
| Castor oil (*Ricinus communis*) | Do not use internally if you have intestinal obstruction or abdominal pain. Do not use for more than 8 to 10 days. |
| Cat's claw (*Uncaria tomentosa*) | Do not use if you have hemophilia. Side effects may include headache, stomachache, or difficulty breathing. |
| Cayenne (*Capsicum annuum*) | When ingested, may irritate the gastrointestinal tract if taken on an empty stomach. Externally, don't use near eyes or on injured skin. |
| Chamomile (*Matricaria recutita*) | Very rarely, may cause an allergic reaction when ingested. Drink the tea with caution if you are allergic to closely related plants, such as ragweed, asters, and chrysanthemums. |
| Chaparral (*Larrea tridentata*) | Do not use internally unless under the supervision of a qualified practitioner. Safe when used topically. |
| Chasteberry (*Vitex agnus-castus*) | May counteract the effectiveness of birth control pills. |
| Chinese herbal formulas | To ensure quality, purchase these products, also known as patent medicines, from a qualified practitioner of Traditional Chinese Medicine. |
| Coleus (*Coleus forskohlii*) | Do not use unless under the supervision of a knowledgeable medical doctor. May negatively enhance the effects of medications for asthma or high blood pressure. |
| Comfrey (*Symphytum officinale*) | For external use only. Do not use topically on deep or infected wounds; may promote rapid surface healing and not allow healing of underlying tissue. |
| Dandelion (*Taraxacum officinale*) | If you have gallbladder disease, do not use root preparations unless under the supervision of a knowledgeable medical doctor. |
| Dang gui (*Angelica sinensis*) | If you have a condition that involves heavy menstrual bleeding, such as endometriosis, do not use unless under the supervision of a qualified practitioner. |

| Herb | Safe Use Guidelines and Possible Side Effects |
|---|---|
| Echinacea (*Echinacea angustifolia*; *E. purpurea*; *E. pallida*) | Do not use if you are allergic to closely related plants, such as ragweed, asters, and chrysanthemums. Do not use if you have tuberculosis or an auto-immune condition such as lupus or multiple sclerosis; stimulates the immune system. |
| Elderberry (*Sambucus canadensis*) | Unripe fruit can cause vomiting or severe diarrhea. |
| Eucalyptus (*Eucalyptus globulus*) | Do not use if you have inflammatory disease of the bile ducts or gastrointestinal tract or severe liver disease. May cause nausea, vomiting, and diarrhea in doses exceeding 4 grams a day. |
| Fennel (*Foeniculum vulgare*) | Do not use medicinally for more than 6 weeks unless under the supervision of a qualified herbalist. |
| Feverfew (*Tanacetum parthenium*) | Chewing fresh leaves may cause mouth sores in some people. |
| Flaxseed (*Linum usitamissimum*) | Do not use if you have a bowel obstruction. Take with at least 8 ounces of water. |
| Garlic (*Allium sativum*) | Do not use supplements if you are taking anticoagulants (blood thinners) or before undergoing surgery; thins the blood and may increase bleeding. Do not use more than two cloves of fresh garlic daily prior to surgery or if you are taking anticoagulants (blood thinners). Do not use if you are taking drugs to lower blood sugar. |
| Ginger (*Zingiber officinale*) | If you have gallstones, do not use therapeutic amounts of dried root or powder unless under the supervision of a knowledgeable medical doctor; may increase bile secretion. |
| Ginkgo (*Ginkgo biloba*) | Do not use with antidepressant MAO inhibitor drugs such as phenelzine sulfate (Nardil) or tranylcypromine (Parnate); aspirin or other nonsteroidal anti-inflammatory medications; or blood-thinning medications such as warfarin (Coumadin). May cause dermatitis, diarrhea, and vomiting in doses exceeding 240 milligrams of concentrated extract. |

| Herb | Safe Use Guidelines and Possible Side Effects |
|------|-----------------------------------------------|
| Goldenseal (*Hydrastis canadensis*) | Do not use if you have high blood pressure. |
| Guggul (*Commiphora mukul*) | Rarely, may cause diarrhea, restlessness, apprehension, or hiccups. |
| Hawthorn (*Crataegus oxyantha*; *C. laevigata*; *C. monogyna*) | If you have a cardiovascular condition, do not take regularly for more than a few weeks unless under the supervision of a knowledgeable medical doctor. You may require lower doses of other medications, such as blood pressure drugs. If you have low blood pressure caused by heart valve problems, do not use without medical supervision. |
| Hops (*Humulus lupulus*) | Do not take if prone to depression. Rarely, may cause skin rash; handle fresh or dried hops carefully. |
| Horse chestnut (*Aesculus hippocastanum*) | May interfere with the action of other drugs, especially blood-thinning medications such as warfarin (Coumadin); may irritate the gastrointestinal tract. |
| Horsetail (*Equisetum* spp.) | Do not use tincture if you have heart or kidney problems. May cause a thiamin deficiency. Do not exceed 2 grams a day of powdered extract or use for prolonged periods. |
| Kava kava (*Piper methysticum*) | Do not use with alcohol or barbiturates. Do not exceed the dosage recommended on the label. Use caution when driving or operating equipment; kava is a muscle relaxant. |
| Kelp (*Nereocystis luetkeana*) | If you have high blood pressure or heart problems, use only once a day or less. Do not use if you have an over-active thyroid. Take with adequate liquid. Long-term use is not recommended. |
| Lotus seeds (*Nelumbo* spp.) | Do not use while constipated or when the stomach is distended. |
| Marshmallow (*Althea officinalis*) | May slow the absorption of medications taken at the same time. |

| Herb | Safe Use Guidelines and Possible Side Effects |
|------|------------------------------------------------|
| Meadowsweet (*Filipendula* spp.) | Do not use if you need to avoid aspirin; the active ingredient, salicin, is related to aspirin. |
| Myrrh (*Commiphora myrrha*) | Can cause diarrhea and irritation of the kidneys if ingested. Do not use if you have uterine bleeding for any reason. |
| Nettle (*Urtica dioica*) | May worsen allergy symptoms; take only one dose a day for the first few days. |
| Oats (*Avena sativa*) | Do not use if you have celiac disease (gluten intolerance); contains gluten, a grain protein. |
| Psyllium seeds (*Plantago ovata*) | Do not use if you have a bowel obstruction. Do not take within 1 hour of taking other drugs. Take with at least 8 ounces of water. |
| Pygeum (*Prunus africanum*) | Consult your doctor if using to treat an enlarged prostate. |
| Rehmannia (*Rehmannia glutinosa*) | Do not use if you have diarrhea, lack of appetite, or indigestion. |
| Sage (*Salvia officinalis*) | In therapeutic amounts, can increase sedative side effects of drugs. Do not use if you have low blood sugar or are undergoing anticonvulsant therapy. |
| St. John's wort (*Hypericum perforatum*) | Do not use with antidepressants unless under the supervision of a knowledgeable medical doctor. Avoid direct sunlight while using; may cause skin sensitivity. |
| Saw palmetto (*Serenoa repens*) | Consult your doctor before using to treat enlarged prostate. |
| Shepherd's purse (*Capsella bursa-pastoris*) | Do not use if you have a history of kidney stones. |
| Terminalia Arjuna (*Terminalia arjuna*) | Do not use unless under the supervision of a qualified Ayurvedic practitioner. |
| Tribulus Terrestris (*Tribulus terrestris*) | Do not use unless under the supervision of a qualified Ayurvedic practitioner. |
| Turmeric (*Curcuma domestica*) | Do not use medicinally if you have high stomach acid or ulcers, gallstones, or bile duct obstruction. |

| Herb | Safe Use Guidelines and Possible Side Effects |
| --- | --- |
| Uva-ursi (*Arctostaphylos uva-ursi*) | Do not use for more than 2 weeks unless under the supervision of a qualified herbalist. Do not use if you have kidney disease; contains tannins, which may cause further kidney damage and may irritate the stomach. |
| Valerian (*Valeriana officinalis*) | May intensify the effects of sleep-enhancing or mood-regulating medications. May cause heart palpitations and nervousness in sensitive individuals; if such stimulant action occurs, discontinue use. |
| White oak (*Quercus alba*) | Do not use externally if you have extensive skin damage. Do not use internally for more than several days at a time. |
| Yarrow (*Achillea millefolium*) | Rarely, handling flowers can cause skin rash. |
| Yellow dock (*Rumex crispus*) | Do not use unless under the supervision of a knowledgeable medical doctor if you have a history of kidney stones; contains oxalates and tannins that may adversely affect this condition. |

## VITAMINS AND MINERALS

Although reports of toxicity from vitamins and minerals are rare, they do occur. This guide is designed to help you use vitamins and minerals safely. The doses mentioned below are not recommendations; rather, they are the levels at which harmful side effects can occur. Some people may experience problems at significantly lower levels, however.

For best absorption and minimal stomach irritation, take most supplements with a meal unless otherwise indicated. It's important to realize that supplements should never be taken as substitutes for a healthy diet, since they do not provide all the nutritional benefits of whole foods. If you have a serious chronic illness that requires continual medical supervision, always talk to your doctor before self-treating. And even if you're perfectly healthy, you should always tell your doctor which supplements you're taking. That way, if you need medication for any reason, your doctor can take your supplements into consideration and avoid dangerous drug combinations. If you are pregnant, nursing, or attempting to conceive, do not take supplements without a doctor's supervision.

| Nutrient | Safe Use Guidelines and Possible Side Effects |
|---|---|
| Vitamin A | Taking more than 10,000 international units (IU) a day may cause vomiting, fatigue, dizziness, and blurred vision. Do not exceed 10,000 IU daily unless under the supervision of a knowledgeable medical doctor. |
| B-complex vitamins | Do not exceed the dosage recommended on the label. |
| Vitamin $B_6$ | Daily doses of more than 100 milligrams may cause nerve damage, resulting in a tingling sensation in the fingers and toes. Other possible side effects include pain, numbness, and weakness in the limbs; depression; and fatigue. Do not exceed 100 milligrams daily unless under the supervision of a knowledgeable medical doctor. |
| Beta-carotene | Doses exceeding 25 milligrams seem to have no benefit and should be taken only under the supervision of a knowledgeable medical doctor. In one study, smokers who received doses of 30 milligrams had an increased risk of lung cancer. |
| Vitamin C | Daily doses exceeding 1,000 milligrams may cause diarrhea. |
| Calcium (all forms) | Do not exceed 2,500 milligrams daily unless under the supervision of a knowledgeable medical doctor. Some natural sources of calcium, such as bone meal and dolomite, may be contaminated with lead. |
| Chromium (all forms) | Do not exceed 200 micrograms daily unless under the supervision of a knowledgeable medical doctor. |
| Copper | Do not exceed 9 milligrams daily unless under the supervision of a knowledgeable medical doctor. |
| Vitamin D | Do not exceed 2,000 IU (50 micrograms) daily unless under the supervision of a knowledgeable medical doctor. |

| Nutrient | Safe Use Guidelines and Possible Side Effects |
| --- | --- |
| Vitamin E | Do not exceed 150 IU daily unless under the supervision of a knowledgeable medical doctor. Because the vitamin acts as a blood thinner, consult your doctor before beginning supplementation in any amount if you're already taking aspirin or a blood-thinning medication such as warfarin (Coumadin), or if you're at high risk for stroke. |
| Iron | For most people, doses exceeding 25 milligrams daily must be taken under medical supervision. The maximum daily dose for men and post-menopausal women is 10 milligrams. |
| Vitamin K | Take only under the supervision of a knowledgeable medical doctor. |
| Magnesium (all forms) | Check with your doctor before beginning supplementation if you have heart or kidney problems. Doses exceeding 350 milligrams a day can cause diarrhea in some people. |
| Manganese (all forms) | Do not exceed 10 milligrams daily unless under the supervision of a knowledgeable medical doctor. |
| Niacin (all forms) | Do not exceed 35 milligrams daily unless under the supervision of a knowledgeable medical doctor. |
| Potassium | Take only under the supervision of a knowledgeable medical doctor. |
| Potassium-magnesium-aspartate | Take only under the supervision of a knowledgeable medical doctor; there is no need to take supplemental potassium unless prescribed by a doctor. |
| Selenium | Do not exceed 200 micrograms daily unless under the supervision of a knowledgeable medical doctor. |
| Zinc | Do not exceed 30 milligrams daily unless under the supervision of a knowledgeable medical doctor. |

# Referrals and Information

A number of organizations provide listings of medical professionals and practitioners who use some or all of the therapies mentioned in this book. For more information, contact the following sources.

## *Directories of Practitioners*

### Alternative Medicine Directory
www.altmedicine.net
*This Web site maintains an international database of practitioners in a wide variety of areas.*

### American College for Advancement in Medicine
23121 Verdugo Drive, Suite 204
Laguna Hills, CA 92653
www.acam.org
*For a state-by-state directory of physicians who may lead you to someone who prescribes natural testosterone, send a stamped, self-addressed envelope containing $1 in postage to the address above. The information is available on their Web site free of charge.*

### American Holistic Medical Association
6728 McLean Village Drive
McLean, VA 22101
www.holisticmedicine.org
*This organization represents M.D.'s and D.O.'s who combine mainstream medicine with complementary therapies. They publish the* National Referral Directory of Holistic Practitioners, *which is available by mail. Referrals are also available on their Web site.*

### EarthMed.com
2009 Renaissance Boulevard,
Suite 100
King of Prussia, PA 19406
www.earthmed.com
*This Web site maintains a directory of more than 100,000 alternative medicine practitioners nationwide. Referrals are also provided by mail.*

### Health World Online
Professional Referral Network
www.healthreferral.com
*This is a compilation of searchable referral databases from member lists of participating associations. The Web site contains referral informa-*

tion for practitioners of acupuncture and Oriental medicine, flower remedies, guided imagery, homeopathy, naturopathic medicine, and vision training.

## Healthy Alternatives
www.health-alt.com
*This site provides referral information for practitioners of aromatherapy, herbal medicine, homeopathy, massage therapy, naturopathy, reflexology, and yoga.*

## Acupressure

### Acupressure Institute
1533 Shattuck Avenue
Berkeley, CA 94709
www.acupressure.com
*Referrals are available only for the northern California area. National referrals may become available in the future.*

### Jin Shin Do Foundation for Bodymind Acupressure
PO Box 416
Idyllwild, CA 92549
www.jinshindo.org
*This organization provides referrals to authorized teachers.*

## Aromatherapy

### National Association for Holistic Aromatherapy
4509 Interlake Avenue North, #233
Seattle, WA 98103
www.naha.org
*There is no standardized certification or registration of aromatherapists in the United States. However,*

you can check with this association to see if the practitioner is registered with it.

## Ayurvedic Medicine

### Ayurveda Holistic Center
82A Bayville Avenue
Bayville, NY 11709
www.ayurvedahc.com
*This center maintains a small list of U.S. Ayurvedic practitioners. They also see patients in the Bayville area of Long Island in New York, and the Web site offers online consultations.*

### Bastyr University
14500 Juanita Drive NE
Kenmore, WA 98028-4966
www.bastyr.edu
*The nation's leading school of naturopathic medicine also provides referral information.*

### The College of Maharishi Vedic Medicine
Maharishi University of Management
Fairfield, IA 52557
www.maharishi-medical.com
*This organization provides referrals to Ayurvedic practitioners. Its Web site lists affiliated Maharishi Medical Centers located nationwide.*

### Maharishi College of Vedic Medicine
2721 Arizona Street NE
Albuquerque, NM 87110
*This organization provides referrals to Ayurvedic practitioners.*

**The Raj Maharishi Ayurveda Health Center**
1734 Jasmine Avenue
Fairfield, IA 52556
*This organization maintains a list of practitioners nationwide, which is available by mail.*

## Breath Therapy

**The International Breath Institute**
5921 East Miramar Drive
Tucson, AZ 85715
www.transformbreathing.com
*This organization provides free referrals—by mail or on their Web site—to breath facilitators who have graduated from their institute.*

## Energy Healing

**American Polarity Therapy Association**
PO Box 19858
Boulder, CO 80308
www.polaritytherapy.org
*This organization accepts requests by mail or via their Web site. Information is sent out by mail.*

## Barbara Brennan School of Healing

500 Spanish River Boulevard, Suite 103
Boca Raton, FL 33481-4559
www.barbarabrennan.com
*This school provides referrals to energy healers who have trained there.*

## International Association for Reiki Professionals

PO Box 104
Harrisville, NH 03450

www.iarp.org
*For a free referral to a Reiki practitioner in your area, visit the Web site or write to the address above.*

**Quantum-Touch**
PO Box 852
Santa Cruz, CA 95061
www.quantumtouch.com
*This organization offers nationwide referrals to practitioners of Quantum-Touch.*

## Flower Essences

**Dr. Edward Bach Centre**
Mount Vernon, Bakers Lane
Sotwell, Oxon, OX10 0PZ
United Kingdom
www.bachcentre.com
*This organization can provide an international listing of flower remedy therapists.*

**Flower Essence Society**
PO Box 459
Nevada City, CA 95959
www.flowersociety.org
*This nonprofit organization maintains a registry of practitioners who use flower essences and will provide names of experts in your area.*

## Herbal Medicine

**American Herbalists Guild**
1931 Gaddis Road
Canton, GA 30115
www.americanherbalistsguild.com
*This organization provides referral information to certified herbalists. You can also obtain referral information on their Web site.*

## Homeopathy

### The American Board of Homeotherapeutics

801 North Fairfax Street, Suite 306
Alexandria, VA 22314
*For the bound Directory of the American Board of Homeotherapeutics, send $10 to the address above.*

### The Homeopathic Academy of Naturopathic Physicians

12132 Southeast Foster Place
Portland, OR 97266
www.healthy.net/pan/pa/homeopathic/hanp
*This organization certifies naturopathic homeopaths and makes referrals by mail or via their Web site.*

### The National Center for Homeopathy

801 North Fairfax Street, Suite 306
Alexandria, VA 22314
www.homeopathic.org
*This organization provides referrals by mail or on their Web site.*

### The North American Society of Homeopaths

1122 East Pike Street, Suite 1122
Seattle, WA 98122
www.homeopathy.org
*This organization provides referrals by mail or on their Web site.*

## Hydrotherapy

*See the entry for Naturopathic Medicine. Naturopathic doctors are the only licensed health care professionals who are trained to use hydrotherapy. You can also find qualified, experienced hydrotherapists in some spas and other health care facilities.*

## Magnet Therapy

*There is no professional certification for individuals practicing magnet therapy; the therapy is usually self-administered.*

## Massage Therapy

### American Massage Therapy Association

820 Davis Street, Suite 100
Evanston, IL 60201-4444
www.amtamassage.org
*The association's locator service provides referrals to certified massage therapists nationwide. Write for information or visit their Web site.*

### Associated Bodywork and Massage Professionals

1271 Sugarbush Drive
Evergreen, CO 80439-9766
www.abmp.com
*This organization provides a complete list of its members by mail or on their Web site.*

### The International Massage Association

25 South Fourth Street, PO Box 421
Warrenton, VA 20188
*This organization provides referrals to massage therapists nationwide. You can obtain information by writing or by visiting their Web site.*

**National Certification Board
for Therapeutic Massage
and Bodywork**
8201 Greensboro Drive, Suite 300
McLean, VA 22102
www.ncbtmb.com
*This organization provides referrals
to certified massage therapists nationwide. You can obtain information by
writing or by visiting their Web site.*

## *Movement Education*

**Alexander Technique
International**
1692 Massachusetts Avenue, 3rd floor
Cambridge, MA 02138
www.ati-net.com
*This organization provides referrals
by mail or on their Web site.*

**The Aston Training Center**
PO Box 3568
Incline Village, NV 89450
www.aston-patterning.com
*This organization provides referrals
by mail or on their Web site.*

**Feldenkrais Guild
of North America**
3611 Southwest Hood Avenue, Suite
100
Portland, OR 97201
www.feldenkrais.com
*This organization provides referrals
by mail or on their Web site.*

**Hellerwork International**
3435 M Street
Eureka, CA 95503
www.hellerwork.com
*This organization provides referrals
by mail or on their Web site.*

## *Music Therapy
and Sound Healing*

**American Music Therapy
Association**
8455 Colesville Road, Suite 1000
Silver Spring, MD 20910
www.musictherapy.org
*This organization can recommend
health professionals in your area
who use this technique.*

## *Naturopathic Medicine*

**The American Association
of Naturopathic Physicians**
8201 Greensboro Drive, Suite 300
McLean, VA 22102
www.naturopathic.org
*This organization has a database at
their Web site for locating N.D.'s in
your area. For a fee, a list is also
available by mail.*

**The Canadian Naturopathic
Association**
1255 Sheppard Avenue East
(at Leslie)
North York, Ontario, M2K 1E2,
Canada
www.naturopathicassoc.ca
*This organization makes referrals to
naturopathic doctors in Canada by
mail or on their Web site.*

**The Council on Naturopathic
Medical Education**
PO Box 11426
Eugene, OR 97440-3626
www.cnme.org
*This is the only accrediting agency
that has been recognized by the gov-
ernment's Department of Education.*

**The Homeopathic Academy
of Naturopathic Physicians**
12132 Southeast Foster Place
Portland, OR 97266
www.healthy.net/pan/pa/
homeopathic/hanp
*This organization certifies naturo-
pathic homeopaths and makes referrals by mail or via their Web site.*

## Qigong

**National Qigong (Chi Kung)
Association USA**
PO Box 540
Ely, MN 55731
www.nqa.org
*This organization provides a free list-
ing of instructors by mail or on their
Web site.*

## Reflexology

**American Academy
of Reflexology**
606 East Magnolia Boulevard,
Suite B
Burbank, CA 91501-2618
*This organization offers referrals to
practitioners trained by the academy.*

**American Reflexology
Certification Board**
PO Box 740879
Arvada, CO 80006-0879
*Write to this organization for a list-
ing of certified reflexologists.*

**International Institute
of Reflexology Inc.**
5650 First Avenue North
PO Box 12642
St. Petersburg, FL 33733-2642

*This organization provides free
referrals by mail.*

**Reflexology Association
of America**
4012 Rainbow, Suite K-PMB #585
Las Vegas, NV 89103-2059
www.reflexology-usa.org
*This organization provides nation-
wide referrals via mail or on their
Web site.*

## Relaxation Therapy

*To find a health professional who
specializes in relaxation therapy,
contact a psychologist or counselor
who is trained in biofeedback or
other relaxation techniques.*

## Traditional Chinese Medicine

**The American Association
of Oriental Medicine**
433 Front Street
Catasauqua, PA 18032
www.aaom.org
*This organization provides referrals
by mail or on their Web site.*

**The National Acupuncture
and Oriental Medicine Alliance**
14637 Starr Road, SE
Olalla, WA 98359
www.acuall.org
*This organization provides referrals
by mail or on their Web site.*

**The National Certification
Commission for Acupuncture
and Oriental Medicine**
11 Canal Center Plaza, Suite 300
Alexandria, VA 22314
www.nccaom.org

*This organization provides referrals by mail or on their Web site. A small fee is charged for referrals sent by mail.*

## Visualization

**The Academy for Guided Imagery**
PO Box 2070
Mill Valley, CA 94942
www.interactiveimagery.com
*Established by visualization pioneer Martin Rossman, M.D., this organization provides referrals by mail or on their Web site. For information by mail, send a stamped, self-addressed envelope to the address above.*

**The American Society of Clinical Hypnosis**
130 East Elm Court, Suite 201
Roselle, IL 60172-2000
*This organization provides referrals by mail. Send a stamped, self-addressed envelope to the address above.*

**The Society for Clinical and Experimental Hypnosis**
PO Box 642114
Pullman, WA 99164-2114

*A professional organization that can refer you to member hypnotherapists around the country. Send a stamped, self-addressed envelope to the address above.*

## Yoga Therapy

**International Association of Yoga Therapists**
2400A County Center Drive
Santa Rosa, CA 95403
www.yrec.org
*Referrals are provided free of charge on their Web site. To receive the list by mail, send a stamped, self-addressed envelope to the address above.*

## Miscellaneous

**International Academy of Oral Medicine and Toxicology**
PO Box 608531
Orlando, FL 32860-8531
www.iaomt.org
*This organization provides free referrals by mail to dentists who use alternative methods.*

# Products

Many of the herbs, supplements, and other health care products recommended in this book are available at local drugstores or health food stores or on the Internet. If you have trouble locating a specific product, however, you may be able to obtain it from one of the following sources.

## Acupressure

### Acupressure Institute
1533 Shattuck Avenue
Berkeley, CA 94709
www.acupressure.com
*Contact this organization for audio and video products and body tools used for acupressure.*

### Jin Shin Do Foundation for Bodymind Acupressure
PO Box 416
Idyllwild, CA 92549
www.jinshindo.org
*This organization provides books, videotapes, audiotapes, acupressure charts, articles, and other materials about Jin Shin Do Bodymind Acupressure.*

## Affirmations

### Brainstickers.com
PO Box 4815
Boise, ID 83711-4815
www.affirmation.com
*Contact this company for information on positive reinforcement stickers for your environment.*

### Castlegate Publishers
25597 Drake Road
Barrington, IL 60010
www.midpointtrade.com/castlegate_publishers.htm
*This company publishes* Spontaneous Optimism: Proven Strategies for Health, Prosperity, and Happiness *by Maryann Troiani, Ph.D.*

## Aromatherapy

### Aroma Land
www.buyaromatherapy.com
*This Web site sells oils, blends, and aromatherapy products with a money-back guarantee.*

### Aroma-Vera
5310 Beethoven Street
Los Angeles, CA 90066

*This company offers more than 100 essential oils, plus a large variety of aromatic soaps, candles, bath and massage oils, and hair and skin care products. You can order a free catalog from the address above.*

**Dhyana Education
and Rejuvenation Centre**
6871 Covey Road
Forestville, CA 95436
www.aromaveda.com
*This Ayurvedic clinic, educational center, and mail-order company offers aromatherapy oils.*

**Leydet Aromatics**
PO Box 2354
Fair Oaks, CA 95628
*This company offers about 150 essential oils, one of the largest selections available in the United States. Contact the address above for information.*

**Santa Fe Botanical Fragrances**
PO Box 282
Santa Fe, NM 87504
*This company carries approximately 75 essential oils. Request a free catalog from the address above.*

## *Ayurvedic Medicine*

**Ayurveda Holistic Center**
82A Bayville Avenue
Bayville, NY 11709
www.ayurvedahc.com
*This center sells Ayurveda-related products on their Web site and by mail.*

**The Ayurvedic Center**
4100 Westheimer, Suite 235
Houston, TX 77027
www.holheal.com
*This company sells a variety of Ayurvedic herbs and herbal formulations.*

**The Ayurvedic Institute**
11311 Menaul NE
Albuquerque, NM 87112
www.ayurveda.com
*This organization sells a variety of items, including Ayurvedic herbs, software, and tapes.*

**Ayush Herbs**
2115 112th Avenue NE
Bellevue, WA 98004
www.ayush.com
*This company offers Ayurvedic herbs formulated in India and clinically tested in the United States at the Ayurvedic and Naturopathic Medical Clinic.*

**Dhyana Education
and Rejuvenation Centre**
6871 Covey Road
Forestville, CA 95436
www.aromaveda.com
*This Ayurvedic clinic, educational center, and mail-order company offers Ayurvedic treatments, Ayurvedic herbs and aromatherapy oils, and classes in Ayurveda and aromatherapy.*

**Sushakti**
1840 Iron Street, Suite C
Bellingham, WA 98225
www.ayurveda-sushakti.com

*This company offers a variety of Ayurvedic items, including bulk herbs, audiotapes, and skin care products.*

## Breath Therapy

### Authentic Breathing Resources
PO Box 31376
San Francisco, CA 94131
www.authentic-breathing.com
*This organization offers books, articles, and tapes about therapeutic breathing, including The Tao of Natural Breathing.*

### The International Breath Institute
5921 East Miramar Drive
Tucson, AZ 85715
*Write this organization for information on tapes, books, and breathing enhancement products.*

### Optimal Breathing
Box 1551
Waynesville, NC 28786
www.breathing.com
*This organization provides education, services, and products for learning breathing techniques that enhance health, performance, and longevity.*

## Energy Healing

### American Polarity Therapy Association
PO Box 19858
Boulder, CO 80308
www.polaritytherapy.org
*This organization offers audiotapes and CDs, videos, charts, and more.*

*Send a request for product information.*

### Barbara Brennan School of Healing
500 Spanish River Boulevard, Suite 103
Boca Raton, FL 33481-4559
www.barbarabrennan.com
*This Web site offers books and audiotapes on energy healing by Barbara Brennan.*

### Quantum-Touch
PO Box 852
Santa Cruz, CA 95061
www.quantumtouch.com
*This organization offers books and tapes by Richard Gordon, the creator of this technique.*

## Flower Essences

### Flower Essence Services
PO Box 1769
Nevada City, CA 95959
www.floweressence.com
*This organization sells flower essence products as well as books and audio- and videotapes on the subject.*

### Nelson Bach USA Ltd
100 Research Drive
Wilmington, MA 01887
www.nelsonbach.com
*This company sells flower essences online or through the mail.*

## Herbal Medicine

### Mothernature.com
www.mothernature.com
*This Web site sells herbal products.*

**Nature's Herbs**
47444 Kato Road
Fremont, CA 94538
*If you can't find medicinal herbs
nearby, you can order from this
company. For a free catalog, write
to the address above.*

**Vitanica**
PO Box 1285
Sherwood, OR 97140
www.vitanica.com
*This company offers a full range
of herbal/nutrient "naturopathic
supplements" for women that are
formulated by Tori Hudson, N.D.,
author of* Women's Encyclopedia
of Natural Medicine.

**Zand Herbal Formulas**
1441 West Smith Road
Ferndale, WA 98248
www.zand.com
*This company offers a variety of clini-
cally developed herbal formulas, single
herb extracts, standardized extracts,
and sugar-free herbal lozenges.*

## Homeopathy

**Homeopathic Educational
Services**
2124 Kittredge Street
Berkeley, CA 94704
*Write to this organization for home-
opathy-related products, such as software, cassettes, videos, and remedies.*

## Hydrotherapy

**Bodywork Emporium**
414 Broadway
Santa Monica, CA 90401
www.bodywork-emporium.com

*This company offers books on alter-
native modalities, including
hydrotherapy, on their Web site.
Their catalog is also available by
mail.*

## Magnet Therapy

**Magnetic Ideas**
125 Industrial Park Drive
Sevierville, TN 37862
www.magneticideas.com
*This company offers a variety of
therapeutic magnets on their Web
site. You can also receive information by writing to the address
above.*

**Theramagnets**
48 Skyline Drive
Coram, NY 11727
www.theramagnets.com
*This company offers a variety of
therapeutic magnets on their Web
site. You can also receive information by writing to the address
above.*

## Massage Therapy

**The International Massage
Association**
25 South Fourth Street, PO Box 421
Warrenton, VA 20188
*This organization sells a variety
of accessories and books related to
massage.*

**SelfCare Catalog**
2000 Powell Street, Suite 1350
Emeryville, CA 94608
*This company offers massage and
self-massage items. For a catalog,
write to the address above.*

**V.I.E.W. Video**
34 East 23rd Street
New York, NY 10010
*For an introduction to Swedish and
shiatsu massage techniques, you can
order "Massage Your Mate," a 92-
minute, color, VHS cassette. Rebecca
Klinger, a licensed massage therapist
in New York, is your guide through
an introduction to massage.*

## Movement Education

**The Aston Training Center**
PO Box 3568
Incline Village, NV 89450
www.aston-patterning.com
*Visit their Web site or write for
information on offerings such as
articles, videos, and ergonomic
products.*

**Feldenkrais Guild
of North America**
3611 Southwest Hood Avenue,
Suite 100
Portland, OR 97201
www.feldenkrais.com
*Visit their Web site or write for infor-
mation on video- and audio-cassettes.
Educational material is also available for children.*

## Music Therapy
## and Sound Healing

**Inner Peace Music**
PO Box 2644
San Anselmo, CA 94979-2644
www.innerpeacemusic.com
*This company provides tapes by
Steven Halpern for relaxation and
enjoyment, plus a wide variety of*

*subliminal tapes for better perfor-
mance, deeper sleep, safer driving,
increased creativity, and other self-
help areas.*

**Sound Healers Association**
PO Box 2240
Boulder, CO 80306
www.healingsounds.com
*Visit their Web site or write for
information on audiotapes, CDs, and
tuning forks.*

## Naturopathic Medicine

**The American Association of
Naturopathic Physicians**
8201 Greensboro Drive, Suite 300
McLean, VA 22102
www.naturopathic.org
*This organization maintains a title
index of recommended books and
software.*

## Qigong

**National Qigong (Chi Kung)
Association USA**
PO Box 540
Ely, MN 55731
www.nqa.org
*This organization provides a free
resource list of recommended books
and videos on qigong.*

**Qi Journal Catalog**
Insight Publishing
PO Box 18476
Anaheim Hills, CA 92817
www.qi-journal.com
*This catalog contains a variety of
qigong and alternative medicine
products.*

**Wayfarer Publications**
PO Box 39938
Los Angeles, CA 90039
*This company sells videos on qigong and the martial arts.*

## Reflexology

**American Academy of Reflexology**
606 East Magnolia Boulevard, Suite B
Burbank, CA 91501-2618
*This organization offers educational materials and courses on foot, hand, and ear reflexology.*

**Bodywork Emporium**
414 Broadway
Santa Barbara, CA 90401
www.bodywork-emporium.com
*This company offers books for reflexology for sale on their Web site. Their catalog is also available by mail.*

**International Academy of Advanced Reflexology and Advanced Reflexology Complementary Health Center**
2542 Easton Avenue, PO Box 1489
Bethlehem, PA 18016
www.reflexology.net
*This organization offers videos and charts for sale on their Web site or by mail.*

## Traditional Chinese Medicine

**Blue Poppy Press**
5441 Western Avenue, #2
Boulder, CO 80301
www.bluepoppy.com

*This company publishes a number of items on Traditional Chinese Medicine. Write to the address above for a list of products, or visit their Web site. It contains free articles to download and an online book catalog.*

**Redwing Book Company**
44 Linden Street
Brookline, MA 02445
www.redwingbooks.com
*This company publishes books on alternative medicine, including Traditional Chinese Medicine.*

## Visualization

**The Imagery Store at the Academy for Guided Imagery**
PO Box 2070
Mill Valley, CA 94942
*This company offers visualization tapes for specific health and behavior problems, including "Mind-Controlled Anesthesia for Systemic Pain," "Restful Sleep," "Chest Pain, Anxiety, and Heartbreak," and "Forgiveness in Healing."*

**Source Cassette Learning System**
131 East Placer Street, PO Box 6028
Auburn, CA 95603
*Psychiatrist Emmett Miller, M.D., a pioneer in visualization cassettes, offers tapes for specific health and behavior problems, including "Smoke No More," "The Sleep Tape," "Imagine Yourself Slim," "Letting Go of Stress," "Freeing Yourself from Fear," "Successful Surgery and Recovery," "Power Vision," and "The Source Meditation."*

## *Vitamin and Mineral Therapy*

### Body Language Vitamin Company

www.bodylangvitamin.com
*This Web site offers a number of high-potency nutritional formulas created by anti-aging expert Michael Seidman, M.D., including anti-aging formulas, formulas for children, cold and flu treatments, and a multivitamin, among others.*

### Mothernature.com

www.mothernature.com
*This Web site sells vitamin and mineral supplements.*

### Safe and Sound

5343 Tallman Avenue NW
Tallman Medical Center, Suite 208
Seattle, WA 98107
www.nwnaturalhealth.com
*This company has a line of nutritional supplements for cancer and HIV patients.*

### Simone Protective Health Care

123 Franklin Corner Road
Lawrenceville, NJ 08648
www.drsimone.com
*This site sells a range of doctor-formulated nutritional products, including a multivitamin, a mineral supplement, a children's supplement, a fiber supplement, a pet supplement, an energy supplement, and others.*

### Total Health Nutrients

PATH Medical
185 Madison Avenue, 6th floor
New York, NY 10016
www.pathmed.com

*This company offers doctor-formulated vitamins and supplements for improved brain health and function, sexual performance, prostate health, energy, and anti-aging.*

### Vitamins.com

2924 Telestar Court
Falls Church, VA 22042
www.vitamins.com
*This company provides a wide range of nutritional, herbal, and other supplements.*

### Vitamin Shoppe

www.vitaminshoppe.com
*This company sells more than 17,000 products. Write for a catalog or visit their Web site.*

## *Yoga Therapy*

### International Association of Yoga Therapists

2400A County Center Drive
Santa Rosa, CA 95403
www.yrcc.org
*Send a stamped, self-addressed envelope to this organization for a flyer on product resources.*

### Yoga Accessories

PO Box 13976
New Bern, NC 28561
www.yogaaccessories.com
*This company offers yoga mats and straps for sale. Write for a catalog or visit their Web site.*

### Yoga Zone

3342 Melrose Avenue
Roanoke, VA 24017
www.yogazone.com

*This company offers a wide variety of yoga products. Write for a catalog or visit their Web site.*

## Miscellaneous

**Apollo Light Systems**
369 South Mountain Way Drive
Orem, UT 84058

**Bio-Brite**
4340 East West Highway, Suite 401S
Bethesda, MD 20814

**Enviro-Med**
1600 SE 141st Avenue
Vancouver, WA 98683

**The SunBox Company**
19217 Orbit Drive
Gaithersburg, MD 20879
*These four companies sell light boxes for SAD treatment.*

**Earthpulse Press**
PO Box 201393
Anchorage, AK 99520
www.earthpulse.com
*To learn about the Pointer Plus stimulator for auricular therapy, visit the Earthpulse Web site. You can order the product or get more information by writing to the address above.*

# Panel of Experts

**Pamela Adams, D.C.,** is a chiropractor and yoga instructor in Larkspur, California.

**Lauri Aesoph, N.D.,** is a naturopathic doctor in Sioux Falls, South Dakota, and author of *How to Eat Away Arthritis.*

**Rosemary Agostini, M.D.,** is a physician at the Virginia Mason Sports Center and clinical associate professor at the University of Washington, both in Seattle.

**Edward M. Arana, D.D.S.,** is a retired dentist in Carmel Valley, California, and past president of the American Academy of Biological Dentistry.

**Joan Arnold** is a certified teacher of the Alexander Technique in New York City.

**Guillermo Asis, M.D.,** is director of Path to Health in Burlington, Massachusetts, board-certified in intravenous chelation therapy, and founder of three integrative medicine centers in New England, including the Marino Center in Cambridge, Massachusetts.

**James F. Balch, M.D.,** is director of Health Counseling in Trophy Club, Texas, and author of *Heartburn and What to Do about It* and *Prescription for Dietary Wellness*.

**Adela T. Basayne** is a licensed massage therapist and Gestalt therapist in Portland, Oregon, and past president of the American Massage Therapy Association.

**DeAnna Batdorff** is a clinical aromatherapist, Ayurvedic practitioner, nutritional counselor at Dhyana Meditation in a Bottle, and founder and director of the Dhyana Education and Rejuvenation Centre in Forestville, California.

**Seth J. Baum, M.D.,** is an integrative cardiologist and founder of the Baum Center for Integrative Heart Care in Boca Raton, Florida.

**Paul Beals, M.D.,** is a naturally oriented physician in Laurel, Maryland.

**Barry L. Beaty, D.O.,** is an osteopathic physician, medical director of the DFW Pain Treatment Center and Wellness Clinic in Fort Worth, Texas, and president of the American College of Osteopathic Pain Management and Sclerotherapy.

**Brenda Beeley** is a licensed acupuncturist and director of the Menopause and PMS Options for Women health center on Bainbridge Island, Washington.

**Peter Bennett, N.D.,** is a naturopathic and homeopathic physician; acupuncturist; founder and medical director of the Helios Clinic in Victoria, British Columbia; and author of *The 7-Day Detox Miracle*.

**Johnathan Berent** is a psychiatric social worker and director of Berent Associates Center for Social Therapy in Great Neck, New York.

**Kenneth Blanchard, M.D., Ph.D.,** is an endocrinologist in Newton, Massachusetts.

**Mary Ann Block, D.O.,** is an osteopathic physician in Dallas-Fort Worth, specializing in preventive medicine, ADHD, learning differences, and allergies; founder and director of the Block Center in Hurst, Texas; and author of *No More Ritalin: Treating ADHD without Drugs*.

**Kenneth A. Bock, M.D.,** is codirector of the Rhinebeck Health Center in Rhinebeck, New York, and the Center for Progressive Medicine in Albany, New York, and author of *The Road to Immunity: How to Survive and Thrive in a Toxic World*.

**Steven J. Bock, M.D.,** is a family practitioner; acupuncturist; codirector of the Center for Progressive Medicine in Rhinebeck, New York; and author of *Stay Young the Melatonin Way*.

**Bradley Bongiovanni, N.D.,** is a naturopathic physician at Wellspace, a complementary health care center in Cambridge, Massachusetts.

**Tammy Born, D.O.,** is an osteopathic physician and director of the Born Preventive Health Care Clinic in Grand Rapids, Michigan.

**Joan Borysenko, Ph.D.,** is a licensed clinical psychologist, president of Mind/Body Health Sciences in Boulder, Colorado, and author of *Guilt Is the Teacher, Love Is the Lesson*.

**James Braly, M.D.,** is an allergy specialist in Boca Raton, Florida; medical director of the Web site www.drbralyallergy-relief.com; author of *Food Allergy Relief Now!*; and editor of the e-mail newsletters "Allergy in the News" and "Food Allergy and Nutrition Update."

**Alan Brauer, M.D.,** is a psychiatrist; sex therapist; founder and director of the TotalCare Medical Center in Palo Alto, California; and coauthor of *ESO (Extended Sexual Orgasm).*

**Eric R. Braverman, M.D.,** is an alternative medicine specialist, director of the Place for Achieving Total Health in New York City, and author of *Hypertension and Nutrition.*

**Peter R. Breggin, M.D.,** is director of the International Center for the Study of Psychiatry and Psychology in Bethesda, Maryland, and author of *Your Drug May Be Your Problem: How and Why to Stop Taking Psychiatric Medications* and *Talking Back to Ritalin: What Doctors Aren't Telling You about Stimulants for Children.*

**Doug Brodie, M.D.,** is an alternative physician in Reno.

**Pierre Brunschwig, M.D.,** is a member of the American Holistic Medical Association who practices at the Helios Health Center in Boulder, Colorado.

**Jane Buckle, R.N.,** is a nurse and aromatherapist in Albany, New York.

**Nancy Buono** is a registered Bach flower practitioner in Tempe, Arizona.

**Kathryn Burgio, Ph.D.,** is director of the continence program at the University of Alabama at Birmingham and author of *Staying Dry: A Practical Guide to Bladder Control.*

**Dawn Burstall, R.D.,** is a dietitian in the gastroenterology program at Queen Elizabeth II Health Sciences Center in Halifax, Nova Scotia, and coauthor of *I.B.S. Relief.*

**Sharon Butler** is a certified Hellerwork practitioner in Paoli, Pennsylvania, and author of *Conquering Carpal Tunnel Syndrome and Other Repetitive Strain Injuries.*

**Rashid Ali Buttar, D.O.,** is an osteopathic physician who practices emergency and preventive medicine in Charlotte, North Carolina.

**Richard Carmen** is a clinical audiologist, director of the Northern Arizona Speech and Hearing Center in Sedona, and author of *Consumer Handbook on Hearing Loss and Hearing Aids.*

**Donald Carrow, M.D.,** is founder and director of the Florida Institute of Health in Tampa.

**Hyla Cass, M.D.,** is assistant professor of psychiatry at the University of California, Los Angeles, School of Medicine.

**Miranda Castro** is a certified homeopath based in Seattle; president of the North American Society of Homeopaths; a fellow of the Society of Homeopaths in the United Kingdom; and author of *The Complete Homeopathy Handbook, Homeopathy for Pregnancy, Birth, and Your Baby's First Year,* and *Homeopathic Guide to Stress.*

**James Clay** is a certified clinical massage therapist in Winston-Salem, North Carolina, and author of *Clinical Massage Therapy: Integrating Anatomy and Treatment.*

**Barbara Close** is an aromatherapist; herbalist; president and founder of the Naturopathica Holistic Health Spa in East Hampton, New York; and author of *Well-Being: Rejuvenating Recipes for the Body and Soul.*

**Misha Cohen, O.M.D.,** is a doctor of Oriental medicine and licensed acupuncturist at Paths to Wellness, clinical director of Chicken Soup Chinese Medicine, and research and education chair at Quan Yin Healing Arts Center, all in San Francisco; research associate at the University of California, San Francisco, School of Medicine; and author of *The Chinese Way to Healing, The HIV Wellness Sourcebook,* and *The Hepatitis C Help Book.*

**William Cone, Ph.D.,** is a geriatric psychologist in Pacific Palisades, California, and author of *Stop Memory Loss: How to Fight Forgetfulness over Forty.*

**Elizabeth Cornell** is a licensed massage therapist and craniosacral therapist in New York City.

**Dennis Courtney, M.D.,** is director of the Courtney Clinic for Pain Relief and the Center for Complementary Health, both in McMurray, Pennsylvania.

**Amanda McQuade Crawford** is a medical herbalist and nutritionist in Ojai, California; founder of the National College of Phytotherapy in Albuquerque, New Mexico; and author of *The Herbal Menopause Book* and *Herbal Remedies for Women.*

**Walter Crinnion, N.D.,** is a naturopathic doctor; director of the Healing Naturally clinic in Kirkland, Washington; and a faculty member at Bastyr University in Kenmore, Washington; the National College of Naturopathic Medicine in Portland, Oregon; and the Southwest College of Naturopathic Medicine and Health Sciences in Tempe, Arizona.

**David A. Darbro, M.D.,** is a physician in Indianapolis.

**Carolyn Dean, M.D.,** is a physician in New York City and a consultant in the field of integrative medicine.

**Sandra Denton, M.D.,** is a naturally oriented physician in Anchorage, specializing in diet, nutritional therapy, exercise, and removing toxic heavy metals.

**Kathleen DesMaisons, Ph.D.,** is president and CEO of Radiant Recovery in Albuquerque, New Mexico, a treatment program for alcoholism, drug addiction, and other types of compulsive behavior, and author of *Potatoes, Not Prozac.*

**Leah J. Dickstein, M.D.,** is professor and associate chair for academic affairs in the department of psychiatry and behavioral sciences, director of the division of attitudinal and behavioral medicine, and associate dean for faculty and student advocacy at the University of Louisville School of Medicine in Kentucky, and past president of the American Medical Women's Association

**Ben Dierauf** is a licensed acupuncturist and practitioner of Traditional Chinese Medicine in San Francisco and vice president of the California Association of Acupuncture and Oriental Medicine.

**Daniel John Dieterichs, O.D.,** is an optometrist in Belen, New Mexico.

**Colleen Dodt** is an aromatherapist in Rochester Hills, Michigan, and author of *The Essential Oils Book: Creating Personal Blends for Mind and Body.*

**Alice Domar, Ph.D.,** is director of the Mind/Body Center for Women's Health and director of the behavioral medicine program for infertility, both at Beth Israel Deaconess Medical Center in Boston; assistant professor of medicine at Harvard Medical School; and author of *Healing*

*Mind, Healthy Woman: Using the Mind-Body Connection to Manage Stress and Take Control of Your Life* and *Self-Nurture: Learning to Care for Yourself as Effectively as You Care for Everyone Else.*

**Patrick Donovan, N.D.,** is a naturopathic physician in Seattle.

**John Douillard, D.C.,** is a chiropractor; expert in Ayurveda; director of LifeSpa in Boulder, Colorado; and author of *Body, Mind, and Sport.*

**Nedra Downing, D.O.,** is an osteopathic physician who practices alternative medicine in Clarkston, Michigan.

**Robert Dozor, M.D.,** is president and chief executive officer of the California Institute of Integrative Medicine in Calistoga.

**Edward Drummond, M.D.,** is associate medical director of the Seacoast Mental Health Center in Portsmouth, New Hampshire, and author of *Benzo Blues: Overcoming Anxiety without Tranquilizers* and *The Complete Guide to Psychiatric Drugs.*

**Eric P. Durak** is director of Medical Health and Fitness in Santa Barbara, California, and an expert on exercise and diabetes.

**David Edwards, M.D.,** is a nutritionally oriented physician in Fresno, California.

**Ted L. Edwards Jr., M.D.,** is a physician in Austin, Texas; adjunct professor in the department of pharmacology at the University of Texas at Austin; and former chairman of the Texas Governor's Commission on Physical Fitness.

**Jason Elias** is a licensed acupuncturist; practitioner of Traditional Chinese Medicine; director of Integral Health

Associates in New Paltz, New York; and coauthor of *Chinese Medicine for Maximum Immunity, Feminine Healing,* and *The A-Z Guide to Healing Herbal Remedies.*

**Rita Elkins** is a master herbalist in Orem, Utah, and author of *The Complete Home Health Advisor.*

**William Faber, D.O.,** is director of the Milwaukee Pain Clinic in Wisconsin.

**David Filipello** is a licensed acupuncturist in San Francisco.

**Richard Firshein, D.O.,** is an osteopathic physician, founder and director of the Firshein Center for Comprehensive Medicine in New York City, and author of *Reversing Asthma* and *The Nutraceutical Revolution.*

**Pamela Fischer** is a former wilderness guide, an herbalist, and founder and director of the Ohlone Center for Herbal Studies in Concord, California.

**Bob Flaws** is a licensed acupuncturist and expert in Chinese medicine in Boulder, Colorado, and author of *Curing Insomnia Naturally with Chinese Medicine.*

**Bill Flocco** is founder and director of the American Academy of Reflexology in Burbank, California, and past president of the International Council of Reflexologists.

**Albert Forgione, Ph.D.,** is chief clinical consultant and founder of the TMJ/TMD pain center at the Gelb Orofacial Pain Center at Tufts University School of Dental Medicine in Boston.

**James Forsythe, M.D.,** is medical director of the Cancer Care Center in Reno.

**Therese Francis, Ph.D.,** is an herbalist in Santa Fe, New Mexico, and author of *20 Herbs to Take Outdoors: An Herbal First-Aid Primer for the Outdoor Enthusiast.*

**Scott M. Fried, D.O.,** is an osteopathic physician and orthopedic surgeon in East Norriton, Pennsylvania; a fellow of the American Osteopathic Academy of Orthopedics; and author of *Light at the End of the Carpal Tunnel.*

**Alan Gaby, M.D.,** is a nutritionally oriented physician in Seattle, author of *Preventing and Reversing Osteoporosis,* and coauthor of *The Patient's Book of Natural Healing.*

**Andrew Gaeddert** is a professional member of the American Herbalists Guild, director of the Get Well Clinic in Oakland, California, and author of *Healing Digestive Disorders.*

**Steve L. Gardner, N.D.,** is a naturopathic doctor in Milwaukie, Oregon.

**Hope Gillerman** is a certified Alexander Technique instructor in New York City, media spokesperson for the American Society for the Alexander Technique, and a former faculty member in the graduate acting program at Harvard University.

**Ann Louise Gittleman, N.D.,** is a naturopathic physician and certified nutrition specialist in Bozeman, Montana, and author of *Eat Fat, Lose Weight.*

**Betty Sy Go, M.D.,** is a naturally oriented doctor in Bellevue, Washington.

**Herbert A. Goldfarb, M.D.,** is director of the Montclair Reproductive Center in New Jersey and Minimally Invasive Gynecology in New York City and author of *The No-Hysterectomy Option: Your Body—Your Choice.*

**Tara Skye Goldin, N.D.,** is a naturopathic physician in Boulder, Colorado.

**Lawrence Green, M.D.,** is assistant professor of dermatology at George Washington University in Washington, D.C., and author of *The Dermatologist's Guide to Looking Younger.*

**Ted Grossbart, Ph.D.,** is a clinical psychologist in Boston, faculty member at Harvard Medical School, and author of *Skin Deep: A Mind/Body Program for Healthy Skin.*

**Marc Grossman, O.D.,** is an optometrist; licensed acupuncturist; codirector of the Integral Health Center in Rye and New Paltz, New York; and author of *Natural Eye Care.*

**Gerard Guillory, M.D.,** is a physician in Denver and author of *IBS: A Doctor's Plan for Chronic Digestive Troubles.*

**Elson Haas, M.D.,** is director of the Preventive Medical Center of Marin in San Rafael, California, and author of seven books, including *The False Fat Diet* and *The Staying Healthy Shopper's Guide.*

**Linaya Hahn** is a licensed nutrition counselor; director of Hahn Holistic Health Centers in Buffalo Grove, Illinois; and author of *PMS: Solving the Puzzle.*

**Steven Halpern, Ph.D.,** is a composer, recording artist, author, and educator and founder of Steven Halpern's Inner Peace Music record company in San Anselmo, California.

**Jesse Lynn Hanley, M.D.,** is a physician in Malibu, California.

**James Hardy, D.M.D.,** is a holistic dentist in Winter Park, Florida, and author of *Mercury-Free: The Wisdom behind the Global Consumer Movement to Ban "Silver" Dental Fillings.*

**Thom Hartmann** is a psychotherapist in Montpelier, Vermont, and author of *Healing ADD: Simple Exercises That Will Change Your Life.*

**Ross A. Hauser, M.D.,** is director of physical medicine and rehabilitation at the Caring Medical Rehabilitation Service in Oak Park, Illinois, and coauthor of *Prolo Your Pain Away!*

**J. P. Heggers, Ph.D.,** is professor of surgery (plastic) and of microbiology and immunology at the University of Texas Medical Branch in Galveston and director of clinical microbiology at the Galveston Shriners Hospital.

**Roger C. Hirsh, O.M.D.,** is a doctor of Oriental medicine, licensed acupuncturist, and specialist in herbal medicine in Beverly Hills.

**Christopher Hobbs** is a fourth-generation herbalist; a licensed acupuncturist and expert in Chinese medicine in Santa Cruz, California; and author of *Natural Liver Therapy: Herbs and Other Natural Remedies for a Healthy Liver.*

**Stephen Hochschuler, M.D.,** is an orthopedic surgeon, founding member of the American Board of Spinal Surgery, cofounder of the Texas Back Institute in Plano, and author of *Treat Your Back without Surgery* and *Back in Shape.*

**Kevin Hogan, Ph.D.,** is a psychologist and doctor of clinical hypnotherapy in Burnsville, Minnesota, and author of *Tinnitus: Turning the Volume Down.*

**Jay M. Holder, M.D., D.C., Ph.D.,** is a chiropractor and addiction specialist in Miami and Miami Beach.

**Julie Claire Holmes, N.D.,** is a naturopathic physician and clinical hypnotherapist in Kula, Hawaii.

**Peter Holyk, M.D.,** is a board-certified ophthalmologist, specializing in macular degeneration, and director of Contemporary Health Innovations in Sebastian, Florida.

**Judy Howard** is a nurse, director of training at the Bach Centre in Sotwell, England, and author of *Bach Flower Remedies for Women.*

**Tori Hudson, N.D.,** is a naturopathic physician; medical director of A Woman's Time clinic and professor of gynecology at the National College of Naturopathic Medicine, both in Portland, Oregon; and author of *Women's Encyclopedia of Natural Medicine.*

**John D. Huff, M.D.,** is an ophthalmologist and codirector of the Prather-Huff Wellness Center in Sugarland, Texas.

**John Hughes, M.D.,** is medical director of the Hilton Head Longevity Center in Bluffton, South Carolina.

**Stanley W. Jacob, M.D.,** is professor of surgery at Oregon Health Sciences University in Portland, director of the DMSO clinic at the university, and coauthor of *The Miracle of MSM: The Natural Solution for Pain.*

**Gregg Jacobs, Ph.D.,** is assistant professor of psychiatry at Harvard Medical School, an insomnia specialist at the sleep disorders center at Beth Israel Deaconess

Medical Center in Boston, and author of *Say Goodnight to Insomnia*.

**Michael Janson, M.D.,** is past president of both the American College for Advancement in Medicine and the American Preventive Medical Association; a consultant physician at Path to Health in Burlington, Massachusetts; and author of *The Vitamin Revolution in Health Care*, *All about Saw Palmetto and Prostate Health*, *Chelation Therapy and Your Health*, and *Dr. Janson's New Vitamin Revolution*.

**Mary Beth Janssen** is an aromatherapist; cosmetologist; owner of the Janssen Source, a beauty consulting firm in Chicago; and author of *Naturally Healthy Hair*.

**Pamela Sky Jeanne, N.D.,** is a naturopathic doctor; adjunct clinical professor at the National College of Naturopathic Medicine in Portland, Oregon; and owner of Mount Hood Holistic Health in Gresham, Oregon.

**Keith W. Johnsgard, Ph.D.,** is professor emeritus of psychology at San Jose State University in California.

**Debbie Johnson** is author of *Think Yourself Thin* and *Think Yourself Loved*.

**Ramona Jones** is a certified nutritional consultant in Shawnee, Oklahoma, and has a nutritional consulting service on the Internet.

**Jon Kaiser, M.D.,** is director of the Jon Kaiser Wellness Center in San Francisco.

**Patricia Kaminski** is cofounder and co-director of the Flower Essence Society in Nevada City, California.

**Emily A. Kane, N.D.,** is a naturopathic physician and licensed acupuncturist in Juneau, Alaska.

**Catherine Karas** is a a physical therapist and energy healer in Tiburon, California, and a former teacher at the Barbara Brennan School of Healing in East Hampton, New York.

**Shoshanna Katzman** is a certified acupuncturist, director of the Red Bank Acupuncture and Wellness Center in New Jersey, cofounder of the Feeling Light weight-management program, and co-author of *Feeling Light: The Holistic Solution to Permanent Weight Loss and Wellness*.

**David Kennedy, D.D.S.,** is a dentist in San Diego and author of *How to Save Your Teeth with Toxic-Free Preventive Dentistry*.

**James Kennedy, D.D.S.,** is a dentist in Littleton, Colorado, specializing in conditions such as temporomandibular disorder.

**Dharma Singh Khalsa, M.D.,** is president and director of the Alzheimer's Prevention Foundation in Tucson and author of *Brain Longevity*.

**Linda Kingsbury** is an herbalist, holistic nutritionist, and director of Earth Wisdom Holistic Services in Keene, New Hampshire.

**Douglas Klappich** is a reflexologist, yoga teacher, expert in Ayurvedic medicine, and director of the Wellth Health Alternative Center in Columbus, Ohio.

**Spencer David Kobren** is a New York City–based consumer advocate for people with hair loss, author of *The Bald Truth* and *The Truth about Women's Hair Loss*, and host of a nationally syndicated radio program about hair loss.

**Kal Kotecha** is an aromatherapist and founder and president of the Academy of Aromatherapy in Waterloo, Ontario.

**Jacqueline Krohn, M.D.,** is an environmental medicine physician in New Mexico and author of *Allergy Relief and Prevention: A Doctor's Complete Guide to Treatment and Self-Care.*

**Esta Kronberg, M.D.,** is a dermatologist in Houston, specializing in cosmetic and dermatological surgery.

**Dana Laake** is a nutritionist in Rockville, Maryland.

**Dan Labriola, N.D.,** is a naturopathic physician in Seattle and director of the Northwest Natural Health Specialty Care Clinic.

**Tai Lahans** is an acupuncturist and practitioner of Traditional Chinese Medicine in Seattle.

**Ahnna Lake, M.D.,** is a physician in Stowe and Burlington, Vermont, specializing in burnout and stress-related issues.

**Susan Lark, M.D.,** is a physician in Los Altos, California.

**John Lee** is director of the Facing the Fire Institute in Asheville, North Carolina, and author of *Facing the Fire: Experiencing and Expressing Anger Appropriately.*

**John Lee, M.D.,** is a retired physician in Sebastopol, California, and author of *What Your Doctor May Not Tell You about Menopause.*

**Ralph Lee, M.D.,** is a family physician specializing in preventive medicine and nutritional therapy in Marietta, Georgia.

**Richard Leigh, M.D.,** is a former gynecologist in Fort Collins, Colorado.

**David Lerner, D.D.S.,** is a holistic dentist and founder of the Center for Dental Wellness in Cold Spring, New York, who has a Web site at www.holisticdentist.com.

**Dennis Lewis** is a certified Chi Nei Tsang practitioner, who teaches natural breathing, qigong, tai chi, and meditation in San Francisco, and author of *The Tao of Natural Breathing* and the audio program *True Breathing as a Metaphor for Living.*

**Michael Lipelt, N.D., D.D.S.,** is a naturopathic physician, dentist, licensed acupuncturist, and expert in Traditional Chinese Medicine in Sebastopol, California.

**Elizabeth Lipski** is a certified clinical nutritionist in Kauai, Hawaii, and author of *Digestive Wellness* and *The Complete Guide to Natural Digestive Health.*

**JoAnne Lombardi, M.D.,** is a board-certified internist and pulmonologist in Belmont, California.

**Joni Loughran** is an esthetician, cosmetologist, and aromatherapist in Petaluma, California; a consultant to many natural cosmetics manufacturers; and author of *Natural Skin Care: Alternative and Traditional Techniques.*

**Elizabeth Ann Lowenthal, D.O.,** is an osteopathic physician and cancer specialist in Alabaster, Alabama.

**Ruth Luban** is a counselor in Santa Monica, California, and author of

*Keeping the Fire: From Burnout to Balance.*

**Jerome F. McAndrews, D.C.,** is a chiropractor in Claremore, Oklahoma, and national spokesperson for the American Chiropractic Association.

**Carole Maggio** is an esthetician in Scottsdale, Arizona, and author of *Facercise: The Dynamic Muscle-Toning Program for Renewed Vitality and a More Youthful Appearance.*

**Alexander Majewski** is a certified Oriental body therapist and founder and director of the Acupressure Institute of Alaska in Juneau.

**Samuel J. Mann, M.D.,** is associate professor of clinical medicine at the hypertension center at New York Presbyterian Hospital-Cornell Medical Center in New York City and author of *Healing Hypertension.*

**Robert E. Markison, M.D.,** is a hand surgeon; associate clinical professor of surgery at the University of California, San Francisco; and cofounder of the UCSF Health Program for Performing Artists.

**Brigitte Mars** is a professional member of the American Herbalists Guild; a nutritional consultant in Boulder, Colorado; and author of *Natural First Aid: Herbal Treatments for Ailments and Injuries, Emergency Preparedness, Wilderness Safety,* and *Herbs for Healthy Skin, Hair, and Nails.*

**Alexander Mauskop, M.D.,** is director of the New York Headache Center in New York City, a licensed acupuncturist, and author of *The Headache Alternative.*

**Joseph L. Mayo, M.D.,** is cofounder of A Woman's Place Medical Center in Healdsburg, California, and coauthor of *The Menopause Manager: A Safe Path for a Natural Change.*

**James Medlock, D.D.S.,** is a mercury-free dentist in West Palm Beach, Florida.

**Gerald Melchoide, M.D.,** is professor of psychiatry and lecturer at the University of Texas Southwestern Medical Center in Dallas and author of *Beyond Viagra.*

**Harold Mermelstein, M.D.,** is a dermatologist in Westchester County and Riverdale, New York, and assistant clinical professor of dermatology at New York University Medical Center in New York City.

**Genevieve M. Messick, M.D.,** is a physician in Columbus, Ohio, specializing in urinary incontinence and pelvic floor dysfunction.

**Deborah Metzger, M.D., Ph.D.,** is medical director of Helena Women's Health in San Francisco and Palo Alto, California.

**Burton Miller, D.D.S.,** is director of the Health Center Dentistry Clinic in Anchorage.

**Emmett Miller, M.D.,** is medical director of the Cancer Support and Education Center in Auburn, California.

**Light Miller, N.D.,** is a naturopathic doctor and Ayurvedic practitioner in Sarasota, Florida.

**Philip Lee Miller, M.D.,** is a specialist in anti-aging medicine and founder and director of the Los Gatos Longevity Institute in California.

**Dixie Mills, M.D.,** is breast specialist at Women to Women in Yarmouth, Maine, and president of the Association of Women Surgeons.

**Earl L. Mindell, Ph.D.,** is a pharmacist and nutritionist in Beverly Hills, professor of nutrition at Pacific Western University in Los Angeles, and author of *Earl Mindell's Supplement Bible* and *Earl Mindell's Vitamin Bible for the 21st Century.*

**Phillip Minton, M.D.,** is a homeopathic physician in Reno.

**David Molony, Ph.D.,** is director of the Lehigh Valley Acupuncture Center in Catasauqua, Pennsylvania; executive director of the American Association of Oriental Medicine; and author of *The American Association of Oriental Medicine's Complete Guide to Chinese Herbal Medicine.*

**Anu de Monterice, M.D.,** is a practitioner of holistic medicine and psychiatry in Cotati, California.

**Kate Montgomery** is a licensed massage therapist in San Diego and author of *End Your Carpel Tunnel Pain without Surgery.*

**Terri Moon** is a certified massage technician and director of Touched by the Moon holistic health center in Santa Rosa, California.

**Martin Moore-Ede, M.D., Ph.D.,** is a former professor of physiology at Harvard University and president of Circadian Technologies in Cambridge, Massachusetts.

**Ralph Moss, Ph.D.,** of New York City, is director of "The Moss Reports," a series of comprehensive guides to cancer treatment.

**Charles Muir** is director of the Source School of Tantra Yoga in Wailuku, Hawaii, and coauthor of *Tantra: The Art of Conscious Loving.*

**Andrea Murray** is a certified reflexologist and herbalist in Portland, Maine.

**Steve Nenninger, N.D.,** is a naturopathic physician in New York City.

**Diane Kaschak Newman** is a nurse practitioner in Philadelphia specializing in incontinence and urology nursing.

**Maoshing Ni, O.M.D., Ph.D.,** is a doctor of Oriental medicine and director of the Tao of Wellness Center and cofounder of Yo San University of Traditional Chinese Medicine, both in Santa Monica, California.

**Thomas O'Bryan, D.C.,** is a chiropractor; certified clinical nutritionist; director of Omnis Chiropractic Groups in Glenview, Illinois; past president of the Chicago Chiropractic Society; and a director of the Illinois Chiropractic Society.

**Michael Olmsted, D.D.S.,** is a dentist in Del Mar, California, and a member of the International Academy of Oral Medicine and Toxicology.

**John O. A. Pagano, D.C.,** is a chiropractor in Englewood Cliffs, New Jersey, and author of *Healing Psoriasis: The Natural Alternative.*

**Edward L. Paul Jr., O.D., Ph.D.,** is an optometrist, holistic nutritionist, and director of Atlantic Eye Associates in Hampstead, North Carolina.

**William Payne, D.D.S.,** is a dentist in McPherson, Kansas.

**Michael D. Pedigo, D.C.,** is a chiropractor in San Leandro, California, and past president of the American Chiropractic Association.

**Reneau Z. Peurifoy** is a marriage and family therapist and anxiety specialist in Sacramento, California, and author of *Anxiety, Phobias, and Panic* and *Anger: Taming the Beast.*

**Robbie Porter** is a hydrotherapist and certified massage therapist in Albany, Oregon.

**Deirdra Price, Ph.D.,** is a psychologist in San Diego, president of Diet Free Solution, and author of *Healing the Hungry Self: The Diet-Free Solution to Lifelong Weight Management.*

**James Privitera, M.D.,** is an allergy and nutrition specialist in Covina, California.

**Gus Prosch, M.D.,** is a physician in Birmingham, Alabama, and coauthor of *Arthritis.*

**Seth Prosterman, Ph.D.,** is a sex therapist and licensed marriage and family therapist in San Francisco.

**Patrick Quillin, R.D., Ph.D.,** is director of the Rational Healing Institute in Tulsa, Oklahoma, and former consultant to the National Institutes of Health in Bethesda, Maryland; the Scripps Clinic in San Diego; and La Costa Resort and Spa in Carlsbad, California.

**Pratima Raichur, N.D.,** is a naturopathic physician and esthetician in New York City, director of Tej Ayurvedic Skin Care, and author of *Absolute Beauty: Radiant Skin and Inner Harmony through the Ancient Secrets of Ayurveda.*

**Simone Ravicz, Ph.D.,** is a licensed clinical psychologist and consultant in Pacific Palisades, California, and author of *High on Stress: A Woman's Guide to Optimizing the Stress in Her Life* and *Thriving with Your Autoimmune Disorder: A Woman's Mind-Body Guide.*

**Harold Ravins, D.D.S.,** is director of the Center for Holistic Dentistry in Los Angeles.

**Barbara Bailey Reinhold, Ed.D.,** is director of the career development office at Smith College in Northampton, Massachusetts, and author of *Toxic Work: How To Overcome Stress, Overload, and Burnout and Revitalize Your Career.*

**Rich Rieger** is a licensed massage therapist in Morgantown, West Virginia.

**Andrew Ries, M.D.,** is professor of medicine and director of pulmonary rehabilitation at the University of California, San Diego, and coauthor of *Shortness of Breath: A Guide to Better Living and Breathing.*

**Teresa Rispoli, Ph.D.,** is a nutritionist, licensed acupuncturist, and founder of the Institute for Health in Agoura Hills, California.

**Lawrence Robbins, M.D.,** is director of the Robbins Headache Clinic in Northbrook, Illinois, and coauthor of *Headache Help.*

**Joel Robertson** is president of the Robertson Institute in Saginaw, Michigan.

**Aviva Jill Romm** is a midwife and herbalist in Bloomfield Hills, Michigan; a professional member and secretary of the American Herbalists Guild; and author of *The Natural Pregnancy Book, Natural*

*Healing for Babies and Children*, and *Pocket Guide to Midwifery Care*.

**Kitty Gurkin Rosati, R.D.,** is a licensed dietitian; nutrition director for the Rice Diet Program at Duke University in Durham, North Carolina; and author of *Heal Your Heart: The New Rice Diet Program for Reversing Heart Disease through Nutrition, Exercise, and Spiritual Renewal*.

**Paul Rosch, M.D.,** is president of the American Institute of Stress, clinical professor of medicine and psychiatry at New York Medical College in Yonkers, and coauthor of *Magnet Therapy*.

**Edward Rosen** is a physical therapist in Cotati, California.

**Michael Rosenbaum, M.D.,** is an alternative physician in Corte Madera, California, and author of *Super Supplements: Your Guide to Today's Newest Vitamins, Minerals, Enzymes, Amino Acids, and Glandulars*.

**Norman E. Rosenthal, M.D.,** is clinical professor of psychiatry at Georgetown University Medical School in Washington, D.C., and author of *The Winter Blues: Seasonal Affective Disorder—What It Is and How to Overcome It*.

**Julia Ross** is executive director of Recovery Systems, a clinic for chronic dieters and those with serious food addictions or eating disorders, in Mill Valley, California, and author of *The Diet Cure*.

**Geneen Roth** is an expert on the relationship between emotions and overeating in Santa Cruz, California, and author of *When You Eat at the Refrigerator, Pull Up a Chair* and *When Food Is Love: Exploring the Relationship between Eating and Intimacy*.

**Amy Rothenberg, N.D.,** is a naturopathic physician in Enfield, Connecticut, and editor of the *New England Journal of Homeopathy* at the Faculty National Center of Homeopathy summer school in Amherst, Massachusetts.

**Glenn S. Rothfeld, M.D.,** is regional medical director of American WholeHealth in Arlington, Massachusetts, and author of *Natural Medicine for Heart Disease: The Best Alternative Methods for Prevention and Treatment*.

**Robert Rountree, M.D.,** is cofounder of the Helios Health Center in Boulder, Colorado.

**Andrew Rubman, N.D.,** is a naturopathic physician and founder of the Southbury Clinic for Traditional Medicine and professor of clinical medicine at the College of Naturopathic Medicine at the University of Bridgeport, both in Connecticut.

**Melanie Sachs** is an Ayurvedic lifestyle counselor in San Luis Obispo, California; cofounder of Diamond Way Ayurveda; and author of *Ayurvedic Beauty Care: Ageless Techniques to Invoke Natural Beauty*.

**William B. Salt II, M.D.,** is clinical associate professor of medicine at Ohio State University College of Medicine and Public Health in Columbus and author of *Irritable Bowel Syndrome and the Mind-Body/Brain-Gut Connection*.

**Arthur Samuels, M.D.,** is medical director of the Stress Treatment Center of New Orleans, associate professor of psychiatry at Louisiana State University School of Medicine, a member of the American Psychiatric Association, and author of *Creative Grieving*.

**Elizabeth Sander, M.D.,** is an internist in Los Angeles.

**Michael Schachter, M.D.,** is director of the Schachter Center for Complementary Medicine in Suffern, New York.

**David and Carol Schiller** are certified aromatherapy instructors in Phoenix and coauthors of *500 Formulas for Aromatherapy.*

**Rosa Schnyer** is an acupuncturist in Tucson.

**Mona Lisa Schultz, M.D., Ph.D.,** is a neuropsychiatrist and neuroscientist in Yarmouth, Maine.

**Erika Schwartz, M.D.,** is a former trauma specialist and head of emergency medicine for Westchester County Medical Center in New York; an internist in Irvington, New York; and author of *Natural Energy.*

**Othniel Seiden, M.D.,** is a physician in Denver and author of *5-HTP: The Serotonin Connection.*

**Michael D. Seidman, M.D.,** is an ear, nose, and throat specialist; medical director of the tinnitus center at the Henry Ford Health System in West Bloomfield, Michigan; and regional coordinator of otolaryngology and head and neck surgery and co-chair of the complementary and alternative medicine initiative for the Henry Ford Health System.

**Jamie Shaw** is a certified teacher of Kripalu yoga in Westlake Village, California, and associate director of the International Association of Yoga Therapists.

**Fred D. Sheftell, M.D.,** is director and cofounder of the New England Center for Headache in Stamford, Connecticut; president of the American Council for Headache Education; and coauthor of *Conquering Headache* and *Headache Relief for Women.*

**Sylla Sheppard-Hanger** is an aromatherapist and principal instructor at the Atlantic Institute of Aromatherapy in Tampa, Florida.

**Eugene Shippen, M.D.,** is a physician in Shillington, Pennsylvania, and author of *The Testosterone Syndrome.*

**Jade Shutes** is director of the Institute of Dynamic Aromatherapy in Seattle.

**Alan B. Siegel, Ph.D.,** is a psychotherapist in San Francisco and Berkeley, California; president of the Association for the Study of Dreams; and coauthor of *Dreamcatching: Every Parent's Guide to Exploring and Understanding Children's Dreams and Nightmares.*

**Paul and Marilena Silbey** of American Tantra in Fairfax, California, are creators of the video "Intimate Secrets of Sex and Spirit."

**David Simon, M.D.,** is a neurologist; medical director of the Chopra Center for Well-Being in La Jolla, California; and author of *The Wisdom of Healing.*

**Charles B. Simone, M.D.,** is a medical oncologist, radiation oncologist, and tumor immunologist; a former researcher at the National Cancer Institute; and director of the Simone Protective Cancer Center in Lawrenceville, New Jersey.

**Stephen T. Sinatra, M.D.,** is a cardiologist; director of the New England Heart Center in Manchester, Connecticut; assistant clinical professor of medicine at the

University of Connecticut School of Medicine in Farmington; director of medical education at the Eastern Connecticut Health Network in Manchester; author of *The Coenzyme $Q_{10}$ Phenomenon*; and editor of the monthly newsletter *HeartSense*.

**Sydney Ross Singer and Soma Grismaijer** are a husband-and-wife medical anthropology team, coauthors of *Dressed to Kill: The Link between Breast Cancer and Bras*, and codirectors of the Institute for the Study of Culturogenic Disease in Hilo, Hawaii.

**Deborah Valentine Smith** is a licensed massage therapist and senior teacher of Jin Shin Do Bodymind Acupressure in West Stockbridge, Massachusetts.

**Pamela Smith, R.D.,** is a nutritionist in Orlando, Florida, and author of *The Energy Edge*.

**Duane Smoot, M.D.,** is associate professor of medicine in the department of gastroenterology at Howard University College of Medicine in Washington, D.C.

**Virender Sodhi, M.D. (Ayurved), N.D.,** is an Ayurvedic and naturopathic physician and director of the American School of Ayurvedic Sciences in Bellevue, Washington.

**Gregory W. Spencer, D.P.M.,** is a podiatrist and director of the Renton Foot Clinic in Renton, Washington.

**Jill Stansbury, N.D.,** is chair of the botanical medicine department at the National College of Naturopathic Medicine in Portland, Oregon.

**Carol Staudacher** is a grief consultant in Santa Cruz, California, and author of *A Time to Grieve, Men and Grief,* and *Beyond Grief.*

**Flora Parsa Stay, D.D.S.,** is a dentist in Oxnard, California, and author of *The Complete Book of Dental Remedies*.

**David Steenblock, D.O.,** is an osteopathic physician in Mission Viejo, California.

**Wynne A. Steinsnyder, D.O.,** is an osteopathic physician and urologist in North Miami Beach and professor of urology at Nova Southeastern University in Fort Lauderdale.

**Mark Stengler, N.D.,** is a naturopathic physician in San Diego and author of *The Natural Physician, Virus Killers, Drink Your Greens, Echinacea,* and *Your Child's Health.*

**Ralph R. Stephens** is a licensed massage therapist and instructor of sports massage and neuromuscular therapy with Ralph Stephens Seminars in Cedar Rapids, Iowa.

**Elaine Stillerman** is a licensed massage therapist in New York City and author of *Mother Massage: A Handbook for Relieving the Discomforts of Pregnancy*.

**Steven Subotnick, D.P.M., N.D., D.C., Ph.D.,** is a podiatrist, naturopathic doctor, and chiropractor in Berkeley and San Leandro, California, and author of *Sports and Exercise Injuries: Conventional, Homeopathic and Alternative Treatments* and *Sports Medicine of the Lower Extremity: An Integrative Approach.*

**John M. Sullivan, M.D.,** is a physician in Mechanicsburg, Pennsylvania.

**Gerard Sunnen, M.D.,** is associate clinical professor of psychiatry at New York

University–Bellevue Medical Center in New York City, an expert on medical hypnosis, and author of *Primer of Clinical Hypnosis*.

**Robert E. Svoboda** is a faculty member at the Ayurvedic Institute in Albuquerque, New Mexico, and a visiting faculty member at Bastyr University in Kenmore, Washington.

**Shawn M. Talbott, Ph.D.,** is adjunct assistant professor in the department of food and nutrition at the University of Utah in Salt Lake City and executive editor for Supplement Watch in Provo, Utah.

**Jacob Teitelbaum, M.D.,** is a physician in Annapolis, Maryland; director of the Annapolis Research Center for Effective Fibromyalgia and Chronic Fatigue Syndrome Therapy; and author of *From Fatigued to Fantastic!*

**Susan Thys-Jacobs, M.D.,** is an endocrinologist at St. Luke's–Roosevelt Hospital in New York City.

**Swami Sada Shiva Tirtha** is director of the Ayurveda Holistic Center in Bayville, New York, and author of *The Ayurveda Encyclopedia*.

**Stephanie Tourles** is a licensed esthetician, reflexologist, and herbalist in West Hyannisport, Massachusetts, and author of *Natural Foot Care: Herbal Treatments, Massage, and Exercises for Healthy Feet* and *Naturally Healthy Skin*.

**Maryann Troiani, Ph.D.,** is a clinical psychologist in Barrington, Illinois, and author of *Spontaneous Optimism: Proven Strategies for Health, Prosperity, and Happiness*.

**Eva Urbaniak, N.D.,** is a naturopathic physician, director of Alternative Medical Arts Associates in Seattle, and author of *Healing Your Prostate: Natural Cures That Work*.

**David S. Utley, M.D.,** is clinical instructor at Stanford University Medical Center.

**Gary Verigin, D.D.S.,** is a dentist in Escalon, California.

**Vijay Vijh, M.D., Ph.D.,** is director of the Cherry Hill Wellness Center in New Jersey.

**Morton Walker, D.P.M.,** is a former podiatrist in Stamford, Connecticut, and coauthor of *The Complete Foot Book: First Aid for Your Feet*.

**Susun Weed** is an herbalist; founder of the Wise Woman Center in Woodstock, New York; and author of *Healing Wise, Wise Woman Herbal for the Childbearing Year, Breast Cancer? Breast Health! The Wise Woman Way,* and *Menopausal Years: The Wise Woman Way*.

**Norma Pasekoff Weinberg** is an herbalist in Cape Cod, Massachusetts, and author of *Natural Hand Care: Herbal Treatments and Simple Techniques for Healthy Hands and Nails*.

**Skye Weintraub, N.D.,** is a naturopathic physician in Eugene, Oregon, and author of *Allergies and Holistic Healing*.

**Julian Whitaker, M.D.,** is founder and director of the Whitaker Wellness Institute in Newport Beach, California; author of *Reversing Heart Disease* and *Is Heart Surgery Necessary?*; and coauthor of *Reversing Health Risks* and *The Pain Relief Breakthrough: The Power of Magnets*.

**Glen P. Wilcoxson, M.D.,** is director of the New Beginnings Medical Group in Gulf Shores, Alabama, and coauthor of *Cook in the Fourth Dimension*.

**Carla Wilson** is executive director of the Quan Yin Healing Arts Center in San Francisco.

**Roberta Wilson** is an aromatherapist in Albuquerque, New Mexico, and author of *Aromatherapy for Vibrant Health and Beauty*.

**Reid Winick, D.D.S.,** is an alternative dentist in New York City.

**Jonathan Wright, M.D.,** is a nutritionally oriented physician; director of the Tahoma Clinic in Kent, Washington; and author of *Natural Hormones for Women over 45*, *Maximize Your Vitality*, and *Potency for Men Over 40*.

**Kenneth Yasny, Ph.D.,** is a nutritionist in Beverly Hills, founder of the Colon Health Society, and author of *Put Hemorrhoids and Constipation behind You*.

**Beverly Yates, N.D.,** is a naturopathic physician, director of the Natural Health Care Group in Seattle, and author of *Heart Health for Black Women*.

**Melanie von Zabuesnig** is an aromatherapist in Murietta, California.

**Janet Zand, O.M.D.,** is a doctor of Oriental medicine and licensed acupuncturist in Austin, Texas, and coauthor of *Smart Medicine for Healthier Living: A Practical A-to-Z Reference to Natural and Conventional Treatments for Adults*.

**Holly Zapf, N.D.,** is a naturopathic physician in Portland, Oregon, specializing in classical homeopathy, botanical medicine, and nutrition.

**Elke Zuercher-White, Ph.D.,** is a psychologist at Kaiser-Permanente in the San Francisco area and author of *An End to Panic* and *Treating Panic Disorder and Agoraphobia*.

**Jonathan Zuess, M.D.,** is a psychiatrist at the Good Samaritan Regional Medical Center in Phoenix.

# *Index*

Underscored page references indicate boxed text and tables. **Boldface** references indicate illustrations.

## N

treating, with
  aloe, 612
  antioxidants, 614
  green tea, 613
  homeopathy, 613–14
  hydrotherapy, 613–14
  lavender essential oil, 613
  yogurt, 613
Sun exposure, age spots from,
  10
Sunlight, for treating
 insomnia, 429–30
 jet lag, 444
 premenstrual syndrome, 556
 seasonal affective disorder,
  583–85
 thyroid problems, 622
Supplements. *See also specific sup-*
  *plements*
 safety guidelines for, 704,
  704–10
Swimmer's ear, 248

# T
Tapotement, for osteoporosis
 prevention, 509–10, **510**
Taurine, for treating
 arrhythmia, 44
 emphysema and chronic bronchitis, 255–56
 macular degeneration, 459
Tea
 black, for toothache, 630
 citrus peel, for belching, 90
 clove, for belching, 90
 green
  for hair loss, 332–33
  for limiting side effects of
   chemotherapy and radiation,
   161
  for sunburn, 613
 herbal, as caffeine alternative, 144
 umeboshi, for limiting side effects
  of chemotherapy and radiation, 161

Tea tree oil, for treating
 plantar warts, 530
 shingles, 588
Temporomandibular disorder
  (TMD), 615–20
 professional care for, <u>616</u>
 treating, with
  acupressure, 618, 619–10
  ice and stretch, 616–17
  isometric exercise, 619
  stretching, 617–18, **617**
  TMD mantra, 618–19
Tendinitis. *See* Bursitis and tendinitis
Testosterone, for male menopause,
  <u>462</u>
Thiamin, for treating
 Parkinson's disease, 522–23
 tooth sensitivity, 641
Thin Oil, for limiting side effects of
  chemotherapy and radiation,
  159–60
Thyme essential oil, for treating
 athlete's foot, 68
 bronchitis, 124
 foot odor, 293
Thymus extract, for treating
 colds, 178
 flu, 285
 pneumonia, 533
Thyroid problems, 620–24
 at-home test for detecting, 623
 professional care for, <u>621</u>
 treating, with
  diet, 623
  energy exercise, 621–22
  fatty acids, 624
  progesterone, 623–24
  sunlight, 622
  tyrosine, 624
Tinnitus, 625–27
 professional care for, <u>626</u>
 treating, with
  auditory habituation, 626–27
  B vitamins, 625
  diet, 627